Gerontological Nursing

Gerontological Nursing
A Holistic Approach to the Care of Older People

CAROLINE VAFEAS, PhD, BSc (Hons), MA Nurse Education, RN
Director Undergraduate Nursing Studies
School of Nursing and Midwifery
Edith Cowan University, Joondalup
Western Australia, Australia

SUSAN SLATYER, PhD, BNurs (Hons), RN
Associate Professor of Nursing
College of Science, Health, Engineering and Education
Murdoch University, Murdoch
Western Australia, Australia

ELSEVIER

ELSEVIER

Elsevier Australia. ACN 001 002 357
(a division of Reed International Books Australia Pty Ltd)
Tower 1, 475 Victoria Avenue, Chatswood, NSW 2067

ISBN: 978-0-7295-4367-5

Notice
This publication has been carefully reviewed and checked to ensure that the content is as accurate and current as possible at time of publication. We would recommend, however, that the reader verify any procedures, treatments, drug dosages or legal content described in this book. Neither the author, the contributors, nor the publisher assume any liability for injury and/or damage to persons or property arising from any error in or omission from this publication.

National Library of Australia Cataloguing-in-Publication Data

 A catalogue record for this book is available from the National Library of Australia

Senior Content Strategist: Melinda McEvoy
Content Project Manager: Sukanthi Sukumar
Edited by Margaret Trudgeon
Proofread by Tim Learner
Cover Designer: Georgette Hall
Index by SPi Global
Typeset by New Best-set Typesetters Ltd
Printed in Singapore by KHL

Last digit is the print number: 9   8   7   6   5   4   3   2   1

About the Authors

THE EDITORS

Caroline Vafeas, PhD, BSc (Hons), MA Nurse Education, RN
Director Undergraduate Nursing Studies
School of Nursing and Midwifery
Edith Cowan University, Joondalup
Western Australia, Australia

Susan Slatyer, PhD, BNurs (Hons), RN
Associate Professor of Nursing
College of Science, Health, Engineering and
    Education
Murdoch University, Murdoch
Western Australia, Australia

OTHER CONTRIBUTORS

Agathe Daria Jadczak, PhD
Postdoctoral Research Fellow
Adelaide Geriatrics Training and Research with Aged
    Care Centre and National Health and Medical
    Research Council Centre of Research Excellence in
    Frailty and Healthy Ageing
Adelaide Medical School,
University of Adelaide, Adelaide
South Australia, Australia

Aisling Smyth, BSc, MSc, PhD, RN
Lecturer
School of Nursing and Midwifery
Edith Cowan University, Perth
Western Australia, Australia

Andrew Stafford, BPharm (Hons), MBA, PhD, MPS, AACPA
Senior Lecturer
Curtin Medical School
Curtin University, Perth
Western Australia, Australia

Anne-Marie Holt, Bsc Human Movement, MHealth Promotion, PhD
School of Medicine
University of Notre Dame, Fremantle
Western Australia, Australia

Christine Stirling, PhD, MPA, BN Nur
Associate Head of School
School of Nursing, College of Health and Medicine
University of Tasmania, Hobart
Tasmania, Australia

President
Australian Association Gerontology, Melbourne
Australia

Dana Dermody, BSN, MSN, PHD, RN, CNL, GAICD
Senior Lecturer
University of the Sunshine Coast
School of Nursing, Midwifery and Paramedicine
Australia

David Betts, PhD
Lecturer
Humanities and Social Science
The University of Newcastle, Newcastle
NSW, Australia

Davina Porock, PhD, RN
VC Professorial Research Fellow
Director
Centre for Research in Aged Care
School of Nursing and Midwifery
Edith Cowan University, Joondalup
Western Australia, Australia

Deborah Sundin, RN, RM, BN (Hons), PhD
Senior Lecturer
School of Nursing and Midwifery
Edith Cowan University, Joondalup
Western Australia, Australia

Elisabeth Jacob, PhD, MEd, GradDipCritCare, DipAppSci(Nsg), RN, FACN
Associate Professor
School of Nursing, Midwifery and Paramedicine
Australian Catholic University, Melbourne
Victoria, Australia

Emma Chaffey, BSc (Hons) UWA, MClinAud (UWA), MAudA CPP
Senior Audiologist
Fremantle Hearing Centre
Hearing Australia, Perth
Western Australia, Australia

Chapter Chair
WA Chapter
Audiology Australia
Western Australia, Australia

Helena Halton, RN, PG Cert Emer., PG Dip NP, MNNP, PhD Candidate
Director of Post Graduate Nursing Studies
School of Nursing and Midwifery
Edith Cowan University, Perth
Western Australia, Australia

Helene Metcalfe, RN, BEd, MSc, EdD
Lecturer
School of Nursing and Midwifery
Edith Cowan University, Perth
Western Australia, Australia

Adjunct Associate Professor
School of Medicine
University of Western Australia, Perth
Western Australia, Australia

Helga Merl, MHSc (Aged Care Serv), MN (NP), GradCertPallCare, BN, MRN, RN
Nurse Practitioner Academic
Wicking Dementia Research and Education Centre
University of Tasmsnia, Hobart
Tasmania, Australia

Jacqueline Allen, RN, PhD
Senior Lecturer
School of Nursing and Midwifery
Monash University, Clayton
Victoria, Australia

Karen Heslop, PhD, MEd, Grad Dip Soc Sci, BN, RN
Associate Professor
School of Nursing, Midwifery and Paramedicine
Curtin University, Perth/Bentley
Western Australia, Australia

Keith Hill, PhD, Grad Dip Physio (Neuro), BAppSc (Physio)
Director
Rehabilitation, Ageing and Independent Living (RAIL) research centre
School of Primary and Allied Health Care
Peninsula Campus, Monash University, Frankston
Victoria, Australia

Lauren Entwistle, BSc (Nursing)
Registered Nurse
Ophthalmology
Royal Perth Hospital, Perth
Western Australia, Australia

Lily Dongxia Xiao, PhD
Professor
College of Nursing and Health Sciences
Flinders University, Adelaide
South Australia, Australia

Lisa Whitehead, PhD, MA, BSc (Hons)
Professor
School of Nursing and Midwifery
Edith Cowan University, Joondalup
Australia

Margaret Sealey, PhD, BPsych (Hons), GradDipCouns, FT, FHEA
Lecturer
College of Science, Health, Engineering and Education
Murdoch University, Murdoch
Western Australia, Australia

Martinique Louise Sandy, MLM, PGCCN (Emerg), BN, RN
Lecturer, Nursing
College of Science, Health, Engineering and Education
Murdoch University, Murdoch
Western Australia, Australia

Natalie Luscombe-Marsh
Senior Research Scientist
The Commonwealth Scientific Industrial Organisation (CSIRO)
Canberra, Australia

Norman Davies, DipMedTech, MMedSc, PGCertHMQL
Casual lecturer
Murdoch University
Perth, Australia

Renuka Visvanathan, PhD, MBA, Grad Cert Higher Ed, MBBS
Head of Unit
Aged and Extended Care Services
The Queen Elizabeth Hospital, Central Adelaide Local
    Health Network, Adelaide
South Australia, Australia

Project Lead
Adelaide Geriatrics Training and Research with Aged
    Care Centre and National Health and Medical
    Research Council Centre of Research Excellence in
    Frailty and Healthy Ageing
Adelaide Medical School
University of Adelaide, Adelaide
South Australia, Australia

Robyn Rayner, BSc (Nursing), Masters of Wound Care, PhD
Sessional Academic
School of Nursing, Midwifery and Paramedicine
Curtin University, Bentley
Australia

Roger Goucke, FANZCA, FFPMANZCA
Clinical Associate Professor
Faculty of Health and Medical Sciences
University of Western Australia, PERTH
Western Australia, Australia

Ruth Wei, PhD
Lecturer in Nursing
SHEE, Murdoch University
Western Australia, Australia

Sheridan Read, BSc (Nursing)
Lecturer
School of Nursing and Midwifery
Edith Cowan University, Joondalup
Western Australia, Australia

PhD Candidate
School of Nursing Midwifery and Paramedicine
Curtin University, Bentley
Western Australia, Australia

Vicki Ellen Patton, PhD, MN (hons), BaHealth (Nursing), RN
Adjunct Lecturer
Nursing and Midwifery
Edith Cowan University, Joondalup
Western Australia, Australia

Preface

This first edition of *Gerontological Nursing: A Holistic Approach to the Care of Older People* appreciates the specialist role of the nurse in the care of older people. Over the past few decades, as life expectancy has increased, the number of people reaching very old age has increased year on year. This ageing population brings challenges and opportunities, especially for the nursing workforce. Increasing numbers of older people are living with chronic health problems, disability, and frailty. Nurses work with older people across the care continuum, from primary care to acute care, rehabilitation, community and residential aged care settings. Gerontological nursing recognises the complexity of older persons' healthcare, and the critical role of nurses in promoting healthy ageing, supporting older people to navigate life transitions and enabling people to live well despite limitations. Nurses who are skilled in gerontological care take a holistic and person-centred approach to addressing the older person's physical, mental, emotional, social and spiritual needs. As the population continues to grow and age, nurses will increasingly lead care that identifies and responds to deterioration and decline in older individuals, integrates family into comprehensive care, and reduces health disparities in diverse communities.

This specialist text on gerontological nursing highlights the need for nurses to have knowledge on the ageing process, from undergraduate to postgraduate level to be able to provide the level of care required within today's healthcare domain. It brings together topic experts from around Australia to provide an evidence-based, holistic approach to nursing older people in contemporary society.

This book identifies healthy ageing, risk factors for illness and functional decline, and evidence-based care. It also incorporates the Australian and New Zealand, as well as the international, standards and current guidelines at the time of writing. Chapter 1 gives an overview of each of the 28 chapters to follow and covers all aspects of person-centred care of older people.

Chapters also feature boxes relating to the following subject areas:
- Promoting Wellness
- Research Highlights
- Tips for Best Practice
- Practice Points
- Safety Alerts
- Case Studies
- Multiple Choice Questions or Review Questions

Finally, we hope you enjoy this text as much as the editors and authors did putting it together. We hope we have captured every aspect required to ensure that holistic, knowledgeable, evidence-based care is provided to every older person.

Dr Caroline Vafeas
Dr Susan Slatyer

Contents

CHAPTER 1

Gerontological Nursing in Australia and New Zealand

CAROLINE VAFEAS • SUSAN SLATYER

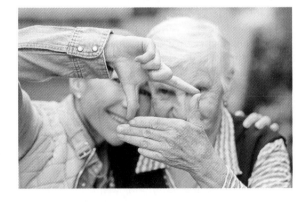

This chapter will explore the unique role of the nurse within the speciality of gerontology. The term 'gerontology' describes the study of ageing and older people, and has become an acceptable term to cover this specialised area of nursing. This chapter will explore the history of the gerontological nurse to give an understanding of the development of this unique role in today's healthcare system. The hospital, community and residential settings will all be considered in relation to aged care leadership and research. Current challenges faced in light of funding and public expectation will also be addressed. This chapter concludes by providing an overview of the whole book, setting the scene for the reader. This text is suitable for use in the undergraduate curriculum and will assist students to understand the unique needs of older people.

The global population is growing older as fertility rates fall and life expectancies increase (United Nations, Department of Economic and Social Affairs [UN] 2019). People over the age of 65 years account for the fastest growing demographic, with one in six people anticipated to be in this age group by 2050 (UN 2019). An estimated 15–20% of the populations of Australia and New Zealand were aged 65 years and older in 2020. By the end of the 21st century, 25–30% of Australians and 30–35% of New Zealanders will be older than 65 years (UN 2019). Older people today are generally more educated and well-travelled than previous generations and expect a higher quality of life. While many will realise the goal of healthy ageing, others will live longer while managing chronic diseases that are more common in later age, including frailty, functional decline and an increasing dependence on caregivers. The healthcare of the older person is complex, requiring a holistic approach that considers their physical, psychological, social and spiritual wellbeing, as well as the inclusion and support of family.

Nurses, as the largest proportion of the healthcare workforce, are at the frontline of caring for older people across the continuum of healthcare. In 2016–17 in Australia, people aged 65 years and older accounted for 1.6 million presentations to emergency departments and 1.8 million (41%) overnight hospitalisations (Australian Institute of Health and Welfare [AIHW] 2018). Over 1.2 million people received aged care services in Australia, ranging from support to remain independent at home through to full-time care in a residential aged care facility (AIHW 2019). Apart from multiple chronic diseases and related symptom exacerbation, many older people develop frailty, defined as 'an age-related state of decreased reserves characterised by a weakened response to stressors and increased risk of poor outcome' (Apóstolo et al 2019:149).

Frailty is regarded as a syndrome characterised by at least three of the following markers:
- weight loss
- globalised weakness and muscle strength
- overall slowness
- fatigue
- decreased balance and mobility
- low physical activity.

The presence of only one or two markers is considered to be an indicator of 'pre-frailty' (Apóstolo et al 2019). Far from a benign condition, frailty puts the older person at risk of falls, hospitalisation and disability, and ultimately leads to death. Nurses lead care that ensures safe physical and social environments for frail older people and work with multidisciplinary teams to implement interventions to prevent progression of frailty and pre-frailty (Apóstolo et al 2019; Craig 2019), thereby taking a central role in reducing poor outcomes and health crises.

In the past, 'aged care' was often regarded as an unpopular branch of nursing, thought to require fewer capabilities than acute care and specialty settings. In reality, the nursing care of older people is multifaceted, requiring knowledge and skills which include (but are not limited to):
- chronic disease management
- pharmacology
- comprehensive assessment
- critical analysis and decision-making
- complex communication

- end-of-life care
- advance care planning
- person-centred care (Wyman et al 2019).

Nurses apply these skills across healthcare settings to promote the health and safety of older people of all ages and cultures. Additionally, most registered nurses working in residential aged care facilities do so autonomously, providing leadership and mentorship to a large, mostly multicultural care workforce. Gerontology recognises the specialised knowledge and skills required to provide high-quality care responsive to the individual and complex needs of older people. Gerontological nursing captures the complexity of assessment and care planning required to address and prevent health crises that enable older people to live well at all ages and stages of later life.

INTERNATIONAL CONTEXT OF GERONTOLOGY

The term gerontology is widely used internationally. Gerontology is the study of ageing and older people and includes the study of processes associated with bodily changes from middle age through to later life. Practitioners and researchers in the field of gerontology apply this specialised knowledge to policies and programs to benefit the older population (AAG 2019). Gerontology can be considered a multidisciplinary approach to ageing and the care of older people. The nurse often takes a primary role in this field, but is likely to work in collaboration with gerontologists, occupational therapists, physiotherapists, dietitians, podiatrists and social workers to ensure quality care for older people.

THE STUDY OF AGEING WITHIN THE INTERNATIONAL CONTEXT

The British Society of Gerontology was founded in 1971 with members who shared an interest in the understanding of ageing and the life course and who had a commitment to promoting wellbeing in later life (British Society of Gerontology 2020). The Australian Association of Gerontology (2020) has existed since 1964 and consists of members with a keen interest in evidence-based care for the older population and an aim to improve the experience of ageing through research, policy improvement and education. The Gerontological Society of America (GSA 2020) was created in 1949 by scientists and has provided visionary leadership for health professionals over the past 70 years. The GSA published the first edition of the *Journal of Gerontology* in 1946 and *The Gerontologist* in 1961. It was also instrumental in the founding of The National Institute of Aging in 1974 with *Innovation in Aging* being their first online, open access journal, established in 2017. The New Zealand Association of Gerontology (NZAG) was founded in 1981 with the primary aims of promoting quality research on ageing and encouraging education and training in relation to ageing, to stimulate debate on the wellbeing of older people, to contribute to public discussion and policy development, as well as providing a forum for networking and the sharing of ideas (NZAG 2020). These associations often work collaboratively and internationally for the wellbeing of older people, and all are members of IAGG – the International Association of Gerontology and Geriatrics.

THE ROLE OF THE NURSE

The privilege of being able to care for someone in the later years of their life cannot be underestimated. The care of the older person needs to be considered as a holistic approach, taking into consideration physical, psychological, social and spiritual wellbeing. The nurse must know the person or take time to learn who they are and where they have come from, what their life means to them and to their friends and family. All too often the older person is ignored or seen as a nuisance in a general acute ward, a drain on resources and not deserving of care or time. Terminology when addressing an older person must be carefully considered so as to not cause offence (Gendron et al 2016). It is vital to ensure that the older person is both seen and heard, and treated with the dignity and respect they deserve within a person-centred model of care.

Person-Centred Care

The concept of person-centred care (PCC) was first articulated by James Kitwood (Kitwood & Bredin 1992; Kitwood 1997). The key principles include:

1. Older people must be treated with dignity, compassion and respect.
2. The nurse must provide coordinated care, support and treatment.
3. The nurse will offer personalised care, support and treatment.
4. Person-centred care will enable service users to recognise and develop their strengths and abilities, so they can live an independent and fulfilling life.

Person-centred care was originally applied to the care of the person living with dementia, with Kitwood arguing that the limitations of a medical diagnosis could reduce the complexity of a person, resulting in a loss of personhood. The uniqueness of a person in relation to their thoughts, memories, values and interconnections with friends and family needs deeper consideration to create individual care options. Davis and colleagues (2005) identified that PCC should be considered across eight dimensions, including:

1. an awareness and respect of the person's values and needs as they identify them
2. the information required by the person to be educated and empowered to make informed decisions
3. equal and fair access to care
4. psychosocial support
5. the involvement of people the person considers important to their own wellbeing; for example, family and loved ones
6. consistent transition through the required healthcare settings
7. physical comfort
8. the coordination of all the above.

To be able to achieve a true PCC approach, the nurse requires expert, multifaceted knowledge and skills (Phelan & McCormack 2016). The individual and the team require an advanced level of interpersonal skills to develop collaborative sharing relationships with the older person and the family (McCormack et al 2010). Therefore, without a sense of purpose or dedication to the older person and their lives, aspiring to person-centred care will not be successful (Phelan & McCormack 2016). The key to PCC is communication: with the older person, with the family and within the healthcare team.

Communication

The family must be involved in all plans regarding the older person, as they are often the primary caregivers. The issue of shared decision-making and informed choice is further explored in Chapter 7. The care given to younger people must also be extended to others, regardless of age. Ageism is still an area for concern and older people must not be invisible.

Communication skills are vitally important and the older person must be addressed with respect. If a first name is preferred, this can be used, but must never be assumed. The use of first names may be earned through respect and/or permission. The use of terms such as *love, doll, pet, honey, hun* must be avoided and do not offer any respect within a professional therapeutic relationship (Avers et al 2011; Gendron et al 2016).

Age-related changes in older people can develop gradually, and with healthy ageing these changes may not develop until very old age. It must never be assumed that age equals a hearing and vision deficit prior to a full holistic assessment. Hearing and vision issues are key to effective communication and the sharing of information (see Chapters 20 and 21). The need for hearing aids to be maintained and in good working order is a daily requirement to ensure effective communication.

The person who knows the older person best is the family or friend, and this detail must be included in an initial assessment. It is of vital importance that the next of kin are able to be contacted at any time so that communication can be effective and timely. It should never be assumed that family/next of kin contact details are the same as those used during a previous assessment/admission.

A nurse with specialist knowledge in older people will take time to get to know the person, understand age-related changes that may occur and develop plans of care to continue to promote independence when they are able. The life and relationships of the older person need to be acknowledged and considered during assessment and care planning.

Within the context of gerontology, it is important to understand the national and international profile of ageing (see Chapter 2). Every nurse needs to be an expert in the care of older people; someone who acknowledges the need for an individualistic approach to ensure effective care always.

CHALLENGES OF GERONTOLOGICAL NURSING CARE

The challenges of providing specialised gerontological nursing care to older people in the current healthcare context is complicated by the funding of services and the constant changing landscape of care. Challenges include the following:

- The need for further education and specialist qualifications in gerontology.
- Recruitment and retention of appropriate registered/enrolled nurses.
- A fast-changing landscape of policy and practice.
- Gerontological nursing being prominent in the undergraduate nursing curriculum.
- The healthcare profession appreciating gerontology as a specialised area of practice.
- Promotion of gerontology as an attractive option for a career pathway.

Due to the increasing number, globally, of older people living longer (Chapter 2), gerontological nursing can provide an exciting career structure for new graduates. It is imperative that healthcare organisations provide support and education to attract the right people to do this important job. The gerontological nurse needs to be enquiring, adaptable, skilled, knowledgeable and up to date with all current and new aged care legislation.

The Royal Commission into Aged Care Quality and Safety in Australia

In 2018, the Royal Commission into Aged Care Quality and Safety (Royal Commission) was established in Australia following a public outcry in response to media reports of deficiencies and failings in aged care facilities, many of which were brought to light by families. At the time of writing, in October 2020, the Royal Commission remains in progress. An interim report released in October 2019 and titled *Neglect* found that the aged care system in Australia 'fails to meet the needs of our older, often very vulnerable, citizens … does not deliver uniformly safe and quality care for older people …' (Royal Commission 2019). The report acknowledged that most nurses strive to deliver safe and compassionate care in a challenging environment. Yet results of surveys undertaken by the National Ageing Research Institute (NARI) and released by the Royal Commission in October 2020 revealed that about one-third (33.4%) of people in residential aged care report that their care needs are met only 'sometimes', 'rarely' or 'never' (Batchelor et al 2020). Nurses will be crucial to the forthcoming recommendations for 'fundamental reform and redesign' (p. 12) in the Royal Commission's final report scheduled for 2021 (Royal Commission 2019). The commissioners acknowledge that aged care, whether in residential facilities or home-based community care, is integral to the national social support system and required to deliver care responsive to older people's needs that achieves the best quality of life possible. Nurses skilled in gerontological care, who understand and address the complex needs of older people, are well placed to lead more person-centred, safe, responsive and accountable care delivery.

Future Education of the Aged Care Workforce

A taskforce is currently exploring the future of aged care educational preparation (The Centre for Workforce at Macquarie University and SkillsIQ Limited 2020). An initial discussion document titled *Pathways and tertiary education in aged care* highlights the needs for the educational preparation of the aged care workforce moving into the next decade. An increase in the workforce is anticipated due to the increase in life expectancy and corresponding health care needs of an older population.

Gerontological Research and the Nurse

Research and the care of older people is important in today's health care context. The need to identify best practice and explore the perceptions of nurses in relation to providing specialised care to older people will help to improve care for this population. Three key recent research studies are detailed below:

- Mueller and colleagues (2020) explored the development and growth of advanced practice registered nurses (APRNs), who specialised in the care of older people in the United States. They found that having extra knowledge and qualifications specifically in gerontology had a significant positive impact on the care of older people in all settings.
- Garbrah and colleagues (2017), in an integrative review, explored why student nurses did not pursue a career in gerontological nursing. The review of 21 papers identified the need for an age-friendly curriculum with a focus on the speciality of gerontological nursing. The issues of witnessing poor practice in the aged care environment was also highlighted. One other key finding was the need to improve the mentorship and support during gerontological nursing placements to provide a positive learning experience.
- Fulmer (2020), in a recent paper, provided the history of gerontological nursing over 40 years, identifying the key themes as:
  - a shortage of trained geriatric healthcare professionals
  - a shortage of academic staff
  - a paucity of research funding
  - an increased need for interdisciplinary care
  - the meaningful use and integration of technology
  - a current lack of research funding
  - a general lack of interest in geriatrics as a specialty.

The paper also highlighted that the demand for specialist gerontological nursing is growing in line with an increased older population and nurses are ideally placed to fill any gaps in care. Leadership qualities were also identified as essential in moving the aged care agenda forwards. Fulmer also praised the visionary work of The John A. Hartford Foundation in raising the profile of gerontological nursing.

SUMMARY

This chapter has highlighted the burgeoning demand for older persons' healthcare as the global population ages. While healthy ageing is a goal that many older people will realise, others will spend their final years with multiple chronic illnesses, frailty, disability and increasing dependence on caregivers. Nurses care for older people across the spectrum of care settings and are central to preventing poor outcomes and promoting quality of life until the end of life. Gerontology recognises the specialised knowledge and skills required to deliver high-quality care responsive to the individual and complex needs of older people. Gerontological nursing integrates a holistic, comprehensive and person-centred approach to care where respectful communication and the expertise of family are valued. Older people are frequent consumers of healthcare and most nurses will care for an older person at some point in their career. Nurses skilled in gerontological care currently provide multifaceted care to address the older person's needs across healthcare settings, and will be even more instrumental as leaders of safe, quality and compassionate care for older people into the future.

Tips for Best Practice
Nursing the Older Person in All Care Settings

- Address the older person with dignity and respect
- Practise person-centred care
- Maintain clinical assessment skills and currency in practice
- Stay up to date with research, policy directions and national frameworks for practice
- Perform a head-to-toe physical assessment
- Take a full history
- Conduct a psychosocial assessment
- Ensure prompt and ongoing assessment of the older person along the care continuum
- Record any/all medications
- Source evidence-based practice information and updates from specialised healthcare organisations
- Maintain consistent and regular communication with the older person and their family
- Document all findings, discussions and observations.

SUMMARY OF CHAPTERS

The following chapters contain up-to-date information relating specifically to the care of the older person. Promoting wellness, best practice, research highlights, safety alerts and practice scenarios underpins the content of all chapters.

Chapter 2: Contemporary Ageing

This chapter considers the changing demographic profile and the impact on an ageing population in Australia and New Zealand. The diversity of the ageing population and the impact on older Australians and New Zealanders and their health needs, including an Indigenous and Pacific peoples' perspective, is discussed. Current policy and strategies to ensure social participation, good health and security as 'pillars' to ageing well is also explored.

Chapter 3: Cross-Cultural Ageing

Cultural diversity in older people in Australia and New Zealand, including an explanation of cultural competence and cultural safety, is covered in this chapter. Challenges and opportunities in promoting healthy ageing for older people from Indigenous and culturally and linguistically diverse backgrounds are explored. Useful tools and resources are also identified to achieve healthy ageing for older people from Indigenous and culturally and linguistically diverse backgrounds.

Chapter 4: Promoting Healthy Ageing

The importance of exploring the concepts and determinants of healthy ageing is discussed. Understanding the key factors and strategies that underpin health promotion for older people cannot be underestimated. The Transtheoretical model of health promotion, as well as the application of Miller's functional consequences theory, are addressed as frameworks to promote healthy ageing across clinical settings.

Chapter 5: Navigating the Healthcare System

Navigating aged care services within the Australian and New Zealand context needs to be clearly understood by all nurses, older people and their families. This chapter also highlights key quality and safety issues in health and aged care, including clinical governance frameworks.

Chapter 6: Gerontological Nursing Across the Continuum of Care

This chapter describes the different care options, including community-based and residential care, available to the older person within the Australian and New Zealand context. The importance of thorough holistic assessment of the older person in relation to accessing services is discussed, as well as the process of transitioning into permanent residential aged care.

Chapter 7: Communication and Shared Decision-Making

This chapter identifies the legal and ethical principles that underpin shared decision-making for older people. Communication strategies to facilitate shared decision-making

for older people, and the ability to establish decision-making capacity and identify appropriate substitute decision-makers, are addressed.

Chapter 8: Comprehensive Health Assessment

The physiological and functional changes of the ageing process are discussed. A range of assessment tools offering the nurse options for a holistic assessment are explored. Techniques used to assess the older person and the importance of documentation in providing quality care in a range of settings are highlighted.

Chapter 9: Living With Chronic Conditions

Chapter 9 discusses the prevalence of chronic disease among older people and the types of chronic diseases experienced, including the concept of multimorbidity. The drivers of the increase in chronic disease among older people are outlined, as well as the reasons why older people are vulnerable to developing chronic conditions. The role of the nurse in supporting the older population to age well through prevention and management of chronic disease is explored.

Chapter 10: Infection Prevention and Control

The measures taken to reduce infection in older people in Australia and New Zealand are defined in relation to infection control principles. The challenges and opportunities to prevent norovirus and influenza in the older population are explored. The issue of presenteeism and the effects on the older population are also discussed.

Chapter 11: Safe Use of Medications

This chapter discusses the legislation relevant to medication safety in Australia and New Zealand. It examines the pharmacokinetic and pharmacodynamic changes that influence the safe use of medications, and how multimorbidity and polypharmacy increase the risk of adverse outcomes associated with medication use in older people. The consequences of non-adherence with medication regimens and the appropriateness of medications used for older people with limited life expectancy are also explored.

Chapter 12: Nutrition and Hydration

This chapter highlights the importance of monitoring and managing the nutritional status of older people. The causes, risks and consequences of weight loss, malnutrition and obesity in older people are discussed. The importance of oral health and how it might affect the nutritional status of older people, as well as understanding the risks and consequences of dehydration and recommended intervention strategies, are also explored. The most common screening tools to assess the nutritional status of older people and recommended nutritional and activity therapies are explained.

Chapter 13: Elimination

This chapter explores the misconception of incontinence being a normal part of ageing. The most common types of bladder and bowel dysfunction and the nursing interventions that can improve the older person's bladder and bowel function are discussed.

Chapter 14: Sleep and Rest

Chapter 14 highlights the physiology of sleep and the age-related changes which impact on sleep. The most common sleep disorders and the appropriate nursing care strategies to promote sleep in the older population are discussed.

Chapter 15: Promoting Healthy Skin

This chapter explores age-related skin changes in older people and distinguishes between intrinsic and extrinsic ageing. The three most common age-related skin manifestations are highlighted, as well as the management of skin tears and venous, arterial and neuropathic ulcers.

Chapter 16: Falls and Falls Prevention

Chapter 16 identifies the risk factors for falls among older people and explores the cumulative impact of multiple risk factors. The importance of a medical review for older people if they are unsteady or have falls is highlighted. The difference between falls risk screening and falls risk assessment and examples of evidence-based tools are explored. Interventions to reduce the risk of falls in the older population are also discussed.

Chapter 17: A Palliative Approach

Chapter 17 discusses the role of palliative care for older people with life-limiting conditions, recognition of the dying older person, symptom management, and the nurse's role in communication and decision-making in end-of-life care. The elements of a 'good death' are highlighted. Three recognised trajectories of chronic illness are discussed, along with application of a palliative approach in residential aged care settings. There is a discussion of the role of nurses in facilitating the process of advance care planning to ensure an older person's choices for end-of-life care are known and documented.

Chapter 18: Safety and Security

Common safety and security issues of concern in older people are explored in this chapter. Natural disasters and implications for the safety of older people are highlighted. The risk factors and implications of homelessness in the older population are discussed. Innovative technologies used to facilitate ageing in place and quality of life is also explored.

Chapter 19: Pain Assessment and Management

The biopsychosocial model of pain and the differences between acute and chronic pain in older people are explained in this chapter. The differences between nociceptive and neuropathic pain, as well as the components of a comprehensive pain assessment, are discussed. Common non-pharmacological and pharmacological pain relief measures are outlined. Considerations required of pain management in older people with cognitive and communicative impairments are also explored.

Chapter 20: Hearing

The incidence and risk factors of hearing loss, nursing assessment and health promotion strategies in the older population are identified. The three main types of hearing loss and the implications for communication in older people are explored, as well as the referral pathways for available assistance in Australia and New Zealand.

Chapter 21: Vision

This chapter describes age-related changes and the most common conditions affecting vision in older age. Appropriate nursing interventions for older people with vision impairment and the challenges of vision impairment in later life are also discussed.

Chapter 22: Musculoskeletal Health

Chapter 22 explores the current trends in musculoskeletal disorders in older people and identifies the age-related changes that occur in bones, muscles and connective tissues. The physical changes that occur in inflammatory conditions, including osteoarthritis, rheumatoid arthritis and gout, are highlighted. Nursing assessment, interventions, and management of bone and joint disorders to minimise disability, as well as the consequences associated with traumatic injury and limited mobility in older people, are discussed.

Chapter 23: Cardiovascular Health

Age-related changes of the cardiovascular system associated with normal ageing, as well as common conditions associated with older people, are discussed in this chapter.

Assessment and interventions for maximising health relating to the cardiovascular system in older people are also explored.

Chapter 24: Respiratory Health

The age-related changes of the respiratory system associated with normal ageing are identified, as well as the common conditions associated with older people. Assessment of the respiratory system in older people, interventions and methods for maximising health of the respiratory system are explored.

Chapter 25: Mental Health in Older Age

The factors that contribute to good mental health and poor mental health in older people, including the cultural factors that contribute to mental disorders in older people, are explored in this chapter. The prevalence and clinical features of depression, anxiety and psychosis in older age, as well as alcohol and other substance-use disorders and suicide, are addressed. The specific care and treatment of the older person in relation to mental problems and mental health disorders is also outlined.

Chapter 26: Neurocognitive Disorders

Chapter 26 explores delirium, as well as major and minor neurocognitive disorders, including mild cognitive impairment, dementia and Parkinson's disease. Tools used to assess for dementia and delirium are also highlighted. The importance of the use of language within the context of living with dementia and the inclusion of dementia-friendly environments are considered. Responsive behaviours are discussed in the context of behavioural and psychological symptoms of dementia (BPSD) to identify strategies for a person with dementia to live well.

Chapter 27: Relationships in Later Life

Chapter 27 explores the importance of relationships in later life for older people relating to wellbeing. A range of diverse relationships is considered, as well as the potential obstacles and challenges within relationships in later life. Nursing strategies that recognise and support relationships in later life are also explored.

Chapter 28: The Caregiver

The changing role and recognition of family caregivers within the context of the Australian and New Zealand health systems and policies are considered in this chapter. The knowledge and skills required in assessing family caregiving, including training and education to support the caregivers, are explored. An analysis of the family caregiving experience in relation to developing strategies to improve outcomes and manage barriers is discussed.

Chapter 29: Loss, Grief and Bereavement

Chapter 29 discusses loss, grief, mourning and bereavement, including cultural influences on mourning. The main factors that impact on an older person's risk of developing complicated, prolonged or persistent grief are described. The nursing response to assist older people experiencing ambiguous loss is discussed, as well as appropriate communication strategies to consider when supporting a bereaved older person.

REFERENCES

Apóstolo J, Cooke R, Bobrowicz-Campos E et al (2018) Effectiveness of interventions to prevent pre-frailty and frailty progression in older adults: a systematic review. JBI Evidence Synthesis 16(1). Online. Available: https://journals.lww.com/jbisrir/Fulltext/2018/01000/Effectiveness_of_interventions_to_prevent.15.aspx

Australian Association of Gerontology (2020) Australian Association of Gerontology. Online. Available: www.aag.asn.au/about-us

Australian Institute of Health and Welfare (AIHW) (2019) Aged care. Online. Available: www.aihw.gov.au/reports/australias-welfare/aged-care

Australian Institute of Health and Welfare (AIHW) (2018). Older Australia at a glance. Online. Available: www.aihw.gov.au/reports/older-people/older-australia-at-a-glance/contents/health-aged-care-service-use/health-care-hospitals

Avers D, Brown M, Chui K et al (2011) Use of the term 'elderly'. Journal of Geriatric Physical Therapy 34(4):153–154.

Batchelor F, Savvas S, Dang C et al (2020) Inside the system: aged care residents' perspectives. National Ageing Research Institute, Parkville. Online. Available: https://agedcare.royalcommission.gov.au/sites/default/files/2020-10/research-paper-13.pdf

British Society of Gerontology (2020) British Society of Gerontology. Online. Available: www.britishgerontology.org/

Craig L (2019) The role of the registered nurse in supporting frailty in care homes. British Journal of Nursing 28(13):833–837.

Davis K, Schoenbaum SC, Audet AM (2005) A 2020 vision of patient-centered primary care. Journal of General Internal Medicine 20(10):953–957.

Fulmer T (2020) A retrospective/prospective on the future of geriatric nursing. Geriatric Nursing 41(1):29–31.

Garbrah W, Välimäki T, Palovaara M et al (2017). Nursing curriculums may hinder a career in gerontological nursing: An integrative review. International Journal of Older People Nursing 12:e12152.

Gendron TL, Welleford EA, Inker J et al (2016) The language of ageism: Why we need to use words carefully. The Gerontologist 56(6):997–1006.

Kitwood T (1997) Dementia reconsidered: The person comes first. Open University Press, Berkshire, UK.

Kitwood T, Bredin K (1992) Towards a theory of dementia care: Personhood and well-being. Ageing and Society 12:269–287.

McCormack B, Dewing J, Breslin L et al (2010) Developing person-centred practice: Nursing outcomes arising from changes to the care environment in residential settings for older people. International Journal of Older People Nursing 5(2):93–107.

Mueller C, Burggraf V, Neva L et al (2020) Growth and specialization of gerontological nursing. Geriatric Nursing 41(1):14–15.

New Zealand Association of Gerontology (2020) What is the NZ Association of Gerontology? Online. Available: https://gerontology.kiwi/about-nzag/home/

Phelan A, McCormack B (2016) Exploring nursing expertise in residential care for older people: a mixed methods study. Journal of Advanced Nursing 72(10):2524–2535.

Royal Commission into Aged Care Quality and Safety (2019) Interim report: Neglect. Online. Available: https://agedcare.royalcommission.gov.au/publications/interim-report-volume-1

The Centre for Workforce at Macquarie University and SkillsIQ Limited (2020) Pathways and tertiary education in aged care: discussion paper. Online. Available: www.skillsiq.com.au/site/DefaultSite/filesystem/documents/Research/Pathways%20and%20Tertiary%20Education%20Discussion%20Paper%20Final2.pdf

The Gerontological Society of America (2020) History. Online. Available: www.geron.org/about-us/history

United Nations, Department of Economic and Social Affairs (2019) World population prospects: Ten key findings. Online. Available: https://population.un.org/wpp/Publications/Files/WPP2019_10KeyFindings.pdf

Wyman JF, Abdallah L, Baker N et al (2019) Development of core competencies and a recognition program for gerontological nursing educators. Journal of Professional Nursing 35(6):452–460.

CHAPTER 2

Contemporary Ageing

ANNE-MARIE HOLT

LEARNING OBJECTIVES

After reading this chapter, you will be able to:

- consider the changing demographic profile and the impact on an ageing population in Australia and New Zealand
- consider and discuss the diversity of the ageing population and the impact on older Australians and New Zealanders and their health needs, including Indigenous and Pacific peoples' perspective
- discuss and evaluate the ability of current policy and strategies to ensure social participation, good health and security as 'pillars' to ageing well
- explore and consider the challenges and opportunities that older people in Australia and New Zealand face now and in the future
- consider how some of these challenges and opportunities associated with ageing might be addressed through professional practice and patient-centred care.

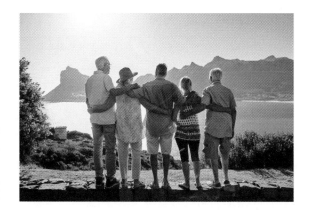

INTRODUCTION

This chapter will focus on the economic and social dimensions of ageing in 21st century Australia and New Zealand and will also examine the current profile of older people. The biological and psychosocial theories of ageing will be explored to create an awareness of the psychological and cognitive aspects of ageing. The trajectory of illness will also be discussed within these theoretical realms.

An overview of the World Health Organisation (WHO) Decade of Health Ageing 2020–2030 initiative (2019) – a global strategy and plan on ageing and health in a rapidly changing society, will be examined within the current healthcare system. This strategy is important when planning and developing systems within countries on all levels to support older populations to maintain and sustain functional ability.

The often-overlooked opportunities that older people present as a solution to ageing in contemporary times will also be discussed. Older people continue to contribute to society in many ways post-retirement, with the knowledge, skills and experiences acquired across their life course, as well as in their capacity as consumers and volunteers. This chapter will also explore the most current developments in ageing in Australia and New Zealand. These developments will be discussed in a constructive and innovative way, allowing development of knowledge and skills to equip the nurse with the capacity to work with older people in a broad scope and capacity.

CURRENT TRENDS AND PATTERNS IN AUSTRALIA AND NEW ZEALAND

This first section explores the changing demographic trends in Australia and New Zealand in population ageing with a special focus on Indigenous Australians and the Māori and Pacific peoples of New Zealand.

The Australian Context

Current trends and patterns

In the past 30 years, life expectancy in Australia has increased at a faster rate than many other developed nations. In 2009, Australia was ranked fifth globally for highest life expectancy. However, over the last decade, life expectancy has changed with Australia now ranked tenth globally, its international ranking set to decrease even further over the next decade (Organisation for Economic Co-operation and Development [OECD] 2018) (see Fig. 2.1).

Initially, growth in life expectancy during the 1990s was due to strong public health policy and legislation (e.g. tobacco control), along with the advent of health screening programs (e.g. breast cancer and bowel cancer) and the promotion of active lifestyles. However, rising rates of obesity and overweight, which are strongly linked to chronic disease and co-morbidity in the ageing population, have contributed to the decline in life expectancy as a nation since then. Middle-age is a critical period for disease prevention via the promotion of healthy lifestyles. With a disproportionate number of older people experiencing poorer outcomes in the last decades of life, it is important to initiate behaviour change during middle-age that will support good healthy ageing in older persons.

Promoting Wellness
Measuring Life Expectancy

Life expectancy is calculated using prevailing mortality rates for a given population in a given period of time. Life expectancy is often viewed from a disease-orientated model that focuses on poor health, pathology and dysfunction.

The Health-Adjusted-Life-Expectancy (HALE) score is an alternative measure of life expectancy. HALE refers to the number of years we spend in full health. It views ageing from an 'asset-based' perspective by taking into consideration the number of years spent in full health rather than poor health.

Tips for Best Practice
How Old Do You Feel?

A recent Council on the Ageing (COTA) study reported that 90% of people surveyed who were 50 years of age felt younger than their actual chronological age. Along with looking after various dimensions of physical health, an older person's attitude to getting older has a direct impact on wellbeing and the capacity to age healthfully (Council on the Ageing 2018).

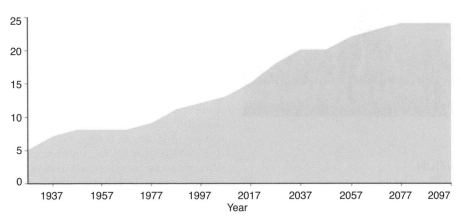

FIG. 2.1 **The percentage of the Australian population aged 65 years and over, 1901–2097.** (ABS 2014.)

Diversity of older Australians

Older Australians are a diverse group emanating from many cultural and linguistic backgrounds. Post-war migration policies contributed to the multicultural profile of older persons in contemporary Australia. Around three out of ten older Australians were born overseas, and two out of every ten older Australians speak a language other than English (Australian Bureau of Statistics [ABS] 2016). About 20% of Australians aged over 65 years were born in a non-English speaking country, primarily from Italy (3%), Greece (2%) and Germany (1%). It is estimated that 10% of older Australians were born in the United Kingdom and Ireland (Australian Institute of Health and Welfare [AIHW] 2018b).

Where do older Australians live?

In Australia, 59% of older people living in urban areas reside in the largest cities, making up 6.3% of the total metropolitan population. It is interesting to note that the other 41%, who live in regional areas, make up a larger proportion (8.1%) of all people living outside Australia's major cities. State by state the highest proportion of older Australians live in the coastal areas of New South Wales and South Australia, along with the more arid farming areas of north-western Victoria, Western Australia and central-western NSW (AIHW 2018b).

Life Expectancy of Older Persons in Rural and/or Remote Communities in Australia

There are fundamental differences between the health of older people living in rural and remote areas of Australia and those living in metropolitan areas. Life expectancy decreases with remoteness and is often up to seven years lower in remote areas, especially for men (AIHW 2018b). Additionally, older people in rural and remote areas report poorer overall health when compared to urban-dwelling older persons.

Higher rates of chronic illness, co-morbidity and poor physical health, particularly reduced mobility, are experienced by older populations in rural and remote communities. Social isolation due to geographical distance is a common feature of living in a rural or remote community and is one of the main contributors to this disparity (AIHW 2018b).

Future Trends

As the Australian population continues to age there will be a higher proportion of people classified as 'old-old', being in the 80–95+ year-old category as opposed to the 'young-old', a term that refers to those aged 65–80 years. Some gerontologists see Australia's population as becoming a super-aged society. With the right support

> ### Research Highlight
> ### *Age Migration: Sea Change/Tree Change*
>
> The characteristics of older persons who live in rural or remote areas vary among communities. There are many people who have worked and lived in these areas for many years, often for most of their lives, whereas others may have moved to the 'country' for retirement, often referred to the 'sea change or 'tree change' phenomenon.
>
> Over the last two decades, rural Australia has experienced a steady increase in the number of older people moving from urban areas to rural towns. More recently there has been an increase in the number of older people choosing to retire in remote communities.
>
> National statistics on people making a sea change or tree change are scarce. In 2014, the ABS released results of a study on Queenslanders aged over 55 years and their migratory patterns to coastal areas for the period 2006–2011 (ABS 2014). Most of these older Queenslanders moved from Brisbane, and the major cities of NSW. Around 44% had moved from interstate areas, while the rest had come from intrastate areas. Of the top 25 regions for internal migration of older Queenslanders, 13 were either tree-change or sea-change locations (Stokes & Faulkner 2008).

ABS (2014); Stokes & Faulkner (2008).

via age-friendly policies, along with age-friendly communities, there is no reason that longevity and quality of life cannot be maintained in the very late years of life.

Current Health Profile of Older Australians

In 2018, life expectancy for Australians was 82.6 years, with average life expectancy at 80.5 years for males and 84.6 years for females (OECD 2018). The four leading causes of death for older Australians are: coronary heart disease; lung cancer; dementia and Alzheimer's disease; and chronic obstructive pulmonary disease (COPD). Colorectal cancer is the fifth leading cause of death for people aged 65–74 years, while influenza and pneumonia are ranked fifth for the very old (people aged 95+ years) (see Fig. 2.2). The most recent data show that coronary heart disease was the leading cause of death in all older Australians in the period 2014–2016 (AIHW 2018b). As the proportion of people aged over 65 continues to grow there will be an increase in the number of people with dementia and Alzheimer's disease and is set to surpass coronary heart disease in the coming years (AIHW 2018b).

It is estimated that 80% of Australians aged over 65 have three or more co-morbidities. Many older Australians with arthritis also have hypertension, cardiovascular

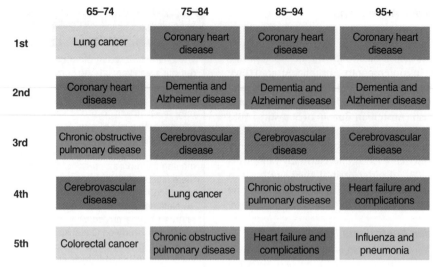

	65–74	75–84	85–94	95+
1st	Lung cancer	Coronary heart disease	Coronary heart disease	Coronary heart disease
2nd	Coronary heart disease	Dementia and Alzheimer disease	Dementia and Alzheimer disease	Dementia and Alzheimer disease
3rd	Chronic obstructive pulmonary disease	Cerebrovascular disease	Cerebrovascular disease	Cerebrovascular disease
4th	Cerebrovascular disease	Lung cancer	Chronic obstructive pulmonary disease	Heart failure and complications
5th	Colorectal cancer	Chronic obstructive pulmonary disease	Heart failure and complications	Influenza and pneumonia

FIG. 2.2 **Five leading causes of death for older Australians, by age group 2014–2016.** (AIHW 2018b.)

disease and diabetes (AIHW 2018b). The presence of multiple chronic conditions can have profound impacts on the older person's quality of life, activities of daily living (ADLs), mobility and levels of psychological stress. This in turn leads to higher use of health services, putting increasing pressure on federal and state health budgets (see Chapter 9).

Research Highlight
Homelessness

More older Australians have become homeless in recent years. The proportion of homeless older Australians increased by 30% in the period between 2011 and 2016 (Thredgold et al 2019). Poverty and the lack of affordable housing is the root cause of homelessness, which has a major impact on all components of the older person's health, including physical, mental and spiritual health.

Older women (55+ years) are becoming the fastest growing cohort of homeless Australians in current times. Older women in these situations are less visible and are becoming an emerging vulnerable population. The homeless situation is a contemporary ageing issue that requires immediate action through a strong healthy ageing policy that supports longevity and overall wellbeing. Having safe, affordable and sustainable housing is a fundamental principle of the WHO Decade of Healthy Ageing 2020–2030, discussed later in this chapter.

Thredgold et al (2019); WHO (2019).

The Indigenous Perspective

Remote areas make up about 78% of Australia's landmass and are home to a large proportion of Indigenous Australians. Older Indigenous Australians who live remotely are at higher risk of many of the determinants associated with ageing poorly.

The Aboriginal and Torres Strait Islander peoples' perspective

Aboriginal and Torres Strait Islander peoples do not age at an accelerated rate, but face a greater burden of disease at an earlier age due to the premature onset of age-related health conditions. By the time they reach their mid-40s, Indigenous Australians are more likely than non-Indigenous Australians to face premature death. There is a higher incidence of chronic disease, such as heart disease, kidney disease, lung disease and diabetes (see Chapter 3). Dementia rates are also increasing in this population. The higher rates of chronic disease and the discrepancy in health status means life expectancy *still* remains 10 years less than for the rest of the Australian population (Commonwealth of Australia 2020).

While many of the determinants of poor health are specifically related to lifestyle factors such as alcohol use, smoking and poor diet, trauma has recently been acknowledged as a root cause of the age gap in life expectancy between Indigenous and non-Indigenous Australians (AIHW 2018a; Menzies 2019). The biopsychosocial factors that impact on the ageing process for older Indigenous

Australians living in remote communities are substantially different to those of older non-Indigenous Australians. This includes higher rates of incarceration, unemployment, domestic violence and homelessness, along with substance abuse. They experience overall poorer mental health, higher levels of discrimination and have poor self-assessed health (AIHW 2018c). These factors influence and accelerate conditions normally not seen in non-Indigenous Australians (AIHW 2018c). Despite this, there is evidence that many Indigenous Australians live healthy lives well into their 80s (AIHW 2018c).

The factors contributing to this phenomenon of ageing in the Indigenous population need to be identified more clearly.

Early British settlement in Australia marked a significant period in Australia's history where the British Crown claimed possession and established the east coast of Australia as a penal colony (Maxwell-Stewart & Oxley 2020). This early colonisation of Australia had a devastating impact on Indigenous Australians. There is now a strong ongoing precedent to improve and build relationships between Indigenous Australians and the Australian nation state by approaching the de-colonisation of Australia through a formal reconciliation process (Dodson & Cronin 2011; Paradies 2016). The process of de-colonisation aims to recognise Indigenous rights by empowering change and transformation via strong public policy (Dodson & Cronin 2011; Paradies 2016).

However, colonisation and de-colonisation are more than just historical processes – they are still ongoing. Colonisation included the severance of connection to the land for many Indigenous people, and the removal of Indigenous people from their own ethnic groups. This has led to the destruction of many economic and social practices, resulting in a loss of cultural heritage, such as native languages. Ongoing social exclusion and racism established through policies of assimilation have compounded the effects of colonisation and de-colonisation on the First Nations people in many countries (Dodson & Cronin 2011; Paradies 2016).

The Australian Government's main focus for improving the health of older Australians is to prevent or reduce chronic disease. The government seeks to enable healthy ageing by maintaining and improving the health and quality of life among *all* older Australians – even more so for Indigenous Australians (AIHW 2018a).

THE NEW ZEALAND CONTEXT
Current Trends and Patterns

New Zealand's older population is increasing in line with global trends. It is predicted that by 2036 around 1,258,500 people will be over the age of 65, equating to one in every 4.5 New Zealanders. Currently 15% of New Zealanders are over 65 years old (Ministry of Health NZ 2018).

In New Zealand, life expectancy mirrors that of Australia. In the 1970s, New Zealand experienced a growth in life expectancy ranking followed by a gradual decline, and it now ranks 15th in the world (OECD 2018). New Zealand also experiences very high levels of obesity and overweight within the older population, contributing to declining life expectancy rates. And also, similarly to Australia, while life expectancy is decreasing overall, the number of older New Zealanders aged 65+ years is increasing (see Fig. 2.3).

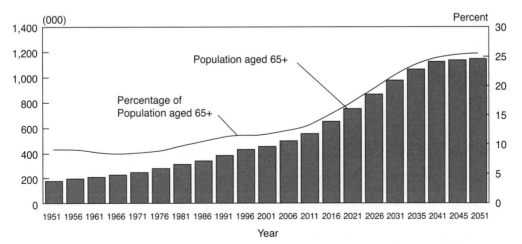

FIG. 2.3 **New Zealand's population 65+, 1951–2051** (Statistics New Zealand 2007.)

Future Trends
Diversity of older New Zealanders
Presently, older New Zealanders are largely of European background. However, as New Zealand's population continues to age, other ethnic groups will increase proportionally in the older cohort. It is predicted that there will be a 60% rise in older Europeans aged 65 and over, while those of Māori ethnicity will increase by 115%, Pacific peoples will increase by 160% and people of Asian descent (who have migrated or were born in New Zealand) will increase by 260%. Older New Zealanders are set to become one of the most culturally diverse groups in the world (Ministry of Health NZ 2019a).

Where do older New Zealanders live?
Many older New Zealanders live in regional and rural areas. In around 41% of regional towns and 29% of rural centres more than 20% of the population is over the age of 65. However, similarly to Australia, the four main cities in New Zealand have the largest number of older people aged 65 years and over (ABS 2017; Ministry of Health NZ 2019a).

Health Profile of Older New Zealanders
Average life expectancy in New Zealand for males is 80.5 years and for females is 82.2 years (WHO 2019). Latest New Zealand Health Survey data state that higher rates of diabetes, high blood pressure and colorectal cancer are contributing to poor health in many older New Zealanders (Ministry of Health NZ 2019a). Cancer is the leading cause of premature death in older New Zealanders, accounting for nearly one-third of all deaths (Ministry of Health NZ 2019a). The Global Burden of Disease Study (Institute for Health Metrics and Evaluation [IHME] 2018) reported that 'in terms of numbers of years of life lost due to premature death in New Zealand, ischaemic heart disease, trachea, bronchus and lung cancers, and cerebrovascular disease were the highest-ranking causes in 2016–17'.

Multimorbidity is common in older New Zealanders, particularly for those living in areas of high social and economic deprivation, and even more so among Māori and Pacific peoples. For older Māori males and females, ischaemic heart disease was the leading cause of death in 2018 (Ministry of Health NZ 2019a).

The Māori and Pacific peoples' perspective
Health inequalities persist and continue to affect the health of older New Zealanders, particularly older Pacific peoples of New Zealand. Older Māori and Pacific peoples have poorer health outcomes compared to people from other ethnic groups in New Zealand. There are higher rates of chronic disease, such as diabetes, stroke and chronic kidney conditions (see Chapter 3). Older Māori and Pacific peoples have lower income, wealth and assets contributing to poor health outcomes experienced by this group of New Zealanders (Ministry of Health NZ 2019b).

The health gradient is strongly reflected in the social gradient and social structure in which older Māori and Pacific peoples live. Social gradient is best explained as those people who are less advantaged in socioeconomic status, with poorer health and life expectancy than those who are more advantaged (WHO 2008). These factors underlie health inequalities and health disparity in these cultural groups.

A study conducted by Lotoala and colleagues (2014) found that across four different ethnic groups in New Zealand (Pacific, Māori, European and Asian), Pacific and Māori older persons had poorer physical and mental health than the other ethnic groups. These findings were attributed to lower socioeconomic status and found that this health disadvantage was due to differences in access to the resources needed for good health. Lifetime poverty accumulates to produce inequalities in mortality in older age. As such, the life expectancy of Māori and Pacific peoples in New Zealand is not dissimilar to that of Indigenous Australians – lower than that of people of European descent. Addiction (cigarette smoking, alcohol consumption), education, employment and income, along with deprivation, are some of the social determinants that are strong contributing factors to health disparities in older Māori and Pacific peoples in New Zealand (Ministry of Health NZ 2019b).

THEORIES ON AGEING
Compression of Morbidity Theory
The future health of the ageing population depends on the interplay between two critical periods in a person's lifetime – the first being onset of major disease and/or disability, and the second being time of death. As life expectancy continues to increase in Australia, there is a need to consider whether advances in medical technology will produce less disease and disability for older people. The Compression of Morbidity theory, first proposed by Fries in 1998, envisions a prolonged active life and delayed disability for older people who 'do the right things'. According to this theory, it is not inevitable that the population must become sicker as it becomes older. It is worth noting that '80% of the years of life lost to non-traumatic, premature death have been eliminated,

Ageism, much like sexism and racism, is a process of discriminating and stereotyping older persons because they are old! Ageism is a barrier to many things as a person gets older including good quality healthcare.

We often see ageism in the way we communicate with older people. At times we can be unaware of how we reinforce stigma around ageing and older persons. Often there is a specific language used to communicate attitudes and perceptions of older people, and this is where it begins – the seeding of attitudes and, thus, communication. A study by Williams and Giles in the 1990s discovered (not surprisingly) that communication to older people was often patronising, depersonalised and disrespectful. Unfortunately not much has changed since then in so many ways.

We need to be mindful of the effects of ageism, whether it is institutionalised, internalised (by the older person themselves) or personally mediated; these overwhelmingly underlie how effective our communication is with the older people we come into contact with as a nurse. Good and positive communication ensures that we do not over-accommodate or adjust too much, so that we as nurses remain respectful and do not appear to be condescending.

Gendron et al (2016).

and most premature deaths are now due to the chronic diseases of the later years' (Fries 1980:130).

In a nutshell, Fries proposed, and later confirmed through a 20-year longitudinal study, that compressing the number of years in which people are ill (morbidity) into a smaller time period can increase longevity, with the direct result that the older population is relatively healthy and independent for most of their years of life.

Compression of morbidity is the key goal of healthy ageing, achieved through delaying the onset of chronic disease and disability to lessen the burden of illness over a person's lifetime. In essence, the idea is to live disease-free for as long as possible by incorporating the lifestyle changes that are needed early on.

Compression of morbidity and age-related changes to body systems

Disability in older people results from three key factors:
- the impact of chronic disease (especially co-morbidity)
- lifestyle factors that influence risk of disease
- the biological changes that occur with ageing.

Of course, it is now known that the rate of physical ageing is not determined by genetics alone. Lifestyle factors

that can be changed or modified have a very powerful influence, and include the following (see Chapter 4):
- physical inactivity
- hypertension
- obesity
- high blood cholesterol
- diabetes
- poor diet
- alcohol overuse
- mental inactivity
- smoking.

A person's ability to function productively as they become older is as much about the lifestyle choices they make as it is about how they perceive their own health status (see Chapter 4).

Biological ageing is determined to a certain extent by the reduction in reparative and regenerative potential in tissues and organs. Individuals who are of the same chronological age can exhibit wide differences in trajectories of age-related decline. Postponing biological changes that are associated with ageing offer the potential to extend fitness, vitality and years lived free of morbidity and frailty.

Biological Theories of Ageing

Ageing brings about the slowing down of many biological and physiological functions. Modern biological theories of ageing no longer support the notion that ageing is determined by genetic predisposition or adaptation (Kunlin 2010). Contemporary theories consider the ageing process to be either programmed or caused by damage or error at the cellular level (Williams 2016).

Programmed cell death considers the ageing process to be a consequence of changes in gene expression that influence maintenance, repair and defence mechanisms within the body. It includes three sub-categories:
- programmed longevity
- endocrine theory
- immunological theory.

These theories are often interrelated. The sequential switching off and on of certain genes is associated with age-related deficits. Ageing is hormonally regulated, with insulin playing a major role in the regulation of ageing via each subcategory (Williams 2016). For example, the effectiveness of the immune system declines with increased age after peaking at puberty, and antibodies begin to lose their effectiveness. A dysregulated immune response has been linked to inflammation and infection. This in turn affects the ageing process.

Damage or error theories focus on environmental determinants that can act to stimulate cumulative damage across many different body systems. Wear and tear theory,

TABLE 2.1
Theories on Ageing From a Biological Perspective

Theory	Significance in the Ageing Process
Neuroendocrine theory	Loss of neurons and hormones influence the ageing process
Autoimmune theory of ageing	Compromised immune system associated with ageing
Free radical theory of ageing	Free radical production creates damage that causes ageing
Cross-linkage theory of ageing	Cross-links impair cell function and cause physical signs of ageing
Genetic control theory of ageing	Genes are programmed for a set number of divisions from birth
Somatic mutation theory of ageing	Harmful mistakes occur in the body and may lead to disease associated with ageing
Wear-and-tear theory of ageing	Initial theory postulates that the body simply wears out and ageing occurs

Adapted from Williams (2016).

Research Highlight
Telomere Theory – the Science Around Telomeres and Healthy Ageing

Telomeres lie at the end of chromosones, much like the protective strips (aglets) the end of a shoelace. They protect the chromosome from wear and tear and function to make sure that DNA gets copied when cells divide. Over time they fray, wear down and cannot protect chromosomes, leading to increased risk of major disease such as cancer, diabetes or cardiovascular disease. An enzyme called telomerase can mitigate this process and slow down the rate at which this occurs, preventing the telomeres from shortening.

There is some evidence to support the notion that incorporating positive lifestyle changes such as healthy eating, exercise, smoking cessation and alcohol reduction can stop the telomeres from shortening and may reverse ageing by taking care of your telomeres through increasing telomerase. However, this has been contested as much as it has been supported.

Lara et al (2019); Shammas (2011).

rate of living theory and cross-linking theory are all part of this perspective on biological ageing. More recently, the 'free radicals' theory has gained popularity. Free radicals act at the molecular level giving rise to accumulated damage causing cellular dysfunction at the organ level (Kunlin 2010).

Table 2.1 summarises theories on ageing from a biological perspective.

It is important to note that there is no single theory that can explain why the human body ages. Each theory provides insight into the multifaceted process of ageing. Ageing follows a trajectory and is a highly individual process.

Psycho-Social Theories on Ageing

There are three main psychosocial theories on ageing, which are described and summarised below.

Activity theory

This theory is based on the notion that high levels of social interaction and participation with family, friends and the community in which one lives are necessary to inhibit the negative effects of ageing. Activity theory is most often linked to life satisfaction and an individual's societal role. For example, retirement for many older persons can bring about a loss of identity or reduced sense of self because of no longer having an occupational role, and disengagement because of decreased social interaction that accompanies their withdrawal from participating in the workforce. However, withdrawal from the workforce can lead to new roles and social participation in other areas of society, as long as the older person actively seeks out these new experiences (Kunlin 2010; Williams 2016).

Disengagement theory

This theory is based on the idea that ageing is inevitable as it is accompanied by the linear withdrawal of the self from society and society from the individual. Disengagement follows the life course and is a universal phenomenon where the older person retreats from the social world, but may do so at different timings. This theory views ageing as an organic process where it is natural and acceptable for older adults to withdraw from society (Kunlin 2010; Williams 2016).

Continuity theory

During middle-age and early older-hood the adaptation to the 'normal' ageing process is supported by relying on existing resources and coping strategies brought about

Tips for Best Practice
Cognition and Ageing

Cognitive abilities have different developmental trajectories across the lifespan, with neurological maturation occurring by the mid-20s, followed by a very gradual decline up until the 60s, after which a more rapid decline occurs. Overall, the cognitive changes that occur with ageing are often more subtle than the accompanying physical changes.

The cognitive changes that occur with advancing age happen in many but not all individuals. The changes that occur are often subtle and result in the slowing down of certain processes. For example, in a task that asked people to substitute symbols for numbers, on average the 20-year-olds in the group performed this task 75% faster than the 75-year-old participants. It is important to note that cognitive slowing does not translate to functional decline.

Attention is one of the most prominent examples of cognitive slowing. For example, the capacity to multi-task becomes impaired. Processing information rapidly and distributing attention across many tasks peaks in early adulthood. Being able to hold multiple pieces of information in your mind at the same time is affected with advancing age. However, memory decline depends upon the type of memory being used. The ability to recall a person's name becomes more difficult after age of 70. For example, we may hear an older person say, 'her name is on the tip of my tongue'. The ability to recall new information peaks early, and slowly declines after age 40 (see Chapter 26).

Murman (2015).

by past experiences, decisions and behaviours that form the foundations for present behaviour. This is known as 'continuity of self' that happens in both the internal and the external domains of the whole person. Personality and behaviour patterns remain unchanged over the life-course and of importance is the idea that self-identity is maintained and continued by preserving roles and capacity over the ageing process (Kunlin 2010; Williams 2016).

WHO Decade of Healthy Ageing 2020–2030

The WHO views health as more than just the absence of disease. People need more than just information to remain and stay healthy over the lifespan. Its Healthy Ageing Framework (WHO 2019) provides clear direction for planning and strategies:
- To develop and maintain functional ability as one ages

- To support physical and mental capacity
- To develop resilience that enables wellbeing, life satisfaction and fulfillment and enjoyment.

The framework takes a lifespan approach to ageing that is holistic in nature and realises the value that both the physical (built) and other environments can bring to this. It also strongly advocates for the individual's relational connection to these elements in ageing in a healthy manner (WHO 2019).

The WHO Decade of Healthy Ageing (2020–2030) is a global initiative that supports an intersectoral approach to bring together governments, international agencies, civil societies, academia and various health professionals, along with the media and private corporations, to make healthy ageing a priority on the world's health agenda (WHO 2019). Its primary aim is to initiate collaborative efforts to improve the lives of all older people in the communities in which they live and exit. It takes an intergenerational approach by bringing families and communities together to develop autonomy in maintaining good health across the lifespan. It plans for a decade of concerted global action on healthy ageing. This includes improving access to the most basic resources necessary for a meaningful life that is inclusive, so that older persons are supported in achieving their full potential with dignity and equity, no matter what environment they live in (WHO 2019).

There are ten areas of action that have been nominated as a priority under this WHO initiative:
1. Build a platform for innovation and change
2. Support country planning and action
3. Collect better global health data on healthy ageing
4. Promote research that addresses the needs of older people
5. Align health systems to the needs of older people
6. Lay the foundations for long-term-care systems in every country
7. Ensure the human resources necessary for integrated care
8. Undertake a global campaign to combat ageism
9. Make the economic case for investment in healthy ageing
10. Develop the global network for age-friendly cities and communities (WHO 2019).

These are *concrete* actions that support the WHO global strategy and action plan on ageing and health. Each area of focus is critical to create a shift in the world where ageing, and specifically healthy ageing, becomes a priority for action. These ten areas of action provide the roadmap for societies, communities and the individual, and require the collaboration of key partners to push forward this agenda.

SUMMARY

The growth of the older population in Australia has directly parallelled New Zealand proportionally for over 25 years. Both countries are similar in age structure and rate of population ageing, and both countries face similar issues regarding caring for their older citizens. As this rate of population ageing continues steadily over the next two decades, focus on health and social policy needs to be at the forefront of government planning at both the macro and the micro level.

The theories that currently underpin contemporary ageing allow for new approaches to practice to be developed. Their relevance to nursing may provide a base of support and guidance on how to care for older persons. Nursing practice to support the care of older persons may be quite different depending on the theoretical perspective taken.

There is a need to recognise and harness the potential of the increasing numbers of older people in the community. Ageism based on archaic concepts that, for example, infantilise older persons as 'cute, little or adorable' are outdated and perpetuate myths around getting older, and older persons. Contemporary times and a new way of thinking about ageing and older people need to be put forward to promote ageing and working with older people in new and innovative ways.

This may mean utilising a model of interprofessional practice to coordinate health, medical and social services to support older patients more effectively. Many hospital re-admissions are preventable and enabling older patients to live in their own homes for longer is desirable. Reducing hospital re-admissions of older patients once they have been discharged is more effective if access to gerontology-trained providers is coordinated by gatekeepers such as nurses, whose strengths lie in the unique knowledge and skills in caring for older persons.

REVIEW QUESTIONS

1. What factors have contributed to the change in life expectancy over the last two decades?
2. What are the key components of the theories on ageing presented in this chapter?
3. The WHO Decade of Healthy Ageing 2020–2030 focuses on a multi-sectoral approach to population ageing. There are ten areas of action put forward as a framework in response to this. Choose three of these and identify areas within your own community or workplace that you can apply these to.
4. Reflect on your own experience in engaging with an older person. How do you feel you communicate with them? How do your own personal attitudes and feelings towards getting older influence the way you communicate with an older person?

REFERENCES

Australian Bureau of Statistics (ABS) (2017) ABS Census of population and housing. ABS Canberra. Online. Available: www.abs.gov.au/ausstats/abs@.nsf/Lookup/by%20Subject/2071.0~2016~Main%20Features~Ageing%20Population~14

Australian Bureau of Statistics (ABS) (2016) Ageing population 2016, ABS, Canberra. Online. Available: www.abs.gov.au/ausstats/abs@.nsf/Lookup/by%20Subject/2071.0~2016~Main%20Features~Ageing%20Population~14

Australian Bureau of Statistics (ABS) (2014) Australian historical population statistics 2014, ABS, Canberra. Cat No. 3105.0.65.001. Online. Available: www.abs.gov.au/AUSSTATS/abs@.nsf/DetailsPage/3105.0.65.0012014?OpenDocument

Australian Institute of Health and Welfare (AIHW) (2018a) Aboriginal and Torres Strait Islander Stolen Generations and descendants: numbers, demographic characteristics and selected outcomes. Cat. No. IHW 195. AIHW, Canberra.

Australian Institute of Health and Welfare (AIHW) (2018b) Australia's health 2018. Australia's health series. no 16. AUS 221. AIHW, Canberra.

Australian Institute of Health and Welfare (AIHW) (2018c) Older Australians at a glance. Cat. No. Age 87.

Commonwealth of Australia, Department of the Prime Minister and Cabinet (2020) Closing the Gap Report 2020. Commonwealth of Australia, Canberra.

Council on the Ageing (2018) State of the older nation report. Newgate Research. Project reference number: NGR18010008.

Dodson P, Cronin D (2011) An Australian dialogue: decolonising the country. In Maddison S., Brigg M. (eds) Unsettling the settler state. Creativity and resistance in Indigenous settler-state governance, Federation Press, Alexandria NSW.

Fries J (1980) Aging, natural death and the compression of morbidity. New England Journal of Medicine 303:130–135.

Gendron TL, Welleford EA, Inker J et al (2016) The language of ageism: why we need to use words carefully. The Gerontologist 56(6):997–1006.

Institute for Health Metrics and Evaluation (IHME) (2018) Findings from the global burden of disease study 2017. IHME, Seattle.

Kunlin J (2010) Modern biological theories of aging. Aging and Disease 1(2):72–74.

Lara MC, Puhlmann SL, Valk VE et al (2019) Association of short-term change in leukocyte telomere length with cortical thickness and outcomes of mental training among health adults. JAMA Network Open 2(9):e199687.

Lotoala F, Brehney M, Alpass F et al (2014) Health and wellbeing of older Pacific Peoples in New Zealand. The New Zealand Medical Journal 127(1407):1–13.

Maxwell-Stewart H, Oxley D (2020) Convicts and the colonization of Australia, 1788–1868. Digital Panopticon. Online. Available: www.digitalpanopticon.org/Convicts_and_the_Colonisation_of_Australia,_1788-1868

Menzies K (2019) Understanding the Australian Aboriginal experience of collective, historical and intergenerational trauma. International Social Work 62(6):1522–1534.

Ministry of Health NZ (2019a) Annual update of key results 2018/2019: New Zealand Health Survey. MOH, Wellington.

Ministry of Health NZ (2019b) Maori health data and stats. Online. Available: www.health.govt.nz/nz-health-statistics/health-statistics-and-data-sets/maori-health-data-and-stats?mega=Health%20statistics&title=Māori%20health.

Ministry of Health NZ (2018) Older people's health data and stats. https://www.health.govt.nz/nz-health-statistics/health-statistics-and-data-sets/older-peoples-health-data-and-stats.

Murman DL (2015) The impact of age on cognition. Seminars on hearing 36(3):111–121.

Organisation for Economic Co-operation and Development (OECD) (2019). Health at a glance 2019: OECD Indicators, OECD Publishing, Paris.

Paradies Y (2016). Colonisation, racism and indigenous health. Journal of Population Research 33(1):83–96.

Shammas MA (2011) Telomeres, lifestyle, cancer and ageing. Current Opinion in Clinical Nutrition and Metabolic Care 14(1):28–34.

Statistics New Zealand (2007) New Zealand's population: A statistical volume, Wellington.

Stokes A, Faulkner S (2008) National Sea Change Taskforce: the challenge of coastal infrastructure. Submission 239. Parliament of Australia: Canberra.

Thredgold C, Beer A, Zufferey C et al (2019) An effective homelessness services system for older Australians. AHURI Final Report No. 322, Australian Housing & Urban Research Institute Limited, Melbourne.

Williams AM (2016). Helping relationships with older adults. From theory to practice. SAGE Publications, California.

Williams A & Giles H (1998) Communication of ageism. In: Hecht ML (ed.) Communicating prejudice. Sage Publications, New York.

World Health Organisation (WHO) (2019) Decade of healthy ageing 2020–2030. WHO: Geneva.

World Health Organisation (WHO) (2008) World Health Report. Key concepts. WHO: Geneva.

CHAPTER 3

Cross-Cultural Ageing

LILY DONGXIA XIAO

LEARNING OBJECTIVES

After reading this chapter, you will be able to:

- describe cultural diversity in older people in Australia and New Zealand
- define and explain cultural competence and cultural safety
- discuss challenges and opportunities in promoting healthy ageing for older people from Indigenous and culturally and linguistically diverse backgrounds
- identify useful tools and resources to achieve healthy ageing for older people from Indigenous and culturally and linguistically diverse backgrounds.

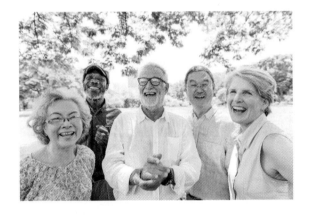

INTRODUCTION

Aboriginal and Torres Strait Islander peoples are First Australians while Māori people are First New Zealanders. As of 2016, people who migrated to Australia since colonisation came from over 190 countries, 300 different ancestries, and spoke over 300 languages at home (Australian Bureau of Statistics [ABS] 2017). In New Zealand, 27% of the population were born

overseas in 2018 (Stats New Zealand 2019). In this chapter, the terms culturally and linguistically diverse (CALD) groups and ethnic minority groups are used interchangeably. Research evidence has found that older people from Indigenous and CALD backgrounds experience poorer health, have more barriers in accessing care services, and have suboptimal health outcomes across the whole care spectrum (promotion, prevention, treatment, rehabilitation and palliation), compared to those from the dominant mainstream culture. The lack of culturally competent and culturally safe care for these populations at policy, organisation and individual levels have contributed to this situation. Achieving healthy ageing for these populations requires nurses to demonstrate culturally competent and culturally safe care and to critically reflect on their own practice.

OVERVIEW OF CULTURAL DIVERSITY IN OLDER PEOPLE
Australian Aboriginal and Torres Strait Islander Older People

Aboriginal and Torres Strait Islander peoples have very rich cultural heritages. They make up 2.8%

(649,171) of the Australian population and speak over 150 languages (ABS 2017). Approximately 10% of Aboriginal and Torres Strait Islander peoples speak an Australian Indigenous language at home. Of those, 85% indicated that they spoke English well or very well in the 2016 census. Older people from Aboriginal and Torres Strait Islander backgrounds aged 50 or over comprised 16% of the Indigenous population and 1.5% of the total Australian population in 2016 (ABS 2017). The geographic locations of Aboriginal and Torres Strait Islander peoples are presented in Table 3.1.

In Australia, life expectancy for Aboriginal and Torres Strait Islander populations, a crucial indicator of health equity, is 10.6 years less for males and 9.5 years less for females, than for the non-Indigenous population (Australian Institute of Health and Welfare [AIHW] 2018). In 2016, only 4.8% of the Indigenous population were aged over 65 years, compared to 15.9% in the non-Indigenous population. Reflecting this disparity in life expectancy, the eligibility for aged care services for older people from an Indigenous background is currently 50 years of age (Australian Government Department of Health 2019).

Older Australians From Culturally and Linguistically Diverse Backgrounds

The term 'culturally and linguistically diverse' (CALD) describes people who differ in culture and language from the mainstream Australian population (ABS 2017).

In 2016, overseas-born people made up 26% of the population and people who speak languages other than English at home made up 21% of the population (ABS 2017). The main religions identified were Christianity (47%), Buddhism (6.5%), Islam (6.0%), Hinduism (5.8%), and Sikh (1.6%) (ABS 2017).

According to the 2016 census, approximately 37% of older Australians were born overseas (ABS 2017). Their regions of birth were mainly in European countries. Nearly a quarter (24.1%) of older people speak a language other than English at home. The three most common languages spoken at home other than English are Italian, Chinese and Greek. Table 3.2 presents the top 16 languages older Australians spoke at home in 2016. Family-based care for older people is common in CALD communities and older people from CALD backgrounds are more likely to utilise community aged care services (up to 26%), but less likely to utilise residential aged care services (19%) (Productivity Commission 2019).

Older Māori People in New Zealand

Māori people (Tangata Whenua – people of the land) have a rich culture and heritage. Māori language is one of the official languages in New Zealand and is used in government documents. The number of Māori people in 2018 was 775,836, making up 16.5% of the total population (Stats New Zealand 2019). In Māori cultural norms, whānau (family or extended family) plays a key role in caring for older Māori at home (Ministry of

---

TABLE 3.1
Aboriginal and Torres Strait Islander Peoples by State and Territory

State or Territory	Urban Areas (%)	Rural Areas (%)	Total (no.)	People 65+ in the Total Australian Population (%)
New South Wales	85.5	14.1	216,176	5.4
Victoria	86.8	12.6	47,788	5.3
Queensland	81.2	18.4	186,482	4.4
South Australia	80.7	18.5	34,184	4.6
Western Australia	72.6	26.6	75,978	4.2
Tasmania	72.3	27.5	23,572	6.2
Northern Territory	50.0	48.8	58,248	3.8
Australian Capital Territory	99.3	0.3	6,508	3.1
Australia	79.0	20.4	649,171	4.8

ABS (2017).

TABLE 3.2
The Top 16 Languages Spoken at Home Among Older People 65+

Rank	Language Spoken at Home	Persons	Proportion of 65+ (%)
1	English	2,790,607	75.9
2	Italian	109,831	3.0
3	Chinese	79,762	2.2
4	Greek	72,893	2.0
5	South Slavic	51,375	1.4
6	Middle Eastern Semitic Languages	32,140	0.9
7	Iberian Romance	26,359	0.7
8	German and Related Languages	25,831	0.7
9	Mon-Khmer	21,622	0.6
10	Indo-Aryan	20,320	0.6
11	Southeast Asian Austronesian Languages	18,525	0.5
12	West Slavic	16,612	0.5
13	Dutch and Related Languages	16,050	0.4
14	Maltese	15,945	0.4
15	East Slavic	12,321	0.3
16	French	10,752	0.3

Total older people 65+ years = 3,676,765; Total population = 23,401,892.
ABS (2017).

Health NZ 2016). Older Māori value spiritual health (taha wairua), even in advanced age, and engage in community activities via the marae, a communal or sacred place (Dyall et al 2013). The life expectancy at birth in 2013 for Māori people was 73 and 77 years of age for males and females respectively, a seven-year difference compared to the non-Māori population (Ministry of Health NZ 2015). The proportion of Māori people aged 65 or over was 6.2% of the total Māori population, which was lower than the general population, at 15.2%. Māori older people are currently defined as those aged 50 or over to reflect the shorter life expectancy compared to the non-Māori population (Ministry of Health NZ 2011). The distribution of the population by District Health Board is presented in Table 3.3.

Older People From Ethnic Minority Groups in New Zealand

The total New Zealand population was 4,699,755 in the 2018 Census, with 1,271,775 (or 27%) born overseas. People born overseas were from over 248 countries or regions over the world (Stats New Zealand 2019). The word ethnicity describes 'a person who identifies with or has a sense of belonging to independent of birthplace' (Stats New Zealand 2019) and is used interchangeably with CALD in New Zealand. In the 2018 census, there were 180 ethnic groups and 176 different languages spoken at home. The main ethnic groups were European (70.2%), Māori (16.5%), Asian (15.1%), Pacific peoples (8.1%) and Middle Eastern/Latin American/African (1.5%). The top three Asian ethnic groups were Chinese (4.9%), Indian (4.7%) and Filipino (1.5%), with two-thirds of ethnic groups residing in Auckland. The main ethnic groups in New Zealand are presented in Table 3.4. Older people from ethnic minority groups are usually cared for by family carers or whānau carers (extended family carers) at home.

CULTURAL COMPETENCE AND CULTURAL SAFETY

Culture

Culture is defined as 'the shared, overt and covert under-standings that constitute conventions and practices, and

TABLE 3.3
Māori People by District Health Board

District Health Board	Total Māori Population	People 65+	People 65+ in the Total New Zealand Population (%)
Northland	63,249	5,304	0.7
Waitemata	59,040	2,868	0.4
Auckland	39,432	2,316	0.3
Counties Manukau	87,375	4,287	0.6
Waikato	96,882	5,841	0.8
Lakes	40,116	2,811	0.4
Bay of Plenty	61,062	4,653	0.7
Tairawhiti	24,807	2,100	0.3
Taranaki	23,223	1,422	0.2
Hawke's Bay	45,168	3,141	0.4
Whanganui	17,886	1,386	0.2
MidCentral	35,916	2,154	0.3
Hutt Valley	26,217	1,347	0.2
Capital and Coast	35,841	1,824	0.3
Wairarapa	8,136	546	0.1
Total - New Zealand by District Health Board	777,195	48,369	6.8

Total population 65 or over = 715,167.
Stats New Zealand (2019).

TABLE 3.4
Main Ethnic Groups in New Zealand in 2018 Census

Ethnic Groups	Persons	Proportion of Total Population (%)	Persons 65+	Proportion of 65+ (%)
European	3,297,864	70.2	613,140	18.6
Māori	775,836	16.5	48,252	6.2
Asian	707,598	15.1	45,462	6.4
Chinese	231,387	4.9		
India	221,916	4.7		
Filipino	72,612	1.5		
Pacific peoples	381,642	8.1	20,232	5.3
Middle Eastern/ Latin American/ African	70,332	1.5		
Other ethnicity	56,397	1.2		

A person might report more than one ethnic group; total population = 4,699,755; population 65 years of age or over = 715,167.
Stats New Zealand (2019).

the ideas, symbols, and concrete artefacts that sustain conventions and practices, and make them meaningful' (Napier et al 2014:1610). This definition reveals that culture is not only formed on the basis of ethnicity and language used, but could be identified based on personal and social factors, such as age, gender, religion, socioeconomic background, sexual orientation and lived experiences. People from the same ethnic group may differ culturally, as diversity exists in a cultural group. Moreover, a culture held by a person is not stable, but changes over time and is influenced by the person's experiences through their life course. Older people from migrant and CALD backgrounds may or may not have adapted to the culture in their host countries. Nurses will need to assess each older person during their clinical encounters using a person-centred approach, rather than basing practice on presumptions or stereotypical views. This chapter focuses on cultural diversity of older people from Indigenous and CALD backgrounds. Other culturally diverse groups, i.e. based on rural/remote locations or sexual orientation, are discussed in Chapters 6 and 27 respectively.

Cultural Competence

Most definitions of cultural competence focus on the individual level. In a healthy ageing context, we embrace culture competency which was described by Cross and colleagues as 'a set of congruent behaviours, attitudes, and policies that come together in a system, agency or among professionals and enable that system, agency or those professionals to work effectively in cross-cultural situations' (1989:7). This definition emphasises a systemic approach to achieving healthy ageing by developing culturally competent health and social care systems, requiring action to be taken by policymakers, health organisations, social care facilities and individual healthcare providers. Nurses are required not only to demonstrate culturally competent care for older people, but also to engage with them in developing, implementing and evaluating care plans and services; and advocating on their behalf for policy, resources and practice developments to promote healthy ageing.

Cultural Safety

Cultural safety in a nursing context is defined as 'the effective nursing practice of a person or family from another culture, and is determined by that person or family' (Nursing Council of New Zealand 2011:7). This definition articulates the power imbalance between nurses and clients from Indigenous and CALD backgrounds and the need for the clients or their family carers to decide whether or not the care services are culturally safe for them.

Cultural safety addresses colonial history as the root cause of health inequity for Indigenous and CALD people, and as accounting for the presence of different forms of colonisation in the contemporary health and social care environments (Curtis et al 2019). At the governmental and organisational levels, the achievement of culturally safe care for older people requires co-design, co-implementation and co-monitoring of healthcare policies, services and resources with Indigenous and CALD people. At an individual level, providing culturally safe care requires nurses not only to learn and apply knowledge, skills and attitudes in cross-cultural care, but also to perform critical self-reflection on their own assumptions, biases, prejudices and power relationships including the impact of these on clients from Indigenous and CALD backgrounds.

CHALLENGES IN PROMOTING HEALTHY AGEING
Social Determinants of Health

The social determinants of health are defined as 'conditions in which people are born, grow, work, live and age, and the wider set of forces and systems shaping the conditions of daily life' (World Health Organisation [WHO] 2017). Social determinants include, but are not limited to, racism, discrimination, poverty, education, employment and access to healthcare services (Ministry of Health NZ 2015; AIHW 2018). Older people from Indigenous backgrounds have been exposed to many social disadvantages as a consequence of colonisation, and the manifestations of this history still exist today via the unequal distribution of power, resources and services in society (Bourke et al 2019; Curtis et al 2019). Living in disadvanted areas is an indicator of social disadvantage. A higher proportion of Indigenous Australians (37% *vs* 9% of non-Indigenous) and Māori people in New Zealand (23.5% *vs* 6.8% of non-Māori) live in more deprived areas (AIHW 2018; Ministry of Health NZ 2015). The social determinants largely account for 34% of the gap in health outcomes in Australia between Indigenous and non-Indigenous peoples (AIHW 2018).

Racism and discrimination towards Indigenous and CALD people contribute to their poor mental health and reduced health-seeking behaviours. This contributes to an increase in unhealthy lifestyles, such as an unhealthy diet, high smoking rates and an increase in alcohol and drug use (AIHW 2018; Harris et al 2018; Ministry of Health NZ 2015). In a national survey in New Zealand, a higher proportion of people from Asian and Māori backgrounds reported that they encountered racism in the past 12 months and such experiences were related to a poorer quality of life, unmet care needs and low satisfaction with care services compared with other ethnic groups (Harris et al 2018, 2019). Institutional racism is defined as:

> the collective failure of an organisation to provide an appropriate and professional service to people because of their colour, culture, or ethnic origin. It can be seen or detected in processes, attitudes and behaviour which amount to discrimination through unwitting prejudice, ignorance, thoughtlessness and racist stereotyping which disadvantage minority ethnic people (Macpherson 1999:49).

Racism plays a major role in perpetuating inequitable healthcare for people from Indigenous backgrounds and ethnic minority groups (Bourke et al 2019).

Chronic Disease Burden

In Australia, Indigenous older people continue to experience a higher burden of chronic disease than non-Indigenous older people (AIHW 2018). In 2011, the top five disease burdens in the 65–74 age group for Indigenous older people were coronary heart disease (16%), lung cancer (10%), diabetes (9.2%), chronic obstructive pulmonary disease (COPD) (9.0%) and chronic kidney disease (4.6%). The top five diseases of burden in the 75+ age group were coronary heart disease (16%), stroke (8.9%), diabetes (8.0%), dementia (7.7%) and COPD (7.6%).

In New Zealand, the top five diseases contributing to the years of life lost in the 70+ age group were cardiovascular disease, cancers, neurological disorders, COPD and diabetes (Ministry of Health 2018). Dementia rates in Māori and non-Māori aged 80–90 years were similar and estimated at 16%. The Māori population living with dementia were identified as having complex care needs. In Māori and non-Māori older people, falls contribute to nearly 75% of hospital trauma admissions and 18.5% of older people aged 85 or over who fell sustained at least one fracture. Around 35% of older people took five or more medications (polypharmacy) in New Zealand, and polypharmacy was more prevalent for Māori (Ministry of Health NZ 2018) (see Chapter 11).

Gaps in Dementia Care

Older people living with dementia from Indigenous and CALD communities are less likely to be diagnosed or are diagnosed later compared to those from the mainstream culture. This is attributed to lower dementia literacy, the stigma attached to dementia, barriers to seeking help, a lack of access to health services and other social determining factors (AIHW 2012). Carers of people with dementia from Indigenous and CALD backgrounds experience a high level of burden as they receive little or no dementia education and cannot access dementia care services due to undiagnosed dementia and other barriers, including language barriers (AIHW 2012). Older people living with dementia for whom English is a second language may lose their ability to use English to communicate (Tipping & Whiteside 2015). Additionally, older people living with dementia who do not speak English well or cannot speak English at all are at risk of social isolation, loneliness and unmet care needs in the mainstream aged care homes and hospitals (Mbuzi et al 2017; Runci et al 2012).

Research Highlight
Gaps in End-of-Life Care

Culture and religion have a profound influence on people's attitudes, preferences and approaches to a 'good death' (Australian Government Department of Health and Ageing 2011; Ohr et al 2017). People from Indigenous and CALD communities may not be familiar with, or accept, the Western concept of palliative care. They may show a low rate of advanced care planning and misunderstandings of palliative care, have unmet communication needs, as well as unmet care needs at end of life across care settings (Green et al 2019; Kirby et al 2018). Inequitable palliative care for these populations is attributed to a lack of partnership with clients, families and communities, as well as institutional racism and low levels of cultural competence and safety. The deficit is also due to a lack of culturally and linguistically appropriate education and resources.

Australian Government Department of Health and Ageing (2011); Green et al (2019); Kirby et al (2018); Ohr et al (2017).

OPPORTUNITIES IN PROMOTING HEALTHY AGEING

Demonstrating Culturally Competent and Culturally Safe Care

Nurses have an obligation to demonstrate culturally competent and culturally safe care, as described in the Code of Conduct for Nurses (Nursing and Midwifery Board of Australia [NMBA] 2018); and in the Registered Nurses Standards for Practice (NMBA 2016). In addition, nurses have an obligation to report 'behaviour that may be interpreted as bullying or harassment and/or culturally unsafe' (NMBA 2018:10).

Healthy ageing is defined as 'the process of developing and maintaining the functional ability that enables well-being in older age' (WHO 2015:28). Older people from Indigenous CALD backgrounds may have low physical and mental capabilities (intrinsic capacity) due to poor health developed through their life course. Greater effort is needed to create caring environments to develop and maintain activities that are culturally appropriate, meaningful and improve physical, psychological, spiritual and social wellbeing (functional ability) for Indigenous and CALD older people. A caring environment has the characteristics of cultural competence and cultural safety at policy-making, organisational and individual levels.

Promoting Wellness
Aboriginal and Torres Strait Islander Peoples

- Older people and their family in remote areas prefer residential aged care facilities that are on Country or close to their families and communities.
- The National Aboriginal and Torres Strait Islander Flexible Aged Care Program is provided to enable older people to receive aged care services in locations that are close to their families and on country in remote areas.
- Families should be encouraged to engage in care planning.
- Residential aged care homes should provide spaces, resources and flexible visiting times for residents and families in order to promote wellbeing.
- Enabling older people to continue engaging in activities they enjoy, e.g. deciding their preferred foods and daily leisure activities, promotes wellbeing.

Australian Government Department of Health (2018).

Promoting Wellness
Māori Older People

- Māori older people experience a high burden of chronic disease due to the social determinants of health.
- Improving social assistance, access to primary healthcare and home and community services are ways to improve their wellbeing.
- Supporting whānau carers to help older people manage their chronic diseases at home reduces the care burden and improves wellbeing for the family.

Ministry of Health NZ (2016).

Effective Cross-Cultural Communication

Effective cross-cultural communication is both an attitude and an action that overcomes communication barriers.

It is about exchanging information and negotiating shared meanings between individuals from two (or more) cultures or linguistic backgrounds in the interests of the care recipient. It is a prerequisite for timely detection of patient deterioration; for identifying and meeting care needs; and building a therapeutic relationship with older people for optimal care outcomes. Language barriers and ageing or disease-related impairments affect older people's capability for cross-cultural communication; therefore, their participation in care plans, their understanding and compliance with following up treatment regimens and health promotion activities may be impaired. Inadequate cross-cultural communication has a detrimental effect on the health and wellbeing of older people, including medication errors, adverse events, unmet care needs and dissatisfaction with care services (Suurmond et al 2010; van Rosse et al 2016). Evidence consistently shows that older people who request interpreter services are often ignored and are not offered these services when they are in the hospital setting (Green et al 2019; Mbuzi et al 2017).

The principles of effective cross-cultural communication reflect cultural competence and cultural safety requirements. First, nurses need to critically reflect on their own culture, assumptions, prejudices and biases and the influence these have on communication with older people and their families from Indigenous and CALD backgrounds. Second, nurses need to be empathetic and/or culturally humble to demonstrate understanding for what the older person is expressing or feeling, and to empower the older person to participate in communication, including those with dementia or cognitive impairment, and to engage and communicate with families or carers. Third, nurses need to let clients and their carers determine whether the cross-cultural communication is being effective. See *Tips for best practice: Cross-cultural communication* and *Tips for best practice: Using interpreters.*

Tips for Best Practice
Cross-Cultural Communication

- Smile and be friendly.
- Make eye contact, if appropriate.
- Listen.
- Be self-aware of your own biases and prejudices and the influence of these on your communication.
- Do not allow cultural differences (preferences) to become the basis for criticism and judgements.

Giger (2013); Ziaian & Xiao (2014).

Tips for Best Practice
Using Interpreters

- Use qualified language interpreters during formal assessment, meetings or other events for communication with older people and their carers.
- Use translation as necessary in seeking feedback from older people, their families and communities.
- Work with bilingual staff and relatives for communication with older people from the same culture for day-to-day problems with activities.

Giger (2013); Ziaian & Xiao (2014).

SUMMARY

Cultural and linguistic diversity are significant in older people in Australia and New Zealand. Promoting healthy ageing in this social context requires nurses to demonstrate culturally competent and culturally safe care. Nurses have an obligation to advocate for appropriate policy, resources and practices that ensure a systemic approach to healthy ageing for all. This includes an obligation to eliminate racism and discrimination from policy, in organisations and at the individual level. Empowering older people, their families and communities to participate in developing and monitoring care services to reduce health inequity and to tackle racism and discrimination is a way to let them determine whether care services are culturally competent and culturally safe for them. Effective cross-cultural communication enables nurses to build therapeutic and trusting relationships with older people and their families to achieve healthy ageing outcomes.

Practice Scenario
Promoting Wellness for Rosa

Rosa is an 82-year-old Italian woman who has pneumonia. She is admitted to a geriatric ward in a tertiary hospital from a residential aged care facility. Rosa was diagnosed with dementia three years ago. She migrated to Australia 60 years ago from Italy with her husband and as a housewife raised three children. Her husband passed away five years ago. She is supported by her family and extended family. She cannot speak English and relies on her family to assist her in communication with health professionals. Since day one of her admission, Rosa has been restless, calling out and wandering as she tries to find her way to go home. A care needs assessment is undertaken by her primary nurse, Mary, with the assistance of a professional Italian interpreter. Mary recalls her own learning experience in a cross-cultural dementia care training program and applies the Italian version of RUDAS (Rowland Universal Dementia Assessment Scale, highlighted in *Clinical Practice Guidelines and Principles of Care for People with Dementia* (Australian Government NHMRC 2019)) to assess cognitive function for Rosa (Dementia Australia 2019). Rosa records a score of 18 on the assessment form. Mary organises a case conference with her team and invites Rosa's daughter and Ying, a registered nurse from the residential aged care facility where Rosa lives, to the meeting via the Zoom interactive platform. Ying suggests that the change of environment and routine might be contributing to Rosa's changed behaviours. Rosa's daughter shares that her mother enjoys the daily volunteer visitor from an Italian background very much. A care plan that reflects Rosa's routine is developed and implemented. The change of care approach improves Rosa's wellbeing, as evidenced by a reduction in restless behaviours and an increased engagement with the volunteer and staff.

MULTIPLE CHOICE QUESTIONS

1. The possible causes of Rosa's changed behaviours are:
   a. pneumonia
   b. unfamiliar hospital environment
   c. loneliness
   d. failure to maintain routine activities

2. The Italian version of RUDAS was used because it is:
   a. culturally appropriate
   b. linguistically appropriate
   c. recommended in the Australian Clinical Practice Guidelines and Principles of Care for People with Dementia
   d. possible for nurses to administer it without assistance from an Italian interpreter

3. Social support for people with dementia in a hospital setting:
   a. can be a non-pharmacological intervention to prevent and treat changed behaviours
   b. can improve social wellbeing
   c. can reduce adverse events associated with changed behaviours
   d. can improve older people and their family's satisfaction with hospital care.

USEFUL RESOURCES

Australian Government and Department of Health (2019) Actions to support older Aboriginal and Torres Strait Islander people. Commonwealth of Australia, Canberra.

Ministry of Health NZ (2016) Healthy Ageing Strategy. MOH, Wellington.

Ministry of Health NZ (2015) Tatau Kahukura: Māori Health chart book 2015. MOH, Wellington.

Xiao D, Willis EM, Harrington AC, et al (2017) Cross-cultural care program for aged care staff: An online self-directed learning program. Online. Available: www.flinders.edu.au/cross-cultural-care

REFERENCES

Australian Bureau of Statistics (ABS) (2017) 2071.0 Census of population and housing: Reflecting Australia – stories from the Census, 2016. Australian Bureau of Statistics, Canberra.

Australian Government Department of Health (2019) What is aged care? Online. Available: www.health.gov.au/health-topics/aged-care/about-aged-care/what-is-aged-care

Australian Government Department of Health (2018) National Aboriginal and Torres Strait Islander Flexible Aged Care Program. Commonwealth of Australia, Canberra.

Australian Government Department of Health and Ageing (2011) Guidelines for a palliative approach for aged care in the community setting – best practice guidelines for the Australian context. Commonwealth of Australia, Canberra.

Australian Government, National Health and Medical Research Council (NHMRC) (2019) Clinical practice guidelines and principles of care for people with dementia. Online. Available: www.clinicalguidelines.gov.au/portal/2503/clinical-practice-guidelines-and-principles-care-people-dementia

Australian Institute of Health and Welfare (AIHW) (2018) Closing the Gap targets: 2017 analysis of progress and key drivers of change. AIHW, Canberra.

Australian Institute of Health and Welfare (AIHW) (2012) Dementia in Australia. AIHW, Canberra.

Bourke CJ, Marrie H, Marrie A (2019) Transforming institutional racism at an Australian hospital. Australian Health Review 43(6):611–618.

Cross T, Bazron B, Dennis K et al (1989) Towards a culturally competent system of care. Washington, DC, National Technical Assistance Center for Children's Mental Health, Georgetown University Child Development Center.

Curtis E, Jones R, Tipene-Leach D et al (2019) Why cultural safety rather than cultural competency is required to achieve health equity: a literature review and recommended definition. International Journal for Equity in Health 18(174). https://doi.org/10.1186/s12939-019-1082-3

Dementia Australia (2019) Rowland Universal Dementia Assessment Scale (RUDAS). Online. Available: www.dementia.org.au/resources/rowland-universal-dementia-assessment-scale-rudas

Dyall L, Kepa M, Hayman K et al (2013) Engagement and recruitment of Māori and non–Māori people of advanced age to LiLACS NZ. Australian and New Zealand Journal of Public Health 37(2):124–131.

Giger JN (2013) Transcultural nursing: assessment and intervention. Elsevier Mosby, St Louis.

Green A, Jerzmanowska N, Thristiawati S et al (2019) Culturally and linguistically diverse palliative care patients' journeys at the end-of-life. Palliative & Supportive Care 17(2):227–233.

Harris RB, Cormack DM, Stanley J (2019) Experience of racism and associations with unmet need and healthcare satisfaction: the 2011/12 adult New Zealand Health Survey. Australian and New Zealand Journal of Public Health 43(1): 75–80.

Harris RB, Stanley J, Cormack DM (2018) Racism and health in New Zealand: Prevalence over time and associations between recent experience of racism and health and wellbeing measures using national survey data. Plos One 13(5) e0196476.

Kirby E, Lwin Z, Kenny K et al (2018) 'It doesn't exist…': negotiating palliative care from a culturally and linguistically diverse patient and caregiver perspective. BMC Palliative Care 17(90). https://doi.org/10.1186/s12904-018-0343-z

Macpherson W (1999) Report of The Stephen Lawrence inquiry. Home Office, London.

Mbuzi V, Fulbrook P, Jessup M (2017) Indigenous peoples' experiences and perceptions of hospitalisation for acute care: A metasynthesis of qualitative studies. International Journal of Nursing Studies 71:39–49.

Ministry of Health NZ (2018) Health and independence report 2017: The Director-General of Health's annual report on the state of public health. MOH, Wellington.

Ministry of Health NZ (2016) Healthy ageing strategy. MOH, Wellington.

Ministry of Health NZ (2015) Tatau Kahukura: Māori health chart book 2015. MOH, Wellington.

Ministry of Health NZ (2011) Tatau Kura Tangata: Health of older Māori chart book 2011. MOH, Wellington.

Napier AD, Ancarno C, Butler B et al (2014) Culture and health. Lancet 384(9954):1607–1639.

Nursing and Midwifery Board of Australia (NMBA) (2018) Code of conduct for nurses. Online. Available: www.nursingmidwiferyboard.gov.au/Codes-Guidelines-Statements/Professional-standards.aspx

Nursing and Midwifery Board of Australia (NMBA) (2016) Registered Nurses Standards for Practice. Online. Available: www.nursingmidwiferyboard.gov.au/codes-guidelines-statements/professional-standards/registered-nurse-standards-for-practice.aspx

Nursing Council of New Zealand (2011) Guidelines for cultural safety, the Treaty of Waitangi and Māori Health in nursing education and practice. Nursing Council of New Zealand, Wellington.

Ohr S, Jeong S, Saul P (2017) Cultural and religious beliefs and values, and their impact on preferences for end-of-life care among four ethnic groups of community-dwelling older persons. Journal of Clinical Nursing 26(11–12):1681–1689.

Productivity Commission (2019) Report on government services 2019: part F, chapter 14, aged care services report and attachments. Canberra.

Runci SJ, Eppingstall BJ, O'Connor DW (2012) A comparison of verbal communication and psychiatric medication use by Greek and Italian residents with dementia in Australian ethno-specific and mainstream aged care facilities. International Psychogeriatrics 24(5):733–741.

Stats New Zealand (2019) New Zealand's population reflects growing diversity. Online. Available: www.stats.govt .nz/news/new-zealands-population-reflects-growing -diversity.

Suurmond, J, Uiters E, de Bruijne MC et al (2010) Explaining ethnic disparities in patient safety: a qualitative analysis. American Journal of Public Health 100:S113–S117.

Tipping SA, Whiteside M (2015) Language reversion among people with dementia from culturally and linguistically diverse backgrounds: the family experience. Australian Social Work 68(2):184–197.

van Rosse F, de Bruijne M, Suurmond J et al (2016) Language barriers and patient safety risks in hospital care. A mixed methods study. International Journal of Nursing Studies 54:45–53.

World Health Organisation (WHO) (2017) What are the social determinants of health? WHO. Online. Available: www.who.int/social_determinants/en/

World Health Organisation (WHO) (2015) World report on ageing and health. WHO, Geneva.

Ziaian T, Xiao L (2014) Cultural diversity in health care. In: M. Fedoruk, A Hofmeyer, Becoming a nurse: transition to practice. Oxford University Press, Melbourne.

CHAPTER 4

Promoting Healthy Ageing

HELGA MERL

LEARNING OBJECTIVES

After reading this chapter, you will be able to:
- explore the concepts and determinants of healthy ageing
- understand the key factors and strategies that underpin health promotion for older people
- understand the Transtheoretical model of health promotion and its use by nurses in promoting healthy ageing
- explore and apply Miller's functional consequences theory as a nursing framework to promote healthy ageing across clinical settings.

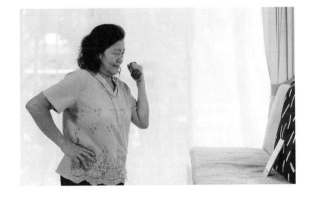

INTRODUCTION

Advances in public health and medicine have seen tremendous gains in life expectancy over past decades. Ideally, longevity would be accompanied by good health, but unfortunately this is not always the case. Most Australians and New Zealanders over the age of 65 have, and will die from, chronic health conditions (Australian Institute of Health and Welfare [AIHW] 2018; Ministry of Health NZ 2020). Healthy ageing as a concept has emerged to address the growing chronic disease burden associated with ageing by promoting wellbeing through developing and maintaining functional ability of the older person. A healthy ageing approach achieves improved health outcomes by moving away from the biomedical model of health to a more integrated, person-centred, health promotion model. This approach requires nurses to understand factors that influence both healthcare and the health of older people (World Health Organisation [WHO] 2015). This chapter will explore the necessary concepts, principles, theories and frameworks that enable nurses to promote healthy ageing.

DEFINITION OF HEALTHY AGEING

The World Health Organisation argues that all people can achieve healthy ageing despite the presence of illness and chronic conditions. The WHO defines healthy ageing as 'the process of developing and maintaining the functional ability that enables wellbeing in older age' (WHO 2015).

This definition challenges all nurses to engage in health promotion across all care settings, to empower older people by facilitating choice and control over health and social care in order to develop functional ability, experience wellbeing and achieve healthy ageing. It is important to understand the drivers of this increased ageing population.

The biggest drivers of aged care need in Australia and New Zealand include:

- a rapidly expanding aged population
- workforce pressures related to the resultant epidemic of chronic disease
- inequities in access to services and health outcomes.

These conditions have caused an explosion in direct aged health and social care costs, and indirect costs, including care provided by families and informal care networks (AIHW 2018). The population therefore needs to be encouraged to participate in health promotion to keep well and reduce the need for healthcare services.

Promoting Wellness
An Example of Healthy Ageing

Allan is a good example of healthy ageing. Allan had a military background (WWII), multiple chronic conditions and lived in a residential aged care facility. With the support of the registered nurse, Allan achieved his long-term goal 'to sky dive again'. Remarkably, at age 86, Allan went on a tandem skydiving experience. In Allan's words 'for the first 20 feet I felt numb, then I opened my arms and soared. I felt ageless'. It is easy to see how Allan achieved wellbeing, which comprises components of positivity, happiness, activity and productivity, satisfaction and fulfilment.

Uniting Care Ageing (2014); WHO (2015).

FUNCTIONAL ABILITY AND HEALTHY AGEING

In the case of Allan (see *Promoting wellness*: *An example of healthy ageing* above), the registered nurse (RN) coordinated responses to these determinants by partnering with Allan to understand his health, and to facilitate person-centred goal attainment. Care plan strategies included: increasing Allan's health literacy level regarding the health requirements and risks of skydiving; a family conference providing information on decision-making capacity and dignity of risk; optimal chronic condition management and an exercise program; all of which resulted in Allan living life his way.

Nurses promote functional ability by enabling older people to be and do what they value. Functional ability includes having the capacity to perform activities of daily living (ADLs), as well as developing and maintaining instrumental activities of daily living (IADLs), as

TABLE 4.1

Supporting Activities of Daily Living (ADLs) and Instrumental Activities of Daily Living (IADLs)

ADLs – self-care	• Hygiene (bathing, grooming and oral hygiene) • Dressing • Toileting • Nutrition (self-feeding) • Mobility (getting from one place to another to perform ADLs)
IADLs	• Telephone use (other communication) • Cleaning and home maintenance • Laundry • Transport and travel (within the community) • Shopping • Food preparation (cooking, serving and cleaning up) • Medication management • Finance management • Relationships • Decision making • Care of others and pets • Religious observances • Safety and emergency responses

Green et al (2006); Shah et al (1989).

identified in Table 4.1. The intrinsic capacity to meet basic and higher-level needs is unique to each individual, and results from the interaction between an individual's physical and mental capabilities and the environmental determinants of healthy ageing, as shown in Fig. 4.1 (WHO 2015) (see Chapter 8 for further detail).

ENVIRONMENT AND HEALTHY AGEING

The environment affects behaviour to either support or hinder healthy ageing. The environment can include a residential aged care facility, home, the community, geographical location and the make-up of society. The interplay of the components within the environment establishes the potential for healthy ageing for the individual, as shown in Fig. 4.1.

The environmental determinants of healthy ageing include:

- societal attitudes such as ageism
- health and social care availability

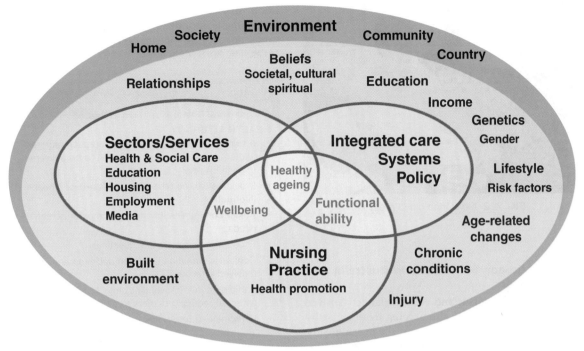

FIG. 4.1 **Environmental determinants of healthy ageing: nursing model**

- formal and informal relationships
- systems and policies
- the built environment.

The evidence shows that integrated care, which coordinates these environment components for health benefit, is an effective approach to healthy ageing (Harvey et al 2018). An integrated care approach can be demonstrated when an RN supports an older person to navigate the complexities of the aged care system.

The value and importance of the nursing role in promoting healthy ageing links to both prevention and management of health conditions. Nurses promote the health literacy of older people to adopt health behaviours in preventing chronic conditions, such as cardiovascular disease, and avoid exacerbation and improve self-management of existing chronic conditions, such as diabetes.

HEALTH LITERACY

As one of the key elements of health promotion, health literacy can be understood as the level to which systems in the environment enable individuals to obtain, understand and evaluate the information required to make relevant health choices (Ministry of Health NZ 2015) (Fig. 4.2).

Low health literacy is caused by the complexities and unfamiliarity of health situations in which people have trouble understanding and applying complex health information and concepts. Low health literacy can also be attributed to systems, services and individual nurses, when they do not provide or present health information in ways that are easy to understand and meaningful. Additionally, older people may lack the necessary skills and capacity to locate, navigate and interpret information to make informed choices (Australian Commission on Safety and Quality in Health Care [ACSQHC] 2018a).

Low health literacy results in more frequent adverse outcomes and increased use of health services, including hospital and emergency care. Low health literacy is a barrier to engagement in health promotion strategies such as health checks and vaccinations. For older people, low health literacy is associated with higher morbidity and mortality rates (De Wit et al 2017).

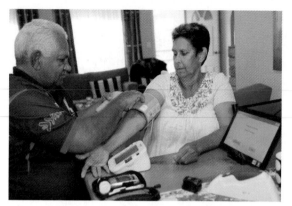

FIG. 4.2 Monitoring blood pressure

Health Literacy Skill Levels in Australia and New Zealand

While older Australians and New Zealanders wish to achieve wellbeing and healthy ageing by being active participants in their own healthcare, the prevailing low levels of health literacy limit their ability to do so (Ding et al 2016). The 2006 Adult Literacy and Life Skills Survey in New Zealand and Australia highlighted that 56% of New Zealanders and 59% of Australians had low health literacy and, therefore, were less able to obtain and understand the health information required to make informed decisions (AIHW 2018; Ministry of Health NZ 2015). Indigeneity and older age further increased the likelihood of low health literacy, occurring in approximately 80% of Māori men and 75% of Māori women (Ministry of Health NZ 2010).

Over a decade later, the 2018 National Health Survey to identify health literacy, conducted by the Australian Bureau of Statistics (ABS), demonstrated that self-reported health literacy rates have improved. However, older people and Aboriginal and Torres Strait Islander people remain less likely to have a positive view of their health literacy skills (ABS 2018a).

Promoting Health Literacy in Older Persons

The more people learn about a health event, its impact on their health and response options, the higher their health literacy becomes. Raising levels of health literacy can be achieved quite quickly. To do this the RN must provide health information that is clear, correct, evidence-based and practical in meeting the older person's perceived needs and healthy ageing goals (see *Tips for best practice*: *Nursing actions to promote healthy ageing*). When older people are educated and empowered, they become

true partners in care, capable of acting on health information to make informed decisions that reflect their own values for healthy ageing, and those they care for (ACSQHC 2018a).

Tips for Best Practice
Nursing Actions to Promote Healthy Ageing

HEALTH LITERACY
- A universal precautions-based approach requires written and verbal communication to be delivered in plain English.
- Provide clear, correct and evidence-based health information.
- Adjust communication style to the older person's needs.
- Encourage people to ask questions.
- Confirm information has been delivered and received effectively.
- Participate in improvement projects, e.g. policies aimed at reducing barriers to health literacy.
- Participate in health literacy education and training.

To tailor programs for healthy ageing across care settings, nurses must also understand how health literacy fits within the discipline of health promotion.

HISTORY OF HEALTH PROMOTION AND HEALTHY AGEING

The inception of the public health movement can be traced back to the early part of the 19th century, in response to epidemics such as the 'Black Death' (third plague pandemic), the result of industrialisation and associated overcrowding. Major improvements in public health were made through provision of adequate housing, sanitation and safe water.

By 1916, the germ theory of disease heralded a new era of preventative medicine and gave rise to 'the new public health'. Major increases in health and life expectancy were achieved through population-based immunisation and vaccination. The biomedical model of health became the dominant health paradigm, attributing illness and dependence to individual failings (WHO 1986).

It was not until the 1970s that public health and health systems were reviewed to combat rising demand for healthcare and its associated costs. In 1978, the WHO endorsed the Alma Ata Declaration to achieve health for all. Three years later, in 1981, the resultant WHO landmark document titled *A global strategy of health for all by the year 2000* became policy.

In 1986, the WHO international conference on health promotion endorsed the Ottawa Charter (WHO 1986). The Ottawa Charter prioritised health promotion, not only as a mechanism to achieve public health, but also as a discipline, distinct from public health and health education in its holistic approach to address the determinants of health, including the behaviour change necessary to achieve healthy ageing. As such, health promotion represented a significant departure from the traditional biomedical model of health.

HEALTH PROMOTION

Health promotion enables people to increase control over their own health and its determinants, in order to improve health outcomes (WHO 1986). The Ottawa Charter outlines five health promotion principles:
- building healthy public policy
- creating supportive environments
- strengthening community action
- developing personal skills
- reorientating health services (WHO 1986).

Health Promotion Response

In Australia and New Zealand, there are two main perspectives of health promotion: Western and Indigenous. From a Western perspective, health promotion is a public health discipline. It is the process of enabling people and communities to take greater control of their health. From an Aboriginal and Torres Strait Islander and Māori viewpoint, health promotion enables greater control of the determinants of health and therefore Indigenous people's future. A third, Pasifika perspective in New Zealand requires the empowering of Pasifika (Pacific Islander) peoples to control their wellbeing and their future (Hauora 2014; Pasifika Futures 2017).

Since the Ottawa Charter, public health policy in Australia and New Zealand has been transitioning beyond the biomedical model to more social models in order to address the environmental determinants of health shown in Fig. 4.1. This transition has proved slow and has not kept pace with the increased demands and costs of aged care.

INTEGRATED PERSON-CENTRED FRAMEWORK

In 2015, building on the Ottawa Charter and with the aim of meeting the global demands of aged care, the WHO published the first *World report on ageing and health* and the *Global strategy on people-centred and integrated health services*. In 2016, the World Health Assembly adopted a *Global strategy and plan of action on ageing and health*. These documents provide the framework for countries to address the determinants of healthy ageing; ensure that health promotion is a primary consideration for all nurses and health staff; and enable older people to receive the care and support required to live a meaningful life.

Requiring a whole-of-system approach, this new paradigm places integrated person-centred care of the older person within a health promotion framework. Both Australia and New Zealand are using these documents along with the Ottawa Charter (1986), and in New Zealand the Treaty of Waitangi 1840, to develop plans to reorientate and achieve integrated person-centred care for older people. These documents include:
- Australia's 2020 *National preventive health strategy*; the 2013 *National Aboriginal and Torres Strait Islander health plan 2013–2023*, with the vision to close the gap in health inequality (see Chapter 3); and state health plans, including the 2019 *Healthy Ageing: A strategy for older Queenslanders*.
- *The New Zealand Healthy ageing strategy* (Ministry of Health NZ 2016) and the *Matariki* (2019). 'Matariki' is the health promotion framework for Māori and other Indigenous peoples. A notable recommendation of the Indigenous viewpoint is an urgent paradigm shift in the way all people see themselves in relationship with the living planet.

Person-Centred Care

As a cheaper and more effective approach, person-centred care principles are now core to all models of aged care nursing. Research shows that person-centred care improves health experience, promotes self-care practices and wellbeing and improves physical and mental health outcomes with lower service utilisation and lower cost (ACSQHC 2018b).

The goal of person-centred care is a meaningful life, using:

> a person-centered approach to care [that] puts persons in the centre with their context, their history, their family, and individual strengths and weaknesses. It also means a shift from viewing the patient as a passive target of a healthcare system to another model where the patient is an active part in his or her care and decision-making (Håkansson Eklund et al 2019:4).

Biological Determinants of Health

In this decade, biological or genetic determinants such as sex, age and inherited conditions, including carrying the ApoE4 gene which increases the risk of heart disease and dementia, account for only 25% of intrinsic capacity of individuals to experience healthy ageing. The other 75% is linked to the cumulative impact of behaviours and experiences across the lifespan. These experiences are influenced by factors such as the environment and the person's social position, reflecting the powerful impact of the social determinants of health on function in older age (WHO 2015).

Social Determinants of Health

The social and environmental determinants of healthy ageing are the conditions in which people are born, grow, live, work and age, including cultural context (see also Chapter 3) and the health and social care system. These circumstances are shaped by the distribution of money, power and resources at global, national and local levels. The social determinants of health are mostly responsible for inequities in health status seen within and between countries (AIHW 2018).

The Social Gradient

Currently good and bad health are unevenly distributed. There is a social gradient, which means that those with less money, less education and insecure working conditions are more likely to have lower health literacy levels and poor access to services, resulting in morbidity and premature death. This inequity is evident in older people and Aboriginal and Torres Strait Islander and Māori people (AIHW 2018; Ministry of Health NZ 2016).

Importantly, older people may already be educated and aware of health supports, but unable to access services or participate safely. For example, 29% of Australians and 27% of New Zealanders were born overseas. Older migrants face language and cultural barriers to accessing healthcare. The social gradient dictates that older Indigenous and non-English speaking migrants experience some of the poorest health in our communities (AIHW 2018; Statistics NZ 2019).

HEALTH PROMOTION AND SOCIAL DETERMINANTS

A health promotion approach categorises the determinants of healthy ageing as either social and environmental, or behavioural, often referred to as lifestyle or risk factors.

Risk Factors

Risk factors can be either non-modifiable, including the biological characteristics of age, sex and genetic make-up, or modifiable factors, such as smoking, inactivity or obesity. At any age, modifying risky behaviour will improve health (WHO 2015) (see *Practice point: Risk factors for dementia*).

Practice Point
Risk Factors for Dementia

NON-MODIFIABLE

- Older age
- Genetics – accounts for less than 1% of all dementias, e.g. Huntington Disease

MODIFIABLE

- physical inactivity
- hypertension
- obesity
- high blood cholesterol
- diabetes
- poor diet
- alcohol overuse
- mental inactivity
- smoking

WHO (2019).

Prevention

Prevention strategies to reduce the burden of disease and improve wellbeing are grouped as below (Daly et al 2019):

1. **Primary prevention**: addressing the social determinants of health and modifiable risk factors to prevent chronic conditions.
2. **Secondary prevention**: directing strategies to early detection of health conditions, treatment and cure, and addressing risk factors to reverse symptoms and prevent condition progression.
3. **Tertiary prevention**: aimed at modifying determinants of healthy ageing to improve wellbeing, reduce symptoms and delay progression of existing chronic conditions.

These three levels of prevention can be illustrated using the example of dementia, a major global health issue as the population ages (see Table 4.2). Dementia is the second leading cause of death of older Australians (ABS 2018b), with older people fearing a diagnosis of dementia more than any other chronic condition (Pfizer Australia 2010). There are nine known modifiable risk factors for dementia, as summarised in *Practice point: Risk factors for dementia* above.

Primary prevention aimed at preventing new cases includes health promotion programs to reduce dementia risk, thereby reducing the incidence rate and impact of dementia. If such a risk reduction program delayed the onset of dementia symptoms by 5 years, the incidence of dementia would halve (Shah et al 2016).

Secondary prevention aimed at early detection requires nurses to screen older people for known risk factors for

TABLE 4.2
Adopting a Prevention Approach in Nursing Practice

Questions to Ask and Actions to Take	

Primary Prevention	• Was this event or condition preventable?
	• How?
	  • Lifestyle/behaviour change
	  • Change to environmental or social determinants – housing
	  • Vaccination or safety precaution – equipment

Secondary Prevention	• Can it be prevented from happening again or worsening? • How? • Screen, manage and monitor risk factors

Tertiary Prevention	• Can function, wellbeing and health be restored or maximised?
	• How?
	  • Rehabilitation
	  • Risk factors management

Ministry of Health NZ (2016); Office of Disease Prevention and Health Promotion (2020).

dementia and implement risk management programs. Facilitating early diagnosis of dementia also allows for treatment of modifiable causes, and the opportunity to self-manage risky behaviours while decision-making capacity is retained. Effective secondary prevention may slow the progression of dementia (Ng & Ward 2019).

Tertiary prevention aimed at managing the effects of the condition involves coordinating environmental factors to reduce the burden of behavioural and psychological symptoms and improve functional capacity. Rehabilitation and wellness options for people diagnosed with dementia can delay high-level service supports such as entry to residential care (Ng & Ward 2019).

MODELS OF HEALTH PROMOTION
Transtheoretical Model
There are a number of behaviour change models that assist nurses to understand health behaviour change.

The transtheoretical model (Prochaska & DiClemente 1983) provides a framework that integrates change-enabling factors from a range of theories. The Transtheoretical model shows good evidence for positive behaviour change in mental health and chronic conditions such as diabetes; modifiable risk factors such as

hypertension and smoking; and in the prevention of cancer and chronic conditions such as osteoporosis. Additionally, the Transtheoretical model is cheap and time efficient as part of routine nursing practice (Hashemzadeh et al 2019).

Also known as the stages of change model, the transtheoretical model hinges on the concept that changing behaviour is a process of different stages of readiness and change that older people pass through and return to on the road to sustained change.

Six stages of the transtheoretical model
1. Pre-contemplation – not yet ready to make a change, lack awareness or denial
2. Contemplation – problem awareness, considering impact of making change
3. Preparation – planning, steps taken towards change
4. Action – making the change
5. Maintenance – converting change into routine habit, relapse minimisation
6. Termination – no relapse or temptation.

The likelihood of change is greater in older people who have low pre-contemplation levels and high levels of other stages. In smoking cessation, interventions which support people move up a stage, doubling the likelihood that the person will quit smoking. Different strategies are used in the different stages to enable permanent behaviour change.

For example, the key to moving on from a relapse is self-re-evaluation by the person to identify strengths and weaknesses at that point. A plan to address a weakness could include: consciousness-raising by providing information on risk and action options; environmental re-evaluation to identify and minimise triggers; and/or engaging helping relationships to support sustained change. Evidence suggests that promoting a higher health literacy level improves the likelihood of future sustained behaviour change (Hashemzadeh et al 2019).

Miller's Functional Consequences Theory
The Functional consequences theory for promoting wellness in older adults model pulls together many concepts and theories to explain age-related changes and determinants that negatively impact on healthy ageing.

Functional consequences
Older people experience age-related changes and cumulative risk factors. Miller (1990:2018) described this as the experience of *functional consequences*. The functional consequences theory directly attributes the interplay of

the determinants of health to the older person's level of function. Functional consequences can be either negative or positive.

- Negative functional consequences: impair functional ability.
- Positive functional consequences: promote functional ability, wellness and healthy ageing.

The Functional consequences theory identifies the following determinants of healthy ageing that can be targeted by nursing interventions to achieve positive functional consequences:

- Aged-related changes: 'normal ageing changes' occur over the life course. Without nursing intervention, physiological age-related changes often have negative functional consequences. Psychological and spiritual changes may have positive functional consequences.
- Risk factors: include environmental, social and biological determinants of health.

Aligning with nursing theories and the domains of the code of conduct for Australian and New Zealand nurses (Nursing Council of New Zealand [NCNZ] 2012; Nursing and Midwifery Board of Australia [NMBA] 2017), such as to promote wellbeing, Miller's model is underpinned by the following four concepts (Gouveia et al 2011; Miller 2018):

1. **Older person:** the interplay of risk factors and age-related changes unique to the individual. The person and their carer are the focus of nursing interventions supporting positive consequences.
2. **Nursing:** nursing approach can reduce negative functional consequences of age-related change and risk factors, to promote wellbeing and healthy ageing, e.g. person-centred care to partner with older people and co-design care plans.
3. **Health:** Capacity of the individual for functional ability that takes account of risk factors and age-related change plus their own healthy ageing goals, e.g. everyone is different.
4. **Environment:** The external conditions that impact on the older person's experience of wellbeing, such as society. Can have negative functional consequences as a risk factor, e.g. ageism, or positive functional consequences as a supportive intervention e.g. safe, accessible, inclusive, 'age friendly environments'.

Functional consequences theory is implemented differently depending on the clinical setting. In the emergency department, the goal is often to save life and interventions are aimed at the older person regaining function. Rehabilitation goals are more likely to focus on achieving prior levels of function by preventing negative and supporting positive functional consequences. The goals of care in residential aged care and community settings often pertain to maintenance of function and improved wellbeing.

By incorporating the Transtheoretical model and functional consequences theory into routine practice, nurses can facilitate healthy ageing for all older people (see *Promoting wellness: The Transtheoretical model and Functional Consequences theory in routine nursing practice*).

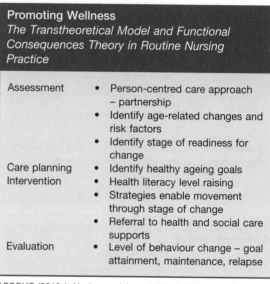

Promoting Wellness
The Transtheoretical Model and Functional Consequences Theory in Routine Nursing Practice

Assessment	• Person-centred care approach – partnership • Identify age-related changes and risk factors • Identify stage of readiness for change
Care planning Intervention	• Identify healthy ageing goals • Health literacy level raising • Strategies enable movement through stage of change • Referral to health and social care supports
Evaluation	• Level of behaviour change – goal attainment, maintenance, relapse

ACSQHC (2018a); Hashemzadeh et al (2019); Miller (2018).

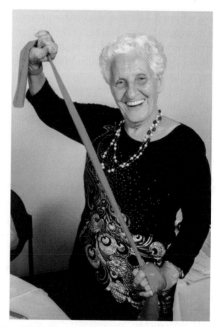

FIG. 4.3 Using a resistance band in a daily routine

EXERCISE AND ACTIVITY

Physical fitness is required for physical function, which is the capacity to undertake physical ADLs. Physical activity includes all movement that expends energy, produced by the individual's skeletal muscles (see Fig. 4.3). Exercise is defined as planned and repeated activity aimed at promoting physical fitness. There is good evidence for the health benefits of physical activity, summarised in the *Research highlight* below. Higher levels of activity are associated with greater health benefit.

Research Highlight
Physical Activity and Healthy Ageing

LOWER RATES OF:

- selected causes of mortality
- cardiovascular disease
- high blood pressure
- type 2 diabetes mellitus (T2DM)
- bowel and breast cancer
- falls

IMPROVED:

- cognition
- biomarkers for prevention of cardiovascular disease and T2DM
- cardiovascular and muscular fitness
- bone health
- body mass index
- functional health
- social roles

Alty et al (2020); Department of Health (2017); Ministry of Health NZ (2013).

How Much is Enough Physical Activity for Healthy Ageing?

The Australian and New Zealand physical activity guidelines for older people recommend:

- engaging in physical activity every day, regardless of age or health conditions
- 30 minutes of moderate intensity physical activity a minimum of 5 days per week
- starting at an easy level and gradually building up activity
- continuing and adapting lifelong vigorous physical activity to capabilities
- undertaking balance training to prevent falls, a minimum of 3 days per week
- undertaking muscle-strengthening exercises a minimum of 2 days per week (Department of Health 2017; Ministry of Health NZ 2013).

Less than one in ten older Australians engage in the recommended amount of physical and strength-based activities. The most common reasons that older people do not engage in health behaviour change is the erroneous belief that nothing can be done, and that it is too late to start (Alty et al 2020).

Practice Point
Preventing Dementia

Recent research shows that approximately one-third of dementia cases can be attributed to modifiable risk factors. One primary prevention strategy is the Preventing Dementia (PD) Mass Open Online Course (MOOC), a short (four-week), online multidomain course that is available free to anyone with an interest in brain health and dementia, from community members to clinicians and aged care providers. The MMOC aims to raise health literacy in this area by presenting the latest evidence on risk factors for dementia and how to interpret them.

With no cure for dementia, the PD MOOC offers a mechanism to reduce the incidence of dementia and its financial and social costs. With over 100,000 enrolments since 2016, it rates highly with global users. This course is free and delivered flexibly online, via computer, tablet or mobile phone. Evaluation demonstrates significant improvement in understanding dementia risk factors and risk-related behaviour change

---

Alty et al (2020); WDREC (2016).

SUMMARY

The paradigm shift from the traditional biomedical model to the more holistic, integrated person-centred approach to the care of older people is urgently required to facilitate healthy ageing and contain the growing demands on and cost of care associated with the ageing population. This transition requires reorientating health and social care systems and nursing practice to focus on addressing the determinants of healthy ageing.

This chapter has outlined the necessary concepts and frameworks for nurses to focus on health promotion and develop practice that supports healthy ageing across all care settings. Key to healthy ageing is the ability of nurses to identify those factors that influence health at an environmental level and the individual level. The powerful role of the social determinants, the social gradient and risk factors in determining healthy ageing requires nurses to keep abreast of current evidence, including risk reduction for prevention and management of chronic conditions and health events.

Nurses who incorporate health promotion into routine care, such as improving health literacy, directing strategies to primary, secondary and tertiary prevention and framing practice on the transtheoretical model and functional consequences theory, offer hope to older people. Proactive, holistic approaches can reduce disease risk and optimise function to improve health outcomes.

In doing so, nurses enable cost effective care, support older people to identify and interpret health information; assist them to make informed choices that reflect their own values; promote wellbeing; and facilitate healthy ageing.

Practice Scenario

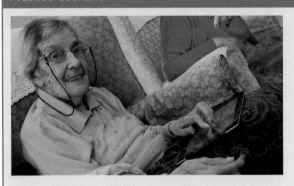

March: Mable is an 81-year-old woman who lives in a residential aged care facility and who wishes to enrol in a dementia prevention program that utilises the PD MOOC. On assessment of her physical activity, she tells the nurse that she used to play tennis with friends three times a week, but gave that up when she developed arthritis in both her knees at the age of 60.

June: Mable is now at the end of the four-week dementia prevention program. On evaluation in the last week of the program, Mable tells the nurse that she is worried about her sedentary lifestyle after learning that inactivity is a risk factor for dementia, and has been trying to do a bit of exercise. She has been for a walk with her husband and is thinking of joining a walking group.

September: Mable has completed the PD MOOC and is responding to the 3-month follow-up questionnaire; she tells the nurse that she joined the walking group and was walking five times a week. However, two weeks ago she tripped on uneven pavement and fell while on one of the walks and has been fearful of walking since. Mable is worried that she has failed to reduce her dementia risk and will probably go back to her previous level of inactivity.

MULTIPLE CHOICE QUESTIONS

1. In March, which stage of readiness for change was Mable in? Circle the correct response.
   a. Pre-contemplation
   b. Contemplation
   c. Preparation
   d. Action

2. What health literacy strategies could assist the nurse progress Mable from one stage to another? Circle the most correct response.
   a. Assume low health literacy level and provide universal precautions with all written and verbal communication delivered in plain English.
   b. Provide clear, correct and evidence-based health information
   c. Encourage Mable to ask questions when in doubt
   d. All of the above.

3. In June, which stage of readiness for change was Mable in? Circle the correct response.
   a. Preparation
   b. Action
   c. Maintenance
   d. Termination

4. What known modifiable risk factors for dementia should Mable also know about to reduce her risk?
   a. Hypertension; obesity and old age
   b. Smoking, alcohol overuse, mental inactivity
   c. High blood cholesterol, being female, hypertension
   d. Diabetes, carrying mutated BRCA1 gene and obesity

5. In September, what actions could the nurse take to assist Mable with a relapse? Circle the most correct response.
   a. facilitate self-re-evaluation to identify strengths and weaknesses at the time of relapse
   b. raise health literacy level of falls risk and risk reduction
   c. refer to falls prevention program
   d. all of the above

USEFUL RESOURCES

Agency for Healthcare Research and Quality (2019) Universal precautions toolkit (US). Online. Available: www.ahrq.gov/qual/literacy/healthliteracytoolkit.pdf

Clinical Excellence Commission (CEC) (2019) NSW Health Literacy Framework. 2019-2024, Sydney: Clinical Excellence Commission

Department of Health (2017) Australia's physical activity and sedentary behaviour guidelines. Canberra: DoH. Online: Available: www1.health.gov.au/internet/main/publishing.nsf/Content/health-pubhlth-strateg-phys-act-guidelines

Reid S, White K (2012) Upfront: Understanding health literacy. Best Practice Journal (NZ). Online. Available: www.bpac.org.nz/magazine/2012/august/upfront.asp

REFERENCES

Alty J, Farrow M, Lawler K (2020) Exercise and dementia prevention. Practical Neurology. Epub ahead of print: doi:10.1136/practneurol-2019-002335

Australian Bureau of Statistics (ABS) (2018a) National health survey: health literacy, 2018 Cat no. 4364.0.55.014. Online. Available: www.abs.gov.au/ausstats/abs@.nsf/mf/4364.0.55.014

Australian Bureau of Statistics (ABS) (2018b) Causes of death, Australia, 2017. Cat. no. 3303.0. Online. Available: www.abs.gov.au/ausstats/abs@.nsf/mf/3303.0

Australian Commission on Safety and Quality in Health Care (ACSQHC) (2018a) National statement on health literacy – Taking action to improve safety and quality. ACSQHC, Sydney.

Australian Commission on Safety and Quality in Health Care (ACSQHC) (2018b) Attributes of person-centred healthcare organisations 2018. ACSQHC, Sydney.

Australian Institute of Health and Welfare (AIHW) (2018) Australia's health 2018. Australia's health series no. 16. AUS 221.

Daly L, Byrne G, Keogh B (2019) Contemporary considerations relating to health promotion and older people. British Journal of Nursing 28(21):1414–1419.

Department of Health (DOH) (2017) Australia's physical activity and sedentary behaviour guidelines. DOH, Canberra.

De Wit L, Fenenga C, Giammarchi C et al (2017) Community-based initiatives improving critical health literacy: a systematic review and meta-synthesis of qualitative evidence. BMC Public Health 17:1–11.

Ding D, Grunseit A, Chau J et al (2016) Retirement – a transition to a healthier lifestyle? Evidence from a large Australian study. American Journal of Preventative Medicine 51:170–178.

Gouveia B, Jardim H, Martins M (2011). Foundation of gerontogical rehabilitation nursing: Applicability of the functional consequences theory. Referência [Suppl] 1(4):475.

Green J, Eager K, Owen A et al (2006) Towards a measure of function for home and community care services in Australia: Part 2. Australian Journal of Primary Health 12(1):82–90.

Håkansson Eklund J, Holmström IK, Kumlin T et al (2019) 'Same same or different?' A review of reviews of person-centered and patient-centered care. Patient Education and Counseling 102(1):3–11.

Harvey G, Dollard J, Marshall A et al (2018) Achieving integrated care for older people: shuffling the deckchairs or making the system watertight for the future? International Journal of Health Policy and Management 7(4):290–293.

Hashemzadeh M, Rahimi A, Zare-Farashbandi F et al (2019) Transtheoretical model of health behavioral change: a systematic review. Iranian Journal of Nursing and Midwifery Research 24(2):83–90.

Hauora (2014). Defining health promotion. Hauora Health Promotion Forum of New Zealand, Auckland.

Miller C (2018) Nursing for wellness in older adults. 8th edn. Wolters Kluwer, Philadelphia.

Miller C (1990) Nursing care of older adults: A concept analysis. Nursing Forum 47(1):39–50.

Ministry of Health (NZ Ministry of Health) (2020) Long-term conditions. MOH, Wellington. Online. Available: www.health.govt.nz/our-work/diseases-and-conditions/long-term-conditions

Ministry of Health NZ (2016) Healthy ageing strategy. MOH, Wellington.

Ministry of Health NZ (2015) Health literacy review: A guide. MOH, Wellington.

Ministry of Health NZ (2013) Guidelines on physical activity for older people (aged 65 years and over). MOH, Wellington.

Ministry of Health NZ (2010) Kōrero Mārama: Health literacy and Māori results from the 2006 Adult Literacy and Life Skills Survey. MOH, Wellington.

Ng N, Ward S (2019) Diagnosis of dementia in Australia: a narrative review of services and models of care. Australian Health Review 43:415–424.

Nurse and Midwifery Board of Australia (NMBA) (2017) Code of conduct for nurses. Nurse and Midwifery Board of Australia, Sydney.

Nursing Council of New Zealand (NCNZ) (2012) Code of conduct for nurses. NCNZ, Wellington.

Office of Disease Prevention and Health Promotion (ODPHP) (2020) Healthy People 2020. ODPHP, Washington.

Pasifika Futures (2017) Pasifika people in New Zealand. How are we doing? Pasifika Futures, Auckland.

Pfizer Australia (2010) Pfizer Health Report Wave 2. Views and understanding of Alzheimer's Disease in Australia. StollzNow Research, Sydney.

Prochaska J, DiClemente C (1983) Stages and processes of self-change in smoking: Toward an integrative model of change. Journal of Consulting and Clinical Psychology 5:390–395.

Shah S, Vanclay F, Cooper B (1989) Improving the sensitivity of the Barthel Index for stroke rehabilitation. Journal of Clinical Epidemiology 42(8):703–709.

Shah H, Albanese E, Duggan C et al (2016) Research priorities to reduce the global burden of dementia by 2025. Lancet Neurology 15(12):1285–1294.

Statistics New Zealand (2019) International migration: November 2019 – Infoshare tables. Online. Available: www

.stats.govt.nz/information-releases/international-migration
-november-2019-infoshare-tables.

Uniting Care Ageing (2014) Finding the why: Enabling active participation in life in aged care [Video file]. https://youtu.be/hZN1CyEiFNM

Wicking Dementia Research and Education Centre (WDREC) (2016) Preventing dementia massive open online course. University of Tasmania, Hobart. Online. Available: www.utas.edu.au/wicking/preventing-dementia

World Health Organisation (WHO) (2019) Risk reduction of cognitive decline and dementia guidelines. WHO, Geneva.

World Health Organisation (WHO) (2015) World report on ageing and health. WHO, Geneva.

World Health Organisation (WHO) (1986) The Ottawa Charter for Health Promotion. WHO, Geneva.

CHAPTER 5

Navigating the Healthcare System

JACQUELINE ALLEN

LEARNING OBJECTIVES

After reading this chapter, you will be able to:

- describe the funding and policy contexts in Australia and New Zealand that shape health and aged care services, and the need for service navigation
- critically appraise aged care service navigation within the Australian and New Zealand context
- evaluate service navigation roles and interventions in improving access to health and aged care services for older people and their families/informal carers
- discuss quality and safety in health and aged care, including clinical governance frameworks, supporting care integration and service navigation for older people and their families/informal carers.

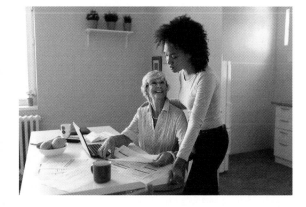

INTRODUCTION

In Australia, New Zealand and internationally, service navigation includes any response to service fragmentation that aims to improve the access of patients and families/informal carers (carers) to services. Service navigation is an evolving area of health services improvement that aims to address service gaps caused by health and aged care service fragmentation. In this way, service navigation is embedded within the health system, funding and

policy contexts at national and program levels. There is debate about service navigation with health and aged care services planners and researchers critiquing service navigation approaches and interventions as surface level solutions to deeper problems within the health system (Carter et al 2018). These deeper systemic problems may result in the fragmentation of health and aged care due to the need for more specialised care for older people and the cost of providing the service. Other commentators consider service navigation as an opportunity for stronger clinical governance and quality improvement directing new models of healthcare and nursing (McMurray et al 2018). This chapter explores service navigation as three main topic areas:

- the healthcare system, including funding and policy contexts
- clinical governance and quality improvement
- accessing and navigating health and aged care in Australia and New Zealand.

NAVIGATING THE SYSTEM

Service navigation on behalf of and by older people and their carers is gaining importance in contemporary health and aged care systems. In all countries, including New Zealand and Australia, communities are ageing because of improved social and environmental determinants of health, reductions in childhood mortality in low- and middle-income countries, and improved public health control of infectious disease (World Health Organisation [WHO] 2015). The ageing population is a major driver of change in the policy and practice orientation of healthcare and aged care services towards improved management of chronic diseases and associated disability (Goncalves-Bradely et al 2016). Older people are users of multiple health and aged care services and require improved access to services.

Approaches to service navigation are evolving and include service system access and self-referral via internet-based and call centre portals, such as the Australian-based My Aged Care, and by coordinated local intake services, such as the New-Zealand-based Needs Assessment Services (Australian Government 2020a; Needs Assessment Service Coordination Association 2020). Additionally, new service models are being researched and evaluated with a focus on how to improve support for older people and their informal carers in service navigation.

Navigator roles are gaining interest for their potential to improve support for older people. In a recent scoping review, Carter and colleagues identified that service navigator roles, including nurse navigators, assist patients and older people to overcome access barriers and improve meeting their care and service needs (Carter et al 2018). A recent project in Queensland implemented a nurse navigator role in general practice and a chronic disease management community coordination centre (McMurray et al 2018). The researchers found that the nurse navigator roles improved care coordination and patients' access to multidisciplinary chronic disease care.

Other models aiming to improve service navigation for older adults are evolving in sub-acute care. A literature review by Hickman and colleagues found that aged care teams and multidisciplinary teams, such as those characterising sub-acute care in Australia and in New Zealand, improved service navigation and reduced unnecessary hospital re-admission rates among older people (Hickman et al 2015). Other research has found that formal transitional care and discharge care interventions improve service navigation and discharge care outcomes for older people (Goncalves-Bradely et al 2016).

AUSTRALIAN PUBLIC HEALTH AND AGED CARE SYSTEMS

Many older people require healthcare and support from multiple areas of the public health and aged care systems.

> ### Research Highlight
> *Navigator Roles*
>
> - Service navigator roles, including nurse navigators, assist older people and their carers to overcome barriers to accessing care and improve meeting their needs for support (Carter et al 2018).
> - Nurse navigator roles improve care coordination and older people's access to multidisciplinary chronic disease care (McMurray et al 2018).
> - Aged care teams and multidisciplinary teams improve service navigation and reduce unnecessary hospital re-admission rates among older people (Hickman et al 2015).

Carter et al (2018); Hickman et al (2015); McMurray et al (2018).

This can range from specialised healthcare, general healthcare and community aged care or residential aged care services (Goncalves-Bradely et al 2016). This care is provided by multiple services funded through a range of Australian federal and state- or territory-administered programs. Policy, funding and program administration in health and aged care at the federal and state and territory government levels are complex. Nationally relevant issues are discussed, debated and negotiated regularly at the intergovernmental forum known as the Council of Australian Governments (COAG) (COAG 2020). New Zealand health ministers are also members of COAG.

In general, the Australian federal government funds or subsidises community and residential aged care (Australian Government Department of Health 2020). The federally funded Medicare universal healthcare insurance scheme partially or fully funds a number of health services in Australia, including general practice and pathology services (Australian Government Department of Human Services 2020). State and territory governments fund local health networks, which provide public inpatient and outpatient services, acute, sub-acute and some community-based health services (Australian Government Department of Health 2019a). Table 5.1 presents a summary of the healthcare system in Australia's states and territories.

Historically, community aged care services were funded by the Australian federal government Home and Community Care (HACC) program (Australian Government Department of Health 2018b). However, the HACC program was discontinued in 2016 as part of significant federal government reforms. As of June 2016, the federal

TABLE 5.1 Summary of the Healthcare System in Australian States/Territories	
Tasmania	In Tasmania, the Tasmanian Department of Health has jurisdiction over the funding, monitoring and performance of the public health system, delivered by the Tasmanian Health Service, as well as human services, including direct service provision for Ambulance Tasmania, child/youth services and housing and disability services (Tasmanian Department of Health 2019). The Tasmanian Health Service is responsible for governing and delivering healthcare in Tasmania through public hospitals, primary care services and community health services.
Victoria	The Department of Health and Human Services is responsible for the funding, regulation and planning of public health services across Victoria (State Government of Victoria 2020). These services include public hospitals and external organisations providing mental health and some community and aged care services.
New South Wales	Public health care in NSW is funded and monitored by the NSW Ministry of Health through NSW Health (New South Wales Government 2018). NSW Health operates public hospitals and community health organisations. It also operates mental health services and some aged care services. NSW Health provides services through a network of local health districts across the state of NSW.
Australian Capital Territory	Public healthcare in the ACT is funded by the ACT Government (ACT Government 2019). These services include public hospitals and community health services.
Queensland	Queensland Health is under the responsibility of the Queensland Minister for Health and Department of Health (Queensland Government 2019). Queensland Health provides health services, including hospital services, community and mental health services, and some aged care services through Queensland's 16 Hospital and Health Boards.
Northern Territory	Healthcare in the NT is provided by Northern Territory Health under the responsibility of the Department of Health Northern Territory Government (Northern Territory Government 2020). NT Health provides direct health care services to the territory through the Top End and Central Australian health services, which include all public hospitals, community health services and mental health services.
Western Australia	WA Health is funded by the Government of Western Australia to provide public health services (Government of Western Australia 2019). WA Health provides public hospital services and community health services, including child and adolescent health and mental healthcare.
South Australia	SA Health is funded by the Government of South Australia to provide public health services to the state of South Australia (Government of South Australia 2019). These public health services include public hospitals, youth services and mental health services.

government initiated the Australian Commonwealth Home Support Program (CHSP), which funds many community aged care services that were formerly funded under the HACC program. Community aged care services funded under CHSP include care provided by local government councils, such as personal care and the Meals on Wheels organisation that provides nutrition to and reduces isolation for older people.

The main difference in federal government policy directing CHSP compared with policy directing the former HACC is the current strong focus on consumer- and family-centred decision-making on their own care. This policy focus is emphasised in the home care packages that run in tandem with CHSP services for older people who require more support at home. Aged care packages are underpinned by a government policy of consumer-directed care (see Box 5.1 for definition) (Australian Government Department of Health 2019b). Eligible older Australians may access different levels of home care packages depending on whether they have high, intermediate or low-level care needs. These home care packages are assigned to the older person, who can then decide for themselves on the mix of in-home services they require, their preferred provider and how to spend their allocated money to support a good quality of life living independently in their own home. The

BOX 5.1
Definition of Consumer-Directed Care

Consumer-directed care is a model of care where the consumer has direct control over their care and services (Laragy & Allen 2015). This typically involves the consumer holding their home care package funding from which they purchase services and care to support their quality of life. Consumer-directed care is increasingly becoming the mainstream approach to care in the community for older people, and also for adults and children living with disability in many western countries including Australia and New Zealand. Consumer-directed care models have a range of program names, including home care packages and the National Disability Insurance Scheme (NDIS) in Australia, Individualised Funding in New Zealand, Individual Budgets in the United Kingdom, and self-directed care in the United States (Laragy & Allen 2015).

federal government requires the consumer to spend their package funds in accordance with legislated guidelines, including the requirement to account for how the funds are disbursed (Australian Government Department of Health 2019b). This is in contrast to the situation prior to the reforms in 2016, when home care packages were allocated to service providers that determined how the funds would be spent together with and on behalf of the older person.

New Zealand Health and Aged Care System
In New Zealand, 75% of health programs are funded through District Health Boards (Ministry of Health NZ 2019). There are 20 District Health Boards (DHBs) and each owns and funds public hospitals within its respective district. The DHBs are structured by the *New Zealand Public Health and Disability Act 2000*. The aims and objectives of the DHBs include:

• to promote and protect health
• to promote integrated health services
• to optimise effective and efficient services targeted to local, regional and national healthcare needs
• to promote care for people requiring health or disability services (Ministry of Health NZ 2019).

Public hospital care, including acute, rehabilitative and outpatient care, is funded through the DHBs. Primary care, including general practice, is partly subsidised through the DHBs with aged care also subsidised through the DHBs (Ministry of Health NZ 2017). Community support for older New Zealanders is funded by the DHBs and provided by a range of government, local district and not-for-profit service organisations (Ministry of

Health NZ 2018a). Older people may access high-, intermediate- and low-level support at home. Consumer-directed care packages are available for New Zealanders living with a disability, although these are not currently widely available to older people (Ministry of Health NZ 2018b).

FUNDING AND CARE OPTIONS
In Australia in 2016–17, AU$181 billion was spent on healthcare (Australian Government Department of Health 2019a). This included 41% spending by the federal government, 27% by state and territory governments, with the remainder spent by individuals, private health insurance companies and non-government companies. Most public clinical healthcare, except for healthcare provided by general practice, is funded by the state and territory governments (Australian Government Department of Health 2019a). Across Australia, general practice is subsidised by the federally funded Medicare scheme. Patients may be required to pay for any gap in fees between the Medicare agreed payment and the fees set by the general practitioner (GP). GPs can elect to 'bulk bill' a patient, whereby the doctor bills Medicare directly for the consultation and accepts the Medicare benefit as full payment, meaning that there is no out-of-pocket cost (Australian Government Department of Health 2018a; Parliament of Australia 2016).

The total amount of New Zealand Government funding spent on the health system in 2016–17 was NZ$16.142 billion (Ministry of Health NZ 2016). Of this funding, more than three-quarters was allocated to the DHBs to fund public clinical health services, such as public hospitals in their respective districts. The Ministry of Health spent the remaining funds on national programs, including disability services, mental health services, screening programs, and child and maternity community health services (Ministry of Health NZ 2016).

The funding arrangements in both Australia and New Zealand, as in other western countries, are complex (Australian Government Department of Health 2018a; Ministry of Health NZ 2016). Numerous care options are available for older people with chronic health and reduced functional abilities. This means that sub-acute and community-based services can be tailored to meet the older person's care needs. More care options means increased choices (and decisions) for older people. Wider choices can be viewed as an improvement in health and aged care services and results in a more personalised and individualised care plan than was formerly available (Fulbrook et al 2017). However, this expanding range of services in health and aged care, and the different funding that supports them, can increase service fragmentation (Carter et al 2018). This can make health and aged care challenging for older people and their carers to navigate and negotiate.

GOVERNMENT POLICY

Government policies relating to health and aged care in Australia and New Zealand, similar to other western countries, are challenged to accommodate the changing healthcare needs of communities in relation to chronic disease and the ageing population (Hickman et al 2015). Decision-makers must develop policy that directs equitable funding of services to support the health and wellbeing of everyone in the population. This requires collective decision-making at all levels of government and health service planning to achieve fair and equal distribution of funding and services (Productivity Commission 2011).

Since the early 1990s, when health services became more formally organised around the need to better care for older people, policymakers and health planners have focused on streamlining care in sub-acute and community services (Allen et al 2017). Their emphasis was and continues to be on 'the right care, at the right time, and in the right place'. This policy shift has seen a burgeoning of sub-acute care services. Examples include the Australian-based Transition Care Program and Geriatric Evaluation and Management, and concomitant programs in New Zealand, being provided both in inpatient settings and in older people's own homes (Australian Government Department of Health 2019a; Ministry of Health NZ 2018a). Other improvements in health services include programs to optimise care transitions and hospital discharge of older people (Robinson et al 2015).

In community aged care, government policies have shifted from organisation-driven care to consumer-directed care models (Laragy & Allen 2015). These policy shifts have seen a concurrent disinvestment in older models of healthcare, for example, those funded through the former Australian-based HACC program, including public district nursing services. Currently in Australia, home care services are largely staffed by personal care workers. There is limited funding to support professional nursing care in the home unless services are provided and funded by sub-acute care programs. Acute care can be provided in the home through the Hospital in the Home program. Professional nurses are employed in general practice; however, at this point in time these nursing roles have only very limited funding to undertake

home visiting. Quality clinical care in the home is dependent on robust clinical governance.

CLINICAL GOVERNANCE

Clinical governance refers to the culture, structures and processes that ensure quality and safe patient care within healthcare services. It includes the design and implementation of policies and procedures within the clinical care setting to optimise patient outcomes (Dragoon et al 2019). Clinical governance emphasises a culture of shared responsibility by all staff, and patients and their carers to maintain and improve high standards of care. In Australia, New Zealand and internationally, registered nurses (RNs) have important roles in clinical governance, including leadership at all levels within healthcare organisations to identify and mitigate clinical risk and prioritise quality care (Sundean et al 2019).

Clinical governance and service navigation for older adults are critically important in contemporary Australian health and aged care, where there are high levels of fragmentation between services. Where care integration and service navigation are ineffective – for example, where discharge planning and transitional care are sub-optimal – older people can experience poor health outcomes and avoidable representations to hospitals (Goncalves-Bradely et al 2016). Within the clinical governance framework, the role of the RN to optimise quality integrated care for older people, including through service navigation, is an expectation of the nursing profession, as well as Australian and New Zealand governments and health services.

QUALITY HEALTH SERVICE STANDARDS

Recent Australian data indicate that 8.9% (AU$4.1 billion) of total hospital expenditure resulted from hospital-acquired complications (Australian Commission on Safety and Quality in Health Care [ACSQHC] 2019). This suggests that quality and safety in healthcare are significant problems that require improvement. The COAG established the Australian Commission on Safety and Quality in Health Care (ACSQHC) in 2006 to coordinate and to provide national leadership in improving quality and safety in healthcare. The federal Parliament passed two laws to structure governance of the ACSQHC. These two laws are the *National Health Reform Act 2011* and the *Public Governance, Performance and Accountability Act 2013* (ACSQHC 2019). The ACSQHC works together with a range of stakeholders to achieve the aims. These stakeholders include patients, carers, healthcare practitioners and health services.

BOX 5.2
NSQHS Standards

1. Clinical governance
2. Partnering with consumers
3. Preventing and controlling healthcare-associated infection
4. Medication safety
5. Comprehensive care
6. Communicating for safety
7. Blood management
8. Recognising and responding to acute deterioration

ACSQHC (2017).

In order to provide quality and safe healthcare to all patients and carers, including older people, Australian health services are required to meet the National Safety and Quality Health Service (NSQHS) Standards (ACSQHC 2017). The NSQHS Standards were developed by the ACSQHC as the national benchmark of quality healthcare provision and to protect the public from harm related to health service provision. NSQHS Standards 1, 2, 4, 5 and 6 are pertinent to the nursing role of service navigation, which aims to address service gaps caused by fragmented health and aged care systems. This is because service navigation enhances patients' and carers' access to services and improves quality of integration between all services resulting in safer care for patients. The eight NSQHS Standards are listed in Box 5.2.

In New Zealand, quality and safety in healthcare is the remit of the Health Quality and Safety Commission New Zealand (HQSCNZ), a crown entity linked to the Ministry of Health NZ (HQSCNZ 2019). The aim of the HQSCNZ is to reduce harm related to healthcare with a focus on reducing hospital acquired infections, risks associated with surgery, risks related to medications and falls prevention.

HEALTH AND AGED CARE STANDARDS, AUDIT AND BENCHMARKING

Australian and New Zealand health services are required to meet expected standards within each country including care integration and service navigation. Australian health services are assessed against the eight NSQHS Standards every four years by the Australian Council on Health Care Standards (ACHCS) as the authorised accreditation organisation with the Australian Commission on Safety and Quality in Health Care (ACHCS 2019). Accreditation by the ACHCS is operationalised within the Evaluation and Quality Improvement Program (EQuIP). Across a four-year cycle, the EQuIP program directs healthcare services to undertake:

- self-assessment
- organisation-wide survey
- review by accreditors of the ACHS.

The accreditors review and audit each health service against the eight NSQHS Standards to identify which standards are being met, and to identify any service gaps (ACHCS 2019).

Australian and New Zealand aged care services are also expected to meet quality and safety standards in order to ensure high quality outcomes for all older people and their carers. The ACHCS implements a number of other accreditation programs following a similar process for organisations not covered by the NSQHS standards. These include the EQuIP6 Aged Care Services accreditation, in which aged care service providers participate in a 3-year assessment and improvement accreditation program that supports excellence in aged care service provision (ACHCS 2019). Currently, further standards are being developed with a focus on quality and safety in primary care.

The HQSCNZ monitors and reports on quality and safety in health services following similar processes (HQSCNZ 2019). For example, the HQSCNZ is also involved in leadership and accreditation to build safe quality health services, including care integration through improved service navigation for older adults.

Tips for Best Practice

- Health practitioners and health services should aim to reduce service fragmentation.
- Health practitioners and health services should aim to improve service navigation.
- Nurses should take active leadership roles to improve health and aged care service navigation for older people and their carers.

Promoting Wellness

- Older people should be supported towards independence in service navigation.
- Families and informal carers require support to independently navigate service systems with older people.
- Older people and carers should be informed how to access public aged care services.

Accessing the Aged Care System: My Aged Care and New Zealand Systems

Safety and quality in health and aged care are vitally important to the nursing and other healthcare professions in Australia and in New Zealand. Timely access to appropriate services, a core principle of service navigation, is integral to mandated standards that ensure high quality and safe care provision in Australasia. Australia and New Zealand have somewhat different access systems into aged care. In Australia, older adults must access publicly-funded aged care through a website and call centre known as 'My Aged Care' (Australian Government 2020). My Aged Care is the system that provides information about formal aged care supports, including finding locally-based services, and eligibility criteria and assessments. This access portal was introduced following the recommendations of the Productivity Commission Report (2011) and calls from consumer advocacy groups (Productivity Commission 2011; Royal Commission into Aged Care Quality and Safety 2019).

Only the older person or their family member/informal carer may make a referral (self-referral) to My Aged Care (Australian Government 2020). When contacted, call centre staff request details on how the older person manages at home and their general health. This information helps to determine the next step in the system and whether the older person requires a more formal assessment of their care needs. An older person who requires more comprehensive care assessments will be referred to the regional Aged Care Assessment Team (Australian Government 2020). Depending on the complexity of the older person's care needs, a range of care options may be suggested, including more support at home (ranging from low- to high-level care) or admission to a residential aged care facility (also ranging from low support to higher-level care). The referral pathway is summarised in Fig. 5.1.

Access to the aged care system in New Zealand occurs at the local level of the DHBs, which contract services for older people needing support through the local Needs Assessment Service Coordination organisation (Needs Assessment Service Coordination Association 2020). These services are 'not-for-profit' organisations based locally in each region of New Zealand. The Needs Assessment Service Coordination organisation arranges focused care needs assessment, and the planning and coordination of services from low- to high-level care depending on the older person's needs.

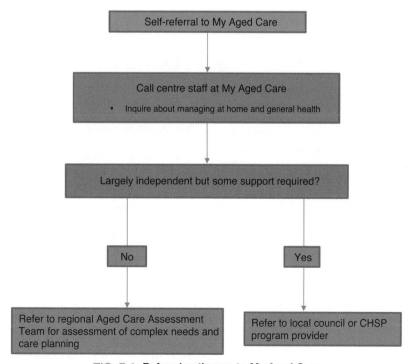

FIG. 5.1 **Referral pathways to My Aged Care**

Practice Scenario

Otto, aged 84 years, lives at home in a suburb of the Australian regional city of Geelong with his spouse Martha aged 80. Family is very important to Otto and Martha and they have daily contact with their daughter and grandchildren. Otto lives with chronic heart failure and takes medications. Recently, Otto was hospitalised in an acute medical ward because he had 'fluid on his lungs'. He was discharged home, but now Otto needs help to have a shower and he requires a walking frame. Otto and Martha are determined to stay living in their own home and be independent. Otto believes that he can look after himself. Otto and his family are unsure about where to access assistance.

MULTIPLE CHOICE QUESTIONS

1. A registered nurse on an acute care ward is:
   a. not required to assist Otto and his family after discharge care as this is beyond the remit of hospital care
   b. legally mandated to assist Otto and his family to navigate the services he will require after discharge
   c. not required to assist Otto and his family with discharge care because allied health staff are responsible
   d. Required to assist Otto and his family as part of a multidisciplinary team
   e. All of the above

2. Which of the following is <u>not</u> part of the role of a nurse navigator?
   a. Assists older people to navigate the healthcare system
   b. Organises healthcare appointments
   c. Reduces service fragmentation
   d. Takes a leadership role in healthcare
   e. Improves care coordination

3. Which of the following is involved in service navigation?
   a. Otto
   b. The general practitioner
   c. Martha
   d. My Aged Care
   e. All of the above

SUMMARY

This chapter has introduced service navigation in terms of three main topic areas: 1) health systems, funding and policy contexts; 2) accessing and navigating health and aged care services; and 3) clinical governance and national health standards. It is argued that quality service navigation is essential in contemporary health and aged care to reduce barriers to service access created by service fragmentation. Improved service navigation is vital to strengthen and support access to health and care services, better health and care outcomes for older people and to improve service efficiency. Nursing has a pivotal role in leading effective service navigation with and on behalf of older people and their carers.

REFERENCES

Allen J, Hutchinson AM, Brown R et al (2017) User experience and care integration in transitional care for older people from hospital to home: A meta-synthesis. Qualitative Health Research 27:24–36.

Australian Capital Territory (ACT) Government (2019) Services and programs. Online. Available www.health.act.gov.au/

Australian Commission on Safety and Quality in Health Care (ACSQHC) (2019) The state of patient safety and quality in Australian hospitals. Online. Available: www.safetyandquality.gov.au/sites/default/files/2019-07/the-state-of-patient-safety-and-quality-in-australian-hospitals-2019.pdf

Australian Commission on Safety and Quality in Health Care (ACSQHC) (2017) The National Safety and Quality Health Service Standards. Second edition. Online. Available: https://www.safetyandquality.gov.au/standards/nsqhs-standards

Australian Council on Health Care Standards (ACHCS) (2019) Overview of programs and services. Online. Available: www.achs.org.au/programs-services/overview/

Australian Government (2020) My Aged Care. Online. Available: www.myagedcare.gov.au/

Australian Government Department of Health (2020) Ageing and Aged Care. Online. Available: https://agedcare.health.gov.au/

Australian Government Department of Health (2019a) The Australian health system. Online. Available: www.health.gov.au/about-us/the-australian-health-system

Australian Government Department of Health (2019b) Home Care Packages Program. Online. Available: https://agedcare.health.gov.au/programs/home-care-packages-program

Australian Government Department of Health (2018a) Aged care funding. Online. Available: https://agedcare.health.gov.au/aged-care-funding

Australian Government Department of Health (2018b) The Commonwealth Home Support Programme Guidelines.

Online. Available: https://agedcare.health.gov.au/programs-services/commonwealth-home-support-programme/the-commonwealth-home-support-programme-guidelines

Australian Government Department of Human Services (2020) What's covered by Medicare. Online. Available: www.humanservices.gov.au/individuals/subjects/whats-covered-medicare

Carter N, Valaitis R, Lam A et al (2018) Navigation delivery models and roles of navigators in primary care: A scoping literature review. BMC Health Services Research 18:1–13.

Council of Australian Governments (COAG) (2020) COAG Health Council. Online. Available: www.coaghealthcouncil.gov.au/

Dragoon N, Nadeau M, Toolin S et al (2019) Nursing professional governance: patient and family centred design. Nursing Management (Springhouse) 50(10):15–19.

Fulbrook P, Jessup M, Kinnear F (2017) Implementation and evaluation of a 'Navigator' role to improve emergency department throughput. Australasian Emergency Nursing Journal 20:114–121.

Goncalves-Bradely C, Lannin NA, Clemson LM et al (2016) Discharge planning from hospital. Cochrane Collaboration, London.

Government of South Australia (2019) Department for health and wellbeing. Online. Available: www.sahealth.sa.gov.au/wps/wcm/connect/public+content/sa+health+internet/about+us/department+of+health

Government of Western Australia (2019) Department of Health About Us. Online. Available: ww2.health.wa.gov.au/About-us

Health Quality and Safety Commission New Zealand (HQSCNZ) (2019) About us. Online. Available: www.hqsc.govt.nz/about-us/

Hickman LD, Phillips JL, Newton PJ et al (2015) Multidisciplinary team interventions to optimise health outcomes for older people in acute care settings: A systematic review. Archives of Gerontology and Geriatrics 61:322–329.

Laragy C, Allen J (2015) Community aged care case managers transitioning to consumer directed care: More than procedural change required. Australian Social Work 68(2):212–227.

McMurray A, Ward L, Johnston K et al (2018) The primary health care nurse of the future: preliminary evaluation of the Nurse Navigator role in integrated care. Collegian 25:517–524.

Ministry of Health NZ (2019) District Health Boards. Online. Available: www.health.govt.nz/new-zealand-health-system/key-health-sector-organisations-and-people/district-health-boards?mega=NZ%20health%20system&title=District%20health%20boards

Ministry of Health NZ (2018a) Health of older people. MOH, Wellington. Online. Available: www.health.govt.nz/our-work/life-stages/health-older-people

Ministry of Health NZ (2018b) Individualised funding. MOH, Wellington. Online. Available: www.health.govt.nz/your-health/services-and-support/disability-services/types-disability-support/individualised-funding

Ministry of Health NZ (2017) Overview of the health system. MOH, Wellington. Online. Available: www.health.govt.nz/new-zealand-health-system/overview-health-system

Ministry of Health NZ (2016) Funding. MOH, Wellington. Online. Available: www.health.govt.nz/new-zealand-health-system/overview-health-system/funding

Needs Assessment Service Co-ordination Association (2020) About us. Online. Available: www.nznasca.co.nz/about-us/

New South Wales Government (2018) New South Wales Health. Online. Available: www.health.nsw.gov.au/about/nswhealth/Pages/structure.aspx

Northern Territory Government (2020) Wellbeing. Online. Available: https://nt.gov.au/wellbeing

Parliament of Australia (2016) Aged care: A quick guide. Online. Available: www.aph.gov.au/About_Parliament/Parliamentary_Departments/Parliamentary_Library/pubs/rp/rp1617/Quick_Guides/Aged_Care_a_quick_guide

Productivity Commission (2011) Caring for Older Australians. Productivity Commission, Canberra.

Queensland Government (2019) Queensland Health organisational structure. Online. Available: www.health.qld.gov.au/system-governance/health-system/managing/org-structure

Robinson TE, Zhou L, Kerse N et al (2015) Evaluation of a New Zealand program to improve transition of care for older high risk adults. Australasian Journal of Ageing 34:269–274.

Royal Commission into Aged Care Quality and Safety (2019) Interim Report. Online. Available: https://agedcare.royalcommission.gov.au/publications/Pages/interim-report.aspx

State Government of Victoria (2020) About us. Online. Available: www2.health.vic.gov.au/about

Sundean LJ, White KR, Thompson LS et al (2019) Governance education for nurses: preparing nurses for the future. Journal of Professional Nursing 35:346–352.

Tasmanian Department of Health (2019) About us. Online. Available: www.dhhs.tas.gov.au/about_the_department

World Health Organisation (WHO) (2015) World report on ageing and health. WHO, Geneva.

CHAPTER 6

Gerontological Nursing Across the Continuum of Care

MARTINIQUE LOUISE SANDY

LEARNING OBJECTIVES

After reading this chapter, you will be able to:
- describe the different care options available to the older person
- discuss how community-based and residential care delivery services can meet the needs of the older person
- discuss the importance of thorough holistic assessment of the older person in relation to accessing services
- outline the process of transitioning into permanent residential aged care.

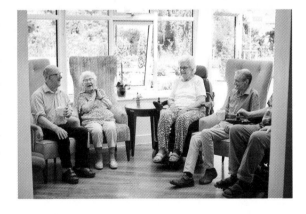

INTRODUCTION

This chapter aims to provide an understanding of the different types of care that an ageing population can access in Australia and New Zealand. With a fluctuating decline in health, the older person will at times require a range of clinical care and care delivery options. The aged care industry intersects with the acute care sector to provide comprehensive care for the older person. The most appropriate care delivery option will be identified through holistic assessment in consultation with the older person. Admission to hospital may be the most appropriate course of action during an acute exacerbation of an illness or through accident or injury. Following an acute admission or through general decline and frailty, an older person may require assistance at home with the activities of daily living (ADLs). This community-based care delivery option provides provisions to help the older person with cooking, cleaning, maintaining social connections, basic care needs and sometimes nursing services. When this community-based delivery of care no longer meets the needs or safety requirements of the older person, then residential aged care is often identified as most appropriate to provide person-centred care, with access to specialised nursing services as required.

There will come a time when the older person will need some level of assistance in maintaining their independence. While family members may be able to assist, there may be times and circumstances where this is not always possible. The Australian Government has created a variety of care packages to address the needs of older people with the goal of helping them stay in their home longer. There are packages that facilitate different levels of community-based care, respite care, as well as transition into permanent residential care.

HOME CARE/RESPITE CARE/ RESIDENTIAL CARE

Home Care

The Australian Government through independent aged care providers helps older people stay in their homes longer through the provision of a suite of home care support options. The Australian Government can support older people with financial assistance under the *Aged Care Act (1997)* and the *Aged Care (Transitional Provisions) Act (1997)*. As of September 2019, over 134,930 older people were in receipt of a home-based care package (Australian Government Department of Health 2019). The support programs offer a variety of benefits to the client dependent upon their assessed needs and funding is allocated accordingly.

Once it is identified that there is a need for an older person to have support at home, an assessment needs to take place. The referral for home-based care can be made by a practitioner, family member or the older person themselves. The assessment is usually completed by a registered nurse (RN) from the Regional Assessment Service and will determine the level of support required to help the client maintain independence and stay at home longer. The two community support programs available are:

- Commonwealth Home Support Program (also see Chapter 7)
- Home Care Program.

Commonwealth Home Support Program

This support package is the entry level package for receiving assistance at home (Australian Government Department of Health 2020g). Services that can be provided under the package are as follows:

- meal preparation
- personal care
- simple nursing services
- allied health and therapy services
- respite care
- domestic assistance
- home maintenance and modifications
- specialised equipment
- transport and social support.

While the services are subsidised by the government, the client must pay a fee for these services. The intention behind the Commonwealth Home Support Package is to provide support structures and services to the older

person who is still high functioning to a degree but requires some support to either maintain independence, stay safe within their home environment, or to stay connected to family and social supports. See *Promoting wellness* box for techniques on how to promote wellness in the older person. Having support structures and services in place early will help to identify any future decline or general frailty in the older person and reassessment and transition to a Home Care Package when the client's needs are no longer being met by the Commonwealth Home Support Package.

In order to facilitate transfer to a Home Care Package, the older person will require reassessment completed by an RN and other allied healthcare professionals as part of the Aged Care Assessment Team (ACAT). ACAT assessments are required for all care packages above the Commonwealth Home Support Package level. The comprehensive assessment is completed in either the home or the hospital setting and looks at the older person's health and medical history, physical requirements and psychosocial needs. Once completed, the ACAT assessment is valid for 12 months and lists the types of care that have been approved for the client (Australian Government Department of Health 2020b).

Promoting Wellness

The following suggestions can help to maintain and promote wellness in the older people with a focus on person-centred care:

- Acknowledge the importance of social connections and help to maintain a level of connectedness.
- Promote the older person's independence as much as is possible at every interaction.
- Value the older person's contribution to society and how they might be able to contribute towards their care.
- Develop a therapeutic rapport with the older person, communicate with the older person and their family regularly.
- Perform routine assessments and after periods of illness or injury.

Home Care Package

The Home Care Package is the next level of home-based support provided by the Australian Government. This package has four different levels of support depending upon the client's needs (Australian Government Department of Health 2020a) (Box 6.1). Each level provides

> **BOX 6.1**
> **Funding Levels for Home Care Packages**
>
> | | |
> |---|---|
> | Level 1 | $8,800 per annum |
> | Level 2 | $15,500 per annum |
> | Level 3 | $33,700 per annum |
> | Level 4 | $51,100 per annum |

Australian Government Department of Health (2020e).

an annual allocation of funds which the client can use to spend on services of their choice and meet different aspects of their care needs (see Chapter 7).

The following list summarises the different services that are available under this package:

- personal care
- more complex nursing services
- allied health and therapy services
- meal preparation
- domestic assistance
- home maintenance and modifications
- specialised equipment
- transport and social support.

The services that are offered through the Home Care Package are similar to those in the entry level Commonwealth Home Support Program. The delineation between the two packages is that Home Care Packages deliver more comprehensive, holistic services for older people with higher level of need, allowing for the provision of high-quality care in the home environment (Australian Government Department of Health 2020d).

This comprehensive approach to the care of the older person in the community allows them to stay in their homes longer, which preserves their connection to their family, community and social supports. While it is important to maintain connection with the community, it is equally important to acknowledge the responsibility of caring and the burden that the older person may feel when receiving care from another family member. Under the community care packages, older people can access respite care in order to address the need for carers to have a break.

Respite Care

Short-term care allows for both the recipient of care and the carer to have a break from the usual routines and responsibilities associated with care delivery by family members (Australian Government Department of Health 2020c). Respite care can vary from a few hours to days or weeks dependent upon the needs of the family and can be arranged on an ad-hoc or regular basis. Older

people with a Commonwealth Home Support Program or Home Care Package in place can access different levels of respite. The level of respite access will be decided during the ACAT assessment process. This assessment can be reviewed as required to meet the needs of the client. Respite care falls into two categories:

- community respite
- residential respite.

Community respite

Community respite provides flexible arrangements to best meet the needs of both the carer and the care recipient. It is available in the following formats:

- Centre-based respite: Community Day Centres provide respite during the day and may include transport to and from the centre. Care staff and allied health professional are based at the centre to meet the needs of daily living and specialised therapy programs.
- Cottage-based respite: This respite service is based in the community, either at a centre or in a host family setting and includes the delivery of comprehensive care overnight or stays of up to a few days at a time.
- Flexible respite: Flexible respite allows the older person to remain in their own home or usual living arrangement and have a paid carer provide care to them during either the day or the night (Australian Government Department of Health 2020c).

Residential respite

Residential respite takes place in a residential aged care facility. Clients usually access respite for a few days or up to several weeks at a time. In order to access residential respite, the older person must have a valid ACAT assessment approving them for respite care. Each client with an approved ACAT assessment can access up to 63 days of respite per year, which can be called upon in an emergency or booked in advance. There is a provision to extend these timeframes in certain circumstances. During a respite stay, the older person is able to access the same support services and care options that are available to the residents of the facility.

For many older people, there comes a time when their needs are not always being met by services available through community-based aged care providers because the person is becoming more dependent, frail, ill or has sustained an injury. It is at this stage that reassessment should occur, which often heralds the transition from home-based care to permanent residential aged care for the provision of more complex and comprehensive care and clinical services.

Residential Aged Care

The transition from living independently to moving into a residential aged care facility is a major life-changing event (McKenna & Staniforth 2017). The transition needs to be handled with sensitivity and expertise, often by a senior RN within the residential aged care facility. An ACAT assessment performed in either the community or the hospital setting will identify if the older adult has low or high care needs in respect to the residential setting. According to the Australian Government Department of Health (2020a), permanent residents of a residential aged care facility have access to the following services:

- accommodation
- hotel/hospitality services
- care services:
  - personal care
  - clinical care.

Accommodation

The resident will be provided with a bedroom, bedroom furniture and associated equipment required to live in the facility.

Hotel/hospitality services

This covers the day-to-day non-care related requirements such as social activities, cleaning, meals, laundry and general maintenance of the buildings, grounds and equipment.

Care services

- *Personal care:* refers to ADLs such as bathing, toileting, medication administration and certain health treatments.
- *Clinical care:* The needs of the resident will determine the level of clinical care and may involve complex nursing services, therapy services, such as physiotherapy, podiatry and speech pathology, as well as specific bedding requirements, e.g. pressure relieving devices, that are related to clinical need.

Funding for residential care is provided by the Australian Government in accordance with the *Aged Care Act (1997)* and the *Aged Care (Transitional Provisions) Act (1997)*. Based on identified needs and through careful assessment, the Aged Care Funding Instrument (ACFI) is the tool that is used to determine what level of care a resident requires and how much funding the residential aged care facility will receive for providing such care (Australian Government Department of Health 2016a). The ACFI program is administered by the Australian Government Department of Health and ensures that residential aged care facilities maintain compliance with the Aged Care Standards in order to facilitate payment and continuation of bed licensure (Australian Government Department of Health 2020b). While residential aged care is subsidised by the government, the resident will need to pay a means-tested fee (the amount the older person pays is calculated according to their income) for the delivery of care.

The ACFI has three broad domains: a) ADLs; b) behaviour; and c) complex healthcare. Each domain comprises three bands of funding allocated according to the resident's care requirement (see Table 6.1). Residents' level of care need in each domain can be reassessed annually, upon discharge from a hospital admission or if there are major changes in their clinical needs and care requirements.

A review of the ACFI was announced in 2017; the Resource Utilisation and Classification Study (RUCS) was created to assess the efficacy of the tool. The preliminary findings of the study recommended the creation of a new funding tool. The *Research highlight: Australian National Aged Care Classification Trial* provides details of the study. It is accepted that a resident's level of care and clinical needs will change over time, either through a general

---

TABLE 6.1
Aged Care Funding Instrument Domains and Funding Levels

Domain	Covers	FUNDING LEVELS		
		Low	*Med*	*High*
Activities of daily living (ADLs)	Nutrition, mobility, personal hygiene, toileting, continence	$37.68/day	$82.05/day	$113.67/day
Behaviour	Cognitive skills, wandering, verbal behaviour, physical behaviour, depression	$8.61/day	$17.85/day	$37.21/day
Complex healthcare	Medication, complex healthcare procedures	$16.71/day	$47.61/day	$68.74/day

Australian Government Department of Health (2016a).

decline and increasing frailty, exacerbation of illness or through injury. It is critically important to ensure prompt reassessment of residents after illness or injury and to maintain routine assessment schedules throughout their stay (Palliative Care Australia 2017). Some acute symptom exacerbations and injuries can be managed within the residential aged care facility. However, there may come a time when acute illness or an injury will warrant transfer and admission to hospital.

TRANSITIONAL CARE

Transitional care is available for the older person with either a Community Home Support Program or Home Care Package to help with the transition of discharge from hospital after an acute admission (Australian Government Department of Health 2020h). Transitional care provides short-term specialised support and care services to help the older person regain functional independence after a hospital admission. Depending upon the older person's level of need, transitional care can be accessed for up to 12 weeks and takes place either in a residential aged care facility, in a community setting or in the client's usual home setting. The services provided through transitional care cover therapy, nursing and personal care services and are described in Box 6.2.

CARING IN THE ACUTE SETTING

In 2016–17, one in five presentations to an emergency department were made by a person aged 65 years or older (Australian Institute of Health and Welfare [AIHW] 2018). Older people accounted for 42% of same-day admissions and 41% of overnight admissions in the same period. It was also found that 90% of older people admitted to a hospital in 2016–17 required care in an acute setting (AIHW 2018). Admission to hospital is usually as a result of an exacerbation of symptoms from

a pre-existing illness or through an injury such as a fall (see Chapter 16). Most older people have more than one co-morbidity and often polypharmacy (see Chapter 11) and other associated medication risks can contribute to a decline in health (LeMone 2017). Special care considerations, specific risk assessments and best practice are required when providing care for an older person in the acute setting as they are exposed to a higher level of risk as an inpatient (see *Research highlight: Australian National Aged Care Classification Trial*).

Research Highlight
Australian National Aged Care Classification Trial

The Australian National Aged Care Classification Trial trial started in November 2019 and builds on the work already completed by the University of Wollongong as part of the Resource Utilisation and Classification Study (RUCS). RUCS investigated the needs and classification of residents and the associated cost drivers involved in delivery care. The Australian National Aged Care Classification (AN-ACC) tool was created as a result of RUCS. It is hoped the AN-ACC will replace the ACFI to alleviate concerns over funding discrepancies identified in the ACFI. The trial will be completed by mid-2020 and looks to test the external assessment modules for aged care funding.

Australian Government Department of Health (2020c).

A thorough risk assessment undertaken at admission can help to identify predictors of future illness, injury and frailty. Assessment tools suitable for acute hospital settings include:

- the Blaylock Risk Assessment Screening Score (BRASS) (Blaylock & Cason 1992)
- Nutritional Screening Tool (see Chapter 12)
- Braden Scale for predicting pressure injury risk (see Chapter 15)
- Falls Risk Assessment and Management Plan (see Chapter 16)
- a Frailty Assessment (see Chapter 8).

Understanding the older person's level of risk enables the RN to develop a plan to prevent adverse events during the admission and identify future needs of the patient upon discharge (Cascio & Logomarsino 2018; Hodgins et al 2018; Lan et al 2020; National Institute for Health and Care Excellence [NICE] 2017). Additionally, the nurse can mitigate the level of identified risk through modification of the physical environment, patient behaviour, increased surveillance, and referral to allied health professionals.

When planning for discharge of an older person, the nurse needs to be aware of the home setting and care

BOX 6.2
Transitional Care Services

Personal care	ADLs, mobility, communication
Nursing services	Wound management, pain management, oxygen therapy medications, catheter and bladder management, and other services
Therapy services	Access to allied health professionals that will improve independence and function

Australian Government Department of Health (2020h).

services in place (see *Tips for best practice: Nursing the older person in all care settings*). If the level of care that the older person is currently accessing in the community is still suitable upon discharge, then discharge should proceed. If the older person's level of function has declined, however, then nurses should consider the need for transitional care or modification of current community care access. This can be coordinated through the hospital via the ACAT team.

Tips for Best Practice
Nursing the older person in all care settings

- Practise person-centred care
- Maintain clinical assessment skills and currency in practice
- Stay up to date with research, policy directions and national frameworks for practice
- Ensure prompt and ongoing assessment of the older person along the care continuum
- Source evidence-based practice information and updates from specialised healthcare organisations
- Maintain consistent and regular communication with the older person and family members

---

RURAL AND REMOTE NURSING

People living in rural and remote areas are reported to have higher levels of risk factors compared to their metropolitan counterparts (AIHW 2019). Higher rates of smoking, alcohol consumption and obesity, along with lower rates of exercise and unhealthy eating habits, place people of all ages living outside major cities at more risk for poorer health outcomes. Life expectancy can vary by as much as five years from metropolitan areas (81 years for males and 84 years for females born in 2015–17) to very remote areas (76 years and 80 years respectively) (AIHW 2019). Despite these setbacks, there are some advantages for those who choose rural living.

Older people living in rural settings have the distinct advantage of having stronger social connections and are generally more likely to participate in society and be self-reliant than their urbanised peers (Menec et al 2015). However, while there are numerous enablers to rural living for older people, there are some concerning barriers that can make this group more vulnerable. Menec and colleagues (2015) identified inadequate infrastructure, geographic distances and the 'out-migration' of younger people, who move out of the community to live elsewhere, as some higher order concerns regarding ageing

in a rural setting. Ideally, older people living in rural and remote locations are able to access appropriate levels of support within their community. This is dependent, however, upon the services and structures offered by local providers. Rural and remote communities depend more heavily on general practitioners for wide-ranging services as there is often little access to specialist care locally (Australian Government Department of Health 2016b). Additionally, older people who find that available levels of care in the local setting no longer meet their needs can face transfer to another area for short-term acute or longer-term sub-acute services.

Metropolitan and regional acute and sub-acute care providers will need to be aware of the special considerations required when caring for the older person from a rural or remote location. Heaton (in LeMone 2017) advocates for the following considerations:

- Isolation: Who is home to help?
- Transport: How is the patient getting home? How long will it take? Can the patient manage this length or type of transport?
- Medications or treatments: Are these readily available in the patient's community?
- Home environment: Is it still safe for the returning patient?
- Current weather patterns: Will local weather forecasts prevent or delay a return home?
- Support: Where will the older person present should problems arise? Is the local GP aware? Is there a requirement for ongoing nursing services or other allied health treatments? What social supports are in place to assist with the transition after discharge?
- Medical review: Is there a need for medical review? Will this take place in person or via teleconference? How will the patient access these resources?

AGED CARE IN NEW ZEALAND

Accessing community-based care and long term care in New Zealand is similar to the Australian setting in that the New Zealand government through their District Health Boards (DHBs) provides access to a Needs Assessment and Coordination Service (NACS) that determines the level of care the older person will require (Ministry of Health NZ 2011). Home support services are provided to eligible New Zealand citizens by the DHBs and include services such as assistance with personal care, help around the home and respite care. Long-term care in a residential facility requires the same NACS assessment, but also includes a financial means assessment to determine if the older person qualifies for subsidised care (Ministry of Health NZ 2019).

Practice Scenario

Phyllis is a 76-year-old widow who lives on her own in a small country town. Her son Mark reports that she is coping well on her own, but is a little isolated now that her friend (who drives her into town for doctor's appointments and weekly grocery shopping) has recently moved into a residential aged care facility after suffering a stroke a few months ago. Mark normally takes his mother shopping and to the doctor when needed, but is finding the additional responsibility a little challenging along with a busy workload both at his office and at home. He tries his best, but is no longer able to keep up with the garden maintenance at Phyllis's and has noticed that Phyllis isn't able to give her house a 'good clean' any more. Phyllis states she can't see the dirt that clearly anymore and it's a bit hard for her to get down low to the floor for scrubbing and picking up small items.

MULTIPLE CHOICE QUESTIONS

1. From the information provided, what is Phyllis's most appropriate level of care?
   a. Transitional Care
   b. Residential Care
   c. Community Care
   d. Respite Care
2. What services would help Phyllis the most from the scenario above?
   a. Personal care, physiotherapy and counselling
   b. Cleaning/home maintenance, transport and social support
   c. Respite care, medication management, podiatry
   d. Social work, specialised nursing services, accommodation
3. Mark is due to go on a holiday in 2 months and he is concerned for his mother's welfare while he is not in the country. Is Phyllis able to access respite care and if so, which is the best option for her and her pet dog?
   a. Yes, cottage-based respite
   b. No, Phyllis can only access respite in an emergency
   c. Yes, centre-based respite
   d. Yes, flexible respite

SUMMARY

With a fluctuating decline in health, the older person at times requires a range of clinical care and care delivery options. This chapter has covered the transition involved for the older person from community-based care into permanent care provided by a residential care facility in the Australian and New Zealand context. The most appropriate care delivery option is identified through thorough holistic assessment and in consultation with the older person and family. The variety of packages offered through community-based care provide services to help the older person with cooking, cleaning, maintaining social connections, basic care needs and simple nursing services. Admission to hospital may be the most appropriate course of action during an acute exacerbation of an illness or through injury. When community-based care no longer meets the needs or safety requirements of the older person, then residential care is identified to provide person-centred care with specialised nursing services as required. Special considerations are required when older people live in a rural and remote location, such as transportation needs, local support services upon discharge, and the need for ongoing review.

REFERENCES

Australian Government (2019) Aged Care (Transitional Provisions) Act (1997) No. 223, 1997. Australian Government, Canberra.

Australian Government (2013) Aged Care Act (1997) No. 112, 1997 as amended. Australian Government, Canberra.

Australian Government Department of Health (2020a) Aged care homes. Australian Government, Canberra. Online. Available: www.myagedcare.gov.au/aged-care-homes

Australian Government Department of Health (2020b) Aged care quality standards. Australian Government, Canberra. Online. Available: www.myagedcare.gov.au/aged-care-quality -standards

Australian Government Department of Health (2020c) Australian National Aged Care Classification (AN-ACC) Trial: Factsheet. Australian Government, Canberra. Online. Available: www.agedcare.health.gov.au/reform/residential -aged-care-funding-reform

Australian Government Department of Health (2020d) Commonwealth Home Support Programme. Australian Government, Canberra. Online. Available: www.myagedcare.gov.au/ help-at-home/commonwealth-home-support-programme

Australian Government Department of Health (2020e) Home Care packages. Australian Government, Canberra. Online. Available: www.myagedcare.gov.au/help-at-home/home-care -packages

Australian Government Department of Health (2020f) Prepare for your assessment. Australian Government, Canberra. Online. Available: www.myagedcare.gov.au/assessment/prepare-your-assessment

Australian Government Department of Health (2020g) Respite care. Australian Government, Canberra. Online. Available: www.myagedcare.gov.au/short-term-care/respite-care

Australian Government Department of Health (2020h) Transition care. Australian Government, Canberra. Online. Available: www.myagedcare.gov.au/short-term-care/transition-care

Australian Government Department of Health (2019) Home Care Packages Program Date Report 1st Quarter 2019–2020. Australian Government, Canberra.

Australian Government Department of Health (2016a) Aged Care Funding Instrument – User Guide. Australian Government, Canberra.

Australian Government Department of Health (2016b) National Strategic Framework for Rural and Remote Health. Australian Government, Canberra.

Australian Institute of Health and Welfare (AIHW) (2019) Rural and Remote Health. Cat. No. PHE 255. AIHW, Canberra.

Australian Institute of Health and Welfare (AIHW) (2018) Australia's health 2018. Australia's health series no.16. AUS 221. AIHW, Canberra.

Blaylock A, Cason CL (1992) Discharge planning predicting patients' needs. J Gerontol Nurs 18:5–10.

Cascio BL, Logomarsino JV (2018) Evaluating the effectiveness of five screening tools used to identify malnutrition risk in hospitalised elderly: A systematic review. Geriatric Nursing 39(1):95–102.

Hodgins MJ, Logan SM, Fraser JM et al (2018) Clinical utility of scores on the Blaylock Risk Assessment Screen (BRASS): An analysis of administrative data. Applied Nursing Research 41:36–40.

Lan X, Hong L, Wang Z et al (2020) Frailty as a predictor for future falls in hospitalised patients: A systematic review and meta-analysis. Geriatric Nursing 41(2):69–74.

LeMone P (2017) Medical – Surgical Nursing: Critical Thinking for Person-Centred Care. 3rd Australian ed. Pearson Australia, Melbourne.

McKenna D, Staniforth B (2017) Older people moving to residential care in Aotearora New Zealand: Considerations for social work at practice and levels. Aotearoa New Zealand Social Work 29(1):28–40.

Menec V, Bell S, Novek S et al (2015) Making rural and remote communities more age-friendly: expert's perspectives on issues, challenges and priorities. Journal of Aging & Social Policy 27(2):173–191.

Ministry of Health NZ (2019) Long-term residential care for older people: What you need to know (revised 2019). MOH, Wellington.

Ministry of Health NZ (2011) Needs assessment and support services for older people: What you need to know. MOH, Wellington.

National Institute for Health and Welfare (NICE) (2017) Falls in older people. Quality Standard (QS86) Guideline. NICE.

Palliative Care Australia (2017) Principles for palliative and end-of-life care in residential aged care. Palliative Care Australia, ACT.

CHAPTER 7

Communication and Shared Decision-Making

CHRISTINE STIRLING

LEARNING OBJECTIVES

After reading this chapter, you will be able to:

- understand the legal and ethical principles that underpin shared decision-making for older people
- identify communication strategies to facilitate shared decision-making for older people
- know how to establish decision-making capacity and appropriate substitute decision-makers.

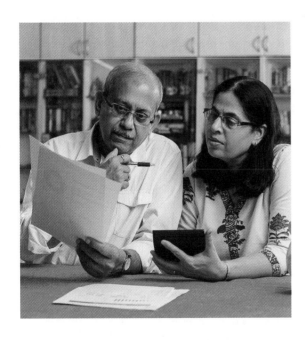

INTRODUCTION

Shared decision-making is increasingly recognised as an important aspect for good quality and safe healthcare in Australia and New Zealand. It is particularly important when providing care and services for older people, as the complexity of decisions increases due to quality of life prerogatives and varied contexts. In addition, shared decision-making with older people who have communication challenges or cognitive decline presents an extra challenge for nurses. Such challenges do not negate the human rights of older people to determine the care and services they wish to receive, even if this brings some risk of harm or even death. Nurses need to understand the capacity of the older person to make relevant decisions. They need to work in partnership with older people and/or any substitute decision-makers and their important 'others' when making healthcare decisions.

Nurses can start by understanding the three key elements of healthcare decisions: choice, capacity and consent. This chapter will help nurses identify the legal and ethical responsibilities that need to be met in any healthcare setting.

AUTONOMY AND SHARED DECISION-MAKING

All older people have the right to autonomy (the right to make decisions), as it is a basic human right. The right to autonomy assumes that everyone is the best judge of their own interests and should therefore make their own choices. Australia and New Zealand are both signatories to the Universal Declaration of Human Rights adopted by the United Nations in 1948, which sets out the right to autonomy. While New Zealand has the *Human Rights Act 1993* and the *Bill of Rights Act 1990* (Human Rights Commission 2008–2020), which legislates the right to autonomy, Australia has no overarching law and instead relies on state and territory laws to address elements of human rights. Regardless of the clarity of the legislation, older people in Australia and New Zealand are entitled to autonomy. Autonomy is a right, regardless of place of residence, such as aged care facility, hospital or in the community.

While autonomy is an important right, healthcare professionals have traditionally been presumed to have better health knowledge and to be best placed to make treatment choices. The healthcare setting was therefore dominated by paternalistic clinician decision-making until the 1990s and many people accepted this situation (Duncan et al 2010). The Control Preference Scale (Degner et al 1997) was developed to assist researchers and clinicians to identify a patient's preference for decision control (see *Research Highlight*).

Research Highlight
The Control Preference Scale

The Control Preference Scale (Degner et al 1997) was developed so that researchers and clinicians could identify the patient's preference for decision control, ranging on a continuum from autonomous to clinician-led.

Research shows that very few patients wish to make completely autonomous decisions, but instead veer towards sharing decision control with health professionals, i.e. shared decision-making.

One study found that 71% of patients preferred shared decision-making (Chewning et al 2012), while other research showed that those patients who are older or have poor health literacy (see Chapter 4) often prefer clinician-led decisions (Mattukat et al 2019).

Chewning et at (2012); Degner et al (1997); Mattukat et al (2019).

Shared decision-making research has mostly related to screening or treatment preferences for choices with clear outcomes, such as cancer and heart disease. The definition of shared decision-making (when healthcare decisions are negotiated between clinicians and patients) reflects this by using clinically-focused language, but there is increasing recognition that shared decision-making is needed to help those with chronic or age-related conditions to make decisions about care services (Duncan et al 2010; Stirling,

Leggett et al 2012) and other lifestyle choices. Shared decision-making is known to improve the quality and safety of patient care and outcomes (National Research Council 2001) and it can be assumed to have a similar impact on care services for older people.

There are several theoretical models that consider shared decision-making as either an outcome or a process (Truglio-Londrigan et al 2012). Regardless, the key elements remain: that the decision is shared between at least a professional and patient, and it respects and responds to best evidence and patient/consumer preferences and values. Shared decision-making is particularly valuable when decisions involve the option of 'doing nothing', where no option is obviously superior, or where the patient's values are highly relevant due to cultural or other factors. Given the increase in chronic illness and longer life spans, the importance of shared decision-making for gerontological nursing has grown.

THREE COMPONENTS OF HEALTHCARE DECISIONS: CHOICE, CAPACITY AND CONSENT
Choice

In order to ensure autonomy and shared decision-making, older people need to have choices in the care and services they receive. Australian policymakers have been embracing the concept of choice through the 2017 National Safety and Quality Health Service [NSQHS] Standards. 'Partnering with Consumers' is a Standard that requires partnering with patients to share decisions and care planning (Australian Commission on Safety and Quality in Health Care [ACSQHC] 2017). Standard 1 of the 2019 Aged Care Quality Standards is 'Consumer Dignity and Choice', which is visually in the centre of a circular pie chart emphasising the importance of consumers making informed choices (Australian Government Department of Health 2019). Consumer-directed care is the model of care adopted by the Australian Government to ensure that older people and their carers have more choice and control over the services they receive. These policy directions put the need for choices and shared decision-making front and centre for all services, not just clinical treatments.

Providing and allowing choice, i.e. autonomy, is a core human right because it is inextricably linked to dignity and personhood. And yet when people want to make choices that create risk and may even result in their own death, nurses can feel there is a clash between the human right to autonomy and a nurse's duty of care. This clash between autonomy and risk may occur when people make big decisions, such as where to live or whether to have a major surgical procedure, but it can also occur when people in long-term care are making smaller decision, such as what to eat or drink. Decisions about food can become high-risk decisions for older people as they may experience increased difficulty chewing and swallowing food. Choking is a serious risk for older people, being responsible for 8% of preventable deaths of older people according to one study (Ibrahim et al 2017). The prevalence of dysphagia can mean that many older people are only allowed to eat puréed diets, but this may represent a serious decrease in quality of life if eating is one of their few remaining pleasures.

The concept of 'dignity of risk' has, therefore, become increasingly important in relation to understanding how to navigate the tension between autonomy and risk when providing care for older people. It has been used with people with disabilities since the 1970s but is gaining recognition in gerontology, which in many ways has erred on the side of duty of care. Dignity of risk is the understanding that individuals have the right to take risks which are important for dignity and self-esteem, and that they should not be prevented by others being overly cautious (Ibrahim & Davis 2013).

Having choice also involves having clarity about the decisions. Dying can be an example of when clinicians may struggle to set out clear choices. Often health professionals avoid giving 'bad news' in order to prevent distress for patients or filter information that they consider too upsetting (Barclay et al 2011; Stirling, Lloyd et al 2012), but this can mean that older people are unaware of the terminal nature of their condition or are not enabled to discuss advance care planning.

Capacity

Capacity to make decisions is the second necessary element for decision-making and an important concept for gerontological nurses to understand if they are engaging in shared decision-making. When working with older people there are likely to be a greater proportion who are facing barriers to capacity, ranging from hearing or vision loss, mild cognitive impairment, delirium to dementia.

Capacity is a legal term for those with the ability to make a decision, which involves:

- being able to understand and retain relevant information (understanding)
- believing and relating the information to oneself (appreciation)
- assessing the information and reaching a decision (reasoning)
- communicating a relatively consistent decision (Moye & Marson 2007).

Among a healthy older population, capacity impairment is low, at around 2.5% (Moye & Marson 2007). However, research has shown that diminished capacity in some settings is likely to be more prevalent than anticipated, with a systematic review suggesting that 34% of patients in a general medical setting lacked capacity, particularly in regard to reasoning, and that up to 58% of these are not recognised (Lepping et al 2015). Between 44% and 69% of older people in long-term care have been found to have capacity impairments (Moye & Marson 2007).

There are many factors that can impact on an older person's capacity and some of them may be time limited. Cognition (the different intellectual activities of the brain) is the main determinant of capacity and includes understanding, appreciation and reasoning. Cognition can be impaired by the neurogenerative decline accompanying conditions associated with ageing (e.g. dementia, delirium, Parkinson's) and mental health problems (e.g. substance abuse, psychosis). Each condition can impact on different aspects of cognition and, therefore, be expressed differently. Research has highlighted the nuanced relationship between capacity and disease, with different dementias impacting on different areas of cognition and being expressed and measured differently (Moye & Marson 2007). Capacity can also vary over time and during the course of an illness. For example, delirium (see Chapter 26) and some forms of mental illness (see Chapter 25) may temporarily impair a person's capacity to make appropriate healthcare decisions. Some conditions may cause difficulty in thinking through complex decisions or a bias in thinking, such as the negative thoughts a person who is suicidal may be feeling. Other conditions that impact on cognition in a chronic or deteriorating manner, such as dementia and Parkinson's disease (see Chapter 26), can also impair decision-making capacity in a variable and fluctuating manner.

The presence of cognitive impairment is not enough to assume lack of capacity, but rather means that further assessment is required to determine the individual's decision-making capacity. If a person is assessed as lacking decision capacity, then they may need supported decision-making or a substitute decision-maker such as a guardian or attorney (Box 7.1). A substitute decision-maker may be guided by the older person's prior written or spoken explanation of their wishes or values, established at an earlier time when they had capacity. In other cases, the guardian may make a substituted judgement, which means making the decision based on the individual's known wishes or values when capable.

The formal appointment of substitute decision-makers is supported by specific laws. In this legal arena,

---

BOX 7.1
Substitute Decision-Makers

Formal substitute decision-makers are legally appointed to make decisions on behalf of someone who lacks capacity.

- **Advance care directives** set out the medical treatment and care a person wishes to have if they no longer have the capacity to make decisions. Values and preferences can be outlined and a substitute decision-maker named.

- **An attorney** is established by the older person when they have capacity through a legal process to establish an Enduring Power of Attorney.

If the older person has not established a substitute decision-maker then they will have a:

- **Statutory health attorney** – the first available and culturally appropriate significant person/relative, such as spouse or de facto, primary carer, close friend or relative.

- **Guardian** – appointed by a statutory authority under law when the older person loses capacity. A public guardian will be appointed if the older person has no suitable relative or significant other available. Different jurisdictions have different laws. In Queensland, for example, the Queensland Civil and Administrative Tribunal would appoint a guardian. In New Zealand the Family Court appoints guardians.

Taken from 'Guardianship and Administration Act (Qld) 2000' and the 'Powers of Attorney Act (Qld) 1998'.

---

lawmakers too have moved to incorporate a stronger focus on autonomy and less paternalism. Guardians and attorneys are able to make decisions on behalf of those unable to make decisions for themselves but this power has been whittled back to a more restricted 'last resort' concept (Australian Law Reform Commission 2014). While substitute decision-makers were always expected to make decisions based on the 'best interests standard', this term was seen as paternalistic. It implied a decision based on what others judge to be in the best interest of an individual, who either never had healthcare wishes or never made them known. However, recent legislation has redefined *best interest standard* to specify previously expressed wishes or known values of the person (Australian Law Reform Commission 2014).

Different jurisdictions will often have different legislation to address the issue of capacity, for example, the Australian state of Victoria has the *Guardianship and Administration Act 1986*, while New Zealand has *The Protection of Personal and Property Rights Act 1988 (PPPR*

Act), but the overall principles listed above remain the same.

Consent

Consent requires evidence that the person has voluntarily chosen among options and agrees to an intervention. Informed consent requires that the person has capacity to make decisions and has been given enough information in order to make an informed decision. In areas of surgical procedures and medical treatments, informed consent is generally well managed, but in other decision areas such as advance care planning or activities of daily living (ADLs), informed consent can often be poorly managed.

Good communication becomes important to ensure informed consent if the older person struggles to understand the information provided because of language barriers, low health literacy and/or hearing or vision impairment. Those with low levels of health literacy (see Chapter 4) are less likely to want involvement in shared decision-making, tend to ask fewer questions, and are more satisfied with the amount of information provided than those with high levels of health literacy (Stacey et al 2017). With up to 80% of people over 80 years of age suffering from hearing loss (see Chapter 20), and only one-fifth of people wearing hearing aids, it is concerning that hearing loss is infrequently accounted for in studies of clinician/patient communication (Cohen et al 2017). The quality of the shared decision-making conversation is also important. Nurses tend to adopt a therapeutic style of communication (Bentley et al 2016), but few shared decision-making studies measure the quality of communication (Kunneman et al 2019). As these possible confounding factors show, making sure that older people can give informed consent requires a skilled communicator.

NURSING SKILLS FOR SHARED DECISION-MAKING

As the previous section has highlighted, capacity and communication are central to shared decision-making. It is important for nurses to have the skills and knowledge to assist shared decision-making for legal and ethical reasons. This next section sets out key nursing skills for assessing capacity and ensuring clear communication with older people.

Assessing Decision-Making Capacity

As life spans extend and more people remain at home as they age, healthcare professionals need to be alert to issues around decision-making capacity, not just for healthcare choices, but also for issues such as driving, and financial and living arrangement choices. The increased risk of elder abuse (see Chapter 27) that accompanies decreased capacity also means that nurses need to understand the key principles around supported and substitute decision-making.

Research into assessment of decision-making capacity is relatively new and results show poor agreement between clinicians when assessing capacity, and poor agreement between formal assessments and clinicians (doctors and nurses) (Moye & Marson 2007; Persoon et al 2012). In the 20th century a person's capacity was judged on a diagnosis, but this approach is no longer acceptable as research has highlighted how capacity can wax and wane over time, can vary within diseases, and that different decisions require different levels of capacity. The following are some general points when considering capacity for decision-making.

- A diagnosis does not equate to incapacity, BUT the likelihood of incapacity does increase with certain illnesses. High-risk diseases that should alert clinicians to consider incapacity include Alzheimer's disease, Parkinson's disease, schizophrenia, complicated or moderate traumatic brain injury, substance abuse and last days of life (Karlawish 2017).
- Cognitive assessment tools such as the MMSE (Mini-Mental State Examination) do not assess capacity, but can alert clinicians to the need for further assessment. For example, MMSE scores of <16 are highly correlated with incapacity and MMSE scores of > 24 are highly correlated with decision-making capacity (Karlawish 2017). Many assessment tools do not adequately account for language and cultural differences, which is just one reason why a 'score' can never be used to measure capacity.
- Not all decisions require the same level of capacity. Treatment decisions require less cognitive skills than financial decisions or choices about living arrangements (Moye & Marson 2007). Financial decisions, for example, require a broader range of cognitive skills, including technical skills, such as using internet banking and factual financial knowledge, as well as judgement. One study found that all levels of dementia had financial decision-making impairment (not to be confused with incapacity), as did mild cognitive impairment (Moye & Marson 2007). This compares with other areas of decision-making capacity where people with early-stage dementia are found to have sufficient decision-making capacity (Kim et al 2002). Choices about living arrangements are also complex and incorporate a broad domain of cognitive functions.

- There is no simple clinical tool for assessing capacity. Clinical assessment remains the key method for capacity assessment, but a structured interview tool can assist with this process. Two capacity assessment tools that guide a structured interview with good validity are the Assessment of Capacity for Everyday Decisions (ACED) and the MacArthur Competency Assessment Tool for Treatment (MacCAT-T) (Karlawish 2017).
- Observation of the older person at different times of the day as they interact with others and undertake different activities helps to assess cognitive abilities (Persoon et al 2011). Observing attention span, orientation to place and time, memory and organising skills are just some of the key domains for observing cognition in the Nurse's Observation Scale of Cognitive Abilities (NOSCA), which provides a tool for nurses to systematically document cognition. Nurses should also be alert to indicators of lack of judgement, which may include frequent changing of opinion, decisions that do not appear to match values or risk-taking that does not appear to appreciate the gravity of the risk.

Tips for Best Practice

The nurse must be aware of the three key elements of healthcare decisions: choice, capacity and consent. These three elements must be considered as part of a holistic assessment in order to plan effective care.

- **Choice:** Consumer Dignity and Choice is a key component of the Aged Care Quality Standards, signifying that consumers need to be assisted to make informed choices.
- **Capacity:** involves being able to understand and retain relevant information, believing and relating the information to oneself, assessing the information and reaching a decision as well as communicating a relatively consistent decision.
- **Consent:** requires evidence that the person has voluntarily chosen among options and agrees to an intervention. Informed consent requires that the person has capacity to make decisions and has been given enough information in order to make an informed decision.

Australian Government Department of Health (2019).

Steps for Nurses to Assist Shared Decision-Making

This chapter has outlined the importance and complexity of decision-making for older people, and the components required for shared decision-making. This section will now outline the skills nurses need for shared decision-making – ensuring that the older person, or their substitute decision-maker, works with the clinician around choice, capacity and informed consent.

Step 1 Preparation

1. Prepare ahead by being clear about the decision choices and the level of capacity these require.
2. Check whether the older person has the capacity to make the decision, checking the health records and/or performing an assessment (using ACED or MacCAT-T, as described above). If the decision is complex and the older person's capacity is under question, refer the person for a more formal assessment of capacity.
3. If the person lacks capacity, identify whether they have a formal substitute decision-maker or a statutory health attorney (spouse, carer, relative). Provide assistance for the older person to identify a substitute decision-maker by listening to the older person's preferences.
4. Help the older person with capacity to decide who they want to be involved in the decision. If there is conflict with or undue pressure from family or a significant other, then the situation may require conflict-resolution support, such as advocacy or social worker input.
5. For the older person with barriers to communication, such as language, hearing loss or speech difficulties, then additional supports such as interpreters or written materials should be used. Hearing aids and glasses should be in place if needed.

Step 2 Communicate decision and choices

1. Good communication is central to ensuring older people have given informed consent and underpins all processes around shared decision-making and consent. The therapeutic relationship is a key strength of nursing communication and nurses are already inclined to use respectful styles of communication that map closely to person-centred care (see Chapter 4) frameworks (Bentley et al 2016). Nurses need to ensure they:
   - use appropriate language
   - practise good listening skills
   - have time to communicate.
2. Clearly explain the decision choices and the relevance of risks and benefits to the older person. It may be useful to use decision support tools such as patient decision aids.

3. Assistance with communication involves hearing what the older person expects and values in relation to the choice to be made, not just providing information. A substitute decision-maker should, where possible, explain how the older person's previously known values and preferences would impact the choice.
4. Answer questions as clearly as possible and seek assistance from others with more knowledge if you are not able.

Step 3 Document

1. Document the process, including those involved and any issues of concern.
2. Major and complex decisions should always involve a multidisciplinary team. For smaller decisions about care and ADLs, even older people with significant impairment are able to indicate preferences. These should be respected as much as possible, keeping in mind the principles of autonomy and dignity of risk. Good documentation of the rationale for allowing a person to engage in possibly 'risky' behaviours provides a clear trail of accountability.

Promoting Wellness

- Shared decision-making is of vital importance when caring for older people, especially those with a cognitive impairment or communication difficulty.
- Older people have the right to decide on their care.
- Many older people prefer shared decision-making.
- Older people may have additional barriers to decision-making due to age-related conditions that must be taken into account.

SUMMARY

Older people have the right to decide on their care, but many prefer shared decision-making. Nurses need to be familiar with the three key components of shared decision-making – choices must be offered, the individual must have capacity or a substitute or support decision-maker and consent must be informed. Older people may have additional barriers to decision-making due to age-related conditions, and decisions may be more complex as they become more relational, quality-of-life focused and values-based. Being clear on the underpinning concepts and legislations allows nurses to take a proactive shared decision-making clinician role.

Practice Scenario

Mrs Caplin, an 86-year-old widow, was admitted to an acute medical ward with a history of falls and self-neglect. She lives alone and has a daughter and son, who both live overseas.

MULTIPLE CHOICE QUESTIONS

1. Which of the following is not a component of healthcare decision-making?
   a. Choice
   b. Consent
   c. Compatibility
   d. Capacity
2. Most older people prefer to make their healthcare decisions without any input or assistance.
   a. True
   b. False
3. Which of the following is true?
   a. Informed consent is when the older adult consents to any treatment or action and places complete trust in the healthcare professional.
   b. Informed consent requires that the older person has capacity to make decisions and has been given enough information in order to make an informed decision.
   c. Following discussion, regardless of diagnosis, the nurse can take the word of the older person as consent.
   d. Health literacy does not affect informed consent.

REFERENCES

Australian Commission on Safety and Quality in Health Care (2017) National Safety and Quality Healthcare Standards 2nd edn. Online. Available: www.safetyandquality.gov.au/standards/nsqhs-standards/partnering-consumers-standard

Australian Government Department of Health (2019) Aged Care Quality Standards. Online. Available: Canberra: https://agedcare.health.gov.au/quality/aged-care-quality-standards

Australian Law Reform Commission (2014) Equality, Capacity and Disability in Commonwealth Laws: Supported and Substitute Decision-Making. Online. Available: www.alrc.gov.au/publication/equality-capacity-and-disability-in-commonwealth-laws-alrc-report-124/2-conceptual-landscape-the-context-for-reform-2/supported-and-substitute-decision-making/

Barclay S, Momen N, Case-Upton S et al (2011) End-of-life care conversations with heart failure patients: a systematic literature review and narrative synthesis. British Journal of General Practice 61(582):e49–62.

Bentley M, Stirling C, Robinson A et al (2016) The nurse practitioner–client therapeutic encounter: an integrative review of interaction in aged and primary care settings. Journal of Advanced Nursing 72(9):1991–2002.

Chewning B, Bylund C, Shah B et al (2012) Patient preferences for shared decisions: a systematic review. Patient Education and Counseling 86(1):9–18.

Cohen JM, Blustein J, Weinstein BE et al (2017) Studies of physician–patient communication with older patients: how often is hearing loss considered? A Systematic Literature Review. Journal of the American Geriatrics Society 65(8):1642–1649.

Degner L, Sloan J, Venkatesh P (1997) The control preferences scale. Canadian Journal of Nursing Research 29(3):21–43.

Duncan E, Best C, Hagen S (2010) Shared decision making interventions for people with mental health conditions. Cochrane Database of Systematic Reviews (1). CD007297 doi:10.1002/14651858.CD007297.pub2

Human Rights Commission (2008–2020) Human rights legislation in New Zealand. Online. Available: www.hrc.co.nz/your-rights/human-rights-legislation-new-zealand/

Ibrahim JE, Bugeja L, Willoughby M et al (2017) Premature deaths of nursing home residents: an epidemiological analysis. Medical Journal of Australia 206(10):442–447.

Ibrahim JE, Davis M-C (2013) Impediments to applying the 'dignity of risk' principle in residential aged care services. Australasian Journal on Ageing 32(3):188–193.

Karlawish J (2017) Assessment of decision-making capacity in adults. Online. Available: www.uptodate.com/contents/assessment-of-decision-making-capacity-in-adults?search=assessment%20of%20decision%20making&source=search_result&selectedTitle=1~150&usage_type=default&display_rank=1

Kim SYH, Karlawish JHT, Caine ED (2002) Current state of research on decision-making competence of cognitively impaired elderly persons. The American Journal of Geriatric Psychiatry 10(2):151–165.

Kunneman M, Gionfriddo MR, Toloza FJK et al (2019) Humanistic communication in the evaluation of shared decision making: A systematic review. Patient Education and Counseling 102(3):452–466.

Lepping P, Stanly T, Turner J (2015) Systematic review on the prevalence of lack of capacity in medical and psychiatric settings. Clinical Medicine (London, England) 15(4):337–343.

Mattukat K, Boehm P, Raberger K et al (2019) How much information and participation do patients with inflammatory rheumatic diseases prefer in interaction with physicians? Results of a participatory research project. Patient Prefer Adherence 13:2145–2158.

Moye J, Marson DC (2007) Assessment of decision-making capacity in older adults: an emerging area of practice and research. The Journals of Gerontology: Series B, 62(1):P3–P11.

National Research Council (2001) Crossing the quality chasm: a new health system for the 21st century. Committee on

Quality of Health Care in America, Institute of Medicine. Washington, DC.

Office of the Public Guardian Queensland (n.d.) Guardianship and decision making. Online. Available: www.publicguardian.qld.gov.au/guardianship

Persoon A, Banningh LJ-W, van de Vrie W et al (2011) Development of the Nurses' Observation Scale for Cognitive Abilities (NOSCA). ISRN Nursing. Art ID:895082.

Persoon A, Schoonhoven L, Melis RJ et al (2012) Validation of the NOSCA – Nurses' Observation Scale Of Cognitive Abilities. Journal of Clinical Nursing 21(21–22):3025–3036.

Stacey D, Hill S, McCaffery K et al (2017) Shared decision making interventions: theoretical and empirical evidence with implications for health literacy. Studies in Health Technology and Informatics 240:263–283.

Stirling C, Leggett S, Lloyd B et al (2012) Decision aids for respite service choices by carers of people with dementia: development and pilot RCT. BMC Medical Informatics and Decision Making 12(1):21.

Stirling C, Lloyd B, Scott J et al (2012) A qualitative study of professional and client perspectives on information flows and decision aid use. BMC Medical Informatics and Decision Making 12(1):26.

Truglio-Londrigan M, Slyer JT, Singleton JK et al (2012) A qualitative systematic review of internal and external influences on shared decision-making in all health care settings. JBI Library of Systematic Reviews 10(58):4633–4646.

CHAPTER 8

Comprehensive Health Assessment

HELENA HALTON

LEARNING OBJECTIVES

After reading this chapter you will be able to:

- explain the physiological assessment of the older person
- discuss the functional assessment of the older person
- examine a range of tools and techniques used in the assessment of older people
- understand the importance of documentation in the provision of quality care in a range of settings.

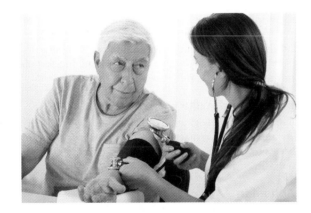

As the older person undergoes the ageing process there are changes to physiological reserves over time which are independent of any disease process. However, optimal ageing occurs in those people who are free from disease and live healthy lives. Ways to delay unnecessary depletion of physiological reserves are to maintain optimal nutrition, daily exercise and day-to-day function in older people. This chapter will also address the importance of accurate documentation in the delivery of quality care.

Promoting Wellness

A comprehensive geriatric assessment is: 'a multidimensional, interdisciplinary diagnostic process to determine the medical, psychological, and functional capabilities of the elderly person, in order to develop a coordinated and integrated plan for treatment and long-term follow-up' (Wieland & Hirth 2003:454–462).

INTRODUCTION

This chapter will examine the techniques used by health professionals to assess the care needs of older people. It will consider the physiological and psychological changes the older person undergoes as a result of the ageing process, and explore how these changes affect an older person's functional ability. A range of tools will be examined, as well as techniques used to perform a comprehensive holistic assessment of an older person.

A SUMMARY OF THE PHYSIOLOGICAL EFFECTS OF AGEING (see Fig. 8.1)

Skin, Hair and Nails (see Chapter 15)

With ageing, the skin wrinkles and begins to sag as it loses turgor, presenting with a loss of vascularity, giving

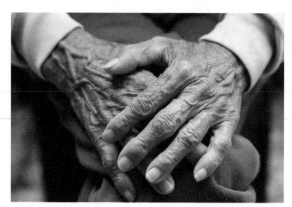

FIG. 8.1 **An older person's hands show the signs of ageing.**

a much paler appearance. The skin may also become dry, flaky and rough with the skin on the back of the hands becoming fragile, loose and transparent. The nails lose lustre and may yellow and thicken.

The hair loses its pigmentation and becomes grey with the number of scalp hairs decreasing. Changes to temperature regulation result in susceptibility to hypothermia.

Head and Neck
Eyes *(see Chapter 21)*
The eyes may appear recessed due to periorbital tissue atrophy. The eyelids may develop ptosis from relaxation of the skin and weakening of the muscles. The lower lids can develop an entropion or ectropion. The sclera becomes yellowish in colour and a white ring may develop around the iris (arcus senilis). The pupils become smaller and slightly irregular. Near vision begins to blur as the lens loses elasticity and the eyes becomes less able to accommodate.

Hearing *(see Chapter 20)*
Hearing generally diminishes with age, beginning with the loss of high-pitched sounds, followed by the lower and middle ranges. Hearing aids may be required to ensure appropriate communication during the assessment process.

Mouth, teeth and lymph nodes *(see Chapter 12)*
In ageing, there is a decrease in salivary secretions and a diminished sense of taste, which is made worse by certain medications and diseases. The older person may lose their sense of smell and is likely to become more sensitive to bitter and salty tastes.

Teeth become worn down, and there is often tooth loss from dental caries or periodontal disease, resulting in a sunken appearance and wrinkles around the mouth. The cervical lymph nodes become harder to palpate, while the submandibular glands become easier to palpate.

Thorax and Lungs *(see Chapter 24)*
Capacity for exercise decreases with age as the chest wall becomes less compliant. The chest muscles weaken, and the lungs lose their elastic recoil, although the respiratory rate remains unchanged. The dorsal curve of the thoracic spine may become more pronounced, resulting in kyphosis in the older person.

Cardiovascular *(see Chapter 23)*
In older people, the heart rate drops while the stroke volume increases in response to the heart's decreased responsiveness to beta-adrenergic catecholamines. The aorta and large vessels can become atherosclerotic, causing an increase in systolic blood pressure and widening pulse pressure. In older people, the pacemaker cells in the sinoatrial nodes decline, resulting in a possible irregular heart rate.

Older people commonly have an aortic murmur due to ageing of the aortic cusps and fibrous tissue build-up and calcification, resulting in aortic stenosis. Similarly, calcification of the mitral valve annulus and ring affecting normal valve closure during systole can result in a systolic murmur, known as mitral regurgitation.

Breasts and Axilla
During ageing, the glandular tissue in the female breast atrophies and is replaced with fatty tissue, causing the breast to become more flaccid and pendulous. Axillary hair diminishes.

Abdomen
In the older person, the abdomen becomes softer and protruding due to the accumulation of fat in the lower abdomen and hips, resulting from weakening abdominal muscles.

Genitalia
In the ageing male, the penis decreases in size and the testicles drop lower and become smaller. There is also an increase in erectile dysfunction.

In the ageing female, the vagina becomes dry as oestrogen levels drop. The vulva and clitoris become smaller and the vagina becomes shorter and narrower. There is an increase in dyspareunia and urinary urgency may be more common.

Musculoskeletal (see Chapter 22)

With ageing, the skeletal muscles decrease in bulk and power. There is also a decrease in the range of motion of the limbs and there is an overall loss of height.

Nervous system (see Chapters 25 and 26)

The ageing brain decreases in volume and in the number of cortical brain cells. There are changes to the biochemistry and the microanatomy. Many older people complain about their memory and may have trouble recalling people's names and details of upcoming events. They also retrieve and process information more slowly and take longer to learn new things. Older people's reaction speed is slower with decreases in motor function and reflexes.

ASSESSMENT OF THE OLDER PERSON

A comprehensive assessment is often initiated by a healthcare professional when problems arise, such as after a fall, incontinence, confusion or periods of immobility. A full comprehensive assessment is also required on admission to hospital or referral to a healthcare professional in the community setting. Older people often present with atypical symptomology to illness compared to a younger person because they have more diseases that are chronic, making assessment more challenging. Therefore, a structured, multifaceted approach to an assessment is recommended.

The assessment is designed to evaluate not only an older person's physical and mental health, but also their functional ability, cognition, along with the environmental, cultural and social influences affecting their health and wellbeing. It is a multidimensional process that includes both medical and non-medical domains, leading itself to the emphasis of the older person's functional capacity and quality of life (Elsawy & Higgins 2011).

Approach to the Older Person's Assessment (see Fig. 8.2)

When conducting an assessment, it is important to consider the environment, ensuring it is well lit, comfortable and free from noise and distraction. Start by establishing rapport with the older person, asking how he or she would like to be addressed and conveying respect, patience and cultural sensitivity. It is also important to balance the assessment of complex problems with the older person's endurance and potential to become exhausted, by pacing the assessment and allowing for regular pauses.

The assessment can be supported with the use of validated screening tools, and input from family members, medical records and other caregivers and allied health professionals. Many older people tend to overestimate their health when affected by disease and disability (Tangarorong 2003). This may occur when the older person disregards new symptoms, thinking the changes are a normal part of ageing. The older person may also have a cognitive impairment; therefore, it may be useful to collect data through other reliable sources and direct observation.

The Health History

The assessment begins by obtaining a history of the presenting complaint. In the older person, this can be vague and may consist of more than one issue. A health history is comprehensive, taking the format of a medical history, social history, family history and a review of body systems. It is considered subjective data and is usually documented in the patient's own words.

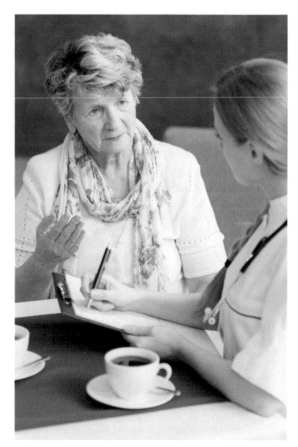

FIG. 8.2 The nurse needs to consider a range of factors when interview the older person.

Tips for Best Practice
Considerations for Communicating With Older Adults During the History-Taking Interview

- Provide a well-lit, quiet room, moderately warm with safe comfortable chairs.
- Make sure any written instructions are in a large font (16 point), which is easy to read.
- Slow down and pace the interview to the stamina of the person.
- Adjust your approach if the person is living with dementia or has a visual or hearing impairment.
- Make sure the older person can see your face and is wearing their glasses and/or hearing aids. Speak in low tones.
- Make use of brief screening instruments, medical records and reports from other healthcare professionals.
- Be respectful and do not patronise the older person.
- Where needed, consider involving a relative or carer to assist with the interview.
- Assess for symptoms of fatigue, loss of appetite, dizziness, loss of weight and pain.
- Allow time for open-ended questions and reminiscing.
- Do not rush.

The assessment does not have to be completed in one day.

Research Highlight

Comprehensive assessments by competent nurses with specialist gerontological skills can reduce length of stay and the incidence of geriatric syndromes. A US study educated nurses and implemented the role of the geriatric nurse consultant over a period of 17 months. The aim was to enable geriatric nurse consultants to complete a comprehensive geriatric assessment in the acute care setting.

This study demonstrated that geriatric nurse consultants practising in the acute care setting can administer a Comprehensive Geriatric Assessment and uncover clinically actionable findings. This study also demonstrated many opportunities to improve evidence-based care of older people.

REFERENCE
Trotta RL, Rao AD, Hermann RM et al (2018) Development of a comprehensive geriatric assessment led by geriatric nurse consultants: A feasibility study. Journal of Gerontological Nursing 44(12):25–34.

BOX 8.1
Special Areas of Concern When Assessing Older People

- Activities of daily living
- Instrumental activities of daily living
- Medications
- Acute persistent pain
- Smoking and alcohol
- Nutrition
- Frailty

Functional Ability

The assessment of functional status is also important when caring for older people. Normal ageing changes, acute illness, worsening chronic illness and hospitalisation can contribute to a decline in the ability to perform tasks necessary to live independently (Graf 2006). The data from a functional assessment can provide objective information to assist with individualised needs or to plan for specific in-home services. A functional assessment can also assist to focus on the person's baseline capabilities, facilitating early recognition of changes requiring further assessment.

A person's functional status relates to their ability to perform the tasks required for living. Learning how older people, especially those with chronic illness, function in terms of daily activities is important as it provides a baseline for future evaluations. It also allows the degree of dependence on others to be assessed.

Assessment of the older person's functional ability begins with a review of the person's activities of daily living (ADL) and instrumental activities of daily living (IADL). The ADLs are self-care activities that a person performs daily (e.g. feeding, bathing, dressing, transferring and controlling bodily functions and using the toilet), while the IADLs are activities needed to live independently (e.g. housework, preparing meals, managing finances etc).

Activities of Daily Living

Living is a complex process and our survival is dependent on undertaking several ongoing activities. These activities of living are influenced by biological, psychosocial, sociocultural, environmental, political and economic factors over the lifespan. There are 12 ADLs that the assessor needs to be familiar with to gain a holistic view of the person's current status. A detailed summary of each activity, as described by the person and the family, needs to be recorded and updated as necessary. The 12 activities of daily living (Roper et al 1996) provide a useful framework to structure this assessment.

1 Maintaining a safe environment

A person's environment relates to both internal (within the body) and external elements. The internal environment is maintained by the body's homeostatic balance. The external environment generally relates to the person's living conditions, presented and observed by the assessor.

2 Communication (see Chapter 7)

As people become older, their ability to socially interact may decrease due to poor mobility and the death of older friends and relatives. It is also often assumed by those caring for older people that the older person's hearing and comprehension is worse than it is. This belief may lead to reduced communication, which, in turn, further isolates the older person, leading to a decline in their psychological and physical wellbeing. Communication can also include the ability to contact others, including verbally or interactively.

3 Breathing (see Chapter 24)

Problems with the respiratory and the cardiovascular system occur more commonly in adults and older people. Breathing difficulties can often be associated with a person's lifestyle rather than age-related changes. It is important to observe the rate of respirations, any breathing difficulties, present and past smoking and exposure to environmental air pollutants.

4 Eating and drinking (see Chapter 12)

A healthy diet in older people is important to maintain an ideal health status. As a person becomes older, they become less active and are likely to lead a more sedentary lifestyle. According to Leslie and Hankey (2015), an older person's ability to maintain an adequate and nourishing diet is associated with ill health, physiological and psychological changes, social isolation and economic and environmental issues. Medications can also influence their nutritional status, as the side effects may cause nausea, constipation or an increased risk of incontinence. An older person experiencing incontinence may lower their fluid intake to avoid needing the toilet, resulting in dehydration and an electrolyte imbalance. Loss of senses, such as taste and smell, along with ill-fitting dentures or poor oral health, can also influence nutritional intake, putting the older person at risk of malnutrition. Hand deformities or weakness from arthritis, along

with a reduction in mental capacity, can result in a decreased ability to shop for food, cook and even use cutlery, again resulting in malnutrition.

5 Eliminating (see Chapter 13)

The inability to control bladder or bowel function is more prevalent in older people, especially in those who are frail. Incontinence can result from a loss in muscular control, changes to the central nervous system (CNS), cerebrovascular disease, medications and constipation. Faecal and urinary incontinence can hugely affect an individual's dignity, health and quality of life and often results in the older person moving into a residential care home. This is highlighted by the fact that there is a higher rate of incontinence in older people residing in residential care homes than those living in their own homes (Wald 2005).

6 Personal cleansing and dressing

According to Roper and colleagues (1996:235):

> Failing eyesight and shaking hands may make it increasingly difficult for older people to retain their independence with conventional clothing. Many older people more readily feel the cold and may wear extra clothing to keep warm.

Independence in personal cleansing and dressing depends on both age and health status. Therefore, an understanding of the ageing process is essential to appreciate the personal cleansing and dressing needs of an older person. It is vital to assess the older person's ability to manage their own personal care before implementing care that might not be required.

7 Controlling body temperature

Older age, along with underlying acute or chronic disease, increase the risk of an older person experiencing a heat- or cold-related illness. This is because the thermoregulation system becomes less efficient due to inability to constrict peripheral blood vessels, resulting in heat loss and the reduction in shivering (Roper et al 1996). Thermoregulation in the older population can also be influenced by medication dependence, obesity, reduced mobility, declining cognitive ability and socioeconomic and environmental factors.

8 Mobilising (see Chapter 16)

There are age-related factors which affect an older person's ability to mobilise. Physiological changes may result in loss of balance and a poorer reaction time, which leads to an increased risk of falls and consequent higher levels of morbidity and mortality (Dionyssiotis 2012). Despite these physiological changes, the impact on function and mobility are modifiable, as is the belief that older people should take it easy – a view that could promote immobility and dependence in the ageing person.

9 Working and playing

Although life expectancy has generally increased over the past 20 years, living a quality healthy life may not necessarily be achieved. Retirement can create more personal leisure time; however, a lack of income or poor physical health can result in more restricted activity (Bowling & Gabriel 2007). It also needs to be acknowledged that many older people work into and past retirement age or provide valuable assistance to the voluntary sector.

10 Expressing sexuality (see Chapter 27)

Given that older people in western society are living longer, second marriages and long-term relationships are more frequent. The image that older people are asexual is now not the case. Expressing sexuality is essential for wellbeing and can be affected indirectly by health problems. Chronic illness, anxiety and depression, along with certain medical treatments, can affect physical capacity and ultimately affect intimacy and sexual activity (Steinke 2013). In some cases, professional counselling can help not only the older person who is experiencing difficulty, but also their partner. Expressing sexuality may also influence the person's personal appearance and how they wish to present themselves in public.

11 Sleeping (see Chapter 14)

Adequate sleep is essential to an older person's functioning and wellbeing. However, older people tend to sleep for shorter periods and wake up more often during the night. This pattern of sleep often results in poor sleep quality and the need for daytime naps (Scullin & Bliwise 2015). Regular night-time awakening can be attributed to changes in bladder function, pain or altered breathing patterns such as in sleep apnoea (see Chapter 24). Sleep can also be affected by depression and anxiety (see Chapter 25) or dementia (see Chapter 26). The older person may sleep less soundly when they are concerned about their personal safety alone in the bed after the death of a spouse or partner.

12 Dying (see Chapter 28)

Death in older age is often viewed as natural and in some cases an older person will lose the will to live. The therapeutic relationship is crucial in communicating with someone who is dying. Cultural preferences and advance care directives need to be considered at this time.

Practice Point
12 Activities of Daily Living

1 Maintaining a safe environment
2. Communication
3. Breathing
4. Eating & drinking
5. Eliminating
6. Personal cleansing & dressing
7. Controlling body temperature
8. Mobilising
9. Working & playing
10. Expressing sexuality
11. Sleeping
12. Dying

Instrumental Activities of Daily Living (IADL)

The Lawton Instrumental Activities of Daily Living Scale (IADL) is an appropriate instrument to assess independent living skills (Lawton & Brody 1969). The instrument is suitable to assess current functional status (Gallo & Paveza 2006) and changes (improvement or deterioration) over time (see Fig. 8.3). Eight domains of function are measured. Domain scores are summed to calculate a total score ranging from 0 (low function, dependent) to 8 (high function, independent). Although developed in 1969, the IADL tool is still relevant in today's health needs context.

Medications (see Chapter 11)

As people age, they are more likely to require medication for multiple medical conditions. Polypharmacy is common in the older population; in fact, 30% of hospital admissions, falls and confusion are related to adverse drug effects (Parameswaran Nair et al 2016). Age-related changes that affect medicines in older people are mainly related to decreased renal and hepatic clearance, due to functional changes and changes in body fat composition (Hunter & Miller 2016). A detailed record of currently used medications is required during initial and ongoing assessments.

Pain (see Chapter 19)

Chronic pain affects physical function in older people, as it does with all age groups. However, assessing pain in older people can be very challenging for all involved, especially during short consultations with clinicians

THE LAWTON INSTRUMENTAL ACTIVITIES OF DAILY LIVING SCALE

Ability to Use Telephone

1. Operates telephone on own initiative; looks up and dials numbers 1
2. Dials a few well-known numbers 1
3. Answers telephone, but does not dial 1
4. Does not use telephone at all 0

Shopping

1. Takes care of all shopping needs independently 1
2. Shops independently for small purchases 0
3. Needs to be accompanied on any shopping trip 0
4. Completely unable to shop 0

Food Preparation

1. Plans, prepares, and serves adequate meals independently 1
2. Prepares adequate meals if supplied with ingredients 0
3. Heats and serves prepared meals or prepares meals but does not maintain adequate diet 0
4. Needs to have meals prepared and served 0

Housekeeping

1. Maintains house alone with occasion assistance (heavy work) 1
2. Performs light daily tasks such as dishwashing, bed making 1
3. Performs light daily tasks, but cannot maintain acceptable level of cleanliness 1
4. Needs help with all home maintenance tasks 1
5. Does not participate in any housekeeping tasks 0

Laundry

1. Does personal laundry completely 1
2. Launders small items, rinses socks, stockings, etc 1
3. All laundry must be done by others 0

Mode of Transportation

1. Travels independently on public transportation or drives own car 1
2. Arranges own travel via taxi, but does not otherwise use public transportation 1
3. Travels on public transportation when assisted or accompanied by another 1
4. Travel limited to taxi or automobile with assistance of another 0
5. Does not travel at all 0

Responsibility for Own Medications

1. Is responsible for taking medication in correct dosages at correct time 1
2. Takes responsibility if medication is prepared in advance in separate dosages 0
3. Is not capable of dispensing own medication 0

Ability to Handle Finances

1. Manages financial matters independently (budgets, writes cheques, pays rent and bills, goes to bank); collects and keeps track of income 1
2. Manages day-to-day purchases, but needs help with banking, major purchases, etc 1
3. Incapable of handling money 0

Scoring: For each category, circle the item description that most closely resembles the client's highest functional level (either 0 or 1).

FIG. 8.3 **The Lawton instrumental activities of daily living scale** (Lawton & Brody 1969.)

(Schofield & Abdulla 2018). To allow for engagement it has been highlighted that older people should be given longer consultation times to aid communication (Macdonald et al 2009). Assessment can be enhanced with the use of simple pain assessment tools (De Rond et al 2000).

Smoking and Alcohol

There is clear evidence for the benefits of quitting smoking in older people. Large-scale studies have found that smokers who quit after the age of 65 years benefit from additional healthy life years and reduced morbidity (Taylor et al 2002). The elderly population is particularly vulnerable to the effects of alcohol, which often results in falls and delirium (Onen et al 2005). The rates of alcohol abuse or misuse among the baby boomer generation has increased compared to previous generations, resulting in increased presentations to the emergency department (ED) (Ouellette et al 2019). Social and health-related reasons for increased alcohol use in older people include social isolation, chronic disease, pain and mental health problems (Choi et al 2015). Evidence indicates that many patients presenting to the ED following a fall after consuming alcohol were also taking prescribed medications, including antidepressants, narcotics, antipsychotics and anxiolytics (Onen et al 2005). Many of these medications react with the alcohol consumed to potentiate the risks of falls in the older population (Onen et al 2005).

Nutrition (see Chapter 12)

Poor nutritional intake is common in older people, resulting in vitamin and mineral deficiencies. It is important to assess the older person's nutritional intake using a checklist (see Fig. 8.4) and record the food consumed over a 24-hour period. It is also important to identify how the older person procures food supplies if living at home and to be aware of personal preferences if eating meals prepared by others, such as people preparing meals in hospital or a residential aged care facility. The older person's weight should be monitored regularly and consistently, and documented, along with other evidence of weight loss, such as poorly fitting clothes or loose skin. General condition of hair and nails can yield clues about the adequacy of nutrition. Good oral health is essential to maintaining an adequate food and fluid intake. Regular observation of the older person's mouth (including checking of dentures) is essential.

Frailty

Frailty in the older population is a condition associated with decreased physiological reserve and increased vulnerability to adverse health outcomes. These outcomes include falls, fractures, disability, hospitalisation and institutionalisation. Frailty has also been shown to be linked to poorer psychological or cognitive outcomes, such as reduced quality of life and dementia (Clegg et al 2013).

Head-to-Toe Physical Examination of the Older Person

A complete head-to-toe assessment of an older person includes the following:

General appearance

Assess for signs of cognitive impairments, including level of alertness, confusion, disorientation and memory loss. Ensure you perform a complete check of vital signs, including blood pressure, pulse, height and weight. Check for weight loss, which is common in the older population.

Hair and skin

Assess skin turgor for signs of dehydration. Look for signs of pressure injuries, bruising and evidence of growths or neoplasms. You are looking for evidence of falls or abuse and signs of skin cancer.

Statement	YES
I have an illness or condition that made me change the kind and/or amount of food I eat.	2
I eat fewer than 2 meals per day.	3
I eat few fruits or vegetables or milk products.	2
I have 3 or more drinks of beer, liquor or wine almost every day.	2
I have tooth or mouth problems that make it hard for me to eat.	2
I don't always have enough money to buy the food I need.	4
I eat alone most of the time.	1
I take 3 or more different prescribed or over-the-counter drugs a day.	1
Without wanting to, I have lost or gained 5 kilograms in the last 6 months.	2
I am not physically able to shop, cook and/or feed myself.	2
Total Score	/21

Nutritional score: 0–2 Low nutritional risk; 3–5 Moderate nutritional risk; 6 or more High nutritional risk

FIG. 8.4 **Nutritional intake checklist** (Sahyoun et al 1997.)

Head – eyes, ears, nose and throat

Check the older person for diminished hearing (see Chapter 20) and vision (see Chapter 21), which may impair independent living. Examine the mouth for dental caries, tooth loss, periodontal gum disease, mouth ulcers and dry mouth. These findings may reflect the older person's nutritional intake or may be a sign of dehydration.

Cardiovascular

If a systolic murmur is heard, consider aortic stenosis. Examine the ankles for swelling, which may indicate venous insufficiency or heart failure.

Breasts and axillae

Perform a breast examination, if appropriate, as the risk of breast cancer increases with age.

Visually inspect the breasts and nipples for size, symmetry, shape, colour texture and discharge, and then palpate using the finger pads, checking for consistency of the breast tissue using one of a variety of palpation techniques. Extend the examination into tissue around each axilla and supraclavicular area and document any tenderness, lumps, open wounds or discharge (Henderson et al 2020).

Abdominal

Observe for abdominal distension or palpable masses and a pulsatile aorta. Pay attention to the signs of a leaking aortic aneurysm, which are back pain, abdominal distension, shock and asymmetrical peripheral pulses in the legs. Older people are also prone to constipation due to decreased food intake, dehydration and medications. The older person may also require a rectal examination. An inspection of the perineal area should follow to observe for any abnormalities, such as rectal prolapse, haemorrhoids, anal skin tags, anal lesions, scarring from episiotomy or tears, gaping anus, bleeding, faecal soiling, infestation, foreign bodies and general skin condition. A digital rectal examination (DRE) is an essential component of bowel assessment (National Institute of Health and Clinical Excellence [NICE] 2007) and nurses should possess the skills and knowledge to assess bowel dysfunction competently, which includes the use of a DRE where appropriate (Kyle 2008).

Musculoskeletal (see Fig. 8.5)

Examine for any deformities and functional disability. Many older people will deny pain or be unable to express it. Observation during movement or change in posture may yield clues that mobility or function may be limited by pain. Using alternative words when assessing movement (e.g. 'stiffness', 'ache') may elucidate further information. Examination of joints commonly affected by osteoarthritis, such as the fingers and knees, with functional observation and gross checking of range of movement/crepitus, is helpful.

Neurological

Perform a mini-mental state examination (MMSE), and if the older person is confused, distinguish between dementia and delirium. Assess the gait for speed, posture, power and balance. Assess getting into and out of a chair. Impaired balance in the older person often presents as increased falls and fall-related injuries. Falls are the leading cause of hospitalisation and injury-related death in older people (Bradley 2013).

Cognitive impairment (see Chapter 26) (see Fig. 8.6)

There is an increased rate of neurocognitive disorders, such as delirium, mild cognitive impairment, dementia

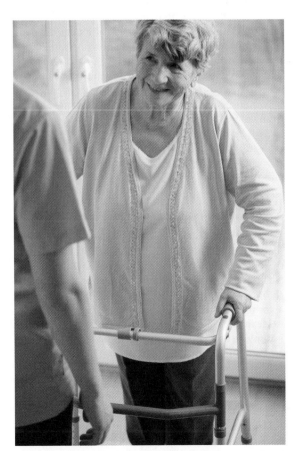

FIG. 8.5 Observing how the older person moves is an important part of the assessment process.

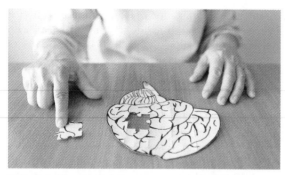

FIG. 8.6 **Neurocognitive disorders can affect many aspects of an older person's health, including gait and balance.**

> **Tips for Best Practice**
> *Reasons for Good Record-Keeping*
>
> Good record-keeping is required for the following reasons:
> - Continuity of care is more effective
> - Promotes better communication and dissemination of information between members of the multidisciplinary team
> - Helps to address complaints or legal processes
> - Supports clinical audit, research, allocation of resources and performance planning
> - Helps to identify risks and enables the early detection of complications
> - Supports patient care and person-centred communication
> - Supports effective clinical judgement
> - Supports delivery of services
> - Helps improve accountability
> - Shows how decisions were made relating to the person's care (Jevon & Ewens 2012).

and Parkinson's disease in the older population. Electrolyte imbalance and acute physiological changes may alter an older person's cognitive ability and may be the first sign of a health problem. Therefore, any change in an older person's health requires an assessment of their mental status. Delirium is a medical emergency with potentially reversible causes, therefore timely identification and intervention are crucial. Early recognition of dementia enables the older person and their family to access care and treatment, practical advice as new challenges arise and to plan ahead while they are still able to make important decisions.

The Mini-Mental state examinations (MMSE) is often used for gross screening of cognition (Folstein et al 1975). It is used to screen attention, memory loss and orientation.

DOCUMENTATION AND RECORD-KEEPING

Documentation is an effective method of sharing information among healthcare professionals and carers of the older person. Nurses, doctors and members of the allied healthcare team can use the older person's medical records as a primary source of data when conducting a comprehensive assessment. Notes can also be used to evaluate whether the older person's condition is improving or deteriorating as an indication of how well a care approach or treatment option is in meeting the person's needs.

An accurate written record detailing all aspects of assessment forms an integral part of the nursing management of the older person. Additionally, this record contributes to the circulation of information between team members providing multidisciplinary care. Reasons for good record-keeping are listed in *Tips for best practice: Reasons for good record-keeping*.

Documentation in Residential Care Facilities and the Hospital Setting

The delivery of effective and suitable care for older people living in residential aged care facilities and hospital settings rests on the quality of care documentation accessible to nurses, care workers and the rest of the multidisciplinary team. The documentation of assessment information, care plans and progress notes are also used in quality improvement audits and to authorise claims for funding. The quality of documentation is a reflection of the standard of care given to aged care residents and hospital patients.

Accurate and comprehensive documentation has legal significance in relation to health records. If an older person or family member lodges a complaint, the nursing notes are the only proof that you have fulfilled your duty of care to the patient. According to the law in many countries, if care or treatment due to a person is not recorded, it can be assumed that it has not taken place (Stevens & Pickering 2010). Poor nursing documentation can therefore mean you are found negligent, even if you are sure you provided the correct care on time.

SUMMARY

Assessment of older people is a highly skilled nursing activity because they often have multiple and complex care needs. Comprehensive nursing assessment of the older person requires applied knowledge of the human anatomy and physiology, supported by use of assessment tools and techniques. Nurses draw on the information gained through observation, questioning, holistic assessment and reviewing medical records. The findings are then documented, and the outcomes communicated to the person, family carers and the members of the multidisciplinary team involved. This information assists in evaluating and monitoring ongoing care and helps in planning future care. A comprehensive assessment requires the nurse to use a person-centred approach to find out what is important to that individual and to maximise their independence in their ADLs while improving their overall quality of life.

Practice Scenario: A True Story

Mrs Jones is a 91-year-old lady who lives alone and has, up until the past four weeks, been extremely independent. She developed backache which did not get any better. Mrs Jones then had a fall, so admission to hospital was arranged. Her past medical history consisted of an overnight stay in hospital for a minor gynaecological procedure in 1974. Blood tests were completed and an abdominal X-ray showing no significant findings. The family were advised to take her home and return with her as an outpatient for a CT scan (categorised as non-urgent). No holistic assessment was performed on admission to the emergency department or on transfer to the ward and no contact details were requested from the family. The family were not included in any assessment or discharge planning. Within 48 hours Mrs Jones was no longer able to walk unaided, was unsteady on her feet and was unable to prepare food or toilet unaided. Her glasses were dirty and her hearing aids had not been charged or removed overnight. The family refused to take her home until the CT scan was performed, which was finally done after 3 days. The scan showed she had cancer of the pancreas, liver and lung metastases, as well as a T12 wedge compression fracture. The family were advised of the findings and that life expectancy was likely to be less than 6 months. The family took Mrs Jones home immediately, only waiting to collect medications. The family were given Oramorph and paracetamol, advised to make contact with the GP and supplied with a kitchen trolley. Mrs Jones died at home 15 days later in the care of her family.

REVIEW QUESTIONS

1. Consider this scenario and using the 12 Activities of Daily Living (ADLs), prepare an assessment based on the information provided.
2. Assess Mrs Jones's situation using the Instrumental Activities of Daily Living 4 weeks before admission and after discharge from hospital.
3. How did the healthcare system fail Mrs Jones?

FURTHER READING

Shantong J, Pinping L (2016) Current developments in elderly comprehensive assessment and research methods. Biomed Research International (2016):3528248.

REFERENCES

Bowling A, Gabriel Z (2007) Lay theories of quality of life in older age. Aging and Society 27:827–848.

Bradley C (2013) Trends in hospitalisations due to falls by older people Australia 1999–2000 to 2010–11, Injury Research and Statistics no. 84. INJCAT 160 Australian Institute of Health and Welfare. Online. Available: www.aihw.gov.au/WorkArea/DownloadAsset.aspx?id=60129543591

Choi N, Marti C, DiNitto D et al (2015) Alcohol risk factors for older adults' emergency department visits: a latent class analysis. The Western Journal of Emergency Medicine 16(7):1146–1158.

Clegg A, Young J, Iliffe S et al (2013) Frailty in elderly people. Lancet 381(9868):752–762.

De Rond MEJ, de Wit R, Van Dam F et al (2000) A pain monitoring program for nurses: effects on communication, assessment and documentation of patient's pain. Journal of Pain Symptom Management 20(6):424–439.

Dionyssiotis Y (2012) Analyzing the problem of falls among older people. International Journal of General Medicine 5:805–813.

Elsawy B, Higgins KE (2011) The geriatric assessment. American Family Physician 83(1):48–56.

Folstein MF, Folstein SE, McHugh PR (1975) 'Mini-mental state'. A practical method for grading the cognitive state of patients for the clinician. Journal of Psychiatric Research 12:189–198.

Gallo JJ, Paveza GJ (2006) Activities of daily living and instrumental activities of daily living assessment. In: JJ Gallo, HR Bogner, T. Fulmer et al (eds), Handbook of geriatric assessment, 4th edn. Jones and Bartlett Publishers, Burlington, MA.

Graf C (2006) Functional decline in hospitalized older adults The American Journal of Nursing 106(1):58–67.

Henderson JA, Duffee D, Ferguson T (2020) Breast examination techniques. In: StatPearls [Internet]. Treasure Island (FL): StatPearls Publishing; 2020. Online. Available: www.ncbi.nlm.nih.gov/books/NBK459179/

Hunter S, Miller C (ed.) (2016) Miller's nursing for wellness in older adults, 2nd edn. Wolters Kluwer/Lippincott Williams & Wilkins, Philadelphia.

Jevon P, Ewens B (2012) Monitoring the critically ill patient, 3rd edn. Wiley-Blackwell, Oxford.

Kyle G (2008) Constipation: an examination of the current evidence. Continence UK 2:61–67.

Lawton MP, Brody EM (1969) Assessment of older people: Self-maintaining and instrumental activities of daily living. The Gerontologist 9(3):179–186.

Leslie W, Hankey C (2015) Aging nutritional status and health. Healthcare 3(3):648–658.

McDonald D, Shea M, Rose L et al (2009) The effect of pain question phrasing on older adult pain information. Journal of Pain Symptom Management 37(6):1050–1060.

National Institute for Health and Clinical Excellence (NICE) (2007) Faecal incontinence: The management of faecal incontinence in adults. Clinical Guideline 49. Online. Available: www.nice.org.uk/guidance/cg49

Onen S, Onen J, Mangeon H et al (2005) Alcohol abuse and dependence in elderly emergency department patients. Archives of Gerontology and Geriatrics 41(2):191–200.

Oulette L, TenBrink W, Gier G et al (2019) Alcoholism in elderly patients: Characteristics of patients and impact on the emergency department. The American Journal of Emergency Medicine 37(4):776–777.

Parameswaran Nair N, Chalmers L, Peterson GM et al (2016) Hospitalization in older patients due to adverse drug reactions – the need for a prediction tool. Clinical Interventions in Aging 11:497–505.

Roper N, Logan W, Tierney A (1996) The elements of nursing: a model for nursing based on a model of living, 4th edn. Churchill Livingstone, Edinburgh.

Rovner BW, Folstein MF (1987) Mini-Mental State Examination in clinical practice. Hospital Practice 22(1A):99–100.

Sahyoun NR, Jacques PF, Dallal GE et al (1997) Nutrition Screening Initiative checklist may be a better awareness/ educational tool than a screening one. Journal of the American Dietetic Association 97(7):760–764.

Schofield P, Abdulla A (2018) Pain assessment in the older population: what the literature says. Age and Ageing. 47(3):324–327.

Scullin M, Bliwise D (2015) Sleep, cognition, and normal aging: integrating a half century of multidisciplinary research. Perspectives on Psychological Science 10(1):97–137.

Steinke E (2013) Sexuality and chronic illness. Journal of Gerontological Nursing 39(11):18–27.

Stevens S, Pickering D (2010) Keeping good records: a guide. Community Eye Health Journal 23(74):44–45.

Tangarorong G, Kerrins G, Besdine R (2003) Clinical approach to the older patient: an overview. In C Cassel, R Leipzig, H Cohen et al (eds), Geriatric medicine, 4th edn. Springer, New York.

Taylor DH, Hasselblad V, Henley SJ et al (2002) Benefits of smoking cessation for longevity. American Journal of Public Health 92:990–996.

Trotta RL, Rao AD, Hermann RM et al (2018) Development of a comprehensive geriatric assessment led by geriatric nurse consultants: A feasibility study. Journal of Gerontological Nursing 44(12):25–34.

Wald A (2005) Faecal incontinence in the elderly: epidemiology and management. Drugs and Aging 22:131–139.

Wieland D, Hirth V (2003) Comprehensive Geriatric Assessment. Cancer Control. November:454–462.

CHAPTER 9

Living with Chronic Conditions

LISA WHITEHEAD

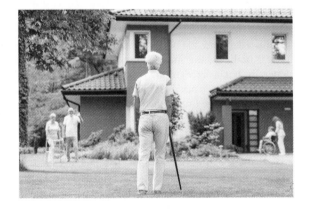

INTRODUCTION

This chapter will describe chronic illness among older adults in Australia and New Zealand and the implications for individuals, families and healthcare delivery. The chapter will outline the drivers behind the increase in chronic conditions, why older people are vulnerable to developing chronic conditions, and the concept of multimorbidity. The challenges of living with and managing type 2 diabetes will be presented to highlight many of the overarching issues facing older people living with chronic conditions. The role of the nurse in supporting the prevention of chronic conditions and in supporting the older population living with chronic conditions will also be described.

AGEING IN AUSTRALIA AND NEW ZEALAND

Australians and New Zealanders are among those with the highest life expectancies in the world. Life expectancy at birth in both countries has risen steadily over time. In 2016, in Australia, life expectancy at birth was 80.4 years for males and 84.6 years for females (Australian Bureau of Statistics [ABS] 2017), and 80.2 years for males and 83.6 years for females in New Zealand (StatsNZ 2019). While many can expect to live a long life, the picture is less certain that it will be a healthy life. Of the life years gained over the last 25 years, 20–30% of them are lived in poor health (Ministry of Health NZ 2014).

Chronic conditions are a substantial global, national and individual health issue, contributing to both premature mortality and premature morbidity. Globally, they are the leading causes of disease burden, and are responsible for around 70% of deaths worldwide (World Health Organisation [WHO] 2017).

The term 'chronic condition' refers to a wide range of health conditions, illnesses and diseases. Chronic conditions are ongoing, long term or recurring conditions that can have a significant impact on people's lives. Chronic conditions are the leading cause of death and ill health worldwide. More than 11 million Australians – almost half of the population – live with one or more chronic conditions, the figure increasing to 87% of people aged 65 years and over (ABS 2017).

For both Australians and New Zealanders aged 65–74 years, an increasing burden from coronary heart disease is reported (see Chapter 23). Lung cancer, chronic obstructive pulmonary disease (COPD) (see Chapter 24) and other musculoskeletal conditions (see Chapter 22) are the most frequently reported chronic conditions. The burden of coronary heart disease is highest among older people aged 75–84 years, followed by dementia, COPD, stroke and lung cancer. These diseases are also the five leading causes of death in Australia. Dementia (see Chapter 26) is more prominent among older people aged 85–94 years. The leading causes of burden among very old people (aged 95 years and over) are dementia, coronary heart disease and stroke.

In Australia and New Zealand, mortality rates have continued to decline. The age-standardised death rate in Australia fell by 69% between 1910 and 2015 for males and by 73% for females. Changes over time have seen the leading causes of death shift from diseases of the circulatory system in the early 1900s to the following picture:

- Coronary heart disease is the leading cause of death in males, although rates are decreasing.
- Dementia and Alzheimer disease among both men and women have increased.
- Cancer of an unknown or ill-defined primary site moved out of the ten leading causes of death for females in 2006 to be replaced by influenza and pneumonia in 2016 (ABS 2017; Ministry of Health NZ 2020).

Multimorbidity, that is, living with two or more chronic conditions, is rising in prevalence (National Academy of Science 2018; National Institute for Health and Care Excellence [NICE] 2016). Multimorbidity is associated with:

- reduced quality of life
- higher mortality
- polypharmacy (see Chapter 11)
- high treatment burden
- higher rates of adverse drug events
- greater health services use
- greater use of unplanned care (NICE 2016).

Around one in four (23%) Australians were living with two or more chronic conditions in 2014–15 (ABS 2015), with the same picture in New Zealand (Ministry of Health NZ 2014).

The increase in longevity, especially in high-income countries, has been largely due to the decline in deaths from cardiovascular disease (stroke and ischaemic heart disease) through the reduction in tobacco use, management of blood pressure and greater reach and effectiveness of health interventions. However, the changes in the wealth and health of developed countries have also shaped the current healthcare problems faced by populations. The reduction in deaths related to childbirth, poor nutrition, infectious diseases and injury mean that older people now account for a larger proportion of the population and as people age they become more vulnerable to developing chronic conditions.

Prevalence of Type 2 Diabetes

Diabetes is a chronic condition marked by high levels of sugar (glucose) in the blood. The body is unable to produce insulin (a hormone made by the pancreas to control blood glucose levels) or to use insulin effectively, or both (Diabetes Australia 2020). Type 2 diabetes, the most common form of diabetes, generally has a later onset. Type 2 diabetes is largely preventable and is often associated with lifestyle factors such as inactivity, unhealthy diet, obesity and tobacco smoking. Based on self-reported estimates from the ABS 2014–15 National Health Survey, more than one in 20 (6.1%, or 1.2 million) Australian adults are living with diabetes. However, self-reported data are likely to underestimate the prevalence. An estimated one in five (19%) Australians aged 75 years and over are living with diabetes compared with 1.3% of people aged 18–44 years (ABS 2017). Type 2 diabetes is a chronic condition that is on the rise. The age-standardised rate of self-reported diabetes has more than tripled over 25 years, from 1.5% in 1989–90 to 4.7% in 2014–15 (ABS 2017).

Older people are at high risk for the development of type 2 diabetes due to the combined effects of genetics, lifestyle and physiological ageing. The direct effect of ageing on diabetes pathophysiology is through impairment of beta-cell function, resulting in a decline in insulin secretion. Type 2 diabetes is by far the most prevalent form of diabetes in older people (see *Promoting wellness* box).

Older Australians and New Zealanders living with diabetes are at risk of many direct complications, including:

- malnutrition
- poor wound healing
- vision impairment
- kidney failure.

Additionally, diabetes puts older people at risk of indirect complications, such as high risk of vascular comorbidities, which can lead to:

- coronary artery disease
- physical and cognitive function impairment
- mortality.

In the United States, people aged 65 years or older are developing diabetes at a rate nearly three times higher than younger adults (Lee & Halter 2017).

Research Highlights

- More than 1 in 20 (6.1%, or 1.2 million) Australian adults is living with diabetes (ABS 2015).
- An estimated 1 in 5 (19%) Australians aged 75 years and over is living with diabetes compared with 1.3% of people aged 18–44 years (ABS 2017).
- Type 2 diabetes is a chronic condition that is on the rise. The age-standardised rate of self-reported diabetes has more than tripled over 25 years, from 1.5% in 1989–90 to 4.7% in 2014–15 (ABS 2017).
- Older people are at high risk for the development of type 2 diabetes due to the combined effects of genetic, lifestyle and physiological ageing.

ABS (2015); ABS (2017).

WHY ARE OLDER PEOPLE MORE LIKELY TO DEVELOP CHRONIC CONDITIONS?

The key areas associated with a decline in health status with age are physiological changes that can lead to frailty. These include sarcopenia, defined as 'progressive and generalised loss of skeletal muscle mass and strength' (Santilli et al 2014:177), which can lead to functional limitations. The strength of the immune system also declines with age. The measurement of the health status of older people has evolved from mortality-oriented measures to measures of life expectancy and quality of life. A wider understanding of older adult health should include not just life expectancy but also healthy life years, prevalence of chronic conditions and the experience of functional limitations.

CHALLENGE OF AGEING HEALTHILY

The challenge of living a longer life is to live as healthy a life as possible. The long-term burden of illness and diminished wellbeing impacts not only on the individual but also their family, health systems and the economy. The prevention of ill health is the first line of action, no matter what the age of the individual. Until recently, older adults were invisible in the health promotion literature. The perception was widespread that it was too late to change the lifestyle of older people, or that changing diet and starting exercise could have a negative impact (Golinowska et al 2016). The WHO highlighted the importance of a healthy lifestyle at every stage of life (WHO 2002). Evidence indicates the key role in preventing many diseases and loss of functional capacity of:

- regular exercise
- giving up smoking

Promoting Wellness

The criteria for diagnosing diabetes is the same for all age groups. However, support to manage type 2 diabetes may include the need to accommodate the co-morbidities and functional impairments associated with ageing in order to self-manage diabetes, for example, weight loss and exercise programs. Nurses play a key role in prevention, early detection and management of type 2 diabetes. It is important that nurses are able to:

- identify risk factors for diabetes, common signs, symptoms and diagnostic criteria
- understand blood glucose monitoring and target ranges
- review common oral and injectable diabetes medications
- consider the impact of exercise and nutrition on blood glucose levels
- recognise and review the management of hypoglycaemia
- identify and consider the impact of long-term complications of diabetes
- identify specialist support services available, e.g. Diabetes Australia and Diabetes New Zealand, and service and support schemes, e.g. The National Diabetes Services Scheme (NDSS).

- limiting alcohol consumption
- participating in learning activities
- community integration.

However, over half (52%) of all adults aged 18–64 years were not sufficiently active to gain a health benefit in 2014–15 and among adults aged 65 and older, 75% were not sufficiently active (ABS 2017).

The key factors underpinning a lifestyle that is as independent and self-sufficient as possible are the maintenance of functional capacity, maintenance or improvement of self-care and the development and maintenance of social networks (WHO 2015). There is much evidence to suggest that social bonds and social activities, including work, life-long learning activities, engagement in cultural and social events and maintaining a social network, are essential for healthy ageing (MOPACT 2016). Therefore, these are important elements to be included in any program developed for older people. Further, the framing of messages around health for the older population is important. Ensuring that health messages reach older people in ways that are acceptable is essential to successfully change attitudes. Examples include:

- targeting messages, for example, the importance of physical activity in later years
- ensuring relevance and appeal, for example, emphasising gains to be achieved in the short and longer term.

Little research to explore the factors that motivate older people to make and sustain positive behavioural changes is available and is an important area for further investigation.

The growing prevalence of chronic conditions increases the pressure on the healthcare system with a rise in emergency department visits, hospital admissions, out-of-hospital services, use of medicines and palliative care. As people are living longer, often with more than one chronic condition, they require treatment and management for longer periods of time. Nationally, programs to promote healthy lifestyles are in place, including a range of tobacco control measures, strategies to reduce harmful levels of alcohol consumption and actions for the early detection of cancer and other chronic conditions. Box 9.1 provides examples of national initiatives in Australia.

In both Australia and New Zealand, national frameworks for chronic condition management have been developed and accepted. In 2017, all Australian health ministers endorsed the National Strategic Framework for Chronic Conditions (the Framework) (Australian Government Department of Health 2017). The framework provides guidance for the development and implementation of policies, strategies, actions and services to tackle

---

> **BOX 9.1**
> **National Chronic Disease Management Initiatives in Australia (Australian Government Department of Health 2017)**
>
> - Access to care plans and assessments through the Medicare Benefits Schedule for the planning and management of chronic conditions
> - Subsidies through the Pharmaceutical Benefits Scheme (PBS) for a range of medicines used in the treatment of chronic conditions
> - Introduction of Health Care Homes where people are enrolled with a specific general practice or Aboriginal Community Controlled Health Service to coordinate their care and to facilitate services by a care team, which can include a range of health professionals (general practitioners, practice nurses, nurse practitioners, allied health professionals).

---

chronic conditions. The framework addresses primary, secondary and tertiary prevention of chronic conditions, recognising that there are often similar underlying principles for the prevention and management of many chronic conditions. It moves away from a disease-specific approach and highlights the shared health determinants, risk factors and multimorbidities across a broad range of chronic conditions. In New Zealand, the Ministry of Health developed a Long Term Conditions Outcomes Framework (Ministry of Health NZ 2017) and a program of work to operationalise this framework. Box 9.2 details the Long-Term Conditions (LTC) Programme in place in New Zealand.

It is important that nurses are not only aware of the national initiatives in place, but also look for opportunities to shape these by:

- providing feedback when calls for consultation are issued
- sitting on committees that develop policies and frameworks
- operationalising policies and frameworks.

National bodies such as the Australian College of Nursing and the College of Nurses New Zealand regularly inform and consult with members on matters of national interest.

Summary

Population ageing is described as one of the greatest challenges of the modern world in both developed and developing countries. In addition to increased life expectancy are the goals of being able to lead active and

Tips for Best Practice

Nurses play an important role in educating and supporting older people and families about chronic health conditions and can connect them with appropriate community resources and services.

In your practice:

- ask older people 'What matters to you?'
- think about an older person's social and mental wellbeing as well as their physical health
- routinely check that older people have a care plan – if not, who in your team is best placed to assist?
- encourage older people to have medications reviewed by their GP or pharmacy at least annually (see Chapter 11) to ensure all medications are still necessary, what might be missing and potential interactions.
- routinely check whether older people have an Advance Care Plan – if not, consider whether advance care planning is appropriate. Who in your team is best placed to assist?

meaningful lives for as long as possible. However, ageing is associated with an increased prevalence of medical conditions and disabilities. Healthcare systems are limited in their capacity to tackle chronic conditions and especially multimorbidity. Healthcare systems need to move from reactive to proactive approaches to enhance the scope of health promotion and disease prevention interventions. Nurses are the key providers of holistic healthcare. Nurses have the skills and experience to promote prevention of ill health as well as to provide treatment for diagnosed conditions and support for older people and their families to self-manage chronic conditions with the goal of promoting the long-term wellbeing of current and future generations.

Practice Scenario

Arthur is a 78-year-old gentleman living in regional Western Australia. He is 180 cm tall and weighs 105 kg. He has recently been diagnosed with type 2 diabetes. He lives with his wife Jean in a bungalow approximately 5 km from the nearest shops. Arthur's GP has asked you to discuss health promotion and lifestyle modification. Identify the key factors to consider, including in the plan.

MULTIPLE CHOICE QUESTIONS

1. Which of the following is not true:
   a. Chronic conditions are ongoing
   b. Chronic conditions are short term
   c. Chronic conditions are recurring conditions
   d. Chronic conditions can have a significant impact on people's lives
2. Which of the following does Arthur need to know about?
   a. Medication management
   b. Exercise planning
   c. Diabetes management
   d. Skin care
   e. All of the above
   f. None of the above
3. Multimorbidity means:
   a. Having a long-term health condition
   b. Having a short-term health condition
   c. Having a few short-term health conditions
   d. Having more than one long-term health condition

REFERENCES

Australian Bureau of Statistics (ABS) (2017) Life tables, states, territories and Australia, 2014–2016. Cat. no. 3302.0.55.001. ABS, Canberra. Online. Available: www.abs.gov.au/AUSSTATS/abs@.nsf/Previousproducts/3302.0.55.001Main%20Features22014-2016?opendocument&tabname=Summary&prodno=3302.0.55.001&issue=2014-2016&num=&view=

Australian Bureau of Statistics (ABS) (2015) National health survey: first results, 2014–15. ABS cat. no. 4364.0.55.001. ABS, Canberra. Online. Available: www.ausstats.abs.gov.au/Ausstats/subscriber.nsf/0/CDA852A349B4CEE6CA257F150009FC53/$File/national%20health%20survey%20first%20results,%202014-15.pdf

Australian Government Department of Health (2017) National Strategic Framework for Chronic Conditions. Online. Available: www1.health.gov.au/internet/main/publishing.nsf/Content/nsfcc

Diabetes Australia (2020) Type 2 diabetes. Online. Available: www.diabetesaustralia.com.au/type-2-diabetes

Golinowska S, Sowa A, Deeg D et al (2016) Participation in formal learning activities of older Europeans in poor and good health. European Journal of Ageing 13:115–127.

Lee PG, Halter JB (2017) The pathophysiology of hyperglycemia in older adults. Clinical Considerations Diabetes Care 40(4):444–452.

Ministry of Health NZ (2020) Annual update of key results 2016/17: New Zealand Health Survey. Online. Available: www.health.govt.nz/publication/annual-update-key-results-2016-17-new-zealand-health-survey

Ministry of Health NZ (2017) Long-term conditions outcomes framework. Online. Available: https://nsfl.health.govt.nz/dhb-planning-package/long-term-conditions-outcomes-framework

Ministry of Health NZ (2014) Health and independence report 2014. Online. Available: www.health.govt.nz/publication/health-and-independence-report-2014

MOPACT (2016) Project MOPACT – Mobilising the potential of active ageing in Europe. Online. Available: www.ncbi.nlm.nih.gov/pmc/articles/PMC6248541/

National Academy of Sciences (2018) Multimorbidity a priority for Global Health Research. Online. Available: https://acmedsci.ac.uk/file-download/82222577

National Institute for Health and Care Excellence (NICE) (2016) Multimorbidity: clinical assessment and management (NG56). Online. Available: www.nice.org.uk/guidance/ng56/resources/multimorbidity-clinical-assessment-and-management-pdf-1837516654789

Santilli V, Bernetti A, Mangone M et al (2014) Clinical definition of sarcopenia. Clinical cases in mineral and bone metabolism 11(3):177–180.

StatsNZ (2019) New Zealand abridged period life table: 2016–18 (final). Online. Available: www.stats.govt.nz/information-releases/new-zealand-abridged-period-life-table-201618-final

World Health Organisation (WHO) (2017) World health statistics 2017: Monitoring health for the SDGs. Online. Available: www.who.int/gho/publications/world_health_statistics/2017/en/

World Health Organisation (WHO) (2015) World report on ageing and health. Online. Available: www.who.int/ageing/events/world-report-2015-launch/en/

World Health Organisation (WHO) (2002) Active ageing: a policy framework. Online. Available: www.who.int/ageing/publications/active_ageing/en/

CHAPTER 10

Infection Prevention and Control

NORMAN DAVIES

LEARNING OBJECTIVES

After reading this chapter, you will be able to:

- describe measures taken to reduce infection in older people in Australia and New Zealand
- define and explain infection control principles
- discuss challenges and opportunities to prevent infection in older people
- understand the challenges of preventing norovirus and influenza in the older population
- understand presenteeism and discuss the effects on the older population.

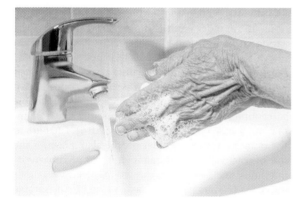

INTRODUCTION

As described in Chapter 2, the world's population is ageing rapidly and estimated to reach two billion people aged 65 years and over by 2050 (Bloom et al 2015; Buckinx et al 2015; World Health Organisation (WHO) 2015). Caring for older people is an expanding speciality, with more people over the age of 65 years now receiving supported care in private homes, as well as in residential aged care facilities. Regardless of the care environment, the older person is more susceptible to infections for a variety of reasons, including reduced immunity and underlying age-related co-morbidities.

Successful infection prevention and control involves implementing work practices that minimise the risk of transmission of infectious agents between staff and the people they care for (National Health and Medical Research Council (NHMRC) 2019). These work practices are known as *standard precautions* and *transmission-based precautions*, and these should be used at all times when providing care.

Standard precautions include:
- hand hygiene
- the appropriate use of personal protective equipment (PPE)
- sharps safety
- environmental cleaning
- spill management
- linen and waste management
- the cleaning of shared equipment
- aseptic technique.

Transmission-based precautions include:

- contact precautions
- droplet precautions
- airborne precautions.

The need to understand the principles of infection prevention and control, therefore, has become more important to both older people and those who provide care. The application of these principles is vital in protecting this cohort and those responsible for their care, as well as reducing the number of infections affecting older people in the community, residential aged care facilities and hospitals. This chapter addresses many of the issues associated with infection prevention and control in the older population.

HAND HYGIENE

Healthcare-associated infections (HAIs) are a global problem which affect hundreds of millions of patients annually worldwide. Hand hygiene has been recognised as the single most important preventative measure to prevent these infections (Russo et al 2012). Hand hygiene should become habitual practice by healthcare workers (Azim & McLaws 2014).

Hand Hygiene Australia (HHA) has adopted the WHO's 'Five Moments of Hand Hygiene' as the best way to minimise the transmission of microorganisms between healthcare workers, those they care for and the environment (Hand Hygiene Australia 2019). The five moments recommended for cleaning hands are:

1. Before touching a patient/resident.
2. Before a procedure.
3. After a procedure or body fluid exposure risk.
4. After touching a patient/resident.
5. After leaving a patient/resident's surroundings.

Hand hygiene can be performed by using alcohol-based hand rubs and should be used for all clinical situations where hands are visibly clean. Alcohol-based hand rubs, which need to contain 60%–80% alcohol, have excellent antimicrobial activity against most bacteria and enveloped viruses (Hand Hygiene Australia 2019). Hands should be washed with soap and water when:

- visibly dirty
- contaminated with proteinaceous material, blood or other body fluids
- exposed to potentially spore forming organisms
- after using the bathroom (Hand Hygiene Australia 2019).

Poor hand hygiene among healthcare workers is associated with infection transmission and is a major factor in the spread of antibiotic resistant organisms (Hand Hygiene Australia 2019). Despite this, the Hand Hygiene Initiative Manual (Australian Commission on Safety and Quality in Health Care (ACSQHC) 2019) notes that there remain barriers to appropriate hand hygiene, which include:

- hand hygiene agents causing skin irritation
- the perception that the patient needs to take priority over hand hygiene
- inconvenient location of handwashing facilities
- high workloads with insufficient time to perform hand hygiene
- inadequate knowledge of policies, guidelines and hand washing techniques
- few positive role models
- often staff simply forgetting to clean their hands.

Other barriers include the presence of jewellery and watches on hands and wrists, and long or artificial fingernails (ACSQHC 2019). As stated, hand hygiene is a vital part of infection prevention and control and is especially important when providing care to older people, who are more vulnerable to diseases for a number of reasons.

AGE-RELATED CHANGES IN THE IMMUNE SYSTEM

As humans age, there are significant changes to both innate and adaptive immunity, and these changes are thought to contribute to the increased frequency of infections in the older adult (Kline & Bowdish 2016). The ageing immune system loses its ability to protect against infections and cancer, and fails to support appropriate wound healing. The inflammatory response mediated by the innate immune system is also of concern as it gains intensity and duration, rendering older people susceptible to tissue-damaging immunity and inflammatory disease (Weyand & Goronzy 2016). Changes to the immune system in older people also increases the risk of reactivation of dormant viral and mycobacterial infections, and predisposes this group to new exogenous infections (Navaratnarajah & Jackson 2017). An example of the reactivation of a dormant virus is the varicella-zoster virus, which initially causes chickenpox and can then reappear as shingles in later life. About half of people who live to 80 years will be affected by shingles and between 13% and 26% of these will develop complications. The most common complication of shingles is post-herpetic neuralgia, which occurs in about 20% of cases of people aged >80 years, which is three times higher in this group when compared with people aged

Research Highlight
New and Emerging Diseases

Greater than 75% of emerging diseases are zoonotic in origin, meaning that they originate in animals and are able to jump the species barrier to humans (Mackenzie & Williams 2020). Over recent decades there has been an increasing number of infectious diseases that have been transmitted from animal hosts to humans, causing disease. The majority of these infections have been viral, one example being HIV/AIDS in the 1980s, which is thought to have originated from the great apes as early as the 1920s (Mackenzie & Williams 2020). Other examples, such as the severe acute respiratory syndrome coronavirus (SARS-CoV) in 2002–03, originated from bats; Middle East respiratory syndrome coronavirus (MERS-CoV) in 2012, originated from dromedary camels, although it is thought to also originate in bats, and more recently, CoV-2 or COVID-19 (corona virus disease 2019), as it has been officially named. This last infection is also thought to have originated in bats, but via a currently unidentified intermediary host such as a pangolin (Mackenzie & Williams 2020).

Coronaviruses are important pathogens for humans and animals, usually associated with respiratory and gastrointestinal infections (Salata et al 2019). Coronaviruses are enveloped viruses which have been considered minor pathogens for humans and are associated with the common cold or minor respiratory infections in immunocompetent people. Severe infections have been reported in infants and older people (Salata et al 2019).

SARS-CoV mainly presented as severe pneumonia with a fatality rate of about 10%, and originated in the Guangdong province of China, affecting 29 countries due to diffusion via travel (Salata et al 2019). Due to strong international action, infections from this virus were limited, and did not reach pandemic proportions.

In 2012, a new lethal zoonotic disease was described in the Middle East, identified in the Kingdom of Saudi Arabia.

The cause of this disease was identified as a coronavirus and has been named MERS-CoV. This illness has a fatality rate of almost 35%, and infections are still occurring (Salata et al 2019).

In December 2019, reports of an outbreak of a new respiratory disease from Wuhan, China, emerged; the origin of the outbreak was traced to a live animal market. Clinical signs of the infection included fever, cough and breathing difficulties, with pneumonia occurring in severe cases. The causative agent was identified as a new or novel coronavirus, provisionally called 2019-nCoV, and later formally named COVID-19 (Salata et al 2019). The first case occurring outside of China was documented in Thailand on 13 January 2020 and human-to-human transmission was confirmed on 21 January 2020. On 30 January 2020, the WHO declared a Public Health Emergency of International Concern.

Australia implemented a number of precautionary measures to limit the spread of infection, which included social distancing, increased hand hygiene awareness, limiting the numbers of people at any public function, and closing borders to international and interstate travel. Some states introduced intrastate travel limitations as well. Limitations on visiting residential aged care facilities were also introduced, however, as at mid-June 2020, 68 residents of care facilities had been infected with the virus resulting in 29 deaths.

It is interesting to note that 62% of all cases in Australia have been acquired overseas, some 28% being contacts of confirmed cases, with less than 10% being locally acquired where a contact has not been identified (Australian Government Department of Health 2020a). This indicates that community transmission is very low in Australia.

Australian Government Department of Health (2020a); Mackenzie & Williams (2020); Salata et al (2019).

20–59 years (Australian Government Department of Health 2020c).

Older people, therefore, are more likely to have age-related co-morbidities, placing them at the forefront of infection statistics. These co-morbidities include conditions such as diabetes mellitus, dementia, atherosclerosis, malnutrition, as well as functional impairment.

Vulnerability to Infection

Older people are more vulnerable to a number of infections, including pneumonia, urinary tract infections, skin and soft tissue infections, as well as latent and reactivated infections, as described above (Kline & Bowdish 2016). The older population are more susceptible to infections for a variety of reasons, such as:

- impaired mental and functional status
- length of stay in hospitals and care facilities
- the emergence of multi-resistant organisms
- antimicrobial prescribing patterns (Bellard-Smith 2013).

Physiological and immunological changes that occur with age compound the presentation and diagnosis of

---

Promoting Wellness
Standard Precautions Should Be Used When Dealing With Every Resident Regardless of Diagnosis

1. Remember the '5 Moments of Hand Hygiene', using either alcohol-based hand rub or soap.
2. Practise good general hygiene
3. Practise physical distancing where possible
4. Follow the limits for public gatherings
5. Understand how to isolate if required
6. If unsure, contact the National Coronavirus Helpline – 1800 020 080
7. Staff immunity assessed and vaccinated against vaccine preventable diseases as recommended.
8. Staff with communicable disease excluded from work in accordance with guidelines.

Australian Government Department of Health (2020a).

---

infectious diseases in older people (Kline & Bowdish 2016). Fevers are often muted and white cells may not increase to the same extent as in younger adults, potentially causing infections to be missed.

Older people may be more susceptible to urinary tract infections due to incomplete bladder emptying and, in the case of older females, recurrent urinary tract infections may be associated with frequent soiling of the perineum or atrophic vaginitis (thinning, drying, inflammation of the vaginal walls due to low oestrogen levels). Therefore, management of these issues should be addressed. In older men, recurrent urinary tract infections are often due to bacterial prostatitis and these issues should be investigated and treated (National Centre for Antimicrobial Stewardship 2019b).

Ageing is a natural process of organismal decay with a decline in cellular function. There is a reduction of bacterial diversity in older people (Bana & Cabreiro 2019). These changes to the gut and respiratory tract microbiome make older people more susceptible to infections such as *Clostridioides difficile* and pneumonia caused by *Streptococcus pneumoniae*. Decreased renal function in older people can alter the pharmacokinetics (see Chapter 11) of antibiotic treatment, which can lead to this treatment being less effective (Kline & Bowdish 2016).

As the older person is more susceptible to infection, it is vital that basic hygiene measures are implemented to minimise the risk of transmission of infectious agents between staff and patients/residents. The basis of good hygiene begins with adequate hand hygiene following the '5 Moments for Hand Hygiene' (Hand Hygiene Australia 2019), previously discussed.

In order to promote optimal management of antimicrobials (antibiotics) and to maximise the effectiveness of treatment, it is vital that antimicrobial therapy is targeted and appropriate. Antimicrobial prescribing should be based on careful clinical assessment and ensure that the benefits of antimicrobial use outweigh potential harm. National guidelines, such as the Therapeutic Guidelines: Antibiotic, should form the basis of prescribing recommendations. These Australian guidelines are the leading source of independent advice on the treatment of infectious diseases (Therapeutic Guidelines 2020). Documentation for all antimicrobial prescriptions should be clear to enable effective communication between all staff members, with the care recipient also receiving clear, easy-to-understand information about their clinical condition and treatment. Antimicrobial prescriptions should be regularly reviewed and refined where necessary, based upon the person's clinical progress and available clinical information, such as pathology results (National Centre for Antimicrobial Stewardship 2019a).

Older people may receive some protection against more common diseases, such as influenza and pneumonia. This protection is through vaccination or immunisation, and specific immunisation schedules are advised for older people (Australian Government Department of Health 2020c).

VACCINATION SCHEDULE FOR OLDER ADULTS

The older person is at increased risk from some vaccine-preventable diseases and serious complications from these diseases, even if they are otherwise healthy. In order to minimise the risk of infection from these diseases, it is recommended that older people be assessed and appropriate vaccines administered (Australian Government Department of Health 2020c). It is recommended in the *Australian Immunisation Handbook* (Australian Government Department of Health 2020c) that adults born during or after 1966 should be assessed as to whether they have received a measles, mumps and rubella (MMR) vaccine. As MMR vaccine was introduced in 1966, any person born prior to that date is assumed to have natural immunity to these diseases. If a person born after this date has not had two doses of MMR vaccine, they should be offered two doses one month apart. In New Zealand, the measles vaccine is recommended and available free for people born in 1969 or later (Ministry of Health NZ 2020c).

Invasive pneumococcal disease is more prevalent in adults over the age of 65 years, as well as in some other groups, such as Aboriginal and Torres Strait Islanders (Australian Government Department of Health 2020b) and Māori and Pacific peoples (Health Navigator New Zealand 2020b). These populations should also be offered pneumococcal vaccine, as well as an annual influenza vaccination. Since 2018, different influenza vaccines have been available for adults over 65 years of age. These vaccines are either a high-dose vaccine (containing four times the amount of each antigen compared with the standard vaccines) or a vaccine containing an adjuvant to improve the immune response in the recipient. As the incidence of shingles increases with age, along with the serious complications such as post-herpetic neuralgia, people aged 70–79 years should also be offered a dose of zoster vaccine. These vaccines are funded under the National Immunisation Program (Australian Government Department of Health 2020c) and under the National Immunisation Schedule in New Zealand (Ministry of Health NZ 2020c). As immunity to some diseases may begin to wane in older people, booster vaccines should also be considered. Adults aged ≥ 65 years should be offered a booster dose of vaccine against diphtheria, tetanus and pertussis (dTpa) if their last dose was more than 10 years ago (Australian Government Department of Health 2020c). The current Australian immunisation guidelines for people aged 65 years and over are available on the Australian Government Department of Health (2020c) website – Immunisation for Seniors. The New Zealand immunisation schedule is available on the Ministry of Health website (2020b).

COMMON INFECTIONS

There are some infections that are not uncommon in older people, especially those living in residential aged care facilities, and can cause outbreaks of disease. The two organisms that are responsible for most outbreaks in residential aged care facilities are norovirus and influenza.

Norovirus

Norovirus infections are caused by a non-enveloped virus and account for over 90% of all gastroenteritis cases and about 50% of outbreaks worldwide (Ong 2013). The incubation period ranges from 10–50 hours and the virus remains communicable, with a significant risk of person-to-person transmission when the person is symptomatic and up to 48 hours after diarrhoea ceases (Ministry of Health NZ 2020c). Symptoms usually begin abruptly and include:
- diarrhoea
- nausea and vomiting
- cramp-like abdominal pain
- low grade fever (Healthdirect 2020).

Symptoms usually last 1–2 days, but can be severe and long-lasting in older people and those with a compromised immune system. The following symptoms warrant referral to a doctor:
- diarrhoea lasting more than 2 days
- signs of dehydration – small amounts of dark urine and/or dry mouth
- high fever
- becoming pale or limp
- unusual fatigue, drowsiness or irritability
- severe pain in abdomen or rectum
- bloody or black diarrhoea (Healthdirect 2020; Health Navigator New Zealand 2020a).

It is estimated that there are 1.8 million cases of norovirus infection in Australia annually, and that cases may be sporadic or part of outbreaks in either the community or healthcare settings. There are also an estimated 50,000 cases in New Zealand each year (Toi Te Ora Public Health 2020). It is estimated that 17% of residential aged care facilities in Australia experience an outbreak of gastroenteritis annually, and that most of these outbreaks occur in Australia's winter (Latta et al 2018). A number of transmission routes were identified by Ong (2013), and these included waterborne (drinking water or recreational), foodborne (contaminated, undercooked food including salads, or improper hand hygiene by an infected food handler) and, probably the most common form of transmission in the elderly, person-to-person (via contamination from faeces or vomitus). Outbreaks of gastrointestinal illness in residential aged care facilities are defined as two or more staff or resident presenting with symptoms of vomiting and/or diarrhoea within 24 hours (NHMRC 2019).

These cases incur substantial costs and can be difficult to control in healthcare institutions or other closed settings. The difficulty in controlling norovirus infections is due to several factors which include the human immune response, environmental survival, multiple transmission routes and the low infectious dose. Ong (2013) notes that the ID_{50} (the dose required to cause infection in 50% of exposed subjects) is as low as 18 virions. Even after symptoms subside, it is recognised that there is often asymptomatic shedding of the virus which can prolong outbreaks where environmental cleaning is inadequate (Ong 2013).

Laboratory studies suggest that alcohol-based hand hygiene products are less active against non-enveloped viruses than washing with soap, followed by a water rinse. Current Australian and New Zealand guidelines recommend that hand hygiene should be performed using soap and water when *C. difficile* or non-enveloped viruses such as norovirus are known or suspected (Healthdirect 2020; Health Navigator New Zealand 2020a).

There is no clinical vaccine available, nor is there any specific antiviral treatment for norovirus infection. Treatment relies on electrolyte replacement, anti-emetics and analgesics, if required (Ong 2013).

Influenza

Influenza is caused by a virus that can affect the respiratory system. It spreads from person to person through coughing, sneezing and close contact, such as kissing and sharing food and drinks (Australian Government Department of Health 2019b). In 2019, there were over 300,000 cases of influenza in Australia. Over the past four years, there have been on average almost 180,000 cases (Australian Government Department of Health 2019a; Immunisation Coalition 2019b). In New Zealand, influenza affects 10–20% of the population each year (Ministry of Health NZ 2020a). Influenza outbreaks usually occur in the winter months; however, unseasonal outbreaks can occur (Davies et al 2019). Outbreaks of influenza-like illness in residential aged care facilities are defined as three or more staff or residents presenting with symptoms of an influenza-like illness within 72 hours (NHMRC 2019).

Influenza symptoms are different to those of a cold. Influenza symptoms include fever, headaches, tiredness and muscle aches. These symptoms are often absent with a cold, start suddenly and can affect people of any age, with infection rates often higher in the young and the older population (Australian Government Department of Health 2019b). In 2019, just over 800 influenza-associated deaths were recorded, with a median age of 86 years; however, these reports do not represent the true mortality associated with the disease (Australian Government Department of Health 2019b).

Currently the single-best prevention is to receive the annual influenza vaccine. This is especially important for those at risk of complications (Immunisation Advisory Centre 2020; Immunisation Coalition 2019a;). Other ways to prevent infection with this virus are to practise good respiratory etiquette, use tissues, which are disposed of in bins, and perform hand hygiene after disposal. Good hand hygiene can limit the spread and

should be performed after contact with someone with influenza, before touching your mouth and face, and before preparing or eating food (Immunisation Coalition 2019a).

Treatment of uncomplicated influenza usually involves bed rest and analgesia for muscle aches and pains. Two main classes of drugs that have been used for treatment and prophylaxis of influenza include neuraminidase inhibitors and adamantanes (Robson et al 2019). Neuraminidase inhibitors prevent the virus escaping from the host cell and should be started within 48 hours of the onset of symptoms, usually being effective within 24 hours. Three neuraminidase inhibitors are registered in Australia – oral oseltamivir, inhaled zanamivir and intravenous peramivir. These drugs have been shown to shorten the duration of symptoms in uncomplicated influenza by approximately one day. The adamantanes are not recommended due to widespread resistance in circulating influenza viruses (Robson et al 2019).

The part played by staff in the transmission of these diseases should not be underestimated, and it is possible for staff to transmit diseases when they attend work while unwell themselves. This phenomenon, known as presenteeism, is not uncommon.

Research Highlights

- It is reported that that between 14% and 23% of healthcare workers in Queensland work while ill with influenza.
- When staff attend work with gastrointestinal symptoms, residents and fellow workers become affected.
- Attending work while unwell, known as presenteeism, is believed to be associated with pressure of work and perceived commitment, with many healthcare workers putting patients' needs first.

Imai et al (2019); Widera et al (2010).

Presenteeism

Presenteeism is when an employee attends work while impaired or may be defined as health-related productivity loss (McGregor 2017). While this phenomenon has been studied in the business and social literature, it carries increased importance in the healthcare setting due to the risk of infectious disease transmission in vulnerable populations, including older people (Widera et al 2010). It was reported by Imai and colleagues (2020) that

---

Tips for Best Practice
Prevention of Infection – Home-Based Care

Standard precautions should be used when dealing with every client, regardless of their diagnosis.

1. Essential infection prevention and control education to be provided for all healthcare workers.

2. Remember the 5 Moments of Hand Hygiene, using either alcohol-based hand rubs or soap and water.

3. Use transmission-based precautions where standard precautions may not be sufficient. These include:

   a. airborne precautions – P2/N95 respirator mask

   b. contact precautions – gloves/gown or apron

   c. droplet precautions – surgical mask and face shield/safety glasses

4. Soap and water must be used if hands are visibly soiled.

5. Preferably use your own hand hygiene products in a client's home.

6. Use personal protective equipment (PPE) appropriately: Perform a risk assessment – ask yourself if you could be contaminated with blood or body fluids; if the answer is yes, what part could be contaminated?

   a. If hands – wear gloves.

   b. If face – wear face protection.

   c. If clothing – wear apron or gown.

7. Use aseptic technique (clean, no-touch technique) when carrying out wound and similar care.

8. Surveillance should be carried out; however, in the home environment this is usually process surveillance rather than outcome surveillance.

9. Be aware of used needles in clients' homes, especially if they self-administer their own insulin.

10. Work with prescribers to comply with the facility's antimicrobial stewardship policy and program.

11. If preparing food for clients in their homes, be familiar with and practise food safety.

12. Encourage clients to be fully vaccinated.

NHMRC (2019), Rhinehart & McGoldrick (2006).

---

between 14% and 23% of healthcare workers in Queensland were working while ill with influenza.

In another study on presenteeism, Widera and colleagues (2010) described an outbreak of gastrointestinal disease in a 100-bed residential aged care facility which resulted in a total of 23 residents, and 18 staff members developing symptoms of nausea, vomiting and diarrhoea. It became obvious that staff members were attending work while unwell, despite recommendations to the contrary. Workers only reported symptoms after they arrived for work, or at the end of a shift. Management instituted a policy of clearance by Employee Health before returning to work, which slowed the outbreak; however, one staff member attended work with symptoms and, following this incident, two further residents presented with symptoms (Widera et al 2010). In the outbreak described by Widera and colleagues (2010), it emerged that if staff attended work with gastrointestinal symptoms, residents were becoming affected, as were fellow workers.

In these cases, it is obvious that when staff attend work while they are unwell themselves, they have the potential to infect not only those they care for, but also fellow workers. This was also emphasised by Chiu and colleagues (2017), who noted that healthcare workers attending work when unwell with influenza-like symptoms in the United States during the 2014–15 influenza season increased the likelihood of transmitting influenza to co-workers and patients.

The reasons for attending work while unwell are not clear; however, it is believed that presenteeism is often associated with pressure of work and perceived commitment to the job, with many healthcare workers putting the patient's needs above their own self-care needs (Imai et al 2020). It is apparent from these studies that the drivers of presenteeism are intricate and multifactorial and that strategies to change ill presenteeism behaviours among healthcare workers must be systematically implemented at institutional levels (Imai et al 2020).

Tips for Best Practice
Prevention of Infection – Residential Aged Care

Standard precautions to be used when dealing with all residents, regardless of diagnosis.

- Essential infection prevention and control education to be provided for all healthcare workers.
- Remember the 5 Moments of Hand Hygiene, using either alcohol-based hand rub or soap and water.
- Use transmission-based precautions where standard precautions may not be sufficient. These include:
  - airborne precautions – P2/N95 respirator mask
  - contact precautions – gloves/gown or apron
  - droplet precautions – surgical mask and face shield/safety glasses.
- Soap and water must be used if hands are visibly soiled.
- Encourage residents to be fully immunised.
- Screen staff for immune status on appointment, and also offer annual influenza vaccination.
- Work with prescribers to implement antimicrobial stewardship.
- Implement a surveillance program to identify and investigate infection trends.
- Be aware of subtle changes in behaviour – these might indicate an infection. Remember signs of infection may not be as clear-cut as in a younger person.
- Be on the lookout for multiple residents with similar symptoms (e.g. vomiting/diarrhoea, influenza-like illness) as these may be the start of an outbreak.
- Outbreaks of gastrointestinal disease are defined as two or more residents/staff presenting with symptoms of vomiting and/or diarrhoea within 24 hours.
- Outbreaks of influenza-like illness are defined as three or more residents/staff presenting with symptoms of an influenza-like illness within 72 hours.
- When an outbreak is suspected:
  - affected residents should be isolated if possible
  - ensure that hand hygiene is optimal; if necessary, provide refresher training for staff
  - implement appropriate transmission-based precautions
  - place a supply of personal protective equipment outside the rooms of affected residents
  - inform families and limit visits to the facility to essential visits only
  - increase environmental cleaning with an appropriate disinfectant, paying attention to high-touch surfaces.
- If the outbreak is widespread, limit communal activities in the facility.
- Inform the local Public Health Unit (PHU) of the possible outbreak, and send them a daily running sheet with details of all residents and staff affected.
- The PHU will advise when the outbreak is over – when no new cases of gastrointestinal disease have occurred for 48 hours, or no new cases of influenza-like illnesses have occurred in the last 5 days.
- If outbreak has been caused by norovirus, continue cleaning with disinfectants due to prolonged shedding of virus even after symptoms have ceased.
- React to possible outbreaks as quickly as possible. Quick reactions = shorter outbreaks.

Kendall (2003); National Centre for Antimicrobial Stewardship (2019a); NHMRC (2019).

Tips for Best Practice
Prevention of Infection – Acute Care

Standard precautions should be used when dealing with every resident, regardless of their diagnosis.

1. Essential infection prevention and control education to be provided for all healthcare workers.
2. Remember the 5 Moments of Hand hygiene, using either alcohol-based hand rub or soap.
3. Use transmission-based precautions where standard precautions may not be sufficient. These include:
   a. airborne precautions – P2/N95 respirator mask
   b. contact precautions – gloves/gown or apron
   c. droplet precautions – surgical mask and face shield/safety glasses.
4. Where transmission-based precautions are required, carry these out with the patient placed in isolation.
5. Soap and water must be used if hands are visibly soiled.
6. Assess staff immunity and vaccinate against vaccine-preventable diseases as recommended.
7. Exclude staff with communicable disease from work in accordance with guidelines.
8. Work with prescribers to comply with the facility's antimicrobial stewardship policy and program.

NHMRC (2019).

SUMMARY

Older people, especially those living in residential care facilities, are at risk of healthcare acquired infections. Contributing factors include shared living conditions, changes to the immune system and comorbidities. Training in infection prevention and control is vital for all staff, who should be familiar with all aspects of standard and transmission-based precautions that are routinely employed as a means of either preventing the transmission of infection or controlling outbreaks in facilities. Other important factors to assist in reducing the transmission of infections in older people include immunisation and the need for symptomatic staff to not attend work until they are well.

Practice Scenario

A care facility resident visited a casino. Shortly after the visit, she vomits and has an episode of diarrhoea. A resident in an adjoining room develops similar symptoms later that day, and by that evening, two further residents have similar symptoms.

MULTIPLE CHOICE QUESTIONS

1. What is the likely situation?
   a. The residents have overeaten
   b. This is a possible outbreak of norovirus
   c. Too many aperients have been given
   d. The residents have eaten food that disagrees with them
2. What initial steps should be taken?
   a. Residents should be isolated
   b. Transmission-based precautions should be implemented with appropriate PPE
   c. Increased environmental cleaning should be commenced
   d. All of the above
3. Normal visiting to the facility should be encouraged.
   a. True
   b. False
4. You are required to inform the local Public Health Unit of the outbreak.
   a. True
   b. False
5. An outbreak of gastrointestinal disease is considered over when:
   a. No new cases have occurred in the past 24 hours
   b. No new cases have occurred in the past 5 days
   c. No new cases have occurred in the past 72 hours
   d. No new cases have occurred in the past 48 hours

REFERENCES

Australian Commission on Safety and Quality in Health Care (ACSQHC) (2019) National Hand Hygiene Initiative Manual. Online. Available: www.safetyandquality.gov.au/publications-and-resources/resource-library/national-hand-hygiene-initiative-manual

Australian Government Department of Health (2020a) Coronavirus (COVID-19) health alert. Online. Available: www.health.gov.au/news/health-alerts/novel-coronavirus

-2019-ncov-health-alert?utm_source=health.gov
.au&utm_medium=redirect&utm_campaign=digital
_transformation&utm_content=health-topics/novel
-coronavirus-2019-ncov#protect-others-and-stop-the-spread

Australian Government Department of Health (2020b) Immunisation for Seniors. Online. Available: www.health.gov.au/health-topics/immunisation/immunisation-throughout-life/immunisation-for-seniors

Australian Government Department of Health (2020c) Vaccination for healthy ageing. Australian Immunisation Handbook 2020. Online. Available: https://immunisationhandbook.health.gov.au/resources/publications/vaccination-for-healthy-ageing

Australian Government Department of Health (2019a) Australian Influenza Surveillance Report, No 12 2019. Online. Available: www1.health.gov.au/internet/main/publishing.nsf/Content/cda-surveil-ozflu-flucurr.htm/$File/flu-12-2019.pdf

Australian Government Department of Health (2019b) The flu vaccine – Information for consumers in 2019 fact sheet. Online. Available: www.health.gov.au/health-topics/flu-influenza

Azim S, McLaws M (2014) Doctor, do you have a moment? National Hand Hygiene Initiative compliance in Australian hospitals. Medical Journal of Australia 200:1–4.

Bana B, Cabreiro F (2019) The microbiome and aging. Annual Review of Genetics 3(53):239–261.

Bellard-Smith L (2013) Infection control and aged care services. Australian Nursing Journal 20(8):44.

Bloom DE, Chatterji S, Kowal P et al (2015) Macroeconomic implications of population ageing and selected policy responses. The Lancet 385:649–657.

Buckinx F, Rolland Y, Reginster J-Y et al (2015) Burden of frailty in the elderly population: perspectives for a public health challenge. Archives of Public Health 73:19.

Chiu S, Black CL, Yue X et al (2017) Working with influenza-like illness: Presenteeism among US health care personnel during the 2014–2015 influenza season. American Journal of Infection Control 45(11):1254–1258.

Davies NJ, Gilles M, Els W et al (2019) Summer influenza outbreaks in two residential aged care facilities in Western Australia – A discussion paper. Unpublished manuscript.

Hand Hygiene Australia (2019) My 5 Moments for Hand Hygiene. Online. Available: www.hha.org.au/hand-hygiene/5-moments-for-hand-hygiene.

Healthdirect (2020) Norovirus infection. Online. Available: www.healthdirect.gov.au/norovirus-infection

Health Navigator New Zealand (2020a) Norovirus. Online. Available: www.healthnavigator.org.nz/health-a-z/n/norovirus/

Health Navigator New Zealand (2020b) Pneumococcal disease. Online. Available: www.healthnavigator.org.nz/health-a-z/p/pneumococcal-disease/#Overview

Imai C, Hall L, Lambert SB et al (2019) Presenteeism among healthcare workers with laboratory-confirmed influenza infection: A retrospective study in Queensland, Australia. American Journal of Infection Control 48(4):355–360.

Immunisation Advisory Centre (2020) Influenza information for health professionals. Online. Available: www.influenza.org.nz/news/ministry-health-immunisation-update-3-april-2020

Immunisation Coalition (2019a) Be smart about the flu. Online. Available: www.immunisationcoalition.org.au/immunisation/be-smart-about-flu/

Immunisation Coalition (2019b) Influenza statistics 2019. Online. Available: www.immunisationcoalition.org.au/news-media/2019-influenza-statistics/

Kendall KJ (2003) Practical approaches to infection control in residential aged care. 2nd edn. Ausmed Publications, Melbourne.

Kline KA, Bowdish DME (2016) Infection in an ageing population. Current Opinion in Microbiology 29:63–67.

Latta R, Eastwood K, Massey PD et al (2018) Outbreak management in residential aged care facilities – prevention and response strategies in regional Australia. Australian Journal of Advanced Nursing 35(3):6–13.

Mackenzie JS, Williams D (2020) Zoonoses. Microbiology Australia 41(1):3–5.

McGregor, A (2017) An investigation into the phenomenon of presenteeism: Examining antecedents and the operationalisation of presenteeism. PhD thesis, School of Psychology, University of Wollongong.

Ministry of Health NZ (2020a) Influenza. Online. Available: www.health.govt.nz/our-work/preventative-health-wellness/immunisation/influenza

Ministry of Health NZ (2020b) Measles. Online. Available: www.health.govt.nz/your-health/conditions-and-treatments/diseases-and-illnesses/measles

Ministry of Health NZ (2020c) National Immunisation Schedule. Online. Available: www.health.govt.nz/our-work/preventative-health-wellness/immunisation/new-zealand-immunisation-schedule

National Centre for Antimicrobial Stewardship (2019a) Australian Aged Care Home: Antimicrobial Stewardship Policy. Online. Available: https://irp-cdn.multiscreensite.com/d820f98f/files/uploaded/AMS%20Policy_PDF_March%2019.pdf

National Centre for Antimicrobial Stewardship (2019b) Urinary tract infection – Frequently asked questions. Online. Available: https://irp-cdn.multiscreensite.com/d820f98f/files/uploaded/Urinary%20Tract%20Infection%20-%20frequently%20asked%20questions.pdf

National Health and Medical Research Council (NHMRC) (2019) Australian guidelines for the prevention and control of infection in healthcare. Online. Available: www.nhmrc.gov.au/about-us/publications/australian-guidelines-prevention-and-control-infection-healthcare-2019

Navaratnarajah A, Jackson SHD (2017) The physiology of ageing. Medicine 45(1):6–10.

Ong CW (2013) Norovirus: a challenging pathogen. Healthcare Infection 18(4):133–142.

Rhinehart E, McGoldrick M (2006) Infection control in home care and hospice, 2nd edn. Jones and Bartlett Publishers, Sudbury, Massachusetts.

Robson C, Baskar SR, Booy R et al (2019) Influenza: overview on prevention and therapy. Australian Prescriber 42:51–55. https://doi.org/10.18773/austprescr.2019.013

Russo P, Pettir D, Grayson L (2012) Australia: a leader in hand hygiene. Healthcare Infection 17:1–2.

Salata C, Calistri A, Parolin C et al (2019) Coronavirus: a paradigm of new emerging zoonotic diseases. Pathogens and Disease 77(9):ftaa006. doi: 10.1093/femspd/ftaa006

Therapeutic Guidelines (2020) Antibiotics. Online. Available: https://tgldcdp.tg.org.au/searchAction?appendedInputButtons=antibiotic

Toi Te Ora Public Health (2020) Norovirus. Online. Available: www.toiteora.govt.nz/norovirus

Weyand CM, Goronzy JJ (2016) Ageing of the immune system, Mechanisms and therapeutic targets. Annals of the American Thoracic Society 13(Supp 5):S422–S428.

Widera E, Chang A, Chen HL (2010) Presenteeism: a public health hazard. Journal of General Internal Medicine 25(11): 1244–1247.

World Health Organisation (WHO) (2015) World report on ageing and health. Online. Available: https://apps.who.int/iris/bitstream/handle/10665/186463/9789240694811_eng.pdf?sequence=1

Safe Use of Medications

ANDREW STAFFORD

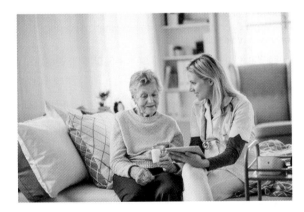

INTRODUCTION

Medication use is ubiquitous among older people living in Australia and New Zealand. While the intention of medication use is to improve quality of life and/or reduce mortality, older people are at a heightened risk of inadvertent medication-related harm. A person's need for medication changes as they age, as does the appropriateness of most medications. Nurses have a crucial role in ensuring that medications used in older people are safe and effective, to optimise benefits and minimise the risk of harm.

THE NEED FOR SAFE MEDICATION USE IN OLDER PEOPLE

Prevalence of Medication Use

The most common intervention in healthcare is the use of medication. Medication use is particularly prevalent in older people, who consume markedly more medication than younger people (Australian Institute of Health and Welfare [AIHW] 2018). Over 85% of Australians aged 50 years or older have reported using at least one medication within the previous 24 hours (Morgan et al 2012). Approximately one-third of Australians aged 65 years or older experience polypharmacy (defined as the use of five or more medications regularly), with the prevalence highest among those aged between 80 and

89 years (Page et al 2019). The situation is similar in New Zealand, where the nationwide prevalence of polypharmacy among people aged 65 years or older increased from 23.4% in 2005 to 29.5% in 2013 (Nishtala & Salahudeen 2015). In both countries, the most commonly used medications groups among older people include antihypertensive agents, lipid-lowering agents and anticoagulants.

Table 11.1 lists medications commonly used in older people living in Australia and New Zealand, and specific considerations for their use in this population.

Text continued on p. 107

TABLE 11.1

Specific Considerations for Medication Classes Commonly Used in Older People in Australia and New Zealand

MEDICATION GROUP		
Body system		
Class	**Examples**	**Specific considerations when used in older people**
Alimentary tract and metabolism		
Proton pump inhibitors	Esomeprazole Lansoprazole Omeprazole Pantoprazole Rabeprazole	Generally safe for short-term use; may alter absorption of medications where this is dependent upon gastric pH Most are metabolised via cytochrome P450 isozymes, and may inhibit 2C19; drug–drug interactions may occur Observational studies have associated long-term use with a number of conditions, e.g. fracture, pneumonia, hypomagnesaemia, vitamin B_{12} deficiency, cognitive decline/dementia, *Clostridium difficile* colitis (Kanno & Moayyedi 2019)
Drugs used in diabetes - biguanides	Metformin	Minimal risk of hypoglycaemia Renally cleared. Dose reduction required in renal impairment; contraindicated if GFR < 30 mL/min/1.73 m^2 Risk of lactic acidosis with chronic heart failure and hepatic dysfunction (Longo et al 2019) Associated with vitamin B_{12} deficiency, particularly when used long term at higher doses (Valencia et al 2018)
Drugs used in diabetes - sulfonylureas	Gliclazide Glibenclamide	Risk of hypoglycaemia; long-acting sulfonylureas (e.g. glibenclamide) are inappropriate in older people due to elevated risk of hypoglycaemia (Longo et al 2019)
Drugs for constipation	Docusate & senna Lactulose Macrogol	Osmotic laxatives are generally the most effective laxative treatment for older people with chronic constipation Macrogol is more effective than lactulose, and may be better tolerated (Emmanuel et al 2017)
Anti-emetics and anti-nauseants	Metoclopramide Prochlorperazine	Increased risk of CNS adverse effects (e.g. sedation, dizziness) Metoclopramide and prochlorperazine may exacerbate Parkinson's disease; domperidone is generally an appropriate alternative (AMH 2018)
Mineral supplements	Calcium carbonate Colecalciferol	Vitamin D and calcium supplementation appear to be most effective for prevention of fracture when used in older, institutionalised people vulnerable to vitamin D deficiency and at a high fracture risk. Supplementation is of questionable benefit in community-dwelling older people for primary prevention of fracture (Bischoff-Ferrari 2019; Cameron et al 2018) Avoid high-dose bolus administration of vitamin D supplements as these may increase falls risk

TABLE 11.1

Specific Considerations for Medication Classes Commonly Used in Older People in Australia and New Zealand—cont'd

MEDICATION GROUP		
Body system		
Class	*Examples*	**Specific considerations when used in older people**
Blood and blood forming organs		
Anticoagulant agents	Apixaban Rivaroxaban Warfarin	Direct oral anticoagulants are renally cleared; most require dose adjustment in older people with renal impairment When used for atrial fibrillation, apixaban and dabigatran are associated with a lower bleeding risk than warfarin and rivaroxaban in older people (Lobraico-Fernandez et al 2019) Many medications may interact with warfarin; check INR regularly when any changes are made to the medication regimen The target INR for older people using warfarin is the same as for younger people; there is no role for low-intensity treatment (SPAF 1996)
Antiplatelet agents	Aspirin (low dose) Clopidogrel	Low-dose aspirin is of minimal benefit for primary prevention of vascular events in people aged ≥ 70 years, but increases the risk of major haemorrhage (hazard ratio 1.38, 95% CI 1.18–1.62, $p < 0.001$) (Patrono & Baigent 2019) Gastrointestinal bleeding associated with low-dose aspirin use for secondary prevention in people aged ≥75 years is markedly more common and disabling or fatal, compared to younger people (Li et al 2017) Clopidogrel use in people aged ≥ 70 years post-acute coronary syndrome is associated with a lower bleeding risk than more potent antiplatelet agents (e.g. ticagrelor or prasugrel) (Gimbel 2019)
Anti-anaemic preparations	Iron sulphate	Once haemoglobin concentration is normal, continue oral iron supplementation for at least 3 months to replenish iron stores (Busti et al 2019) Avoid unnecessary long-term use of iron supplements Iron deficiency in older people is often due to occult gastrointestinal bleeding Concomitant inflammatory disorders may complicate the interpretation of iron stores (i.e. serum ferritin level)
Cardiovascular system		
Agents acting on the renin-angiotensin system	Perindopril Ramipril Candesartan Irbesartan Telmisartan	When used for hypertension or heart failure with reduced ejection fraction, ACE inhibitors and angiotensin receptor blockers confer similar cardiovascular and mortality benefits in older people compared to those aged > 65 years (Osmanska & Jhund 2019; Thomopoulos et al 2018) Adverse effects of hypotension and renal impairment may be more pronounced in older people (Osmanska & Jhund 2019)

Continued

TABLE 11.1

Specific Considerations for Medication Classes Commonly Used in Older People in Australia and New Zealand—cont'd

MEDICATION GROUP		
Body system		
Class	*Examples*	**Specific considerations when used in older people**
Lipid modifying agents	Atorvastatin Rosuvastatin Simvastatin	Statins do not appear to reduce major vascular events in people aged > 75 years without vascular disease, vascular death or death from any cause (Heneghan & Mahtani 2019) For people aged >75 with vascular disease, the number needed to treat (NNT) to reduce one major vascular event is 98 (NNT 54 to 735); statin treatment does not reduce the risk of all-cause mortality (Heneghan & Mahtani 2019) Statins are generally well tolerated by older people; there is limited evidence that the risk of statin-induced myopathy and rhabdomyolysis increases with age (Yandrapalli et al 2019). Monitor creatine kinase and clinically, particularly in people who are frail, of small body frame or with renal impairment
Calcium channel blockers	Amlodipine Lercanidipine	Dihydropyridine calcium channel blockers (e.g. amlodipine, lercanidipine) are generally well tolerated in older people (Pont & Alhawassi 2017) Confer similar cardiovascular and mortality benefits in older people compared to those aged > 65 years when used for hypertension (Thomopoulos et al 2018)
Beta blocking agents	Atenolol Metoprolol	Nebivolol use for heart failure in people aged >70 years was associated with a 14% reduction in all-cause mortality and hospitalisation compared with placebo (hazard ratio 0.86, 95% confidence interval 0.74–0.99, p = 0.039) (Flather et al 2005) Less beneficial than alternative antihypertensives in older people compared to those aged > 65 years when used for hypertension, in terms of cardiovascular and mortality benefits (Thomopoulos et al 2018) Bradycardia and hypotension may be more common in older people (Osmanska & Jhund 2019)
Diuretics	Furosemide (Frusemide) Hydrochlorothiazide	Low doses of thiazide diuretics are equally effective for hypertension as higher doses, with a lower risk of adverse electrolyte and metabolic effects (Sommerauer et al 2017) Confer similar cardiovascular and mortality benefits in older people compared to those aged > 65 years when used for hypertension (Thomopoulos et al 2018)
Genitourinary system and sex hormones		
Urologicals	Oxybutynin Tolterodine	Generally of limited benefit for most people; on average, reduce episodes of incontinence by 0.5 to 0.7 per day (Woodford 2018) Frequently cause dry mouth and constipation Associated with causing or exacerbating cognitive impairment (Woodford 2018)

TABLE 11.1

Specific Considerations for Medication Classes Commonly Used in Older People in Australia and New Zealand—cont'd

MEDICATION GROUP		
Body system		
Class	*Examples*	**Specific considerations when used in older people**
Musculoskeletal system		
Anti-inflammatory and antirheumatic products	Celecoxib Meloxicam	Older people are at an increased risk of gastrointestinal bleeding, acute kidney injury and cardiovascular events due to oral NSAID use (Wongrakpanich et al 2018)
		Should an oral NSAID be required, low-dose, short-term use is recommended. Concomitant administration of proton pump inhibitor or H$_2$ antagonist may reduce the risk of gastrointestinal bleeding (Ali et al 2018)
Drugs for treatment of bone diseases	Alendronate Risedronate Denosumab	Cessation of oral bisphosphonate treatment of osteoporosis may be considered after 5–10 years in postmenopausal women and men over the age of 50 with osteoporosis who have responded well to treatment (T-score ≥–2.5 and no recent fractures) (RACGP 2017)
		Osteonecrosis of the jaw rarely occurs with denosumab or oral bisphosphonate therapy for osteoporosis; it most commonly occurs in people with malignancy-related skeletal conditions receiving high doses of IV bisphosphonates (Alejandro & Constantinescu 2018)
		Long-term use of bisphosphonates and denosumab is associated with an increased, albeit low overall, risk of atypical femoral shaft fractures
		Unlike bisphosphonates, denosumab may be used in people with advanced renal impairment; monitor serum calcium levels and for symptoms of hypocalcaemia
		The effects of denosumab on bone reverse shortly after its cessation, and there is evidence of an increased risk of multiple vertebral fractures after its cessation (Deeks 2018)
Anti-gout preparations	Allopurinol Colchicine	Hypersensitivity reactions to allopurinol appear to be related to higher starting doses; it should be commenced at a low dose and gradually increased (Stamp & Chapman 2014)
		The dose of allopurinol should be increased to achieve a serum urate level of <0.36 mmol/L
		Colchicine clearance is decreased with renal impairment, and the risk of toxicity is increased; should colchicine be used, low doses are recommended to treat gout flares (Abhishek 2017)
Nervous system		
Antipsychotics	Olanzapine Risperidone	Antipsychotics only have evidence for efficacy in treating psychosis, agitation and aggression, but not other behavioural and psychological symptoms of dementia (see Chapter 26). Efficacy is modest for these indications (Bessey & Walaszek 2019)
		Associated with a high risk of serious adverse effects; limit treatment to short-term use at the lowest possible dose

Continued

TABLE 11.1
Specific Considerations for Medication Classes Commonly Used in Older People in Australia and New Zealand—cont'd

MEDICATION GROUP		
Body system		
Class	*Examples*	**Specific considerations when used in older people**
Analgesics – non-opioid	Paracetamol	Use at normal adult doses for most older people In frail older people of low body weight (< 50 kg), or those with renal or hepatic impairment, consider lower doses or reduced frequency of administration (DTB 2018)
Analgesics – opioids	Codeine Oxycodone Tramadol	Lower doses are generally required than those used in younger people; commence at the lower end of the dosing range using a short acting preparation (AMH 2019) Older people are more susceptible to respiratory depression; assess by degree of sedation and not respiratory rate Tramadol also has serotonergic properties and is associated with a risk of seizures and serotonin toxicity when used with antidepressants (Makris et al 2014)
Antidepressants - SSRIs*	Escitalopram Sertraline	SSRIs may cause syndrome of inappropriate antidiuretic hormone (SIADH) and hyponatraemia, particularly people also using diuretics (Sultana et al 2015) Citalopram and escitalopram increase the risk of arrhythmia (Sultana et al 2015); obtain a baseline ECG in people with existing cardiac disease SSRIs are associated with an increased risk of falls and fracture
Antidepressants - other	Amitriptyline Desvenlafaxine Mirtazapine Venlafaxine	Tricyclic antidepressants (e.g. amitriptyline, dosulepin) are sedating and have anticholinergic properties. They are also associated with postural hypotension, falls, arrhythmias and sudden cardiac death (Sultana et al 2015) Desvenlafaxine and duloxetine may cause postural hypotension yet increase blood pressure at high doses; monitor standing and sitting blood pressure
Gabapentinoid antiepileptics	Gabapentin Pregabalin	Excreted unchanged in the urine; dose adjustment required in renal impairment (Motika & Spencer 2016) May cause peripheral oedema and weight gain
Benzodiazepines	Diazepam Oxazepam Temazepam	Associated with a dose-dependent increased risk of falls and fractures (Markota et al 2016) May cause cognitive impairment, which may be irreversible in some patients May be safely withdrawn in long-term users via appropriate tapering regimens; abrupt cessation may cause seizures and rebound anxiety (Markota et al 2016)
Drugs that treat dementia	Donepezil Galantamine Rivastigmine	May be considered for Alzheimer's disease, vascular dementia, dementia with Lewy bodies or Parkinson's disease dementia (Knight et al 2018) Efficacy is modest for most patients (Knight et al 2018); as currently available agents do not modify the underlying disease processes, cease treatment if no benefit is observed Consider a trial of cessation after 12 months' treatment if the condition has deteriorated (Reeve et al 2019)

TABLE 11.1
Specific Considerations for Medication Classes Commonly Used in Older People in Australia and New Zealand—cont'd

MEDICATION GROUP		
Body system		
Class	*Examples*	**Specific considerations when used in older people**
Respiratory system		
Drugs for obstructive airway diseases	Salbutamol Tiotropium	Adverse effects of beta agonists (e.g. salbutamol, salmeterol, eformoterol) may exacerbate coexisting conditions (e.g. tachycardia, tremor)
		Inhaled anticholinergics (e.g. tiotropium, glycopyrrolate) occasionally cause systemic adverse effects
		Administration devices vary in complexity; regularly assess patients' ability to correctly use inhaled medications (Cortopassi et al 2017)
Systemic hormonal preparations		
Corticosteroids for systemic use	Prednisolone	Many co-morbidities that may be exacerbated by oral corticosteroids are more prevalent in older people (e.g. diabetes mellitus, osteoporosis); additional monitoring may be required
		Short-term use (< 30 days) is associated with an increased risk of sepsis, venous thromboembolism and fracture (Waljee et al 2017)
		Oral corticosteroids increase the risk of gastrointestinal bleeding; gastric protection with a proton pump inhibitor may be required
Thyroid therapy	Levothyroxine	Older people are at heightened risk of cardiovascular effects from excessive levothyroxine; commence at low doses (e.g. 25–50 microg/day) and adjust dose every 6 to 8 weeks if necessary (Duntas & Yen 2019)
		Levothyroxine does not appear to be of benefit in older people with subclinical hypothyroidism (Stott et al 2017)

*SSRIs – selective serotonin reuptake inhibitors

Polypharmacy

The term polypharmacy generally has negative connotations, as it has been associated with a broad range of negative health outcomes in older people, including falls, frailty and mortality (Wastesson et al 2018). There are a number of proposed mechanisms by which polypharmacy contributes to adverse outcomes in older people, including:

- an increased risk of clinically significant drug–drug and drug–disease interactions (Koren et al 2019)
- decreased adherence, which negatively affects the likelihood of the sought pharmacological effect being achieved (Koren et al 2019)
- an increased risk of adverse effects, which, if unidentified, may lead to the prescribing of other medications (Alagiakrishnan et al 2018).

However, there is little consistency with such findings between different studies, and there is debate as to the utility of measuring polypharmacy according to arbitrary numeric thresholds (Burt et al 2018). Furthermore, there is a high prevalence of underuse of potentially beneficial medications in older adults (Wright et al 2009), and recognition that certain situations may necessitate the use of multiple medications. Consequently, some authors now differentiate between *appropriate* polypharmacy, and *inappropriate* or *problematic* polypharmacy (Wastesson et al 2018) and advocate for strategies that minimise inappropriate polypharmacy while ensuring continuity of beneficial treatments (Alagiakrishnan et al 2018).

MEDICATION SAFETY IN OLDER PEOPLE

The framework for medication safety in Australia is the National Strategy for Quality Use of Medicines, which is a core component of the National Medicines Policy (Morgan et al 2008). In New Zealand, medication safety activities are led by the Health Quality and Safety Commission and guided by the National Health Strategy (HQSC 2019). The need for such initiatives was in part established by an increasing recognition of the high prevalence of medication-related harm occurring in older people. A 2017 meta-analysis of studies conducted in 21 countries reported that 8.7% (95% confidence interval (CI) 7.6 to 9.8%) of all hospital admissions among people aged 60 years and older were related to adverse drug reactions (Oscanoa et al 2017). It is anticipated that these events will become more frequent in future due to the increased prevalence of older people, increased medication use and better access to medications (Salvi et al 2012).

Issues with medications may occur at any time during their use, such as during prescribing, dispensing, administration and cessation (Salvi et al 2012). Errors that occur during administration are particularly common, accounting for approximately one-quarter of serious medication errors in hospitals and the majority of errors in the community (Salvi et al 2012). Patient non-adherence is also common in older people, and is associated with a range of adverse outcomes. A recent systematic review and meta-analysis reported that medication non-adherence is associated with a 17% increased risk of all-cause hospitalisation in older people, and an increased risk of mortality (Walsh et al 2019).

A high proportion of these events are considered to be preventable if appropriate measures are implemented (Oscanoa et al 2017). In recognition of this, in 2017 the World Health Organisation (WHO) launched its third 'Global Patient Safety Challenge: Medication Without Harm', which aims to reduce severe avoidable medication-related harm by 50% globally in the next 5 years (WHO 2017). The program identifies three priority areas for action: high-risk situations (one of which is medication use in older people), polypharmacy and transitions of care.

Challenges in Medication Use in Older People

There are a number of specific challenges when prescribing medications for older people, particularly those with a limited life expectancy. Older people are poorly represented in clinical trials, with many trials specifically excluding this population, and other trials indirectly through exclusion criteria, such as the presence of co-morbid conditions, cognitive impairment or polypharmacy (Bourgeois et al 2017). Secondly, as most clinical guidelines are only concerned with individual conditions, their application to older people is difficult due to the high prevalence of multimorbidity that occurs with age (McNamara et al 2017). Additional complexity is introduced in situations where limited life expectancy may exceed the time to benefit from many medications (Holmes et al 2013). Finally, for many people, the goals

of treatment may shift from disease prevention to optimising quality of life and minimising treatment burden (Hilmer, McLachlan et al 2007).

AGE-RELATED CHANGES

Ageing is a continuous process that occurs gradually rather than abruptly (Perrie et al 2012). It is the result of a multitude of changes at the molecular, cellular and tissue level, hence there is marked variation between individuals in terms of how ageing influences the effects of medication (Mangoni & Jackson 2004). These changes tend to result in a diminished capacity for each organ system to maintain homeostasis, which may increase the risk of medication-related issues in older people (Dinsmore et al 2018). Consequently, alterations to pharmacokinetics and pharmacodynamics that occur with age should both be considered when selecting and evaluating pharmacotherapy to minimise these risks.

> ### Tips for Best Practice
>
> - Ensure that the older person is aware of the intended duration of any medication that is used, as treatment is not necessarily lifelong.
> - Encourage regular comprehensive review of all medications that an older person is using, particularly when their clinical circumstances change.
> - Regularly monitor older people for both beneficial and adverse effects of medications, especially when any changes are made to the medication regimen.

Pharmacokinetics

Pharmacokinetics refers to the movement of a medication into, through and out of the body. Ageing has variable effects on the four pharmacokinetic processes (absorption, distribution, metabolism and excretion) (Alagiakrishnan et al 2018). A summary of the major changes associated with each process is shown in Table 11.2.

Absorption

While numerous changes to the gastrointestinal tract occur with ageing, absorption generally remains unaffected for most medications (Slattum et al 2017), as the rate of absorption is slower yet the extent is comparable to younger adults (Dinsmore et al 2018). Of greater clinical significance is a decrease in first-pass metabolism

TABLE 11.2
Major Changes to Pharmacokinetics That Occur With Ageing and Disease

Change associated with ageing or disease	Pharmacokinetic effect	Examples of some medications affected
↓ First-pass metabolism	↑ Drug serum concentration	Oral nitrates, beta-blockers, calcium channel blockers, oestrogens
↓ Rate of absorption	↓ Clinical effect	Furosemide (Frusemide)
↓ Lean mass and total body water	↓ Volume of distribution	Digoxin, lithium
↑ Fat content	↑ Volume of distribution	Diazepam, alprazolam
↓ Food intake/catabolic disease states	↓ Serum protein concentration with ↓ binding	Warfarin, phenytoin
↓ Approximately one half of CYP 450 metabolic pathways (Phase I reactions)	↓ Reduction, oxidation, hydroxylation, demethylation →↑ half-life	Diazepam, alprazolam
↓ Renal elimination	↓ Clearance →↑ half-life	Aminoglycosides, vancomycin, digoxin, salicylates

Adapted from Hughes & Beizer (2014).

BOX 11.1
First Pass Effect

A first pass effect is defined as the rapid uptake and metabolism of an agent into inactive compounds by the liver, immediately after enteric absorption and before it reaches the systemic circulation.

Bhosle et al (2017).

(see Box 11.1), which may increase the systemic bioavailability of some medications (e.g. propranolol and labetalol) and decrease the bioavailability of certain prodrugs (e.g. enalapril and codeine).

Distribution

Several physiological changes that occur with age may affect distribution, such as an increase in total fat content and a decrease in body water and lean mass (Dinsmore et al 2018). Changes in serum concentrations of albumin and α_1-acid glycoprotein, two major drug binding proteins, may further influence distribution. The net effect of these changes is reduced volume of distribution (V_d) for hydrophilic medications (e.g. lithium and digoxin), which may produce higher blood levels than anticipated. Conversely, the V_d of hydrophobic medications (e.g. diazepam) may be increased, which may lead to accumulation with continued use (Dinsmore et al 2018).

Metabolism

While changes in metabolism may occur in many organ systems, most of the available data concern the effects of ageing on the liver (Slattum et al 2017). Hepatic metabolism is dependent upon perfusion, liver mass, hepatic enzyme activity, transport activity and protein binding, with age influencing each of these factors to some extent. Additional complexity in evaluating the effect of age on metabolism is created by the marked variability between different medications in terms of the metabolic processes they undergo. Consequently, markers of hepatic function, such as serum transaminase (alanine transaminase [ALT]; aspartate transaminase [AST]) and gamma glutamyl transferase (GGT) levels, cannot reliably be used to predict an individual's response to medication (Alagiakrishnan et al 2018). Increased clinical monitoring for effects and adverse effects may, therefore, be required.

Excretion

Renal excretion is a primary route of elimination for many drugs and their metabolites (Slattum et al 2017). Ageing is associated with reduced renal mass, renal blood flow and tubular secretion, which contribute to a decline in glomerular filtration rate (GFR) in most older people (Slattum et al 2017). This prolongs the plasma half-life of renally excreted medications, particularly those that are entirely dependent upon the kidney for elimination. Table 11.3 lists medications commonly used in older people whose elimination is highly dependent upon

TABLE 11.3
Drugs Highly Dependent on Renal Function for Elimination

Therapeutic class	Examples
Antibiotics	Aciclovir Aminoglycosides Amphotericin B Aztreonam Cephalosporins (most) Fluconazole Fluroquinolones (most) Imipenem Penicillins (most) Sulfamethoxazole Trimethoprim Vancomycin
Cardiovascular	Amiloride Atenolol Captopril Clonidine Digoxin Enalapril Furosemide (Fusemide) Lisinopril Nadolol Procainamide Spironolactone Thiazides Triamterene
Blood and blood-forming	Apixaban Dabigatran Edoxaban Enoxaparin Fondaparinux Rivaroxaban
Neurological	Acetazolamide Amantadine Gabapentin Levetiracetam Pregabalin Pyridostigmine Tramadol
Psychiatric	Duloxetine Lithium
Gastrointestinal	Cimetidine Famotidine Metoclopramide Nizatidine Ranitidine
Rheumatological	Allopurinol Colchicine Methotrexate Probenecid

Adapted from Dinsmore et al (2018).

renal function, and frequently require dose adjustment in this population.

Pharmacodynamics

Pharmacodynamics is concerned with how medications affect the body. There is limited research into the changes in pharmacodynamics that occur with age (Alagiakrishnan et al 2018), and the effect of ageing on pharmacodynamics is highly variable between both individuals and different medications. For example, the anticoagulant activity of warfarin is typically increased in older people, yet the same effect is not observed in heparin (Koren et al 2019). Older people have been reported to be less sensitive to the blood pressure lowering effects of beta blockers, yet cardioselective calcium channel blockers are associated with more bradycardic and hypotensive effects in this population than younger people.

Age-related pharmacodynamic changes may be profound with medications that act on the central nervous system (CNS). Older people are more sensitive to the sedative effects of benzodiazepines and opioids, and are more likely to experience adverse effects from dopamine antagonists (e.g. antipsychotics and metoclopramide), and levodopa (Slattum et al 2017). Medications with anticholinergic effects are much more likely to cause confusion and cognitive impairment in older people, particularly those already presenting with a cognitive impairment (Dinsmore et al 2018). A list of commonly used medications with anticholinergic effects is provided in Table 11.4.

The influence of age on pharmacokinetics and pharmacodynamics is largely unpredictable and varies markedly between individuals. Hence, nurses involved in the care of older people who are using any medication should ensure that these people are monitored closely for both beneficial and adverse effects from medication to optimise benefits and minimise harm. Nurses also have a key role in identifying appropriate and inappropriate medication use in this population.

APPROPRIATE AND INAPPROPRIATE PRESCRIBING

Several tools have been created to assist clinicians in assessing the appropriateness of individual medications for older people (Pazan et al 2019). These are typically created by combining experimental evidence with expert opinion to produce various measures that range in complexity from basic lists to calculated scores. The simplest tools involve lists of medications to avoid (termed potentially inappropriate medications [PIMs]) and necessary medications (potential prescription omissions [PPOs]). Such tools include the Beers criteria

TABLE 11.4
Medications With Anticholinergic Effects

Therapeutic class	Examples
Antimuscarinics	Darifenacin Oxybutynin Solifenacin Tolterodine
Antispasmodic	Atropine Hyoscine Scopolamine
Anti-Parkinson	Benzatropine Trihexyphenidyl
Antihistamine	Brompheniramine Chlorpheniramine Dimenhydrinate Diphenhydramine Doxylamine
Antidepressant	Amitriptyline Clomipramine Desipramine Dosulepin Imipramine Nortriptyline Paroxetine Trimipramine
Antiarrhythmic	Disopyramide Quinidine
Antipsychotic	Clozapine Olanzapine Quetiapine

Adapted from Dinsmore et al (2018).

(AGS 2019), which was first published in 1991, the Medication Appropriateness Index (MAI) (Samsa et al 1994) and the STOPP/START criteria (Screening Tool of Older People's Prescriptions/Screening Tool to Alert to Right Treatment) (O'Mahony et al 2015), first published in 2008. More sophisticated measures also consider additional information such as clinical circumstances, time to benefit and the patient's care goals (Niehoff et al 2019). However, there is currently limited evidence to inform the application of such strategies in practice, and there is considerable research underway in this area (Niehoff et al 2019).

Consistent with international studies, inappropriate prescribing is common among older people living in Australia and New Zealand, with the prevalence dependent upon the specific criteria used. A retrospective cohort study of over 180,000 older Western Australians reported that 74.7% of participants used one or more PIMs, as defined by the 2012 Beers criteria (Price et al 2014).

Using the STOPP criteria, 51% of older people admitted to a Victorian hospital were using a PIM (Manias et al 2015). The most frequently prescribed PIMs were nonsteroidal anti-inflammatory drugs (NSAIDs), benzodiazepines, oestrogen-only hormone preparations and antidepressants. Narayan and Nishtala used the 2012 Beers criteria in a population level evaluation of inappropriate prescribing in New Zealand (Narayan & Nishtala 2015). They identified 40.9% of their cohort as using a PIM, with the most common classes of PIM similar to those seen in Australia. Interestingly, the rate of PIM prescribing by nurse practitioners in New Zealand has been noted to be lower than the rate among other prescribers (Poot et al 2019).

Due to the particularly high risk associated with anticholinergic and sedative medications in older people, a number of tools have been developed to identify and quantify the cumulative exposure of an individual to medications with these effects. Typically, these tools firstly identify specific medications with anticholinergic activity, score each medication according to its specific anticholinergic activity, then sum each medication's score into an overall 'burden' (Villalba-Moreno et al 2016). A 2016 systematic review of these tools identified ten different scales, differing in terms of the medications included and the attributed anticholinergic score (Villalba-Moreno et al 2016). One of the most widely studied is the Drug Burden Index (DBI), which considers medications with sedative activity (e.g. opioids and benzodiazepines), in addition to anticholinergic medications (Hilmer, Mager et al 2007). DBI has been associated with several adverse outcomes for older people, including falls, hospitalisation and cognitive impairment (Wouters et al 2017). While the DBI is available for clinical application (G-MEDSS 2019), there is currently limited data regarding how to effectively use DBI scores in practice to improve patient outcomes.

Neither explicit lists of PIMs nor drug burden scales are intended to be prescriptively applied to individual patients and require clinical judgement in their interpretation. Rather, these tools aim to simplify the process of medication regimen optimisation for individual patients by alerting those involved in the patient's medication management to the potential for medication-related harm (Curtin et al 2019).

MEDICATION REVIEW

There is considerable interest in practices that maximise the benefits of medication use in older people, while minimising the risks of harm (Anderson et al 2019). Worldwide, medication review is one of the most widely implemented interventions, with most reviews being provided by pharmacists or general medical practitioners (GPs) (Jokanovic et al 2016). It is defined by the Pharmaceutical Care Network Europe as being 'a structured evaluation of a patient's medicines with the aim of optimising medicines use and improving health outcomes. This entails detecting drug-related problems and recommending interventions' (Griese-Mammen et al 2018).

Several types of pharmacist-conducted medication reviews are funded in Australia and New Zealand, differing according to patient eligibility criteria, processes and practice settings. Australian pharmacists are remunerated to conduct medication reviews in the community (Home Medicines Reviews and MedsChecks) and in residential aged care facilities (Residential Medication Management Reviews) (Jokanovic et al 2016). In New Zealand, pharmacists provide Medicines Use Reviews, Medicines Therapy Assessments and Comprehensive Medicines Management services (Jokanovic et al 2016). Medication review services are also provided by hospital pharmacists in the provision of clinical pharmacy services (Moles & Stehlik 2015). While the cost-effectiveness of medication reviews is uncertain, they are associated with a range of benefits, particularly in older people with multiple co-morbidities and polypharmacy (Jokanovic et al 2016). This includes:

- reduced number of medications
- reduced medication costs
- improved adherence to treatment regimens
- reduced hospitalisations.

Patient groups that benefit include people with chronic heart failure (Roughead et al 2009), diabetes (Krass et al 2005) and those taking high-risk medications such as anticoagulants (Roughead et al 2011).

Promoting Wellness

- Ensure that older people who may benefit from medication use are provided with the opportunity to choose whether or not to use it.
- Recommend that deprescribing be considered for any older person for whom medication use is burdensome or no longer aligned with their goals of treatment.
- Encourage older people who choose to use complementary and alternative treatments to inform their healthcare team of their decision to do so.

DEPRESCRIBING

A relatively new intervention that seeks to address many of the issues inherent with medication use in older

people is deprescribing. In a systematic review, Reeve and colleagues defined deprescribing as 'the process of withdrawal of an inappropriate medication, supervised by a health care professional with the goal of managing polypharmacy and improving outcomes' (Reeve et al 2015). However, this definition is potentially too narrow, as inappropriate prescribing is not reliant on polypharmacy, and resolving inappropriate polypharmacy may require withdrawing multiple medications (Woodford & Fisher 2019). Deprescribing recognises that the risks and benefits of medication use are not static and vary with time; for example, through the development of new conditions, the resolution of others or changing patient preferences or care goals (Woodford & Fisher 2019). It is a positive, patient-centred activity that is part of the good prescribing continuum (Scott et al 2015). Deprescribing is not dependent upon palliation, and may be undertaken at any stage of medical treatment.

The safety and benefits of deprescribing have been evaluated for several classes of medications that are commonly used in older people. These include:

- antipsychotic use for behaviour associated with dementia (Van Leeuwen et al 2018)
- cholinesterase inhibitors for Alzheimer's disease (Niznik et al 2020)
- proton pump inhibitors for GORD (gastro-oesophageal reflux disease) (Coffey et al 2019; Odenthal et al 2019)
- antihypertensives (Gulla et al 2018)
- bisphosphonates for osteoporosis (Fraser et al 2011)
- benzodiazepines (Tannenbaum et al 2014)
- statins for hyperlipidaemia (Kutner et al 2015).

In general, deprescribing has been found to significantly reduce the prevalence of polypharmacy and PIM use (Shrestha et al 2019; Thillainadesan et al 2018), and does not appear to adversely influence quality of life, hospital admissions, emergency department visits or mortality (Page et al 2016; Pruskowski et al 2019).

A number of deprescribing organisations have been established worldwide to foster collaboration and develop implementation guidance. These include the Ontario Pharmacy Evidence Network, the English Deprescribing Network (EDeN), the Northern European Researchers in Deprescribing Network (NERD), and the Canadian Deprescribing Network (Alagiakrishnan et al 2018; Le Bosquet et al 2019). In Australia, the Primary Health Tasmania Deprescribing Reference Group and Australian Deprescribing Network have published guidelines for several medication groups commonly used in older people (Deprescribing Reference Group 2019; Le Bosquet et al 2019).

BOX 11.2
General Elements of a Deprescribing Process

- Collect a complete and comprehensive medication history
  - Regular, intermittent and 'as required' prescription and non-prescription medications (including vitamins, supplements, 'herbals')
  - Include dose, frequency, duration of use, indication and effectiveness
  - Identify possible adverse drug reactions
  - Assess adherence
- Assess overall risk of harm and benefit and individual patient factors which may affect deprescribing
  - Discuss older person's/caregivers' values, preferences, beliefs and goals of care surrounding continued medication use *vs* deprescribing
  - Drug-related factors: polypharmacy, pill burden (medication regimen complexity), drug–drug interactions, use of 'high risk' drugs
  - Patient-related factors: life expectancy, cognitive and functional impairments, falls risk, co-morbidities multiple prescribers, palliative care
  - Ask 'which medications are most important for you to keep taking? Why?'
- Identify potentially inappropriate medications
  - Consider medications without an indication (condition resolved, unconfirmed, questionable efficacy, altered risk, non-pharmacological alternative), part of a prescribing cascade causing an adverse drug reaction, potential for future harm
  - Use tools such as explicit lists of medications which are inappropriate in older adults, e.g. Beers list, STOPP criteria
  - Use algorithms to determine drug appropriateness, e.g. Medication Appropriateness Index, Good Palliative-Geriatric Practice algorithm

- Decide on medication withdrawal (shared decision-making)
  - If more than one medication identified for withdrawal, prioritise order of drugs for discontinuation (e.g. based on potential for harm, patient preference)
- Plan tapering or withdrawal process and monitoring with documentation and communication to all persons relevant to care
  - Appropriate timing of withdrawal (e.g. consider patient's use of dosage administration aids)
  - Tapering plan – Identify if the medication is commonly associated with an adverse drug withdrawal event (e.g. see online resource medstopper.com). Slow dose reduction prior to discontinuation may also identify lowest effective dose, minimise the impact of return of symptoms if they do occur and increase patient comfort with the process
  - Patient management plan (symptoms to look out for, symptom action plan, monitoring required by a health care professional, person to contact)
- Conduct monitoring and support
  - Monitor for adverse drug withdrawal reactions, return of condition, reversal of drug–drug and drug–disease interactions
  - Monitor for benefits (resolution of adverse drug reactions)
  - Use non-pharmacological approaches to reduce reliance on medication where possible
- Documentation
  - Document reasons for, process and outcome (e.g. medication ceased, dose reduced or withdrawal attempted with reasons for failure) of deprescribing
- Share documentation with all relevant healthcare professionals

Reeve et al (2017).

The main elements of a deprescribing process are outlined in Box 11.2 (Reeve et al 2017). The focus on patient involvement is noteworthy, with the process initially involving:

- raising awareness that options for discontinuing medications exist
- discussing the benefits and harms of these options
- exploring patient preferences to enable an appropriate decision to be made (Woodford & Fisher 2019).

To assist in the decision-making process, many of the deprescribing guidelines that have been developed integrate available evidence from clinical trials with additional tools, such as prescribing appropriateness criteria (e.g. Beers criteria), and risk scores/scales (e.g. anticholinergic burden) (Lee & Kim 2018; Paque et al 2019; Scott et al 2017). Guidelines range from being general, such as a hierarchy of utility of medications (Scott et al 2015), to guidance for specific classes of medications such as anticholinesterase treatment for dementia (Reeve et al 2018).

Despite increasing awareness of deprescribing and the availability of implementation guides, clinicians frequently consider deprescribing challenging (Lundby et al 2019), and deprescribing does not occur as often as it should (Reeve et al 2017). A 2014 systematic review of prescriber-reported attitudes to deprescribing identified four major barriers:

- a lack of awareness
- inertia (a failure to act despite awareness)
- a lack of self-efficacy (including a lack of skills, knowledge and information)
- feasibility (including patient, resource and medical cultural influences) (Anderson et al 2014).

From the patient's perspective, studies indicate that the majority of patients are hypothetically willing to have a medication deprescribed (Galazzi et al 2016; Qi et al 2015; Reeve et al 2013; Sirois et al 2017). This is despite some fear and uncertainty as to how cessation may affect them, or, in the case of caregivers, the person for whom they are caring (Reeve et al 2016).

Nurses are often deeply involved in medication management, and may have a key role in initiating and supporting deprescribing (Reeve et al 2013). Several areas have been identified where nurses may proactively contribute to deprescribing (Wright et al 2019). These include:

- explaining during medication initiation that treatment is not necessarily lifelong
- encouraging the older person to actively discuss medication discontinuation with prescribers
- identifying to prescribers the older people who are likely to be highly receptive to deprescribing, including those who dislike taking medication, have difficulty using medication or are sceptical of benefits
- reinforcing deprescribing activities undertaken by other health professionals.

Deprescribing may be particularly appropriate in older people whose goals of care are palliative. Those with life-limiting illnesses are highly susceptible to adverse drug events, yet polypharmacy and PIM use are highly prevalent (Poudel et al 2017). In a study of New Zealand aged care facility residents, Heppenstall and colleagues (2016) reported that over half of the cohort inappropriately continued to use preventative medications during the last year of life. In Australia, van der Meer and colleagues (2018) reported minimal reduction in the use of preventative medicines in the last year of life. Deprescribing is, therefore, an important consideration for older people with a limited life expectancy to

minimise medication burden and associated adverse outcomes (Thompson 2019).

Research Highlights

- Age affects the pharmacology and pharmacokinetics of many medications; the effects may differ greatly between different people and are highly unpredictable (Dinsmore et al 2018).
- Older people may benefit greatly from the appropriate use of medications, but are also at a markedly elevated risk of medication-related harm. For many older people, the goals of treatment shift from disease prevention to optimising quality of life and minimising treatment burden (Hilmer, McLachlan et al 2007).
- Comprehensive medication reviews reduce medication-related problems and improve health outcomes for older people, particularly those with multimorbidities and polypharmacy (Jokanovic et al 2016).
- Deprescribing, the planned withdrawal of potentially inappropriate medication, provides a means to safely minimise the risk of harm while maximising potential benefits of medication use. It may significantly reduce the prevalence of polypharmacy and potentially inappropriate medication use (Shrestha et al 2019; Thillainadesan et al 2018), and does not appear to adversely influence quality of life, hospital admissions, emergency department visits or mortality (Page et al 2016; Pruskowski et al 2019).

PALLIATIVE CARE

While deprescribing may be valuable during palliation, the main goal of palliative care is to avoid suffering. A key enabler of this is the timely provision of appropriate symptomatic treatment via medication management (Ministry of Health NZ 2017; Palliative Care Australia 2018). Medication is frequently utilised as part of the management plan for many symptoms commonly experienced at the end of life, such as pain, dyspnoea, depression and constipation. Although the focus of this chapter is the use of medications, it must be reinforced that medications are only part of a holistic management plan, and do not substitute for non-pharmacological aspects of care, which should be ongoing (see Chapter 17).

Pain

Pain is associated with many conditions, and people frequently experience more than one type of pain, particularly those who had pre-existing painful conditions (see also Chapter 19). While the principles of palliative analgesia for older people are the same as those for younger people, there are a number of additional considerations for safe analgesic use in older people.

Despite concerns to the contrary, paracetamol may generally be used at normal adult doses in older people. For frail older people of low body weight (< 50 kg) and renal or hepatic impairment, there may be an increased risk of hepatotoxicity at higher doses and lower doses or reduced frequency of administration may be appropriate (DTB 2018).

NSAIDs should be used with caution in older people due to an increased risk of adverse effects, including gastrointestinal bleeding, renal impairment and exacerbation of heart failure (AMH 2018). Diclofenac, low-dose ibuprofen and celecoxib may confer a lower risk of gastrointestinal bleeding than other NSAIDs. For older people with moderate or severe renal impairment, NSAIDs should not be used.

Opioids are frequently used for analgesia in palliative care. Older people generally require lower doses of opioids than younger people (AMH 2018), and initial doses should be at the lower end of the dosing range using a short-acting preparation. Incremental dose increases should be small. Once adequate pain relief is achieved, the short-acting formulation should be converted to a more convenient longer-acting preparation, based on the dose requirements over the previous 24 hours. Additional doses for breakthrough pain are typically one-twelfth to one-sixth of the total regular daily dose, administered every 1–2 hours as required (AMH 2018). It is recommended to use the same opioid for background and breakthrough pain, where possible. Table 11.5 lists additional practice points for individual opioids when used for older people in palliative care. While codeine is sometimes used, it is not preferred as its effects are unpredictable due to genetic variation in its activation to the active metabolite (morphine) (Portenoy & Ahmed 2014).

A variety of adjuvant analgesics may be used when there is only partial response to traditional analgesics, such as antidepressants and anticonvulsants (Palliative Care Expert Group 2016b). Many of these agents require cautious use in older people, particularly the tricyclic antidepressants amitriptyline and nortriptyline, which are strongly anticholinergic (Villalba-Moreno et al 2016). Lower doses of duloxetine, an SNRI (serotonin–noradrenaline reuptake inhibitors) antidepressant, should be used in people with renal or hepatic impairment. The anticonvulsants gabapentin and pregabalin are renally excreted, and require dose adjustment in people

with renal impairment (Palliative Care Expert Group 2016b).

Corticosteroids such as dexamethasone may be used for acute inflammatory pain in cancer, neuropathic pain, cerebral metastases and fatigue (AMH 2018). Older people with specific co-morbidities may be at a greater risk of adverse effects from dexamethasone than younger people, such as hyperglycaemia, gastric irritation and proximal myopathy (Palliative Care Expert Group 2016b). The lowest clinically effective dose should be used and, if possible, the dose tapered to cessation when symptoms are controlled.

Dyspnoea

Pharmacological management of dyspnoea is based on treating the cause; for example, if as a result of an infection, antibiotics may be used. Conversely, should pulmonary oedema be causing dyspnoea (see Chapter 24), diuretic treatment may be required. For symptomatic management, a low-dose opioid may be used without a detrimental effect on respiratory function (AMH 2018), for example 2.5 mg morphine orally, up to every 4 hours. In people for whom anxiety is contributing to dyspnoea, a benzodiazepine may be used (AMH 2018).

Depression

Depression is common in palliative care, for which antidepressants are commonly used. There is no evidence that any one particular antidepressant is more effective than another (AMH 2018), so selection is based on considerations such as:

- previous history of antidepressant use, including effectiveness and adverse effects
- concurrent conditions
- adverse effect profile
- potential for drug interactions.

Older people may respond more slowly to antidepressant treatment than younger people, and an adequate duration should be trialled to assess benefits (e.g. up to 6 weeks) (AMH 2018).

Constipation

Constipation occurs frequently in older people whose care goals are palliative, as exacerbating factors are very common in these people. This includes medications (e.g. opioids, anticholinergics), frailty and inactivity (AMH 2018). Management is invariably multifaceted, and should involve addressing exacerbating factors and the use of laxative treatment. Exacerbating factors include dehydration, hypothyroidism, hypercalcaemia and medications. Deprescribing contributing potentially unnecessary medications (e.g. verapamil, calcium or iron

TABLE 11.5
Practice Points for Opioids Commonly Used in Palliative Care for Older People

Medication	Comments
Buprenorphine	Ceiling effect for analgesia No active renally-excreted metabolites; an opioid of choice in renal impairment Use with caution in hepatic impairment
Fentanyl	No clinically relevant ceiling effect to analgesia Highly potent compared to most other opioids No active renally-excreted metabolites; an opioid of choice in renal impairment
Hydromorphone	No clinically relevant ceiling effect to analgesia More potent than morphine and oxycodone Lower doses may be required in renal and hepatic impairment; not recommended in severe hepatic impairment
Methadone	No clinically relevant ceiling effect to analgesia Complex pharmacokinetics; generally reserved for specialist use May be used in renal impairment (longer dosing intervals required) Lower doses may be required in hepatic impairment; not recommended in severe hepatic impairment
Morphine	No clinically relevant ceiling effect to analgesia First-choice opioid for most people receiving palliative care Lower doses may be required in mild to moderate renal impairment; avoid use in severe renal impairment Avoid use in severe hepatic impairment
Oxycodone	No clinically relevant ceiling effect to analgesia Reduce dose in renal impairment Avoid use in severe hepatic impairment Combination oxycodone/naloxone is contraindicated in moderate and severe hepatic impairment
Tapentadol	Ceiling effect for analgesia Analgesic mechanism is partially related to noradrenergic effects; additional drug interactions are possible Lower doses may be required in renal and hepatic impairment; not recommended in severe hepatic impairment

AMH (2019); Portenoy & Ahmed (2014).

supplements) may improve symptoms while simplifying the medication regimen.

As opioids frequently cause constipation, laxatives should always be considered when opioids are prescribed. Morphine and oxycodone tend to cause more constipation than other opioids, particularly buprenorphine and fentanyl (Wood et al 2018). Oxycodone/naloxone fixed-dose combinations may cause less constipation than oxycodone monotherapy, but should not be used in people with hepatic impairment (AMH 2018). Methylnaltrexone may be beneficial for opioid-induced constipation that is refractory to other laxatives in people receiving palliative care.

Stimulant laxatives (e.g. senna, bisacodyl), with or without softeners (e.g. docusate), are generally used first-line for constipation, and may be used in combination with other laxatives if required. Lactulose should not be used in patients with poor fluid intake as it draws fluid into the intestinal lumen; macrogol 3350 is more appropriate in such situations (Palliative Care Working Group 2016a).

COMPLEMENTARY THERAPY AND SUPPLEMENTS

In addition to conventional medications, there is a high prevalence of use of complementary and alternative medicines (CAMs) among older people. Over half of all Australians report using CAMs, with vitamin and mineral supplements being the most common (Harnett et al 2019). Box 11.3 lists the most commonly used herbal medicines in Australia. While comparable data

BOX 11.3
Most Commonly Used Herbal Medicines in Australia

Aloe vera	Cranberry	Valerian	Black cohosh
Garlic	Peppermint	Liquorice	Bilberry
Green tea	Ginseng	St John's wort	Senna
Chamomile	Ginkgo biloba	Slippery elm	Hawthorn
Echinacea	Evening primrose	Milk thistle	Saw palmetto
Ginger	Dandelion	Dong quai	Chasteberry (vitex)

Barnes et al (2016).

Practice Scenario

FA is an 81-year-old woman (52 kg) with a past medical history of anxiety, atrial fibrillation, chronic kidney disease, hypertension, osteoporosis, osteoarthritis and urge urinary incontinence. Her regular medications include apixaban 2.5 mg twice daily, diazepam 5 mg twice daily, metoprolol 12.5 mg twice daily, oxybutynin 5 mg twice daily, paracetamol 1 g four times daily, paroxetine 20 mg daily, ramipril 2.5 mg daily and rosuvastatin 10 mg daily. She lives independently in a retirement villa with no care assistance, and is comfortable and confident with managing her medications herself.

MULTIPLE CHOICE QUESTIONS

1. Which one of the following age-related changes in pharmacokinetics is MOST likely to account for FA's low dose of metoprolol?
   a. Decreased first pass metabolism
   b. Reduced lean muscle mass
   c. Increased proportion of body fat
   d. Decreased renal elimination

2. In undertaking a medication review for FA, which ome of the following activities is the most appropriate?
   a. Ceasing all medications that appear on Beers' criteria
   b. Changing FA's medication regimen to minimise her drug burden index (DBI) score
   c. Ceasing unnecessary medications until she is using fewer than five regular medications
   d. Ensuring that all medications have an indication and are aligned with her care goals

3. FA expresses an interest in reducing the number of medications she takes. Which one of the following strategies is most consistent with the concept of deprescribing?
   a. Discontinuing all medications with high risk of adverse effects
   b. Ceasing all medications that do not provide symptomatic benefit
   c. Discontinuing medications with an unfavourable risk-to-benefit ratio
   d. Ensure that every medical condition is treated strictly according to current guidelines

4. FA experiences a fall and requires surgery for a fractured neck of femur. Post-surgery she experiences delirium, and her medications are reviewed to minimise potential precipitants. Which one of the following changes to FA's medications is most appropriate at this time?
   a. Increase the diazepam dose to 5 mg three times daily
   b. Temporarily withhold the oxybutynin
   c. Immediately cease the paroxetine
   d. Cease the paracetamol and any recently prescribed analgesia

5. You are the nurse discharging FA from hospital after her recovery from her hip surgery and episode of delirium. You are providing FA with education about her discharge medications. You note that the doctor has prescribed celecoxib 200 mg twice daily in addition to the medications FA was taking before her admission, to help manage her postoperative pain.

   Which ONE of the following nursing actions is the LEAST appropriate for you to undertake to promote FA's safe medication use?
   a. Explain to FA that the celecoxib treatment is not necessarily lifelong.
   b. Tell FA that she already takes too many medications and not to bother with the celecoxib.
   c. Encourage FA to actively discuss medication discontinuation with her GP.
   d. Confirm with the medical team that FA is to use high dose celecoxib in view of her advanced age, low body weight and anticoagulant use.

are not available for New Zealand, it is expected that the prevalence of CAM use is similar to that in other developed countries, such as Australia (Barnes et al 2016).

While CAM use is common among older people, there is often a lack of dialogue between medical professionals and patients regarding use (de Souza Silva et al 2014). This creates the potential for adverse events when CAMs are used with conventional therapies, as potential interactions are unable to be pre-emptively identified. Many older people consider CAMs to be safe as they are obtained from natural sources, and are unaware of the potential for serious interactions with other treatments (Siddiqui et al 2014). For example, ginkgo biloba and garlic may potentiate the effects of conventional antithrombotic treatments (e.g. aspirin and anticoagulants), increasing the risk of bleeding (de Souza Silva et al 2014). St John's wort may interact with numerous conventional medications via its effects on the hepatic cytochrome P450 and P-glycoprotein systems, either increasing or decreasing the effectiveness of interacting medications. Should CAMs be used within an older person's management plan, they should be integrated within the plan to ensure that all members of the person's healthcare team are aware of these additional treatments, to minimise the risk of unintended consequences (Siddiqui et al 2014).

SUMMARY

There are numerous challenges to the safe and effective use of medicines in older people. While age-related changes to pharmacokinetics and pharmacology may predict some of these issues, many others can only be identified through careful assessment of a person's medical history and their current medication regimen. Activities such as medication reviews and deprescribing may alleviate some of the issues associated with medication use in older people, but nurses retain a central role in achieving optimal medication use to support wellness in this population.

REFERENCES

Abhishek A (2017) Managing gout flares in the elderly: practical considerations. Drugs & Aging 34(12):873–880.

Alagiakrishnan K, Mah D, Padwal R (2018) Classic challenges and emerging approaches to medication therapy in older adults. Discovery Medicine 26(143):137–146.

Alejandro P, Constantinescu F (2018) A review of osteoporosis in the older adult: an update. Rheum Dis Clin North Am 44(3):437–451.

Ali A, Arif AW, Bhan C et al (2018) Managing chronic pain in the elderly: an overview of the recent therapeutic advancements. Cureus 10(9):e3293.

American Geriatrics Society (AGS) 2019 Updated AGS Beers Criteria for potentially inappropriate medication use in older adults. Journal of the American Geriatrics Society 67(4):674–694.

Anderson LJ, Schnipper JL, Nuckols TK et al (2019) A systematic overview of systematic reviews evaluating interventions addressing polypharmacy. American Journal of Health-System Pharmacy 76(21):1777–1787.

Anderson K, Stowasser D, Freeman C et al (2014) Prescriber barriers and enablers to minimising potentially inappropriate medications in adults: a systematic review and thematic synthesis. BMJ Open 4(12): e006544.

Australian Institute of Health and Welfare (AIHW) (2018) Australia's health 2018. Australia's health series no. 16. AUS 221. AIHW, Canberra.

Australian Medicines Handbook (AMH) (2018) AMH aged care companion. Australian Medicines Handbook, Adelaide.

Australian Medicines Handbook (AMH) (2019) Analgesics. Australian Medicines Handbook. Australian Medicines Handbook, Adelaide.

Barnes J, McLachlan AJ, Sherwin CMT et al (2016) Herbal medicines: challenges in the modern world. Part 1. Australia and New Zealand. Expert Review of Clinical Pharmacology 9(7): 905–915.

Bessey LJ, Walaszek A (2019) Management of behavioral and psychological symptoms of dementia. Current Psychiatry Reports 21(8):66.

Bhosle VK, Altit G, Autmizguine J et al (2017) Fetal and neonatal physiology, 5th ed. vol 1 pp. 187–200.

Bischoff-Ferrari HA (2019) Should vitamin D administration for fracture prevention be continued? Zeitschrift für Gerontologie und Geriatrie 52(5):428–432.

Bourgeois FT, Orenstein L, Ballakur S et al (2017) Exclusion of elderly people from randomized clinical trials of drugs for ischemic heart disease. Journal of the American Geriatric Society 65(11):2354–2361.

Burt J, Elmore N, Campbell SM et al (2018) Developing a measure of polypharmacy appropriateness in primary care: systematic review and expert consensus study. BMC Medicine 16(1):91.

Busti F, Marchi G, Lira Zidanes A et al (2019) Treatment options for anemia in the elderly. Transfusion and Apheresis Science 58(4):416–421.

Cameron ID, Dyer SM, Panagoda CE et al (2018) Interventions for preventing falls in older people in care facilities and hospitals. Cochrane Database of Systematic Reviews(9) .cd005465

Coffey CP, Barnette DJ, Wenzke JT et al (2019) Implementing a systematic approach to deprescribing proton pump inhibitor therapy in older adults. The Senior Care Pharmacist 34(1):47–55.

Cortopassi F, Gurung P, Pinto-Plata V (2017) Chronic obstructive pulmonary disease in elderly patients. Clinics in Geriatric Medicine 33(4):539–552.

Curtin D, Gallagher PF, O'Mahony D (2019) Explicit criteria as clinical tools to minimize inappropriate medication use and its consequences. Therapeutic Advances in Drug Safety 10: 2042098619829431.

de Souza Silva JE, Santos Souza CA, da Silva TB et al (2014) Use of herbal medicines by elderly patients: A systematic review. Archives of Gerontology and Geriatrics 59(2):227–233.

Deeks ED (2018) Denosumab: a review in postmenopausal osteoporosis. Drugs & Aging 35(2):163–173.

Deprescribing Reference Group (2019) Deprescribing resources. Online. Available: www.primaryhealthtas.com.au/resources/deprescribing-resources/

Dinsmore S, Grams MK, Zimmerman KM (2018) Geriatric drug use. In: Applied therapeutics: the clinical use of drugs. Wolters Kluwer, Philadelphia.

Drug and Therapeutics Bulletin (2018) What dose of paracetamol for older people? Drug and Therapeutics Bulletin 56(6):69.

Duntas LH, Yen PM (2019) Diagnosis and treatment of hypothyroidism in the elderly. Endocrine 66(1):63–69.

Emmanuel A, Mattace-Raso F, Neri MC et al (2017) Constipation in older people: A consensus statement. International Journal of Clinical Practice 71(1):e12920.

Flather MD, Shibata MC, Coats AJ et al (2005) Randomized trial to determine the effect of nebivolol on mortality and cardiovascular hospital admission in elderly patients with heart failure (SENIORS). European Heart Journal 26(3):215–225.

Fraser L-A, Vogt KN, Adachi JD et al (2011) Fracture risk associated with continuation versus discontinuation of bisphosphonates after 5 years of therapy in patients with primary osteoporosis: a systematic review and meta-analysis. Therapeutics and Clinical Risk Management 7:157–166.

Galazzi A, Lusignani M, Chiarelli MT et al (2016) Attitudes towards polypharmacy and medication withdrawal among older inpatients in Italy. International Journal of Clinical Pharmacy 38(2):454–461.

Gimbel ME (2019) Randomized comparison of clopidogrel versus ticagrelor or prasugrel in patients of 70 years or older with non-ST-elevation acute coronary syndrome – POPular AGE. European Society of Cardiology Congress, Paris.

G-MEDSS (2019) Goal-directed Medication review Electronic Decision Support System (G-MEDSS) website. Online. Available: gmedss.com.

Griese-Mammen N, Hersberger KE, Messerli M et al (2018) PCNE definition of medication review: reaching agreement. International Journal of Clinical Pharmacy 40(5):1199–1208.

Gulla C, Flo E, Kjome RL et al (2018) Deprescribing antihypertensive treatment in nursing home patients and the effect on blood pressure. Journal of Geriatric Cardiology 15(4):275–283.

Harnett JE, McIntyre E, Steel A et al (2019) Use of complementary medicine products: a nationally representative cross-sectional survey of 2019 Australian adults. BMJ Open 9(7):e024198.

Health Quality and Safety Commission (HQSC) (2019) Medication safety. Online. Available: www.hqsc.govt.nz/our-programmes/medication-safety/.

Heneghan C, Mahtani KR (2019) Absolute effects of statins in the elderly. BMJ Evidence-Based Medicine 24(5):200.

Heppenstall CP, Broad JB, Boyd M et al (2016) Medication use and potentially inappropriate medications in those with limited prognosis living in residential aged care. Australasian Journal of Ageing 35(2):E18–E24.

Hilmer SN, Mager DE, Simonsick EM et al (2007) A Drug Burden Index to define the functional burden of medications in older people. Archives of Internal Medicine 167(8):781–787.

Hilmer SN, McLachlan AJ, Le Couteur DG (2007) Clinical pharmacology in the geriatric patient. Fundamental and Clinical Pharmacology 21(3):217–230.

Holmes HM, Min LC, Yee M et al (2013) Rationalizing prescribing for older patients with multimorbidity: considering time to benefit. Drugs & Aging 30(9):655–666.

Hughes G, Beizer J (2014) Appropriate prescribing. Ham's primary care geriatrics, 6th edn. Saunders, Philadelphia.

Jokanovic N, Tan ECK, van den Bosch D et al (2016) Clinical medication review in Australia: A systematic review. Research in Social and Administrative Pharmacy 12(3):384–418.

Kanno T, Moayyedi P (2019) Proton pump inhibitors in the elderly, balancing risk and benefit: an age-old problem. Current Gastroenterology Reports 21(12):65.

Knight R, Khondoker M, Magill N et al (2018) A systematic review and meta-analysis of the effectiveness of acetylcholinesterase inhibitors and memantine in treating the cognitive symptoms of dementia. Dementia and Geriatric Cognitive Disorders 45(3–4):131–151.

Koren G, Nordon G, Radinsky K et al (2019) Clinical pharmacology of old age. Expert Review of Clinical Pharmacology 12(8):749–755.

Krass I, Taylor SJ, Smith C et al (2005) Impact on medication use and adherence of Australian pharmacists' diabetes care services. Journal of the American Pharmacists Association 45(1):33–40.

Kutner JS, Blatchford PJ, Taylor DH Jr et al (2015) Safety and benefit of discontinuing statin therapy in the setting of advanced, life-limiting illness: a randomized clinical trial. JAMA Internal Medicine 175(5):691–700.

Le Bosquet K, Barnett N, Minshull J (2019) Deprescribing: practical ways to support person-centred, evidence-based deprescribing. Pharmacy 7(3):129.

Lee SJ, Kim CM (2018) Individualizing prevention for older adults. Journal of the American Geriatric Society 66(2):229–234.

Li L, Geraghty OC, Mehta Z et al (2017) Age-specific risks, severity, time course, and outcome of bleeding on long-term antiplatelet treatment after vascular events: a population-based cohort study. Lancet (London) 390(10093):490–499.

Lobraico-Fernandez J, Baksh S, Nemec E (2019) Elderly bleeding risk of direct oral anticoagulants in nonvalvular atrial fibrillation: a systematic review and meta-analysis of cohort studies. Drugs in R&D 19(3):235–245.

Longo M, Bellastella G, Maiorino MI et al (2019) Diabetes and aging: from treatment goals to pharmacologic therapy. Front Endocrinol (Lausanne) 10:45.

Lundby C, Graabaek T, Ryg J et al (2019) '… Above all, it's a matter of this person's quality of life': health care professionals' perspectives on deprescribing in older patients with limited life expectancy. Gerontologist 60(3):439–449.

Makris UE, Abrams RC, Gurland B et al (2014) Management of persistent pain in the older patient: a clinical review. JAMA 312(8):825–837.

Mangoni AA, Jackson SH (2004) Age-related changes in pharmacokinetics and pharmacodynamics: basic principles and practical applications. British Journal of Clinical Pharmacology 57(1):6–14.

Manias E, Kusljic S, Lam DL (2015) Use of the Screening Tool of Older Persons' Prescriptions (STOPP) and the Screening Tool to Alert doctors to the Right Treatment (START) in hospitalised older people. Australasian Journal of Ageing 34(4):252–258.

Markota M, Rummans TA, Bostwick JM et al (2016) Benzodiazepine use in older adults: dangers, management, and alternative therapies. Mayo Clinic Proceedings 91(11):1632–1639.

McNamara, KP, Breken BD, Alzubaidi HT et al (2017) Health professional perspectives on the management of multimorbidity and polypharmacy for older patients in Australia. Age & Ageing 46(2):291–299.

Ministry of Health NZ (2017) Te Ara Whakapiri: Principles and guidance for the last days of life (2nd ed). Ministry of Health, Wellington.

Moles RJ, Stehlik P (2015) Pharmacy practice in Australia. The Canadian Journal of Hospital Pharmacy 68(5):418–426.

Morgan TK, Williamson M, Pirotta M et al (2012) A national census of medicines use: a 24-hour snapshot of Australians aged 50 years and older. Medical Journal of Australia 196(1):50–53.

Morgan S, McMahon M, Greyson D (2008) Balancing health and industrial policy objectives in the pharmaceutical sector: lessons from Australia. Health Policy (Amsterdam) 87(2):133–145.

Motika PV, Spencer DC (2016) Treatment of epilepsy in the elderly. Current Neurology and Neuroscience Reports 16(11):96.

Narayan SW, Nishtala PS (2015) Prevalence of potentially inappropriate medicine use in older New Zealanders: a population-level study using the updated 2012 Beers criteria. Journal of Evaluation in Clinical Practice 21(4):633–641.

Niehoff KM, Mecca MC, Fried TR (2019) Medication appropriateness criteria for older adults: a narrative review of criteria and supporting studies. Therapeutic Advances in Drug Safety 10:2042098618815431.

Nishtala PS, Salahudeen MS (2015) Temporal trends in polypharmacy and hyperpolypharmacy in older New Zealanders over a 9-year period: 2005–2013. Gerontology 61(3):195–202.

Niznik JD, Zhao X, He M et al (2020) Risk for health events after deprescribing acetylcholinesterase inhibitors in nursing home residents with severe dementia. Journal of the American Geriatrics Society 68(4):699–707.

O'Mahony D, O'Sullivan D, Byrne S et al (2015) STOPP/START criteria for potentially inappropriate prescribing in older people: version 2. Age & Ageing 44(2):213–218.

Odenthal DR, Philbrick AM, Harris IM (2019) Successful deprescribing of unnecessary proton pump inhibitors in a primary care clinic. Journal of the American Pharmacists Association 60(1):100–104.

Oscanoa TJ, Lizaraso F, Carvajal A (2017) Hospital admissions due to adverse drug reactions in the elderly. A meta-analysis. European Journal of Clinical Pharmacology 73(6):759–770.

Osmanska J, Jhund PS (2019) Contemporary management of heart failure in the elderly. Drugs & Aging 36(2):137–146.

Page AT, Falster MO, Litchfield M et al (2019) Polypharmacy among older Australians, 2006–2017: a population-based study. Medical Journal of Australia 211(2):71–75.

Page AT, Clifford RM, Potter K et al (2016) The feasibility and effect of deprescribing in older adults on mortality and health: a systematic review and meta-analysis. British Journal of Clinical Pharmacology 82(3):583–623.

Palliative Care Australia (2018) National Palliative Care Standards 5th ed. Palliative Care Australia, Canberra.

Palliative Care Expert Group (2016) Pain: management in palliative care. Therapeutic Guidelines: palliative care V.4. Therapeutic Guidelines Limited, Melbourne.

Palliative Care Working Group (2016) Gastrointestinal symptoms in palliative care. Therapeutic Guidelines: palliative care V.4. Therapeutic Guidelines Limited, Melbourne.

Paque K, Elseviers M, Vander Stichele R et al (2019) Balancing medication use in nursing home residents with life-limiting disease. European Journal of Clinical Pharmacology 75(7):969–977.

Patrono C, Baigent C (2019) Role of aspirin in primary prevention of cardiovascular disease. Nature Reviews Cardiology 16(11):675–686.

Pazan F, Kather J, Wehling M (2019) A systematic review and novel classification of listing tools to improve medication in older people. European Journal of Clinical Pharmacology 75(5):619–625.

Perrie Y, Badhan RK, Kirby DJ et al (2012) The impact of ageing on the barriers to drug delivery. Journal of Controlled Release 161(2):389–398.

Pont L, Alhawassi T (2017) Challenges in the management of hypertension in older populations. hypertension: from basic research to clinical practice. Advances in Experimental Medicine and Biology 956:167–180.

Poot B, Nelson K, Zonneveld R et al (2019) Potentially inappropriate medicine prescribing by nurse practitioners in New Zealand. Journal of the American Association of Nurse Practitioners 32(3):220–228.

Portenoy RK, Ahmed E (2014) Principles of opioid use in cancer pain. Journal of Clinical Oncology 32(16):1662–1670.

Poudel A, Yates P, Rowett D et al (2017) Use of preventive medication in patients with limited life expectancy: a systematic review. Journal of Pain Symptom Management 53(6):1097–1110.

Price SD, Holman CDAJ, Sanfilippo FM et al (2014) Are older Western Australians exposed to potentially inappropriate medications according to the Beers Criteria? A 13-year prevalence study. Australasian Journal on Ageing 33(3):E39–E48.

Pruskowski JA, Springer S, Thorpe CT et al (2019) Does deprescribing improve quality of life? A systematic review of the literature. Drugs & Aging 36(12):1097–1110.

Qi K, Reeve E, Hilmer SN et al (2015) Older people's attitudes regarding polypharmacy, statin use and willingness to have statins deprescribed in Australia. International Journal of Clinical Pharmacology 37(5): 949–957.

Royal Australian College of General Practitioners (RACGP) (2017) Osteoporosis prevention, diagnosis and management in postmenopausal women and men over 50 years of age. 2nd edn. The Royal Australian College of General Practitioners, East Melbourne.

Reeve E, Gnjidic D, Long J et al (2015) A systematic review of the emerging definition of 'deprescribing' with network analysis: implications for future research and clinical practice. British Journal of Clinical Pharmacology 80(6):1254–1268.

Reeve E, Farrell B, Thompson W et al (2019) Deprescribing cholinesterase inhibitors and memantine in dementia: guideline summary. Medical Journal of Australia 210(4):174–179.

Reeve E, Farrell B, Thompson W et al (2018) Evidence-based clinical practice guideline for deprescribing cholinesterase inhibitors and memantine. The University of Sydney, Sydney.

Reeve E, Low L-F, Hilmer SN (2016) Beliefs and attitudes of older adults and carers about deprescribing of medications: a qualitative focus group study. British Journal of General Practice 66(649):e552–e560.

Reeve E, Thompson W, Farrell B (2017) Deprescribing: A narrative review of the evidence and practical recommendations for recognizing opportunities and taking action. European Journal of Internal Medicine 38:3–11.

Reeve E, Wiese MD, Hendrix I et al (2013) People's attitudes, beliefs, and experiences regarding polypharmacy and willingness to deprescribe. Journal of the American Geriatrics Society 61(9):1508–1514.

Roughead E, Barratt J, Ramsay E et al (2011) Collaborative home medicines review delays time to next hospitalization for warfarin associated bleeding in Australian war veterans. Journal of Clinical Pharmacy and Therapeutics 36(1):27–32.

Roughead EE, Barratt JD, Ramsay E et al (2009) The effectiveness of collaborative medicine reviews in delaying time to next hospitalisation for heart failure patients in the practice setting: results of a cohort study. Circulation: Heart Failure 2:424–428.

Salvi F, Marchetti A, D'Angelo F (2012) Adverse drug events as a cause of hospitalization in older adults. Drug Safety 35 Suppl 1:29–45.

Samsa GP, Hanlon JT, Schmader KE et al (1994) A summated score for the medication appropriateness index: development and assessment of clinimetric properties including content validity. Journal of Clinical Epidemiology 47(8):891–896.

Scott I, Anderson K, Freeman C (2017) Review of structured guides for deprescribing. Eur J Hosp Pharm 24(1):51–57.

Scott IA, Hilmer SN, Reeve E et al (2015) Reducing inappropriate polypharmacy: the process of deprescribing. JAMA Internal Medicine 175(5):827–834.

Shrestha S, Poudel A, Steadman K et al (2019) Outcomes of deprescribing interventions in older patients with life-limiting illness and limited life expectancy: a systematic review. British Journal of Clinical Pharmacology. doi: 10.1111/bcp.14113. Online ahead of print.

Siddiqui MJ, Min CS, Verma RK et al (2014) Role of complementary and alternative medicine in geriatric care: A mini review. Pharmacognosy Reviews 8(16):81–87.

Sirois C, Ouellet N, Reeve E (2017) Community-dwelling older people's attitudes towards deprescribing in Canada. Research in Social and Administrative Pharmacy 13(4): 864–870.

Slattum PW, Ogbonna KC, Peron EP (2017) The pharmacology of aging. In: Brocklehurst's textbook of geriatric medicine and gerontology. Elsevier, Philadelphia.

Sommerauer C, Kaushik N, Woodham A et al (2017) Thiazides in the management of hypertension in older adults – a systematic review. BMC Geriatrics 17(Suppl 1):228.

SPAF (1996) Adjusted-dose warfarin versus low-intensity, fixed-dose warfarin plus aspirin for high-risk patients with atrial fibrillation: Stroke Prevention in Atrial Fibrillation III randomised clinical trial. Lancet 348(9028):633–638.

Stamp LK, Chapman PT (2014) Urate-lowering therapy: current options and future prospects for elderly patients with gout. Drugs & Aging 31(11):777–786.

Stott DJ, Rodondi N, Kearney PM et al (2017) Thyroid hormone therapy for older adults with subclinical hypothyroidism. New England Journal of Medicine 376(26):2534–2544.

Sultana J, Spina E, Trifiro G (2015) Antidepressant use in the elderly: the role of pharmacodynamics and pharmacokinetics in drug safety. Expert Opinion on Drug Metabolism and Toxicology 11(6):883–892.

Tannenbaum C, Martin P, Tamblyn R et al (2014) Reduction of inappropriate benzodiazepine prescriptions among older adults through direct patient education: the EMPOWER cluster randomized trial. JAMA Internal Medicine 174(6): 890–898.

Thillainadesan J, Gnjidic D, Green S (2018) Impact of deprescribing interventions in older hospitalised patients on prescribing and clinical outcomes: a systematic review of randomised trials. Drugs & Aging 35(4):303–319.

Thomopoulos C, Parati G, Zanchetti A (2018) Effects of blood pressure-lowering treatment on cardiovascular outcomes and mortality: 14 – effects of different classes of antihypertensive drugs in older and younger patients: overview and meta-analysis. Journal of Hypertension 36(8):1637–1647.

Thompson J (2019) Deprescribing in palliative care. Clinical Medicine (London) 19(4):311–314.

Valencia WM, Botros D, Vera-Nunez M (2018) Diabetes treatment in the elderly: incorporating geriatrics, technology, and functional medicine. Current Diabetes Reports 18(10):95.

van der Meer HG, Taxis K, Pont LG (2018) Changes in prescribing symptomatic and preventive medications in the last year of life in older nursing home residents. Frontiers in Pharmacology 8(990): doi: 10.3389/fphar.2017.00990. eCollection 2017.

Van Leeuwen E, Petrovic M, van Driel ML et al (2018) Withdrawal versus continuation of long-term antipsychotic drug use for behavioural and psychological symptoms in older people with dementia. Cochrane Database Syst Rev 3: Cd007726.

Villalba-Moreno AM, Alfaro-Lara ER, Pérez-Guerrero MC et al (2016) Systematic review on the use of anticholinergic scales in poly pathological patients. Archives of Gerontology and Geriatrics 62:1–8.

Waljee AK, Rogers MAM, Lin P et al (2017). Short-term use of oral corticosteroids and related harms among adults in the United States: population based cohort study. BMJ 357:j1415.

Walsh CA, Cahir C, Tecklenborg S et al (2019) The association between medication non-adherence and adverse health outcomes in ageing populations: A systematic review and meta-analysis. British Journal of Clinical Pharmacology 85(11):2464–2478.

Wastesson JW, Morin L, Tan ECK et al (2018) An update on the clinical consequences of polypharmacy in older adults: a narrative review. Expert Opinion on Drug Safety 17(12):1185–1196.

Wongrakpanich S, Wongrakpanich A, Melhado K et al (2018) A comprehensive review of non-steroidal anti-inflammatory drug use in the elderly. Aging and Disease 9(1):143–150.

Wood H, Dickman A, Star A et al (2018) Updates in palliative care – overview and recent advancements in the pharmacological management of cancer pain. Clinical Medicine (Lond) 18(1):17–22.

Woodford HJ (2018) Anticholinergic drugs for overactive bladder in frail older patients: the case against. Drugs & Aging 35(9):773–776.

Woodford HJ, Fisher J (2019) New horizons in deprescribing for older people. Age & Ageing 48(6):768–775.

World Health Organisation (WHO) (2017) Medication without harm – global patient safety challenge on medication safety. WHO, Geneva.

Wouters H, van der Meer H, Taxis K (2017) Quantification of anticholinergic and sedative drug load with the Drug Burden Index: a review of outcomes and methodological quality of studies. European Journal of Clinical Pharmacology 73(3):257–266.

Wright DJ, Scott S, Buck J et al (2019) Role of nurses in supporting proactive deprescribing. Nursing Standards 34(3): 44–50.

Wright RM, Sloane R, Pieper CF et al (2009) Underuse of indicated medications among physically frail older US veterans at the time of hospital discharge: results of a cross-sectional analysis of data from the Geriatric Evaluation and Management Drug Study. American Journal of Geriatric Pharmacotherapy 7(5): 271–280.

Yandrapalli S, Gupta S, Andries G et al (2019) Drug therapy of dyslipidemia in the elderly. Drugs & Aging 36(4): 321–340.

CHAPTER 12

Nutrition and Hydration

AGATHE DARIA JADCZAK • NATALIE LUSCOMBE-MARSH •
RENUKA VISVANATHAN

LEARNING OBJECTIVES

After reading this chapter, you will be able to:

- understand the importance of monitoring and managing the nutritional status of older people
- understand the causes, risks and consequences of weight loss, malnutrition and obesity in older people
- understand the importance of oral health and how it might affect the nutritional status of older people
- understand the risks and consequences of dehydration and recommended intervention strategies
- be aware of common screening tools to assess the nutritional status of older people and recommended nutritional and activity therapies.

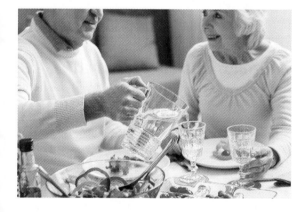

INTRODUCTION

Healthy nutrition and hydration have significant implications for the health and wellbeing of older people. Early identification allows for assessment and proactive management, reducing the risk of poor health outcomes and allowing older people to maintain functional independence, thus promoting healthy ageing and good

quality of life. This chapter provides an overview of the risks, consequences and management strategies for weight loss, malnutrition and obesity, as well as the importance of oral health and dehydration on the nutritional status of older people. It will discuss the healthy body mass index for older people, undernutrition and its contributing factors, as well as screening for obesity, oral health and nutritional status, followed by management strategies and dehydration. It is hoped that this chapter will enable nurses to more effectively determine the nutritional status of older people and develop appropriate management strategies to promote healthy ageing.

NUTRITIONAL HEALTH IN OLDER PEOPLE

Nutritional health is important in achieving healthy ageing. Poor nutritional intake is common among older people and could result in undernutrition or obesity. In Australia, approximately 15–40% of community-dwelling older people aged ≥70 years and up to 80% of nursing home residents are at risk of poor nutrition (Arjuna et al 2017; Visvanathan 2003). This chapter is written with a focus on older people who are frail and thus provides significant attention to the issue of undernutrition, whereby weight loss arising from undernutrition contributes to the development and progression of diseases such as sarcopenia, defined as 'progressive and generalised loss of skeletal muscle mass and strength' (Santilli et al 2014:177), and the geriatric syndrome of frailty.

The Healthy Body Mass Index

Regardless of age, body mass index (BMI) is most commonly used to classify the nutritional status of a person, and to determine whether a person is of a healthy weight for their height. BMI compares a person's weight and height to give an idea of whether they are underweight, healthy weight, overweight or obese for their height, according to their categories. It is calculated by dividing the person's weight (in kilograms) by his or her height (in metres squared). BMI is one type of tool to help health professionals assess the risk for chronic disease. However, there is a risk with applying the same cut-offs across the ethnicity, age and frailty continuum and health practitioners need to be wary.

A healthy BMI for a Caucasian adult is considered to be between 18.5 and 24.9 kg/m^2 (Table 12.1). As people age, these classifications seem to change and weight loss, be it intentional or unintentional, can be harmful as it leads to loss of muscle mass and performance. A meta-analysis of 32 cohort studies, including 197,940 older people aged $\geq$ 65 years, found a U-shaped association between all-cause mortality and BMI, with mortality risk being low at a BMI of 24.0–30.9 kg/m^2 and starting to increase at < 23 kg/m^2 (Winter et al 2014). Consequently, based on these data, the healthy BMI classifications for older people aged $\geq$ 65 years need to be adjusted (Table 12.1).

How much a person weighs is the sum of the amounts of water, bone, cartilage, muscle and fat in the body. A significant change in weight (loss or gain) can therefore relate to a change in any combination of these elements.

For example, weight loss can be seen with dehydration and, conversely, weight gain can be due to water retention. Weight change (loss or gain) of more than 5% over a 6-month period is clinically relevant and reasons for rapid weight change need to be investigated and addressed (Arjuna et al 2017; Miller & Wolfe 2008; Somes et al 2002).

Healthcare professionals need to understand that older people who are malnourished can present as underweight due to loss of muscle and bone mass, or, paradoxically, can carry excess fat, particularly deep visceral fat, and have a relatively low muscle to fat mass ratio. Importantly, the malnourished older person, rather than losing fat, has a greater likelihood of disproportionately losing muscle mass, and maybe even bone mass, leading to conditions such as sarcopenia and osteoporosis (see Chapter 22). It follows, therefore, that any recommendation for weight loss in an obese older person must be carefully considered with attention given to preserving muscle mass and strength, and a focus on protein intake coupled with exercise (Villareal et al 2005).

> **Promoting Wellness**
>
> - Promote good nutrition in combination with multicomponent exercise
> - Promote oral health and seeing the dentist regularly
> - Promote regular fluid intake

UNDERNUTRITION IN OLDER PEOPLE

Malnutrition in older people can lead to various health consequences, including:
- poor wound healing
- a weak immune system, increasing the risk of infection
- muscle weakness and decreased bone mass, increasing the risk of falls and fractures
- a higher risk of hospitalisation
- an increased risk of mortality (Visvanathan 2003).

Undernutrition leading to functional decline and potentially loss of independence (Sanford 2017) is ultimately the consequence of reduced appetite and food consumption, culminating in a failure to meet energy and micro- and macronutrient requirements (MacIntosh et al 2000). The prevalence of malnutrition varies between 10% in community-dwelling people aged 65 years and over, and can affect up to 60% of hospitalised older people and residents of aged care facilities (Elia et al 2005).

TABLE 12.1
Suggested BMI Classifications for Adults Aged < 65 and $\geq$ 65 Years

Classification	Adults Aged < 65 Years BMI (kg/m^2)	Adults Aged $\geq$ 65 Years BMI (kg/m^2)
Underweight	< 18.5	< 23.0
Healthy weight	18.5 – 24.9	23.0 – 30.9
Overweight	$\geq$ 25.0	$\geq$ 31.0

Winter et al (2014).

With increasing age, there are physiological changes that occur which contribute to appetite and weight loss. The 'anorexia of ageing' is defined as the loss of appetite and/or decreased food intake in later life. It is associated with adverse health outcomes (Martone et al 2013), such as poor quality of life, morbidity and mortality (Landi et al 2016). Decreases in the senses of taste and smell with ageing can significantly affect an older person's desire to eat. Additionally, ageing-related increases in pro-inflammatory cytokines are linked to cachexia, excess catabolism and reduced food intake (Minciullo et al 2016). Changes in the production of appetite-regulating hormones and peptides can also affect gastric emptying, satiety and the feeling of satisfaction that dampens hunger (Minciullo et al 2016).

With increasing age, there is a decrease in physical activity; however, the reduction in oral intake is not compensatory (Pilgrim et al 2015). The reality is that when reductions in energy intake exceed reductions in activity, weight loss occurs. Moreover, when weight is lost in the context of more sedentary lifestyle, particularly after the age of 40 years (Keller & Engelhardt 2013), it is disproportionately due to loss of muscle mass and muscle strength, putting the older person at risk of sarcopenia. Weight loss is one of the five criteria to describe physical frailty (Table 12.2).

Weight loss and malnutrition are common in older people, particularly after hospital admissions or bed-rest of more than a few day due to illness (English & Paddon-Jones 2010). The prevalence of unintentional weight loss varies between 15% and 27% in people aged over 65 years and can be as high as 50–60% in residents of aged care facilities (McMinn et al 2011). Weight loss should not be accepted as a normal consequence of ageing, but rather viewed as an indicator of declining health status and an opportunity for early intervention.

Contributing Factors to Undernutrition

Undernutrition is an important issue in the care of older people and can arise from many factors other than reduced oral intake. Therefore, a multidisciplinary approach to the identification, assessment and management is necessary. Nurses have a critical role, along with dietitians and the wider healthcare team, in identifying and intervening in the undernutrition of their older patients.

The mnemonics 'MEALS ON WHEELS' (Morley 2012) is a helpful prompt to assessing potential factors contributing to undernutrition and weight loss, which are amenable to intervention (see Box 12.1).

Psychological factors, including mood disorders such as anxiety or depression (Blazer 2003) can have a significant impact on an older person's appetite and are a common treatable cause of weight loss (Sanford 2017). Social isolation has also been shown to decrease appetite and the perceived pleasure derived from eating (Pilgrim et al 2015). Older people are more vulnerable to feeling isolated, which has a potential impact on nutrition, due to:

- health issues
- cognitive impairment

TABLE 12.2
Criteria and Cut-Offs for Frailty and Sarcopenia

Fried's Phenotype Frailty Criteria & Cut-Offs		EWGSOP2 Sarcopenia Criteria & Cut-Offs	
Weight loss	≥ 4.5 kg or ≥ 5% per year	Low skeletal muscle mass	♂: < 20 kg ♀: < 15 kg
Slow gait speed	♂: ≥ 0.6/≥ 0.7 m/s (≤ 173/> 173 cm) ♀: ≥ 0.6/≥ 0.7 m/s (≤ 159/>159 cm)	Low gait speed	≤ 0.8 m/s
Low grip strength	♂: ≤ 29–32 kg according to BMI ♀: ≤ 17–21 kg according to BMI	Low grip strength	♂: < 27 kg ♀: < 16 kg
Low physical activity	♂: < 383 kcal/week ♀: < 270 kcal/week	Low physical performance	≤ 8 SPPB score ≥ 20 s TUG ≥ 6 min 400 m walk
Exhaustion based on questions from CES-D			

EWGSOP2: European Working Group on Sarcopenia in Older People version 2; ♂: male, ♀: female; CES-D: Centre for Epidemiological Studies Depression Scale; SPPB: short physical performance battery; TUG: Timed Up & Go Test
Cruz-Jentoft et al (2019); Fried et al (2001).

<table>
<tr><td>

BOX 12.1 MEALS ON WHEELS Mnemonic for Treatable Causes of Weight Loss

Medications
Emotional (i.e. depression)
Alcoholism, anorexia tardive, abuse (elder)
Late life paranoia
Swallowing problems

Oral problems
Nosocomial infections, no money (i.e. poverty)

Wandering/dementia
Hyperthyroidism, hypercalcaemia, hypoadrenalism
Enteric problems (malabsorption)
Eating problems (i.e. tremor)
Low salt and low cholesterol diets
Shopping and meal preparation problems, stones (cholecystitis)

Morley (2012).

</td><td>

Promoting Wellness
Strategies to Promote a Healthy Appetite

If you are underweight or have a small appetite
Small regular meals and nutritious snacks are recommended if you are underweight or your appetite is small.

- Thin older women are at greatest risk of bone fractures.
  If you are at risk, have plenty of milk and milk products to keep your bones healthy.
- Eat often – include breakfast, morning tea, lunch, afternoon tea, dinner and supper.
- Nutritious snacks include sandwiches or toast with a topping, yoghurt, milk puddings, a milk drink, soup, a scone or a muffin, a small handful of unsalted nuts or seeds.
- Keep some favourite toppings on hand, such as cheese, peanut butter, eggs, baked beans, avocado or canned fish. These all go well on bread or toast.
- Use standard or full-fat milk and fullcream yoghurts.
- Enjoy desserts such as custard, ice cream, fruit crumble, trifle or rice pudding.

As you get older, there may be times when it's harder to shop for, prepare and cook nutritious foods.
- Use frozen or ready-to-heat dinners (e.g. from the supermarket) for quick and easy meals.
- When you do feel like cooking, make larger meals sometimes and freeze portions for another day.
- Try a protein or milk-based supplementary drink (commercial products are available from a supermarket, chemist or on prescription from your GP).

Reproduced with permission by Ministry of Health NZ (2016).

</td></tr>
</table>

- physical disabilities (i.e. incontinence) (see Chapter 13)
- living alone
- the lack of money
- limited mobility
- transportation barriers that prevent participation in social activities.

Additionally, living and eating alone can lead an older person to eat less due to a lack of support or less motivation to shop, cook and eat well (Pilgrim et al 2015). Environmental and financial barriers are further factors that can affect an older person's nutritional status, such as lack of access to grocery stores due to unsafe terrain, limited transportation or lack of money to buy nutritious food. Older people with medical issues such as dementia or who simply forget to eat will require external support if weight loss is to be prevented and good nutrition achieved (Sanford 2017). Lastly, medication side effects (see Chapter 11), such as constipation, oral dryness and altered senses of smell and taste, can all impact negatively on appetite (Roy et al 2016).

OBESITY IN OLDER PEOPLE

The prevalence of overweight and obesity (BMI > 31 kg/m^2) is increasing in the older population with the average older Australian now 6–7 kg heavier than 20 years ago (AIHW 2004). Overweight and obesity are caused by an energy imbalance, where energy intake

exceeds energy expenditure over a considerable period of time (Visvanathan 2017). The rise in obesity is attributed to numerous factors, including:

- a global trend towards more energy-dense foods that are high in sugar and fat, and low in vitamins, minerals and other micronutrients
- increasingly sedentary lifestyles
- changes in transportation
- increased urbanisation (Visvanathan 2017).

There are many adverse health outcomes associated with obesity in older age. Obesity increases the likelihood of disability, particularly with respect to lower limb arthritis (see Chapter 22), as well as lower muscle mass and strength and, hence, physical frailty (Villareal et al 2004). Obese older people are more likely to:

- experience pain
- have greater limitations of physical function
- be homebound (Chapman 2010)
- be at higher risk of future disability, declining functional status and admission to residential aged care (Baumgartner et al 2004; Villareal et al 2005; Zizza et al 2002).

Obesity also has an impact on respiratory function, affecting overall health. Forced vital capacity, total lung capacity, residual volume and lung compliance decline with increasing BMI and the reduction in respiratory function can develop into obesity hypoventilation syndrome (OHS). Most people with OHS are sleep deprived and drowsy during the day due to obstructive sleep apnoea resulting from OHS (Powers 2008).

There is also a relationship between increasing BMI and urinary incontinence (see Chapter 13) (Hunskaar 2008). Regarding the type, stress incontinence seems to have a stronger association with increasing weight than urge incontinence (Hunskaar 2008). Additionally, weight loss may not only help to reduce the risk of developing urinary incontinence in the first place, but may also help to reduce the symptoms in those already suffering from urinary incontinence (Subak et al 2002).

Obesity has also been associated with late life dementia, especially vascular dementia (Richard et al 2010) (see Chapter 26), highlighting the importance of healthy weight in youth and middle age to reduce the risk of developing dementia in older age. Obese older people have been found to be at a higher risk of developing depression (see Chapter 25), influenced by factors such as reduced physical and social activity (de Wit et al 2010). Obesity is also associated with a 25% increase in mood and anxiety disorders (Simon et al 2006).

ORAL HEALTH IN OLDER PEOPLE

Oral health is particularly important across the lifespan, especially when it comes to ensuring healthy nutrition, and therefore is discussed in detail here. Problems with teeth, gums and dentures can significantly hamper an individual's ability to achieve healthy ageing. For example, pain and difficulty with eating can lead to poor levels of nutrition (Chauncey et al 1984). A dry mouth can be caused by medications and can lead to difficulty in eating, as well as dysphasia (difficulty in speaking) (Narhi et al 1992). Poor appearance and dental incapacity can also lead to low self-esteem and social isolation (Rouxel et al 2016). Poor oral health can also exacerbate a number health conditions, such as diabetes,

cardiovascular disease and aspiration pneumonia, especially where inflammation is present (Aida et al 2011; Azarpazhooh & Leake 2006).

Patterns of oral health in older age are changing with fewer older people relying on complete dentures for function because they have retained some natural teeth due to education in their younger years on better oral hygiene. Nevertheless, there remains a substantial number of older people whose ability to chew is compromised. This results in individuals selecting foods that can be more comfortably chewed, which tends to result in a diet that is low in fruits and vegetables, an associated reduction in both non-starch polysaccharide and micronutrient intakes, and a reduced food intake overall (Walls & Steele 2004). Other factors impacting on the ability to chew and swallow include salivary flow and function related to changes in neurology, gut inflammation or oropharyngeal function (Walls & Steele 2004). These changes fall under the medical condition termed dysphagia (the difficulty of initiating a swallow), which is estimated to be present in 50–60% of individuals in residential aged care facilities and 15–22% in the general population (Attrill et al 2018; Roden & Altman 2013; Sura et al 2012). Changes in oral health status tend to occur gradually.

Nutritional Screening

Early identification that an older person is at risk of poor nutrition allows for earlier assessment and proactive management. Using a screening tool to identify weight change and undernutrition is a fundamental step to good clinical care. There are many screening tools to choose from. It is important to choose one and use it well rather than miss opportunities by debating which tool is the best. Commonly used screening tools include:

- Mini Nutritional Assessment – Short Form (MNA-SF) (Guigoz et al 2002)
- Malnutrition Universal Screening Tool (MUST) (Elia 2003)
- Simplified Nutritional Appetite Questionnaire (SNAQ) (Wilson et al 2005)
- Malnutrition Screening Tool (MST) (Ferguson et al 1999).

The Mini Nutritional Assessment – Short Form is a validated screening tool that can identify people aged 65 and above who are malnourished or at risk of malnutrition. The MNA-SF comprises six questions on food intake, weight loss, mobility, psychological stress, neuropsychological problems and BMI. The MNA-SF can be completed in less than five minutes and is applicable across multiple care settings. The maximum score is 14 and it classifies the older person as malnourished (0–7 points), at risk of malnutrition (8–11 points) and well nourished (12–14 points).

The Malnutrition Universal Screening Tool is a validated five-step screening tool to identify people who are malnourished, at risk of malnutrition or obese, and is applicable across multiple care settings. It also includes management guidelines which can be used to develop a care plan. A total score of ≥ 2 indicates a high risk of malnutrition, a score of 1 indicates a medium risk of malnutrition and a score of 0 indicates a low risk of malnutrition (Elia 2003).

The Simplified Nutritional Assessment Questionnaire is a simple four-item assessment tool to identify people at risk of weight loss (Wilson et al 2005). It consists of four questions relating to taste, appetite, satiety and meal frequency. The SNAQ risk score has a maximum score of 20 and is able to predict future weight loss over a 6-month period with 82% sensitivity and 85% specificity in people aged ≥ 60 years (Wilson et al 2005). A score of <15 indicates a risk for future weight loss and anorexia. The SNAQ is best suited for the primary care setting and can be applied to healthier populations as a strategy for intervening earlier to prevent the onset of undernutrition.

The Malnutrition Screening Tool is a validated tool that is almost universally used in the acute care setting across Australia. It contains only two questions related to weight loss and decreased appetite. A score of ≥ 2 suggests a risk of malnutrition. No training is required to use the tool and it has a simple action pathway. However, the MST does not detect chronically underweight individuals as it only assesses change in weight and appetite. Also, no specific support materials are provided (Chapman 2010).

Besides questionnaires, there is the option to use bioelectrical impedance analyses (BIA) as a tool to measure changes in body composition, including hydration. BIA has emerged as an accurate and consistent tool that is inexpensive, non-invasive, portable and simple to operate (Subak 2002). BIA can be used to measure

---

Tips for Best Practice
The Australian Dietary Guidelines of Most Relevance to Adults (Up to Age 75 Years)

GUIDELINE 1
To achieve and maintain a healthy weight, be physically active and choose amounts of nutritious food and drinks to meet your energy needs.

- Older people should eat nutritious foods and keep physically active to help maintain muscle strength and a healthy weight.

GUIDELINE 2
Eat a wide variety of nutritious foods from these five food groups every day:

- Plenty of vegetables of different types and colours, and legumes/bean
- Fruit
- Grain (cereal) foods, mostly wholegrain and/or high fibre varieties, such as breads, cereals, rice, noodles, polenta, couscous, oats, quinoa
- Lean meats and poultry, fish, eggs, tofu, nuts and legumes/beans
- Milk, yoghurt, cheese and/or their alternatives, mostly reduced fat

  And drink plenty of water.

GUIDELINE 3
Limit intake of foods containing saturated fat, added salt, added sugars and alcohol.

a. Limit intake of foods high in saturated fat such as many biscuits, cakes, pastries, pies, processed meats, commercial burgers, pizza, fried foods, potato chips, crisps and other savoury snacks.

- Replace high fat foods which contain predominantly saturated fats such as butter, cream, cooking margarine, coconut and palm oil with foods which contain predominantly polyunsaturated and monounsaturated fats such as oils, spreads, nut butters/pastes and avocado.

b. Limit intake of foods and drinks containing added salt.

- Read labels to choose lower sodium options among similar foods.
- Do not add salt to foods in cooking or at the table.

c. Limit intake of foods and drinks containing added sugars such as confectionery, sugar-sweetened soft drinks and cordials, fruit drinks, vitamin waters, energy and sports drinks.

d. If you choose to drink alcohol, limit intake.

GUIDELINE 5
Care for your food; prepare and store it safely.

Source: NHMRC, Australian Government Department of Health (2015).

muscle mass, body fat, body fluid, skin hydration and tissue ischaemia (Ricciardi & Talbot 2007). Considering the diversity of available devices, clinics should research which to buy to ensure the device is well validated.

Nursing actions in response to indication that an older person is malnourished or at risk of malnourishment include referral for further assessment and the use of strategies to promote healthy nutrition and optimal weight. Dietitians are allied health professionals who are trained to carry out detailed assessment of changes in nutrition and hydration status. Where possible, referral to dietitians should be recommended. Nurses can also institute simple management strategies while older people are in their care.

Tips for Best Practice

- Nutritional assessments should be undertaken with older people who are at risk of malnutrition
- Older people should be referred to healthcare professionals where needed
- Promoting good oral health, nutrition, exercise and hydration is vital

---

MANAGEMENT FOR MALNUTRITION AND WEIGHT LOSS IN OLDER PEOPLE

Central to the management of malnutrition is exercise and healthy nutrition. In fact, good nutrition combined with multi-component exercise, including aerobic, resistance, balance and flexibility, appear to give older people greater health and wellbeing benefits than nutritional strategies alone (Paddon-Jones & Rasmussen 2009; Phillips 2016).

Other factors contributing to poor nutrition should also be addressed. For example, food palatability and acceptance could be improved by flavour enhancement to counteract the effects of the anorexia of ageing and increase overall quality of life (Guigoz et al 2002). When eating, hearing and intraoral sounds could also compensate for changes in sight, smell and taste (Attrill et al 2018). Exercise has a number of benefits, including increasing the resting metabolic rate, which can stimulate appetite, hence increasing oral intake (English & Paddon-Jones 2010). Exercise also helps to improve mood (Rouxel et al 2016) and build muscle mass and strength, thus reducing the risk of sarcopenia and frailty (Aida et al 2011); it decreases the risk of constipation and, consequently, early satiety that dampens hunger (English & Paddon-Jones 2010).

Regarding nutritional interventions, evidence suggests that older people require higher levels of dietary protein

to counteract age-related changes in protein metabolism (Azarpazhooh & Leake 2006). It is preferable that the recommended intake of dietary protein is achieved through consumption of tailored amounts of:

- lean red or white meat
- fish
- whole grains
- seeds and nuts
- vegetables and fruits
- only limited amounts of highly-processed foods.

However, it might be challenging to meet recommended protein requirements for older people who may not have the appetite and tend to feel satisfied soon after eating (Visvanathan 2015). One strategy to deal with early satiety is to take smaller meals and to snack throughout the day (Roden & Altman 2013). For those individuals, nutritional supplementation with an energy and protein-dense content per serve can ensure that the necessary protein intake is achieved (Sura et al 2012). Apart from protein intake, an adequate caloric intake should also be met (Roden & Altman 2013). For example, a daily supplement of biscuits containing 11.5 g of protein and 244 kcal has been suggested to positively impact on weight and appetite in older people (Attrill et al 2018).

Practice Points

- In older people aged ≥ 65 years, a higher BMI is associated with a lower mortality risk
- Exercise coupled with protein intake is best for preserving muscle mass and strength
- Malnutrition in older people can lead to serious health consequences, making early identification crucial.

Management for Oral Health in Older People

Individuals who lose all of their natural teeth in older age should be given dietary support and advice as the first step in preventing or managing undernutrition. These older people will find using complete dentures a challenge that will often lead to food being liquidised unless positive support and advice are provided. Professional dental help may be required to help older people cope and to maximise efficient oral function (Walls & Steele 2004).

The nurse has an important role to encourage older people to see their dentist regularly in order to maintain good oral health. Further, planning for any dental

---

TABLE 12.3
Overview of the Oral Health Assessment Tool (OHAT) and an Oral Hygiene Care Plan (OHCP)

	OHAT*	OHCP*
Categories	1. Lips	1. Dentist contact details
	2. Tongue	2. Scheduled dental appointments
	3. Gums and oral tissue	3. Existing dentures and/or natural teeth
	4. Saliva	4. Time and frequency of cleaning dentures
	5. Natural teeth	5. Time and frequency of cleaning natural teeth
	6. Dentures	6. Types and frequency of assistance needed
	7. Oral cleanliness	7. List of interventions for oral hygiene care
	8. Dental pain	8. List of regular problems with oral hygiene care

Visual scoring: 0 Healthy, 1 Changes, 2 Unhealthy
If 1 or 2 for any category, dentist referral is suggested
*Table provides an overview of the OHAT and OHCP only. See reference for original tools/plans.
Chalmers et al (2009).

---

treatments needs to take functional dietary issues into account. All who are involved in the healthcare of older people have a responsibility to recognise and promote good nutrition. The use of oral and dental policies and procedures, such as the Oral Health Assessment Tool (OHAT) or an Oral Hygiene Care Plan (OHCP) (Table 12.3) can enhance the involvement of healthcare professionals in the delivery of oral hygiene care to older people and better consequent oral health (Chalmers 2009). The solution to the problem of impaired nutrition related to oral health, however, is much more long term. Nutritional supplementation plays a critical role where oral health status is poor (Walls & Steele 2004).

MANAGEMENT OF OBESITY IN OLDER PEOPLE

As with malnutrition and weight loss, nutrition and exercise play a key role in managing overweight and obesity in older people. Nutritional intervention for obese older people should be considered where the presence of excess fat impacts on function and weight reduction is likely to be of benefit. Standard nutritional interventions would likely consist of a hypocaloric diet with an estimated 500–750 kcal/day deficit while simultaneously providing adequate nutrients. Dietary measures should always be guided by a dietitian, and the most successful weight-loss programs provide ongoing supervision from multidisciplinary health professionals to support life-long behavioural change.

Special considerations for the intake of micronutrients supplementation, vitamins (i.e. Vitamin D), calcium and protein should be taken to prevent the potential acceleration of sarcopenia (Newman et al 2005) and/or

a decrease (1–2%) in bone mass (Villareal et al 2008). To prevent the loss of lean mass in older people ($\geq$ 65 years), consumption of at least 1.0–1.2 g/kg/day of protein is recommended (Bauer et al 2013). For older individuals suffering from acute or chronic disease, it is recommended their daily protein intake is increased to 1.2–1.5 g/kg/day (Bauer et al 2013). It has also been suggested that protein consumed shortly after exercise might have the greatest benefits for muscle retention (Bauer et al 2013). Table 12.4 presents commonly consumed core foods containing relatively moderate to high amounts of protein (compared to other core foods) that can easily be incorporated into a daily menu plan. An older person who weighs 70 kg, for example, and has been advised to lose weight should aim to have approximately 1.4 g/kg/day of protein, which is about 98 g of protein daily. This equates to about three to four serves per day of any lean meat or meat alternative, plus about three serves per day of any dairy or dairy alternative.

Exercise is a main strategy of attenuating loss of muscle mass. A multi-component exercise program (strength, aerobic, balance, flexibility) guided by an exercise physiologist or physiotherapist is recommended, and has been shown to improve physical function. Frailty should not be a contraindication for exercise; in fact it has been shown that more frail older people may show the largest functional improvements with exercise (Sartorio et al 2004).

Therefore, a combination of both nutritional intervention and exercise for older obese Australians and New Zealanders will not only lead to weight loss but perhaps more importantly improve physical function, reduce disease severity and improve quality of life.

TABLE 12.4
Core Foods With Moderate/High Amounts of Protein

Core Foods	Protein (g)	Energy (kcal)	Recommendations
Lean meat – alternatives – typical serve size (3–4 serves per day)			– Meats are a good source of zinc and iron
Chicken: 100 g	22	105	
Pork: 100 g	23	120	– Animal proteins provide Vitamin B_{12}
Turkey: 100 g	22	117	– Oily fish provide healthy fats such as omega-3 and should be consumed twice/week
Beef: 100 g	28	140	
Lamb: 100 g	21	135	– Legumes are a good source of fibre
Fish: 100 g	22	105	
TVP* or soy meat: 170 g	20	204	
Eggs: 2 large	13	132	
Legumes: 150 g (1 cup)	10	153	
Dairy – alternatives – typical serve size (3 serves per day)			– Low-fat varieties can limit unhealthy saturated fats
Low-fat milk: 250 mL (1 cup)	9	105	– Full-fat products are good for those without cardiovascular disease but contain more calories than low-fat choices
Soy milk: 250 mL (1 cup)	8	97	
Evaporated skim milk: 120 mL (1 cup)	11	102	
Unflavoured low-fat/Greek yoghurt: 200 g (1 tub)	15	180	
Low-fat dairy dessert/custard: 200 g (1 tub)	8	165	– Rice/other nut milks are lower in protein than dairy milk, but may be fortified with ~10 g protein powder
Hard cheese: 40 g	10	159	
Soft cheese: 120 g (1/2 cup)	12	151	

*TVP: Textured vegetable protein
Based on the Australian food database FoodWorks®

Safety Alert

Other interventions for obese older people include Very Low Calorie Diets (VLCDs). These diets consist of 3.4 MJ (800 kcal) per day when consumed exclusively (three meals per day) and should contain 0.8–1.5 g/kg/day of high-quality protein, sufficient essential fatty acids and micronutrients. While there is currently no evidence to support the use of these diets in the older population, they may be useful in situations where rapid weight loss is imperative to restore physical function. These diets may be unsafe and are contraindicated in persons with unstable angina, cardiac failure, severe renal or hepatic dysfunction, malignancies and type 1 diabetes.

If an older person has exhausted all other means of managing their obesity, a surgical procedure may be considered. The most common bariatric procedure in Australia is laparoscopic adjustable gastric banding (LAGB). This procedure is recommended for people aged 18–65 (Victorian Government Department of Human Services 2009) and while there is some evidence that LAGB may be performed safely in people aged 65 years and above (Busetto et al 2008; Taylor & Layani 2006), it is only recommended for those with a BMI of > 40 and severe health complications due to their obesity (Yermilov et al 2009).

MANAGEMENT OF DEHYDRATION IN OLDER PEOPLE

Dehydration is often poorly acknowledged as a major contributor to poor health but especially with climate extremes, when older people may experience dehydration. Dehydration reduces the amount of fluid circulating in the blood vessels, which can lower the blood pressure and exacerbate postural hypotension, putting the older person at risk for falls (see Chapter 16) (Wotton et al 2008). During 'heat waves' there is an increase in the number of older people who are hospitialised, as well as an increased rate of mortality (Schols et al 2009).

Indications that an older person may be dehydrated include (Mentes 2006):

- dry mouth
- sunken eyes
- dry, inelastic skin
- drowsiness
- confusion or disorientation
- dizziness
- low blood pressure
- reduced urinary output
- concentrated, strong smelling urine.

While any of these signs can be present in multiple conditions and are rather subjective, they can be simple prompts to initiate nutritional treatment.

With increasing age, there is the physiological change of reduced thirst sensation resulting in older people failing to recognise the need to consume fluids. The recommended daily intake of fluids should be at least 1600 mL/24h in order to ensure adequate hydration (Hodgkinson et al 2003). Dehydration does not need to be severe to affect function. Mild dehydration can affect mental performance, including memory, attention, concentration and reaction time, and increase fatigue (Wilson & Morley 2003).

Dehydration is also a major reason for constipation, which in older people can result in urinary retention or haemorrhoids (Mentes 2006). Encouraging an older person to drink more fluid may therefore increase stool frequency and enhance the beneficial effects of fibre intake. Additionally, increasing fluid intake reduces the risk of urinary tract infection. Poorly hydrated individuals are also more likely to develop pressure injuries and skin conditions (Schols et al 2009). Dehydration is a particular risk for older people living with dementia, who may not recognise the thirst signal, or who are unable to communicate the need for more fluid.

The likelihood of dehydration is also increased when an older person has a restricted fluid intake, for example, to manage heart failure, or is taking medications such as diuretics and laxatives that act by drawing fluid from

---

Practice Scenario

Ms X is 80 years old. She is 165 cm tall and weighs 55 kg (calculated BMI of 20.2 kg/m²). She lives by herself. Her husband recently passed away and her adult daughter is currently on a 2-week summer vacation with her 10-year-old grandson. Ms X is complaining about dizziness and has lately been feeling weak.

MULTIPLE CHOICE QUESTIONS

1. Which of the following is an unlikely cause of her dizziness?
   a. Low blood pressure
   b. Dehydration
   c. Obesity
   d. Hot weather
   e. Changes in medications

2. Is there a reason to be concerned at Mrs X's BMI for her age?
   a. No, a BMI between 18.5 and 24.9 kg/m² is considered to be normal
   b. Yes, for people her age, she may be underweight, which can cause adverse health outcomes. Her weight requires attention.
   c. The BMI does not take water, muscle, bone and fat mass into account, therefore it is not reliable and should be ignored.

3. Which of the following strategies could be applied to Ms X with regards to managing her weakness?
   i   To determine her nutritional status
   ii To determine her social situation, mental state and medical problems
   iii To promote good nutrition, hydration and exercise
   iv To refer to heathcare professionals such as dentists, dietitians, exercise physiologists depending on her needs
   a. Only I
   b. I, II and IV
   c. Only IV
   d. All of the above

4. Which of the following assessments can be recommended to determine the nutritional status of Ms X?
   i   Mini Nutritional Assessment – Short Form (MNA-SF)
   ii Malnutrition Universal Screening Tool (MUST)
   iii Simplified Nutritional Appetite Questionnaire (SNAQ)
   iv Malnutrition Screening Tool (MST)
   a. I and III
   b. Only I
   c. II
   d. All of the above

the kidneys and gastrointestinal systems respectively (Wotton et al 2008). The nurse has an important role in regularly monitoring the older person's fluid status through regular weighing and maintenance of a target weight selected to guide the balance between fluid restriction and adequate hydration. Swallowing difficulties (requiring modified diet such as thickened fluids) and poorly controlled diabetes (see Chapter 9) are prevalent among older people and associated with poor hydration (Wotton et al 2008). Many older people who suffer from incontinence opt to reduce their fluid intake, predisposing them to dehydration and the ensuing adverse consequences (Mentes 2006). In such individuals, it can be difficult to achieve a balance and recommendations such as ensuring adequate fluid intake earlier in the day to minimise urinary frequency at night may be helpful. Strategies to reduce the risk of dehydration might include regular prompting and encouraging wet foods such as puréed fruit, yoghurt, jelly, custard and soup (Wotton et al 2008).

SUMMARY

Maintaining a good nutritional status is crucial for the health and wellbeing of older people. Several age-related changes and multiple factors can affect the nutritional status of this population group and the care provided. Nutritional screening tools can help to identify older people at risk, with strategies available to manage malnutrition, obesity, oral health and dehydration. Nurses need to be aware of those age-related changes and possible management strategies to be able to intervene early and prevent adverse health outcomes.

USEFUL RESOURCES

Australian Government Department of Health (2015) Healthy eating for adults, eatforhealth.gov.au

Ministry of Health NZ (2006, updated 2017). Nutrient reference values: Australia and New Zealand, www.nrv.gov.au/

NSW Government, Central Coast Local Health District (2015) Eating well: A nutrition resource for older people and their carers, www.cclhd.health.nsw.gov.au/wp-content/uploads/EatingWellANutritionResourceforOlderPeople.pdf

REFERENCES

Aida, J, Kondo K, Yamamoto T et al (2011) Oral health and cancer, cardiovascular, and respiratory mortality of Japanese. Journal of Dental Research 90(9):1129–1135.

Arjuna T, Luscombe-Marsh N, Lange K et al (2017) Changes in body weight and nutritional status in South Australian nursing home residents. Innovation in Aging 1(Suppl 1):696.

Attrill S, White S, Murray J et al (2018) Impact of oropharyngeal dysphagia on healthcare cost and length of stay in hospital: a systematic review. BMC Health Services Research 18(1): 594.

Australian Institute of Health and Welfare (AIHW) (2004) Australia's health 2004. AIHW, Canberra.

Azarpazhooh A, Leake JL (2006) Systematic review of the association between respiratory diseases and oral health. Journal of Periodontology 77(9):1465–1482.

Bauer, J, Biolo G, Cederholm T et al (2013) Evidence-based recommendations for optimal dietary protein intake in older people: a position paper from the PROT-AGE Study Group. Journal of the American Medical Directors Association 14.

Baumgartner RN, Wayne SJ, Waters DL et al (2004) Sarcopenic obesity predicts instrumental activities of daily living disability in the elderly. Obesity Research 12(12):1995–2004.

Blazer DG (2003) Depression in late life: review and commentary. Journal of Gerontology. Series A: Biological Sciences and Medical Science 58(3):249–265.

Busetto L, Angrisani L, Basso N et al (2008) Safety and efficacy of laparoscopic adjustable gastric banding in the elderly. Obesity (Silver Spring) 16(2):334–338.

Chalmers JM, Spencer AJ, Carter KD et al (2009) Caring for oral health in Australian residential care. Dental statistics and research series no. 48. Cat. no. DEN 193. AIHW, Canberra.

Chapman IM (2010) Obesity paradox during aging. Interdisciplinary Topics in Gerontology 37:20–36.

Chauncey HH, Muench ME, Kapur KK et al (1984). The effect of the loss of teeth on diet and nutrition. International Dental Journal 34(2):98–104.

Cruz-Jentoft AJ, Bahat G, Bauer J et al (2019) Sarcopenia: revised European consensus on definition and diagnosis. Age and Ageing 48(1):16–31.

de Wit LM, Fokkema M, van Straten A et al (2010) Depressive and anxiety disorders and the association with obesity, physical, and social activities. Depression and Anxiety 27(11):1057–1065.

Elia M (2003) The 'MUST' report. Nutritional screening for adults: a multidisciplinary responsibility. Development and use of the 'Malnutrition Universal Screening Tool' ('MUST') for adults. BAPEN, Malnutrition Advisory Group, a Standing Committee of BAPEN, Redditch.

Elia M, Zellipour L, Stratton RJ (2005) To screen or not to screen for adult malnutrition? Clin Nutr 24(6):867–884.

English KL, Paddon-Jones D (2010) Protecting muscle mass and function in older adults during bed rest. Current Opinion in Clinical Nutrition and Metabolic Care 13(1):34–39.

Ferguson M, Capra S, Bauer J et al (1999) Development of a valid and reliable malnutrition screening tool for adult acute hospital patients. Nutrition 15(6):458–464.

Fried LP, Tangen CM, Walston J et al (2001) Frailty in older adults: evidence for a phenotype. Journal of Gerontology. Series A: Biological Sciences and Medical Science 56.

Guigoz Y, Lauque S, Vellas BJ (2002) Identifying the elderly at risk for malnutrition. The Mini Nutritional Assessment. Clin Geriatr Med 18(4):737–757.

Hodgkinson B, Evans D, Wood J (2003) Maintaining oral hydration in older adults: a systematic review. International Journal of Nursing Practice 9(3):S19–S28.

Hunskaar S (2008) A systematic review of overweight and obesity as risk factors and targets for clinical intervention for urinary incontinence in women. Neurourology and Urodynamics 27(8):749–757.

Keller K, Engelhardt M (2013) Strength and muscle mass loss with aging process. Age and strength loss. Muscles, Ligaments and Tendons Journal 3(4):346–350.

Landi F, Calvani R, Tosato M et al (2016) Anorexia of aging: risk factors, consequences, and potential treatments. Nutrients 8(2):69.

MacIntosh C, Morley JE, Chapman IM (2000) The anorexia of aging. Nutrition 16(10):983–995.

Martone AM, Onder G, Vetrano DL et al (2013) Anorexia of aging: a modifiable risk factor for frailty. Nutrients 5(10):4126–4133.

McMinn J, Steel C, Bowman A (2011) Investigation and management of unintentional weight loss in older adults. BMJ 342: d1732.

Mentes J (2006) Oral hydration in older adults: greater awareness is needed in preventing, recognizing, and treating dehydration. American Journal of Nursing 106(6):40–49; quiz 50.

Miller SL, Wolfe RR (2008) The danger of weight loss in the elderly. The Journal of Nutrition, Health and Aging 12(7):487–491.

Minciullo PL, Catalano A, Mandraffino G et al (2016) Inflammaging and anti-inflammaging: the role of cytokines in extreme longevity. Arch Immunol Ther Exp (Warsz) 64(2):111–126.

Ministry of Health NZ (2016) Eating for healthy older people. MOH, Wellington. Online. Available: www.healthed.govt.nz/system/files/resource-files/HE1145_Eating%20for%20healthy%20older%20people.pdf

Morley JE (2012) Undernutrition in older adults. Fam Pract 29 Suppl 1: i89–i93.

Narhi TO, Meurman JH, Ainamo A et al (1992) Association between salivary flow rate and the use of systemic medication among 76-, 81- and 86-year-old inhabitants in Helsinki, Finland. Journal of Dental Research 71(12):1875–1880.

National Health and Medical Research Council (NHMRC) & Australian Government Department of Health (2015) Australian Dietary Guidelines 1–5. Online. Available: https://www.eatforhealth.gov.au/guidelines/australian-dietary-guidelines-1-5

Newman AB, Lee JS, Visser M et al (2005) Weight change and the conservation of lean mass in old age: the Health, Aging and Body Composition Study. American Journal of Clinical Nutrition 82(4):872–878; quiz 915–916.

Paddon-Jones D, Rasmussen BB (2009) Dietary protein recommendations and the prevention of sarcopenia: Protein, amino acid metabolism and therapy. Current Opinion in Clinical Nutrition and Metabolic Care 12(1):86–90.

Phillips SM (2016) The impact of protein quality on the promotion of resistance exercise-induced changes in muscle mass. Nutrition and Metabolism (London) 13:64.

Pilgrim AL, Robinson SM, Sayer AA et al (2015) An overview of appetite decline in older people. Nursing Older People 27(5):29–35.

Powers MA (2008) The obesity hypoventilation syndrome. Respiratory Care 53(12):1723–1730.

Ricciardi R, Talbot LA (2007) Use of bioelectrical impedance analysis in the evaluation, treatment, and prevention of overweight and obesity. Journal of the American Academy of Nurse Practitioners 19(5):235–241.

Richard E, Ligthart SA, Moll van Charante EP et al (2010) Vascular risk factors and dementia – towards prevention strategies. Netherlands Journal of Medicine 68(10):284–290.

Roden DF, Altman KW (2013) Causes of dysphagia among different age groups: a systematic review of the literature. Otolaryngologic Clinics of North America 46(6):965–987.

Rouxel P, Heilmann A, Demakakos P et al (2016) Oral health-related quality of life and loneliness among older adults. European Journal of Ageing 14(2):101–109.

Roy M, Gaudreau P, Payette H (2016) A scoping review of anorexia of aging correlates and their relevance to population health interventions. Appetite 105:688–699.

Sanford AM (2017) Anorexia of aging and its role for frailty. Current Opinion in Clinical Nutrition and Metabolic Care 20(1):54–60.

Santilli V, Bernetti A, Mangone M et al (2014) Clinical definition of sarcopenia. Clinical Cases in Mineral and Bone Metabolism 11(3):177–180.

Sartorio A, Lafortuna CL, Agosti F et al (2004) Elderly obese women display the greatest improvement in stair climbing performance after a 3-week body mass reduction program. International Journal of Obesity and Related Metabolic Disorders 28(9):1097–1104.

Schols JM, De Groot CP, van der Cammen TJ et al (2009) Preventing and treating dehydration in the elderly during periods of illness and warm weather. Journal of Nutrition Health and Aging 13(2):150–157.

Simon GE, Von Korff M, Saunders K et al (2006) Association between obesity and psychiatric disorders in the US adult population. Archives of General Psychiatry 63(7):824–830.

Somes GW, Kritchevsky SB, Shorr RI et al (2002) Body mass index, weight change, and death in older adults: the systolic hypertension in the elderly program. American Journal of Epidemiology 156(2):132–138.

Subak LL, Johnson C, Whitcomb E et al (2002) Does weight loss improve incontinence in moderately obese women? International Urogynecology Journal and Pelvic Floor Dysfunction 13(1):40–43.

Sura L, Madhavan A, Carnaby G et al (2012) Dysphagia in the elderly: management and nutritional considerations. Clinical Interventions in Aging 7:287–298.

Taylor CJ, Layani L (2006) Laparoscopic adjustable gastric banding in patients > or =60 years old: is it worthwhile? Obesity Surgery 16(12):1579–1583.

Victorian Government Department of Human Services (2009) Surgery for morbid obesity: Framework for bariatric surgery in Victoria's public hospitals. State Government of Victoria, Melbourne.

Villareal DT, Apovian CM, Kushner RF et al (2005) Obesity in older adults: technical review and position statement of the American Society for Nutrition and NAASO, The Obesity Society. American Journal of Clinical Nutrition 82(5):923–934.

Villareal DT, Banks M, Siener C et al (2004) Physical frailty and body composition in obese elderly men and women. Obesity Research 12(6):913–920.

Villareal DT, Shah K, Banks MR et al (2008) Effect of weight loss and exercise therapy on bone metabolism and mass in obese older adults: a one-year randomized controlled trial. Journal of Clinical Endocrinology and Metabolism 93(6):2181–2187.

Visvanathan R (2017) Australian and New Zealand Society for Geriatric Medicine Position Statement Abstract: Undernutrition and the older person. Australasian Journal of Ageing 36(1):75.

Visvanathan R (2015) Anorexia of Aging. Clinics in Geriatric Medicine 31(3):417–427.

Visvanathan R (2003) Under-nutrition in older people: a serious and growing global problem! Journal of Postgraduate Medicine 49(4):352–360.

Walls AW, Steele JG (2004) The relationship between oral health and nutrition in older people. Mechanisms of Ageing and Development 125(12):853–857.

Wilson MM, Morley JE (2003) Impaired cognitive function and mental performance in mild dehydration. European Journal of Clinical Nutrition 57 Suppl 2: S24–29.

Wilson MM, Thomas DR, Rubenstein LZ et al (2005) Appetite assessment: simple appetite questionnaire predicts weight loss in community-dwelling adults and nursing home residents. American Journal of Clinical Nutrition 82(5):1074–1081.

Winter JE, MacInnis RJ Wattanapenpaiboon N et al (2014) BMI and all-cause mortality in older adults: a meta-analysis. The American Journal of Clinical Nutrition 99(4):875–890.

Wotton K, Crannitch K, Munt R (2008) Prevalence, risk factors and strategies to prevent dehydration in older adults. Contemporary Nurse 31(1):44–56.

Yermilov I, McGory ML, Shekelle PW et al (2009) Appropriateness criteria for bariatric surgery: beyond the NIH guidelines. Obesity (Silver Spring) 17(8):1521–1527.

Zizza CA, Herring A, Stevens J et al (2002) Obesity affects nursing-care facility admission among whites but not blacks. Obesity Research 10(8):816–823.

CHAPTER 13

Elimination

VICKI ELLEN PATTON

LEARNING OBJECTIVES

After reading this chapter, you will be able to:
- explain why incontinence is not a normal part of ageing
- identify the different types of bladder and bowel dysfunction common in older people
- identify nursing interventions that can improve the older person's bladder and bowel function.

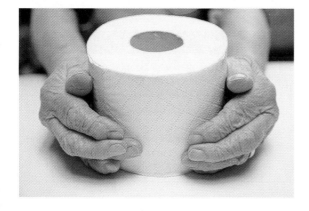

INTRODUCTION

Bowel and bladder issues, such as incontinence, constipation or urinary retention, are common in older people. Contrary to popular belief, incontinence is not an inevitable part of ageing and is usually associated with other disease processes or a potential symptom of more serious medical issues.

Many older people manage incontinence issues for years without sharing or admitting to these problems.

However, with advancing age it becomes more difficult to cope with bowel or bladder issues independently, particularly if the older person is experiencing cognitive decline, functional limitation or increasing co-morbidities.

Bladder and bowel dysfunction are troublesome and costly problems. Apart from the personal experiences of embarrassment and lower quality of life, bowel and bladder management consumes resources, including nursing/carer time. This chapter will address the issues of bladder and bowel function and how to optimise and manage dysfunction in the older person in order to improve quality of life.

AGEING AND URINARY FUNCTION
Age-Related Changes in Renal Function

In normal healthy urinary function, urine production decreases and becomes more concentrated during the night. The body produces increased levels of antidiuretic hormone (ADH) during sleep, stimulating the kidneys to increase water reabsorption, resulting in smaller volumes of more concentrated urine. Production of night-time ADH naturally declines with age, meaning that less water is reabsorbed, but rather is passed as urine. This may be more pronounced in older people with dementia or cognitive impairment (see Chapter 26) due to an added disturbance in the circadian rhythms (Dutoglu et al 2019). Additionally, kidney function in an older person may be increased at night due to decreased demands of other organs that otherwise override the kidneys during the day. The older person may then produce just as much urine at night as they do during the day, if not more.

A 70-year-old kidney has half the filtration rate of a 30-year-old kidney, which results in a less reliable control of serum electrolytes. Older people are less able to concentrate urine in response to dehydration and have a reduced capacity to clear additional fluid overload by diuresis (Tani et al 2008). This means drugs may accumulate in their body leading to toxic effects (see Chapter 11).

Older adults with a cardiac condition such as heart failure (see Chapter 23) may also have increased urine production at night. This is due to the fluid, which is normally circulated through the vascular system, pooling in the lower extremities during the day causing swollen feet and ankles. During the night, when the legs are elevated, fluid moves from the extravascular spaces, such as the lower legs, back into the vascular spaces and is filtered through the kidneys when the renal function is improved (Dutoglu et al 2019).

Bladder Function in Older People

In normal bladder function, the detrusor muscle remains relaxed as the bladder fills to accommodate urine storage. Upon urination, the detrusor muscle then contracts to ensure bladder emptying. In older age, the contractility of the detrusor muscle can become impaired. Firstly, it may become overactive and contract while the bladder is still filling, giving signals of urinary urgency. Secondly, it may not contract fully during urination, resulting in a failed voiding of the bladder with a collection of residual urine remaining (Palmer 2016).

Hormonal Changes and Bladder Function in Older People

The female urinary tract contains oestrogen-receptive tissue, meaning that its health is oestrogen-dependent. Oestrogen maintains the thickness of the lining of the urethra and influences the action of the trigone in the bladder, which, when stretched, triggers the need to urinate (Mannella et al 2013). After menopause, the oestrogen levels reduce and the lining of the urethra thins, leaving older women susceptible to ascending bacteria and also urinary incontinence. Oestrogen has also been shown to influence the strength of detrusor muscle within the bladder (Blakeman et al 2000).

The Prostate

In the older male, the prostate enlarges and may obstruct the flow of urine from the bladder, causing a condition termed bladder outlet obstruction (Palmer 2016). An obstructed outlet combined with impaired contractility of the detrusor muscle leaves the older male at significant risk of having incomplete bladder emptying and the collection of residual urine.

AGEING AND URINARY DYSFUNCTION
Urinary Incontinence

Every older person experiencing bladder dysfunction has the right to be treated with respect and given access to expertise and resources to manage the problem. Too often, nurses accept incontinence as a normal part of ageing when it is often treatable. It is unacceptable to verbally admonish a person for incontinence, or to send a message that an older person is at fault and insisting they wear incontinence pads upon admission to acute care. Unfortunately, these responses are common (Ostaszkiewicz 2018). The nurse has a role in challenging these practices when they occur. Nurses are in a key position to determine and understand the type of urinary incontinence an older person is experiencing in order to provide the most effective management approach.

> **Practice Point**
>
> 1. When an older person is incontinent, how often do you see the nurse accept the incident rather than questioning why has this happened?
> 2. The nurse must consider how to prevent it from happening again.
> 3. Incontinence is **not** an inevitable part of ageing and there are many ways to reduce or treat incontinence episodes in the older person.

TYPES OF URINARY INCONTINENCE
Stress Incontinence

Stress incontinence occurs when abdominal pressure on the bladder increases due to coughing, sneezing, laughing or straining and the pelvic floor cannot provide enough counter-pressure to stop urine from leaking. Many women experience stress incontinence after childbirth, when pelvic ligaments and muscles overstretch and weaken. With age and progressive decline in pelvic floor strength, stress incontinence may become worse. Symptoms of stress incontinence include losses of small amounts of

Research Highlight

Ostaszkiewicz J, Dickson-Swift V, Hutchinson A et al (2020) A concept analysis of dignity-protective continence care for care dependent older people in long-term care settings. BMC Geriatrics 20:266.
This analysis of 18 articles explored and described the concept of dignity in relation to toileting, incontinence, bladder and bowel care for older people living in residential aged care. Six domains were identified, including: respect, empathy, trust, privacy, autonomy and communication. Dignity was found to be a useful guiding principle in the care of older people living in residential aged care who needed assistance with toileting and continence.

Position the patient in a chair and leaning forward with elbows on knees if possible

Ask them to squeeze their bottom as if they are holding in gas.
If female, Then ask them to squeeze as if they are stopping the flow of urine.

If they can do this then ask them to squeeze and hold for three – five seconds.
Repeat this five times in the morning, at lunch and at night.

If they are finding it difficult after one or two squeezes it could be that the muscle is fatigued. Ask them to have a minute rest after two squeezes.

If they can't perform the squeezes ask for a referral to a Nurse Continence Advisor

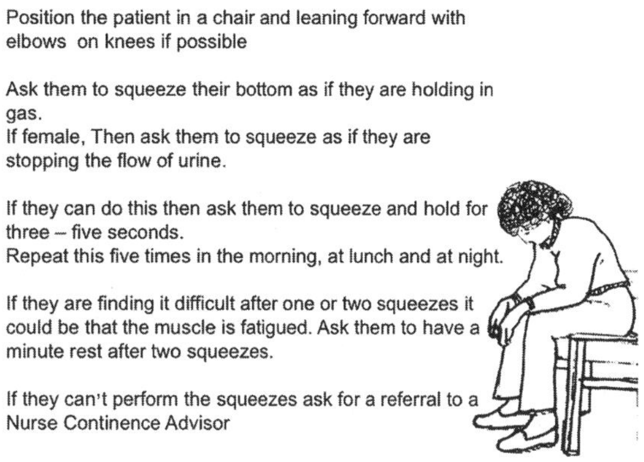

FIG. 13.1 **How to do pelvic floor exercises**

urine during activities that increase abdominal pressure with low post-void residual amounts of urine.

Nursing initiatives
- Local oestrogen cream placed on the vaginal opening and around the labia minora may assist in thickening the urethral lining.
- Pelvic floor exercises that strengthen the pelvic muscles can reduce stress incontinence.
- The older person can learn to squeeze the pelvic floor before coughing.
- Devices such as pessaries can be put inside the vagina to support the bladder neck, often reducing stress incontinence.

Urge Incontinence
Urge incontinence or overactive bladder (OAB) occurs when the detrusor muscle contracts instead of relaxing as the bladder fills. This can affect both males and females. The underlying mechanism may be dysfunction of the nervous system, where incorrect signals stimulate bladder contraction, although the exact cause is unknown. In older people with OAB, small, frequent volumes of urine are passed (Chen et al 2018). Symptoms of urge incontinence include losses of moderate to large amounts of urine while trying to get to the toilet, possible frequency (more than 8 voids in 24 hours) and nocturia, with low post-void residual amounts of urine.

Nursing initiatives
- The first-line treatment for urge incontinence is to ensure the older person does not have a clinically symptomatic urinary tract infection if the urgency has had a sudden onset.
- Behavioural techniques of distraction and trying to extend the time between voiding can be useful.

- Exercises to improve pelvic floor strength can help the older person to feel more confident to extend the time between urinations (see Fig. 13.1).
- Ensure the older person remains well hydrated by drinking sufficient amounts of water to keep the urine less concentrated. The recommended daily intake of fluids should be at least 1600 mL/24h (see Chapter 12). Concentrated urine irritates the bladder wall and may exacerbate symptoms.
- If these initial conservative measures fail and urgency is impacting on the older person's quality of life, refer to a medical practitioner for potential pharmacological management.

Functional Incontinence
Functional incontinence arises from factors outside the urinary tract (see Fig. 13.2). While the older person's urinary tract is intact, there may be limitations and barriers that prevent the person from reaching or using the toilet. These may include:
- mobility problems where the older person cannot get to the toilet in a timely manner
- conditions such as arthritis that cause difficulty releasing buttons on clothing
- environmental barriers, such as poor lighting or clutter
- cognitive impairment
- use of sleeping medication that contributes to disorientation or drowsiness during the night
- lack of assistance.

Nursing initiatives
- May be as simple as replacing buttons or clasps on clothing with Velcro or ensuring trousers have elastic waist rather than zippers and clips.

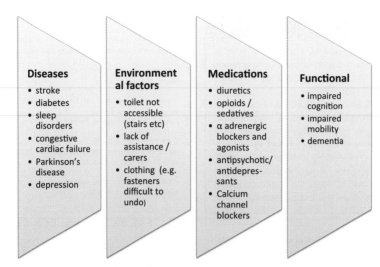

FIG. 13.2 **Factors affecting continence outside the urinary tract**

Practice Point

BLADDER TRAINING
- Suitable for those without cognitive impairment
- The person keeps a record of toileting to identify the pattern
- The person gradually increases the time between toileting
- Uses distraction technique to defer urge
- Uses pelvic floor muscle squeeze to assist with holding on.

PROMPTED VOIDING
- Suitable for the person with some physical/or cognitive impairment
- Carer needs to keep record of incontinence/voids to establish initial timing

- The person is prompted to go to the toilet at regular intervals
- Assisted to the toilet
- Positive reinforcement given.

TIMED VOIDING
- Suitable for those not able to independently toilet – cognitively impaired
- Carer needs to keep record of incontinence/voids to establish initial timings
- Taking the person to the toilet at regular timed intervals, for example, every 2 hours
- Gradually increase the time between voids if possible.

- Ensuring access to the toilet is well lit and there is a clear path.
- Consider placing commode by the bedside at night.
- Scheduled toileting may be useful and remove stressors of urgency.

Nocturia

The International Continence Society (ICS) defines nocturia as 'waking to pass urine during the main sleep period' (Meijlink 2018:1). Nocturia is reported to affect up to 59% of men and 62% of women aged 70 years and older (Weiss et al 2013). Nocturia is not a normal part of ageing. Nocturia can be troublesome as the fluid shift within the night causes the blood pressure to drop, especially when getting up in a hurry trying to make it to the toilet. Older people with nocturia are at an extremely high risk of falling because:

- they are rushing to access the toilet and are likely to trip

- their blood pressure is subject to postural drop and causes dizziness
- if there are existing deficits in mobility the risk of falling will increase (see Chapter 19).

Nocturia is a condition that is frequently ignored and incorrectly considered a minor inconvenience. However, a person woken from sleep several times a night can experience serious consequences in poorer daytime health and wellbeing (Epstein et al 2018). Increased night-time voiding results in the person being fatigued in the day and, as explained above, puts the older person at increased risk of falls and associated mortality (Dutoglu et al 2019).

Management of nocturia

- Administer diuretic medication no later than midday.
- Ensuring a healthy diet (see Chapter 12) and regular exercise assists in maintaining good glycaemic control and has a positive effect in reducing episodes of nocturia (Asplund 2005).
- Promote better sleep generally by identifying and addressing chronic sleep disorders (see Chapter 14).
- Pre-emptive voiding involves going to the toilet immediately before bedtime to ensure there is as little urine in the bladder as possible:
  - There is limited evidence that pre-emptive voiding is useful (Weiss et al 2013). However, most people with nocturia use this as a management strategy.
- Limiting fluids
  - Has been shown to be effective in improving nocturia. One study instructed men (mean age 72 years) to reduce their fluid volume (not the frequency) so they only produced 30mL/kg of urine. They all drank a minimum of 1 litre of fluid per day and limited both day and evening intake, which resulted in a significant improvement in nocturia (Tani et al 2014).
- Behavioural therapy
  - If the urge to urinate is waking the older person, then distraction techniques to remove the sense of urgency can be practised during the day and used during the night to extend the time between needing to void. Referral to a continence specialist nurse for pelvic floor strengthening exercises may assist. Even in the older population, the pelvic floor muscle function can be improved and therefore should be included in a treatment plan.

Urinary Retention

Urinary retention may present as frequent small volumes of urine loss and is commonly dismissed as incontinence. In order to rule out retention, the residual

> **Tips for Best Practice**
>
> **Nocturia** is a common condition that should not be ignored or 'tolerated'. The relationship between nocturia, morbidity and mortality means it should be taken seriously and actively managed.

volume remaining in the bladder after incontinence or voiding should be measured using a bladder scanner or in/out catheter. The urine loss may be due to an overflow. Retention is common in the older person experiencing constipation, especially where there is cognitive decline.

Dementia and Incontinence

Older people living with non Alzheimer's dementias, such as Parkinson's related dementia, dementia with Lewy bodies and vascular dementia, often experience incontinence, which impairs quality of life (Allan et al 2006). Medications needed to reduce the impact of the disease can worsen. In females, continence issues are frequently pre-existing to the onset of dementia. However, as cognition declines, the older person becomes less able to manage absorptive pads, personal hygiene and toileting and becomes more reliant on caregivers.

As toileting is such an ingrained behaviour, it needs to be established whether or not the continence issues are directly related to cognitive decline. It is therefore necessary to eliminate other potential underlying causes.

Urinary Tract Infection (UTI)

In the older female, the presence of bacteria in the urine is common and even thought to be protective of more aggressive bacteria that may cause more serious and even life-threatening infections (Wullt et al 2018). This is called asymptomatic bacteriuria, as the person often does not have any clinical symptoms, such as burning on voiding, flank pain or sudden onset frequency (Echaiz et al 2015).

To confirm the presence of a UTI, the older person *must be clinically symptomatic* AND have a urinalysis showing nitrates with or without blood and protein (Little et al 2006).

> **Promoting Wellness**
>
> Asymptomatic bacteriuria can be a helpful condition and does require treatment! Treating with antibiotics will increase bacterial resistance.

UTI prevention

- Good urine production
  - Plenty of fluids unless contraindicated.
  - Use good lubrication during intercourse to prevent tissue damage.
  - Void after intercourse.
- Maintain good glycaemic control
  - Even without glucose in the urine, older people with unstable blood glucose levels are at a higher risk of developing a UTI.
- Promote bladder emptying and avoidance of urinary retention
  - Sit on the toilet to pass urine.
  - Avoid bedpans and lying in bed to pass urine where possible.
- Perineal hygiene
  - Wipe from front to back after a bowel action.
  - Manage diarrhoea and prevent faecal contamination of urethral opening.
  - Regularly change soiled pads and underwear.

Alternative prevention strategies

Cranberry juice/tablets. Cranberry juice has long been used to prevent UTI and is known to have properties that prevent *Escherichia coli (E. coli)* bacteria from adhering to the bladder wall. However, many studies have been unable to demonstrate its effectiveness in the clinical setting (Duncan 2019), and, despite a small trend suggesting fewer UTIs are experienced by those taking cranberry juice, there is no conclusive evidence that consumption is preventative (Jepson et al 2012).

D-mannose. D-mannose is a complex carbohydrate important in the metabolism of some proteins within the human body. It has been shown to prevent the adherence of *E. coli* bacteria to the lining of the bladder (Schaeffer et al 1984).

Studies using D-mannose as a preventative measure against UTI have been promising (Palleschi et al 2017; Phé et al 2016; Porru et al 2014). D-mannose comes in a powder form that dissolves easily. High doses in the older population may affect renal function in the longer term.

URINARY CATHETERS

The highest risk for UTI is caused by the presence of an indwelling catheter. Therefore, avoid using an indwelling catheter whenever possible. If this is not feasible, adhering to best practice guidelines or using intermittent catheterisation will assist in reducing the risk of developing a UTI (Lo et al 2014).

Catheter Selection Should Be According to Patient Needs

There are several different types of catheter. The two most common are: (i) Foley catheter and (ii) Coudé tip catheter. The Coudé tip catheter has a slightly curved or angled tip and is useful in older male patients with an enlarged prostate as it allows passage of the catheter through a narrowed urethra. Catheters can also be silver-coated, chlorhexidine impregnated or contain other antimicrobial coatings that are designed to reduce infection. The indications for long-term catheterisation include chronic urinary retention, neurogenic injury, such as spinal injury, and bladder outlet obstruction.

Once inserted, an indwelling catheter should be secured to the thigh using a fixation device to prevent unnecessary movement of the tubing and tension on the bladder neck (Chu 2017). The tubing should be visibly clean, and daily perineal hygiene attended to with soap and water. An appropriate catheter drainage bag should be selected, based on the intended duration of catheterisation and the older person's mobility, dexterity and preference. The drainage bag should be changed when the catheter is changed, or when deemed clinically necessary (Andreessen et al 2012), for example, if the bag is stained or emitting an odour. The nurse has a role to ensure that the older person can manage the emptying mechanism on the base of the drainage bag to promote independence.

The drainage bag should be placed below the level of the bladder, but not left lying on the floor (Andreessen et al 2012). A catheter leg bag is a pouch that can be worn on the thigh or calf underneath clothing. It is discrete, enables mobilisation and, therefore, is ideally suited for use by people with long-term catheters. Overnight, when additional urine storage is required, a drainage bag can be connected to the bottom of the leg bag to reduce the need to empty the bag overnight.

> ### Tips for Best Practice
>
> Catheter drainage bags should be changed every 5–7 days. Otherwise they should not be disconnected from the indwelling catheter unless absolutely necessary, and then only using aseptic technique. Additional night bags should only be added to the bottom of leg bags overnight. The leg bag must **NEVER** be routinely disconnected from the catheter. It must remain a closed system.
>
> There is no evidence to suggest that using disinfectants to clean drainage bags prevents UTI (Lockwood et al 2004).

Supra Pubic Catheters

A supra pubic catheter (SPC) is inserted directly into the bladder via the lower abdominal wall. It provides a way to drain urine from the bladder by bypassing the urethra. In some older males with prostatic hypertrophy that is obstructing the urethra and who are unsuitable for surgery, an SPC allows drainage of the urine via an abdominal outlet. In people with neurological disorders, who sit for long periods and require long-term catheterisation, an SPC provides more effective and comfortable urine drainage. The closed system principle applies in the management of SPCs, as with all urinary catheters, meaning the catheter and drainage bag should not be routinely disconnected.

Intermittent Catheterisation

This is referred to as clean intermittent self catheterisation (CISC). In this procedure a person manages their own catheterisation, which involves inserting the catheter into their own bladder, waiting for the urine to drain, and removing the catheter up to six times per day. A clean, but not sterile, technique is used and it requires dexterity and attention to detail to avoid tissue trauma and infection. It is unusual to commence this process with older people, although some older people who have been using this bladder management technique for many years may wish to continue with it. The advantages are that a permanent indwelling catheter can be avoided and the risk of UTI is reduced (Kannankeril et al 2011).

External Catheters

Several devices are available for males that fit over the penis to collect urine and connect to a urinary drainage bag or leg bag. These include the urinary sheath, uridome and urinary pouch (see Figs 13.3 and 13.4). Advantages are that they effectively manage urinary leakage, without the need to insert a catheter into the bladder and the associated risk of UTI. All of these products need changing once per day to ensure penile hygiene.

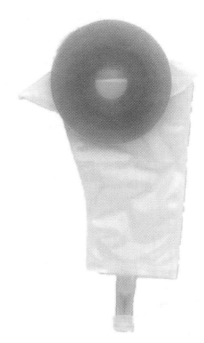

FIG. 13.3 **Urinary pouch** (Hollister Inc.)

> ### Promoting Wellness
> *Where to Get Information*
>
> For information about where to access supplies, government funding and resources for older people, their carers and health professionals contact www.continence.org.au

BOWEL FUNCTION IN THE OLDER PERSON

In keeping with social taboos and attitudes, bowel management is frequently categorised as 'dirty work' that is often left to nurses considered to be on the lower end of the hierarchy (Ostaszkiewicz 2018). Evidence suggests that bowel care in older people could be improved, especially within acute and residential aged care settings (Ostaszkiewicz 2018). There are costly complications of inadequate bowel management, which include:

- urinary retention
- frequent UTI
- confusion
- delirium
- admission to acute care facilities.

Transit time through the colon may be slower in older people and includes those living with Parkinson's disease or stroke, in which the effect of medications and reduced mobility tends to slow bowel motility (Gustafsson et al 2019).

In the older person, the sensation of the urge to empty the bowel may be reduced. Without this stimulus, the older person may miss the signal for bowel elimination, causing constipation to develop. Additionally, the ability to discriminate between urges to pass solids, liquid or gas commonly diminishes. The consequence is that an older person may consciously relax the anal sphincter to expel gas only to be faecally incontinent.

An older person with cognitive impairment may be unable to interpret the urge sensation or communicate

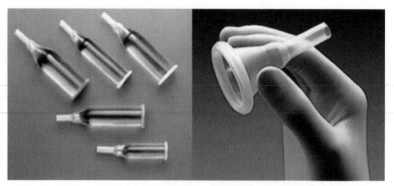

FIG. 13.4 **Urinary sheath and uridome** (Hollister Inc.)

their needs. This may lead to a build-up of faecal matter in the rectum that causes discomfort and behavioural agitation (see Chapter 26), abdominal pain due to gas retention and potentially urinary retention.

Anal Sphincter

Due to ageing, the anal sphincter becomes fibrous and loses tone. This may lead to an inability to control the expulsion of gas or to delay defecation and result in urgency, particularly with liquid stool.

Talking About Bowel Management

Bowel management is a taboo subject that people find embarrassing and difficult to discuss. Finding the words to assist older people and their families to openly discuss bowel issues may be helpful. Here is a list of words that are non-offensive and easily understood by people without nursing experience, which can help communication about bowel function:

1. 'Bowel accidents' or 'bowel leakage', rather than 'faecal incontinence'
2. 'Motions', rather than 'faeces'
3. 'Bottom', rather than 'anus'
4. Passing 'wind' or 'gas', rather than 'flatus'
5. 'Bottom muscles', rather than 'sphincter'
6. 'Pads' or 'tissues' for absorptive pads. Many older people will use toilet paper for protection. Some older people may not class panty liners as pads.

What Is Normal?

Bowel function is considered 'normal' if a bowel motion is passed as often as three times per day or as little as once every three days. The motion should pass without straining and there should be a feeling of complete emptiness.

Promoting Good Bowel Habits in the Older Person

- Exercise is important and even older people who are unable to mobilise independently should be assisted to sit out of bed in the morning.
- Encourage fluid intake, especially earlier in the day (if not contraindicated).
- Avoid high caffeine intake in those with loose stool.
- Encourage good dietary fibre intake.
- Allow time on the toilet in the correct sitting position and in privacy.

AGE-RELATED CHANGES TO THE GASTROINTESTINAL SYSTEM

Types of Faecal Incontinence

Faecal urgency

Faecal urgency is defined as an urge to open the bowels where the person cannot delay for 10–15 minutes. Options to manage faecal urgency are centred around regular toileting and keeping the consistency of bowel motion firm while avoiding constipation.

Nursing initiatives

- Medications that provide soluble fibre supplements (e.g. guar gum, methylcellulose, psyllium) help to bulk up loose stools and sharpen urge sensation.
- Combining fibre supplements with loperamide can help to safely slow bowel transit time while avoiding hard stools.
- Using enemas that wash the bowel out at regular intervals.
- Consider referral for medical review if faecal incontinence is impacting on quality of life. Interventional procedures such as sacral nerve stimulation or formation of a stoma may be warranted. It is worth

investigating the surgical option if this might mean that the older person can remain in their own house or with a carer rather than moving to residential aged care.

Faecal leakage/soiling

Leakage of faecal matter after the person has opened their bowels may be related to incomplete emptying of the rectum or constipation (Carter et al 2019).

Nursing initiatives

- Encourage the older person to discuss the value of soluble fibre supplements with their GP or doctor.
- Advise the older person to put their feet up on a stool during toileting to empty residual faecal matter in the rectum that may leak later.
- Glycerin suppositories may also be useful to assist in emptying the rectum.
- Putting one or two glycerin suppositories into the rectum immediately before defecation may achieve a better rectal emptying.

Types of Constipation

Constipation is common in older adults. The primary causes are medication side effects, reduced mobility, dehydration and underlying conditions such as Parkinson's disease or stroke (Robson et al 2000; Werth et al 2019).

Functional–normal transit constipation

In this type of constipation the colon moves in a normal manner, but there is a problem with the stool being too hard or infrequent. It is commonly seen in older people who take multiple medications (see Chapter 11). This type of constipation is managed by modifying dietary input to increase the fibre content and fluid intake and changing the consistency of the stool. Older people taking opioids, particularly codeine (see Chapter 19), should be routinely commenced on laxative medication (see Table 13.1).

Nursing initiatives

- Use oral laxatives if other medication is the cause of constipation.
- Improve fluid and dietary fibre intake.
- Increase exercise.
- Being active and exercising will assist to improve colonic motility and reduce bloating due to trapped gas.

Obstructive Emptying

This form of constipation occurs in both sexes, but is more common in women who have had children and sustained a pelvic floor injury that obstructs smooth passage of the stool from the rectum through the anal canal. In older people with impaired cognition who may be unable to interpret the urge sensation, the obstruction may be due to hard faeces building up in the rectum. Formations such as rectocele, where the front wall of the rectum bulges into the vagina as a result of tissue damage from childbirth, can cause stool to become trapped in the bulge during a bowel movement, leading to incomplete emptying and constipation (see Fig. 13.5). Rectal prolapse occurs when the rectum descends down towards the anus. Females are more likely to experience rectal prolapse than males. Causes include:

- weakened pelvic floor and anal sphincter muscles
- chronic constipation and straining to pass bowel motions
- weakening of the muscles due to ageing
- conditions that cause increased abdominal pressure, e.g. chronic obstructive pulmonary disease
- prior trauma or disease to the spinal discs.

Nursing initiatives

- Keep consistency of the stool soft but formed, as liquid stool and really hard stool will more easily become trapped in the rectum.
- Use suppositories to improve emptying.
- Encourage the correct sitting position on the toilet to promote good emptying and avoidance of straining.
- Enema and rectal washouts work well for the older population when required.

Safety Alert

Warning: Sometimes increasing soluble dietary fibre in the older population may increase constipation.

Tips for Best Practice

- Laxatives do not make the bowel 'lazy'.
- Laxatives are an effective management strategy for constipation. Stigma around the taking of laxatives should be removed. Far more damage is caused by straining to pass bowel motions and allowing stool to build up than will ever be caused by laxatives.
- If the plan for the older person is to promote a good bowel regimen, sitting on the toilet 30 minutes after breakfast is the optimal time to promote bowel function. This strategy takes advantage of the gastrocolic reflex and so using suppositories at this time may be more effective than other times of the day.

TABLE 13.1
Types of Laxatives, Recommended Dose and Possible Side Effects

Category	Generic Name	Brand Name	Starting Dosage	Ingredients	Contraindications/ Precautions	Comments
Bulking						
	Bran	All Bran (cereal)		Wheat bran	Coeliac disease	Oat bran, wheat bran/high fibre cereals
	Psyllium husk	Metamucil	2 tsps with 250 mL water 1–3/day	Psyllium husk	Can cause bloating – if it does, start with ½ tsp Coeliac disease Absorbs extra water, so encourage oral intake	Bulks stool making it easier to pass; good for FI; lowers cholesterol
	Guar gum	Benefiber	2 tsp twice daily (max 8 tsp/day)	Guar gum	Can cause bloating – if it does, start with ½ tsp Coeliac disease Absorbs extra water, so encourage oral intake	Bulks stool, making it easier to pass; good for FI
	Ispaghula husk	Fybogel	1 tsp with 250 mL of water BD	Ispaghula husk, aspartame	Flatus, bloating, contains phenylalanine, so contraindicated in phenylketonuria	Gluten-free. Bulks stool making easier to pass; good for FI
	Methylcellulose	Normafibe	1–2 heaped tsp 1–2/ daily after meals with 250 mL of water. Do not take just before going to bed or lying down. Do not chew or crush the granules.	Sterculia (also called karaya gum), sodium bicarbonate, sucrose, talc, titanium dioxide, hard paraffin and vanillin	Flatus, bloating, obstruction. If BNO after 4 days contact medical professionals	Can help with IBS pts. Safe for coeliac Dx
	Sterculia & methylcellulose	Normacol plus	1–2 heaped tsp 1–2/ daily after meals with 250 mL of water. Do not take just before going to bed or lying down. Do not chew or crush the granules.	Sterculia 62% and frangula bark powder 8%	Obstruction and impaction	Bulking agent and laxative, good for slow transit constipation resistant to bulk alone; initiating and maintenance of bowel action after rectal surgery and haemorrhoidectomy. Safe for coeliac Dx

Softeners

Sodium docusate	Coloxyl	50 mg tablets: 2 or 3 tablets twice daily; 120 mg tablets: 2 tablets once daily after evening meal	Sodium benzoate, wheat starch	Not recommended for children under 12 years. For infants and young children, Coloxyl drops are preferred Coloxyl tablets should not be taken with prescription medicines or mineral oil. Not recommended in coeliac disease	May be used in conjunction with a stimulant. Only useful alone if transit time is normal
Olive oil	Olive oil	30 mL	Olive oil		Softener only

Stimulants

Bisacodyl	Dulcolax Bisalax	1–2 tablets	Lactose, sucrose, maize starch; gluten-free	Can cause cramps and bloating. Antacids (do not take within 1 hr) Children < 6 yrs (not recommended)	Increases pressure waves in colon and stimulates emptying
Senna	Senna Natrulax Nulax	1–2 tablets	Senna plant	Prolonged use: ileus, intestinal obstruction; undiagnosed abdominal pain; nausea, vomiting	Stimulates colonic movement
Sodium picosulfate	Dulcolax drops Picoprep	Initially 10 drops (5 mg), may increase to 20 drops (10 mg)	Na picosulfate 7.5 mg/mL; Na benzoate, sorbitol	IBD (incl assoc abdominal pain, nausea, vomiting); severe dehydration; electrolyte disturbance; hereditary fructose intolerance; renal, cardiac impairment; dehydration; prolonged, continuous, excessive use; pregnancy; diuretics; adrenocorticosteroids; cardiac glycosides; antibiotics	Stimulates the mucosa of the large intestine, causing colonic peristalsis and promotes accumulation of water and consequently electrolytes, in the colonic lumen. This results in a stimulation of defecation, reduction of transit time and softening of the stool Picoprep – if regularly used ensure to monitor electrolytes Stimulant Can cause dehydration so encourage person to maintain oral intake

Continued

TABLE 13.1
Types of Laxatives, Recommended Dose and Possible Side Effects—cont'd

Category	Generic Name	Brand Name	Starting Dosage	Ingredients	Contraindications/ Precautions	Comments
Osmotic						
	Lactulose	Actilax Dulphalac Lactulose syrup	15–45 mL daily	Lactose, galactose, tagatose & epilactose	Patients who require a low galactose diet, and in patients with galactosaemia or disaccharidase deficiency or who are on a galactose and/or lactose-free diet	Draws fluid into the bowel Can be explosive and windy
	Macrogols (polyethylene glycols)	Osmolax Movicol Clearlax Glycoprep Colonlitely	1–3 sachets daily	Macrogol 3350 13.125 g; Sodium chloride 350.7 mg; Sodium bicarbonate 178.5 mg; Potassium chloride 31.7 mg	Ensure adequate fluid intake; care with electrolyte imbalance and renal function	Triggers colon motility via neuromuscular pathways Effective in resolving faecal impaction, defined as refractory constipation with faecal loading of the rectum and/or colon confirmed by physical examination of abdomen and rectum
	Magnesium sulphate	Epsom salt	1–2 tablets/day	Magnesium sulphate	Care with electrolyte imbalance/dehydration	Works quickly

FI Faecal incontinence; BNO Bowels not opened; BD Twice daily; IBD Irritable bowel disease.

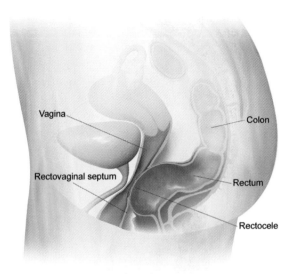

FIG. 13.5 **Rectocele**

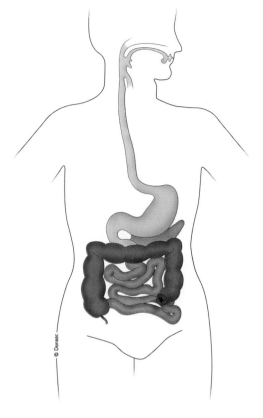

FIG. 13.6 **Colostomy anatomy** (Hollister Inc.)

STOMA

Stoma is the Greek word for mouth or opening. It forms the basis of terms to describe surgically created openings into the body to assist with elimination. A colostomy is an opening into the colon; an ileostomy is an opening into the ileum; and a urostomy, also known as an ileal conduit, is a passage for urine out of the body.

Colostomy (see Fig. 13.6)

A colostomy is usually created on the left side of the abdomen, most commonly when the descending colon is brought out onto the surface. The output from the colostomy is usually a soft formed stool, but it may be softer if more colon has been resected.

The stoma appliance or bag should fit snugly around the stoma. Because the stool from a colostomy is generally formed, the bag is closed on all sides. When full, the bag is removed and replaced rather than emptied.

Ileostomy (see Fig. 13.7)

An ileostomy is most commonly located on the right side of the abdomen. The output is much more liquid as it emanates from the small bowel. This liquid is very corrosive to the skin. It is important that the opening of the bag fits snugly around the stoma to ensure no abdominal skin is exposed. The stoma bag is designed to open at the bottom as it fills much more rapidly than a colostomy and needs to be emptied every 3–4 hours.

The older person with an ileostomy is at risk of dehydration as liquid stool leaves the body before it can be reabsorbed in the colon.

Ileal Conduit (Urostomy) (see Fig. 13.8)

A urostomy is formed when the bladder is removed. A small part of the ileum (small bowel) is used as a conduit into which the ureters are implanted. One side of the ileal conduit is brought out through the abdominal wall, similarly to an ileostomy, and the other end is stitched closed. The urine flows through the conduit and drains into a urostomy bag. The bag for this type of stoma has a tap-like closure on the bottom to allow emptying every 3–4 hours. An additional night bag, the same as that used with a urinary catheter, is connected overnight to allow for extra drainage, negating the need for the older person to get up and empty the bag. As urine flows through this conduit of ileum, it picks up mucus secreted by the bowel, which also flows into

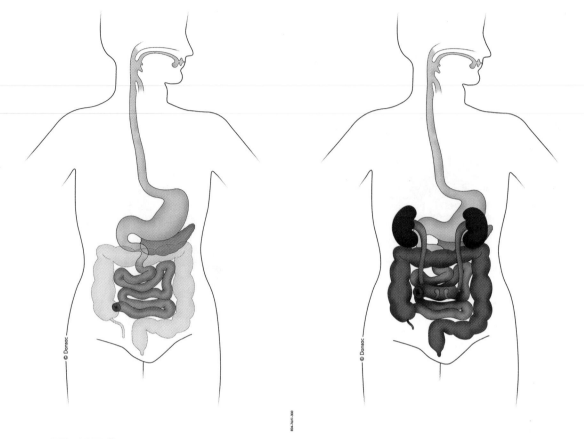

FIG. 13.7 **Ileostomy anatomy** (Hollister Inc.)   FIG. 13.8 **Urostomy anatomy** (Hollister Inc.)

the bag. Taking cranberry tablets thins this mucus and prevents the tap on the urostomy bag from blocking, allowing a longer wear time.

Stoma Care

Stomas are not sterile and do not require a dressing pack or specialised equipment for bag changes. Generally, the older person removes the bag, has a shower and immediately replaces the bag. An older person caring for their own stoma does not require gloves, but must wash their hands after touching the stoma or bag, just as they would after going to the toilet. Nurses, however, must wear protective equipment such as gloves when managing another person's stoma.

Peristomal Skin

It is important the skin around the stoma remains healthy. Incorrect application of the stoma bag can result in bowel contents contacting the skin, causing redness and irritation. Exudate from damaged skin

can prevent the bag from adhering properly, leaving skin exposed and in contact with bowel contents, which increases irritation and exudate. This downward spiral can be averted by paying careful attention to sizing the hole in the stoma bag to exactly fit the stoma and applying the bag so that no skin is left exposed. Stoma bags have a hydrocolloid backin – the same compound used in wound dressings. Applying the bag to damaged skin will protect it from irritant compounds and give it time to heal. It is important to reduce the number of bag changes, except if the bag is leaking (Fig. 13.9).

Stoma observations (see Fig 13.10)

- The stoma should always be pink and moist, like the inside of the mouth.
- The colostomy may be quite flush with the skin, whereas the urostomy and ileal conduit have a spout. This allows the liquid content to drain into the bag rather than sitting on the skin.

1. Closed bag	**2. Drainable bag**	**3. Urostomy bag**

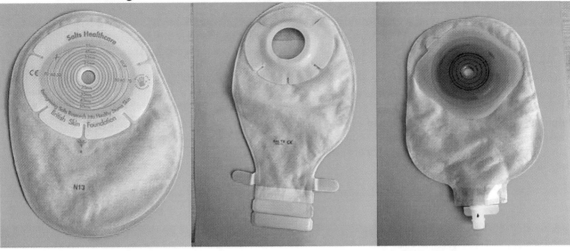

1. Suitable for colostomy. When the bag is full it must be removed and replaced with a new one.

2. Suitable for ileostomy. The bag can be opened to empty loose stool.

3. Suitable for urostomy / ileal conduit. The tap on the bottom allows the urine to be emptied. This bag can connect to catheter drainage bag overnight for additional storage of urine.

FIG. 13.9 **The three most common types of stoma appliances A.** Closed bag **B.** Drainable bag **C.** Urostomy bag

Tips for Best Practice

1. You cannot patch a leaking stoma bag. It must be removed, the skin cleaned with water and a new bag applied.
2. NEVER use anything but water to clean around a stoma.
3. DO NOT use antiseptics, alcohol or detergents, as these will damage the skin.
4. DO NOT use baby wipes as these contain lanolin and will impair the ability of the bag to adhere to the skin.

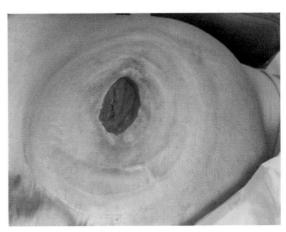

FIG. 13.10 **A mature stoma**

- The stoma should be free of lesions or irregularities.
- It is recommended that a person with a stoma should be seen by a specialist stomal therapy nurse at least every 12 months; more frequently if it is a new stoma.

Supplies

Australian citizens with a stoma receive stoma supplies free of charge under the medical benefit scheme. Each state has an Ostomy Association, which administers funding and provides access to appliances. The older person should also be in contact with a stomal therapy nurse. In New Zealand the stoma supplies are prescribed by the stomal therapy nurse.

Promoting Wellness
Stomal Therapy Nurse

If it is unclear who an older person has seen in the past, you can access the Australian Association of Stomal Therapy Nurses website and find a nurse close to their location. Alternatively, most large tertiary hospitals employ a stomal therapy nurse. In rural or remote areas, a metropolitan stomal therapy nurse should still be able to assist with advice on care either by telephone or via telehealth.

Practice Scenario

Maria is a 75-year-old woman who has presented with voiding small frequent amounts of urine every 45 minutes. She reports her bladder control has been getting worse over the past two months and she needs to get up during the night at least six times. She has arthritis and has recently been started on paracetamol with codeine to assist her with the back pain. Her only other medication is one to reduce hypercholestraemia. She has five children who were all born via vaginal delivery; three were over 4 kg in weight.

MULTIPLE CHOICE QUESTIONS

1. What would be the first action in assessing Maria?
   a. Assist her to the toilet so she doesn't fall.
   b. Assess Maria's abdomen and check the residual urine to see if her bladder is full by either bladder scan, if available, or in/out catheter
   c. Ensure she has had her codeine to assist with her pain
   d. Put a pan by her bed so she can easily pass urine without risk of falling

2. Maria is prescribed codeine; how could this be contributing to her bladder condition?
   a. It negatively affects the bladder emptying
   b. It reduces bladder urge sensation
   c. It may cause severe constipation and impaction, which may impair bladder emptying
   d. It increases bladder urge sensation

3. Maria's bladder scan shows she has a residual urine of 400 mL after voiding 25mL. This demonstrates she is not emptying. A urinary catheter is inserted. The care of the catheter includes:
   a. Fixing the catheter to the upper thigh to ensure no tension on bladder neck
   b. Disconnecting the catheter daily and ensuring the connection is thoroughly cleaned.
   c. Lying the drainage bag on the floor to ensure maximum drainage from the bladder
   d. All of the above

4. Maria reports she hasn't had her bowels open for 10 days. She feels pressure in her back passage. She is given glycerine suppositories followed by oral osmotic agent. An example of an osmotic laxative is:
   a. Senna
   b. Poly ethylene glycol (PEG)
   c. Lactulose also known as Actilax or Duphalac
   d. B and C

5. Maria is instructed to commence on a regular laxative to counteract the codeine and prevent constipation. She is concerned about the laxatives making her bowel lazy. What is the most appropriate response?
   a. You are correct and should get off them as soon as possible.
   b. Laxatives that are osmotic agents are highly addictive and you will need to keep increasing the dose to get them to work.
   c. Laxatives that are osmotic agents are not habit forming and more problems will occur by not taking them.
   d. A and B

SUMMARY

This chapter has outlined the bladder and bowel dysfunction that may be experienced by older people. It is important that the nurse and the older person understand that these issues are not a normal part of ageing. Comprehensive assessment and evidence-based care should be offered or appropriate referrals to a specialist nurse should be made, as many effective treatments can be provided as nursing interventions.

Bladder and bowel dysfunction can be a secretive and embarrassing situation for the older person that they have managed for many years. Having frank and open discussions about these sensitive issues may assist in significantly improving the older person's quality of life.

REFERENCES

Allan L, McKeith I, Ballard C et al (2006) The prevalence of autonomic symptoms in dementia and their association with physical activity, activities of daily living and quality of life. Dementia & Geriatric Cognitive Disorders 22(3):230–237.

Andreessen L, Wilde MH, Herendeen P (2012) Preventing catheter-associated urinary tract infections in acute care: The bundle approach. Journal of Nursing Care Quality 27(3):209–217.

Asplund R (2005) Nocturia in relation to sleep, health, and medical treatment in the elderly. BJU Int 96 Suppl 1:15–21.

Blakeman PJ, Hilton P, Bulmer JN (2000) Oestrogen and progesterone receptor expression in the female lower urinary tract, with reference to oestrogen status. BJU International 86(1):32–38.

Carter D, Bardan E, Maradey-Romero C (2019) Clinical and physiological risk factors for fecal incontinence in chronically constipated women. Techniques in Coloproctology 23(5):429–434.

Chen Z, Phan MD, Bates LJ et al (2018) The urinary microbiome in patients with refractory urge incontinence and recurrent urinary tract infection. Int Urogynecol J 29(12):1775–1782.

Chu WH (2017) Evidence summary. Urinary catheterization: Securement (JBI10308). The Joanna Briggs Institute EBP Database.

Duncan D (2019) Alternative to antibiotics for managing asymptomatic and non-symptomatic bacteriuria in older persons: a review. British Journal of Community Nursing 24(3):116–119.

Dutoglu E, Soysal P, Smith L et al (2019) Nocturia and its clinical implications in older women. Archives of Gerontology & Geriatrics 85:103917.

Echaiz JF, Cass C, Henderson JP et al (2015) Low correlation between self-report and medical record documentation of urinary tract infection symptoms. American Journal of Infection Control 43(9):983–986.

Epstein M, Blaivas J, Wein AJ et al (2018) Nocturia treatment outcomes: Analysis of contributory frequency volume chart parameters. Neurourology and Urodynamics 37(1):186–191.

Gustafsson M, Lamas K, Isaksson U et al (2019) Constipation and laxative use among people living in nursing homes in 2007 and 2013. BMC Geriatrics 19(1):38.

Jepson RG, Williams G, Craig JC (2012) Cranberries for preventing urinary tract infections. Cochrane Database of Systematic Reviews(10).

Kannankeril AJ, Lam HT, Reyes EB et al (2011) Urinary tract infection rates associated with re-use of catheters in clean intermittent catheterization of male veterans. Urologic Nursing 31(1):41–48.

Little P, Turner S, Rumsby K et al (2006) Developing clinical rules to predict urinary tract infection in primary care settings: sensitivity and specificity of near patient tests (dipsticks) and clinical scores. British Journal of General Practice 56(529):606–612.

Lo E, Nicolle LE, Coffin SE et al (2014) Strategies to prevent catheter-associated urinary tract infections in acute care hospitals: 2014 Update. Infection Control & Hospital Epidemiology 35(S2):S32–S47.

Lockwood C, Page T, Conroy-Hiller T et al (2004) Management of short-term indwelling urethral catheters to prevent urinary tract infections. International Journal of Evidence-Based Healthcare 2(8):271–291.

Mannella P, Palla G, Bellini M et al (2013) The female pelvic floor through midlife and aging. Maturitas 76(3): 230–234.

Meijlink J (2018) Nocturia – ICS definition. Online. Available: www.ics.org/committees/standardisation/terminology discussions/nocturia

Ostaszkiewicz J (2018) A conceptual model of the risk of elder abuse posed by incontinence and care dependence. International Journal of Older People Nursing 13(2).

Palleschi G, Carbone A, Zanello PP et al (2017) Prospective study to compare antibiosis versus the association of N-acetylcysteine, D-mannose and Morinda citrifolia fruit extract in preventing urinary tract infections in patients submitted to urodynamic investigation. Archivio Italiano di Urologia e Andrologia 89(1):45–50.

Palmer M (2016) UI and lower urinary tract symptoms in the older adult. In: WOCN Core Curriculum Continence Management, D. Doughty & K. Moore (eds). Philadelphia, Wolters Kluwer.

Phé V, Pakzad M, Haslam C et al (2016) An open label feasibility study evaluating D-Mannose for the prevention of urinary tract infections in patients with multiple sclerosis. Multiple sclerosis (Houndmills, Basingstoke, England) Conference: 32nd Congress of the European Committee for Treatment and Research in Multiple Sclerosis. Neurourology and Urodynamics 2017. 36(7):1770–1775.

Porru D, Parmigiani A, Tinelli C et al (2014) Oral D-mannose in recurrent urinary tract infections in women: a pilot study. Journal of Clinical Urology 7(3):208–213.

Robson KM, Kiely DK, Lembo T (2000) Development of constipation in nursing home residents. Diseases of the Colon & Rectum 43(7):940–943.

Schaeffer AJ, Chmiel JS, Duncan JL et al (1984) Mannose-sensitive adherence of Escherichia coli to epithelial cells from women with recurrent urinary tract infections. Journal of Urology 131(5):906–910.

Tani M, Hirayama A, Torimoto K et al (2014) Guidance on water intake effectively improves urinary frequency in patients with nocturia. International Journal of Urology 21(6):595–600.

Tani M, Hirayama A, Fujimoto K et al (2008) Increase in 24-hour urine production/weight causes nocturnal polyuria due to impaired function of antidiuretic hormone in elderly men. International Journal of Urology 15(2):151–154; discussion 155.

Weiss JP, Blaivas JG, Blanker MH et al (2013) The New England Research Institutes, Inc. (NERI) Nocturia Advisory Conference 2012: focus on outcomes of therapy. BJU International 111(5):700–716.

Werth BL, Williams KA, Fisher MJ et al (2019) Defining constipation to estimate its prevalence in the community: results from a national survey. BMC Gastroenterology 19(1):75.

Wullt B, Sunden F, Grabe M (2018) Asymptomatic bacteriuria is harmless and even protective: don't treat if you don't have a very specific reason. European Urology Focus 5(1):15–16.

CHAPTER 14

Sleep

AISLING SMYTH

LEARNING OBJECTIVES

After reading this chapter, you will be able to:
- describe the physiology of sleep
- identify the age-related changes which impact sleep
- describe common sleep disorders in older people
- describe appropriate nursing care strategies to promote sleep in the older population.

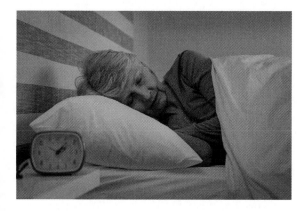

INTRODUCTION

Sleep is a fundamental requirement of life. A recent Australian parliamentary inquiry recommended that sleep health be placed as a national priority due to its pivotal role in maintaining health and wellbeing (Parliament of the Commonwealth of Australia 2019). Sleep is an active process aimed at resting, repairing and rejuvenating the body's cells, tissues and organs.

Sleep affects every cell, tissue, organ and process within the human body. There is not 'one major organ in the body, or process within the brain that is not optimally enhanced by sleep and detrimentally impaired when we do not get enough' (Walker 2017:5). Across the lifetime continuum, sleep quality and quantity alter due to a variety of neurobiological changes. The National Sleep Foundation recommends 7 to 9 hours sleep per night for adults over 65 years of age (Hirshkowitz et al 2015), with a recent Australian survey revealing that older people have an average of 7 hours sleep per night (Adams et al 2017). Sleep disturbances in the older person are common and can result in a bidirectional relationship with other medical illnesses and neurocognitive disorders, whereby, as emerging research is highlighting, sleep is both a risk factor and a symptom of psychiatric, cognitive and medical illnesses in the ageing population. Treatment of sleep disturbances may be pharmacological or non-pharmacological; however, first-line treatment for sleep disturbances in the older person should be non-pharmacological given the potential for adverse effects in this population.

Physiology of Sleep

There are two major stages of sleep: non-rapid eye movement (NREM), and rapid eye movement (REM) sleep. During sleep, an individual will cycle through NREM sub-stages and REM four to five times per night (Gooneratne & Vitiello 2014).

NREM is comprised of four stages (Stages I–IV) with a person becoming increasingly difficult to rouse as they cycle through each stage. During NREM sleep, the parasympathetic nervous system dominates, decreasing blood pressure, pulse rate, respiratory rate, body temperature and metabolic activity. Concurrently, there are increases in growth hormones and thyroid-stimulating hormones during this sleep stage. NREM is important in physical rest and repair. Arousal from sleep in REM is difficult, as such REM sleep is considered 'deep sleep'. REM comprises approximately 20–25% of a person's nightly sleep. During REM sleep, sympathetic nervous system activity increases, which is mirrored by an increase in blood pressure, pulse rate, respiratory rate, body temperature and metabolic activity. REM is also the sleep stage associated with dreaming. Interestingly, there is immobility of large muscle groups via decreased muscle tone and reflexes, resulting in temporary paralysis. This basic structural organisation of sleep is referred to as sleep architecture.

Sleep times are usually aligned with the night phase of a 24-hour period, with wakefulness usually aligned with daytime. This sleep–wake alignment with day–night periods is governed by the body's circadian rhythm. Circadian rhythm refers to the 24-hour internal biological clock which governs every physiological process from cardiac function to body temperature, to mood and metabolism. The 'internal clock' is regulated by the suprachiasmatic nucleus (SCN) within the hypothalamus. Exposure to factors such as light, eating and activity levels can alter the circadian rhythm and therefore impact sleep timings. Ideally, sleep–wake cycles should be synchronised with circadian rhythms, meaning wakeful periods are coupled with high physiological activity and sleeping periods are coupled with decreased physiological activity. Concurrently, several fluctuations of key hormones, namely cortisol and melatonin, act as internal regulators of sleep and wake periods. Cortisol levels tend to peak upon wakening and decrease as the day progresses (Elder et al 2014). Conversely, melatonin levels tend to significantly increase at the time of sleep onset and drop around the time of awakening (Gooneratne et al 2012).

Age-Related Changes to Sleep

Sleep, as with most physiological processes, changes with ageing. Sleep disruption is a normal part of the ageing process with altered sleep quality and quantity (Gulia

& Kumar 2018). Bedtime often shifts to an earlier than usual time, which can dysregulate the internal biological clock (Duffy et al 2015). There is a significant decrease in total sleep time and an increased difficulty in falling asleep and in staying asleep, excessive daytime sleepiness and increased daytime napping (Mattis & Sehgal 2016; Schwarz et al 2017). There are also changes to sleep architecture with a reduction in NREM quality, which is further amplified in older males (Mander et al 2017). In fact, one-third of older people report early morning wakening and/or difficulty maintaining sleep several times per week (Duffy et al 2015). The underlying physiological mechanisms responsible for age-induced sleep alterations include neurobiological changes, hormonal alterations, sleep disorders, medication, nocturnal frequency, chronic pain and medical co-morbidities (Mander et al 2017).

Age-related sleep changes are variable, with some older people significantly affected compared to others who experience minimal sleep changes. However, changes to sleep are not inconsequential. In fact, there is considerable evidence highlighting the negative effects suboptimal sleep has on cognition, mood, quality of life and mortality (Dzierzewski et al 2018; Mander et al 2017; Mattis & Sehgal 2016).

Poor habitual sleep is estimated to increase the risk of developing a chronic health condition by 20–40% (Parliament of the Commonwealth of Australia 2019). Individuals who report sleep disturbances have a higher incidence of all-cause dementia (Shi et al 2018), with a more rapid progression of the disease (Parliament of the Commonwealth of Australia 2019). Both short and long sleep duration are associated with physical frailty (Nakakubo et al 2018).

Increased daytime napping is common among older people compared to their younger counterparts (Mander et al 2017). Daytime sleepiness and napping may be a result of poor overnight sleep. Emerging research suggests that napping in older people may be associated with cognitive impairment, Alzheimer's disease (Leng et al 2019), Parkinson's disease (Leng et al 2018), depression and overall increased medical burden (Cross et al 2015). However, there is also a body of evidence which supports the health-promoting benefits of napping. Effects of naps appear to be dependent on night-time sleep quantity and quality, co-morbidities, age and gender.

SLEEP DISORDERS IN OLDER PEOPLE

As well as normative age-related changes, older people also experience an increased prevalence in sleep disorders

Research Highlights
Sleep and Dementia

- Altered sleep may be both a risk factor for and a symptom of dementia.
- A recent meta-analysis revealed that markers of sleep disturbances, including insomnia, increased wakening and time to fall asleep, are linked to a higher risk of cognitive disorders (Xu et al 2020). Another systematic review found that individuals who reported sleep disturbances also have a higher risk of all-cause dementia, Alzheimer's disease and vascular dementia (Shi et al 2018). Taken together, these results suggest that insufficient sleep quantity or poor sleep quality may predict the risk of dementia development.
- Conversely, it is also accepted that sleep disturbances are a hallmark of dementia as the disease progresses with individuals often waking at night, having trouble getting to sleep and experiencing high levels of daytime sleepiness. Approximately half of all residents in aged care facilities who live with dementia will have disturbed sleep (Capezuti et al 2018).
- Examples of potential non-pharmacological interventions to improve sleep in people living with dementia include increased daylight exposure, supplementation of night-time melatonin and acupressure prior to bed time (Capezuti et al 2018). The effectiveness of these interventions appear variable (Kinnunen et al 2017), thus further research is required to resolve the clinical challenge of treating sleep disturbances in dementia. This is particularly important to address given that improving sleep may slow the progression of dementia and will improve the wellbeing and quality of life of those living with the disease (Holth et al 2017).

(Gooneratne & Vitiello 2014). Sleep disorders can be broadly placed within the following categories:

- insomnias
- hypersomnias
- sleep-breathing disorders
- circadian rhythm disorders
- narcolepsy
- sleep movement disorders.

Common examples of sleep disorders in older people include:

- insomnia
- obstructive sleep apnoea (OSA)

- periodic limb movement disorder (restless leg syndrome).

These disorders are relatively common, with approximately 5% of older people meeting the criteria for insomnia disorder and another 20% for sleep apnoea syndromes (Gooneratne & Vitiello 2014).

Insomnia

Insomnia is the most common sleep disorder and its prevalence increases with age (Brewster et al 2018). Women are twice as likely as men to present with symptoms of insomnia. It may be short-lived, such as during periods of high stress, or more chronic in nature. Insomnia is defined as chronic when symptoms are present three times or more per week for more than 3 months (Australasian Sleep Association 2020a).

Common symptoms of insomnia include:

- difficulty falling asleep
- waking up too early
- difficulty staying asleep
- daytime sleepiness and fatigue
- irritability and/or depression.

Insomnia poses a risk for a myriad of health conditions in older people, including cardiovascular disease, metabolic diseases, cognitive impairment, stroke and depression (Abad & Guilleminault 2018). Acute insomnia does not require treatment and is normally self-resolving. Treatment options for chronic insomnia include sleep hygiene education, cognitive behavioral therapy and relaxation therapy. Pharmacological treatment with sedatives or hypnotics may be used if behavioural modification is unsuccessful, however, these should be a last resort given the potential for adverse effects in the older population (Lam & Macina 2017; Schroeck et al 2016).

Obstructive Sleep Apnoea

Obstructive sleep apnoea (OSA) (see Chapter 24) is a common but potentially dangerous sleep-breathing disorder. The prevalence of OSA increases with age, with approximately 12% of older people diagnosed with OSA (Hirshkowitz et al 2015), and approximately 80% of people with the condition remain undiagnosed (Parliament of the Commonwealth of Australia 2019). OSA is characterised by temporary periods of interrupted breathing lasting 10 seconds or longer which can occur numerous times per hour while asleep. Obesity is one of the most common causes of sleep apnoea as it results in a partial occlusion of the airway by the soft tissues of the mouth and throat. Apnoeic periods result in micro-wakenings, which means a significant reduction of deep REM sleep. In turn, this can result in fatigue and daytime sleepiness.

Common symptoms of sleep apnoea include:

- heavy snoring on inspiration
- awakening with gasping, choking sounds
- delays in breathing while asleep
- morning headaches
- constant fatigue and daytime sleepiness.

OSA causes hypertension and cognitive impairments and may predispose an individual to coronary artery disease, stroke and increased mortality (Australasian Sleep Association 2020b). Treatment plans include:

- management of obesity
- smoking cessation
- alcohol reduction
- dental devices
- potentially, use of continuous positive airway pressure (CPAP) depending upon sleep study outcomes
- in some cases, surgery on the upper airway to aid in opening the airway.

CPAP is administered through a facemask during sleep and is most effective in the treatment of sleep apnoea.

Restless Leg Syndrome

Restless leg syndrome is a neurological disorder characterised by an unpleasant 'creepy-crawly' sensation in the legs. People describe an irresistible urge to move their legs, which disrupts their ability to get a good night's sleep (Gulia & Kumar 2018). The disorder is generally chronic and progressive; however, ongoing research into underlying mechanisms suggests there is a genetic component (During & Winkelman 2019). Massaging the legs and/or moving around may help in reducing symptoms. The incidence of restless leg syndrome increases two to threefold in people aged 60 years and over (During & Winkelman 2019).

SLEEP AND HEALTHY AGEING

While there are normative, age-related changes to sleep architecture and circadian rhythm, older people can attempt to mitigate these changes and preserve optimal sleep health by observing basic sleep hygiene principles (see *Promoting wellness: Sleep hygiene essentials*).

Sleep and Nursing Care

Sleep changes in the older person result in excessive daytime sleepiness. Changes in deep sleep, sleep efficiency and wakefulness all result in decreased physical and psychological wellbeing in the older person. As such, the nurse is strategically placed to assess sleep quality and quantity, and to provide sleep education. Sleep

| **Promoting Wellness** |
| *Sleep Hygiene Essentials* |

- **Keep a regular schedule:** Go to bed and get up at the same time every day, even on weekends.
- **Avoid 'trying' to sleep:** If you are unable to sleep after about 20 minutes, get up and do something calming. Return to bed when you feel sleepy. Avoid clock watching.
- **Avoid stimulants before bed:** Avoid alcohol, caffeine and cigarettes for a minimum of 4 hours before bedtime.
- **Sleep environment:** Maintain a sleep-friendly environment with low lighting, minimal noise distraction, comfortable surroundings and a cooler temperature.
- **Bed is for sleeping:** Keep your bed for just sleeping and sex. Avoid associating bed with other activities.
- **No naps:** If you are having problems sleeping at night, where possible, avoid taking daytime naps to ensure you are tired at bedtime.
- **Sleep rituals:** Implement sleep rituals which signal to your body it is time to go to sleep. These may include reading a book, taking a bath, meditation or stretching exercises.
- **Exercise:** Regular exercise throughout the day can aid with good sleep.
- **Diet:** Eat healthily and avoid eating a heavy meal before bed which can disrupt sleep.

Adapted from Department of Health, Government of Western Australia (n.d.).

disturbances that result from underlying medical conditions require referral and treatment. These may include nocturia, OSA, pain and depression. The recent parliamentary inquiry into sleep health highlighted the important role nurses have in supporting people with sleep issues and delivering interventions to older people to support sleep health (Parliament of the Commonwealth of Australia 2019).

Care settings can also present different sleep-impacting factors. An older person in a hospital or residential aged care facility will have significantly less autonomy over their own sleep environment and patterns. Inpatients identify sleep disruption as one of the main stressors of hospitalisation, citing clinical care requirements and ambient noise as the two primary factors contributing to disturbed sleep (Delaney et al 2018). Given the important role sleep has in rest, repair and rejuvenation, nurses have an important role in preserving sleep in hospital and residential aged care settings. There are numerous pragmatic means of addressing this, as outlined in *Tips for best practice*.

Tips for Best Practice
Optimising Sleep in the Clinical or Residential Aged Care Environment

- **Minimise distractions:** At bed-time, aim for an environment that is conducive to sleep. Turn lighting down low and keep the noise levels as low as possible. Encourage other patients or residents and healthcare professionals to do the same. Suggest ear plugs and eye masks at night.
- **Encourage daytime activity:** Encourage walking during the day and exposure to daylight where possible. This will support a normal circadian rhythm that facilitates night-time sleep.
- **Assess interventions:** Differentiate between essential and non-essential overnight care. Leave non-essential care that may wake the older person until the morning.
- **Older person related factors:** Is the individual unable to sleep due to stress, anxiety and/or pain? Are they taking any medications which may be impacting sleep? If so, can the timing of these medications be altered?

Assessment

Nursing-focused assessment is aimed at identifying the quantity and quality of sleep experienced by the older person. This can be measured by gathering a sleep history, via a sleep diary or with the use of a validated questionnaire such as the Pittsburgh Sleep Quality Index (PSQI) (Buysse et al 1989) (see Fig. 14.1). The PSQI evaluates and scores an individual's sleep in the preceding month, with a score of greater than five indicating clinically significant sleep problems. The Epworth Sleepiness Scale (Johns 1991) is another useful tool which measures daytime sleepiness as a proxy indicator of overnight sleep issues. Reports from the older person of daytime symptoms such as fatigue may also indicate sleep issues. During assessment, the nurse may discuss potential barriers or co-morbidities which may be impeding or interrupting sleep. Examples include:

- nocturia
- pain
- muscle cramping

- stress and anxiety
- use of medications with the potential to interrupt sleep, such as steroids or some antidepressants
- presence of snoring, which, as noted above, may suggest OSA. The STOP-BANG questionnaire is a sleep apnoea screening tool which uses eight questions to assess the risk or presence of OSA (Chung et al 2008).

Care Planning

The following strategies could be included in the nursing care plan:

- Explain the fundamentals of sleep hygiene to the older person and discuss which strategies may be useful and feasible to adopt (see *Promoting Wellness: Sleep hygiene essentials*).
- Support the older person in identifying stress-relieving, rest-promoting activities before bedtime to promote sleep, such as stretching or reading a book.
- Stress the importance of maintaining routine.
- Highlight the importance of trying non-pharmacological and/or lifestyle interventions before resorting to pharmacological interventions.
- Review current medication.

Intervention

Many sleep problems can be adequately addressed by adhering to strict sleep hygiene processes. Non-pharmacological interventions should be exhausted prior to progressing to pharmacological interventions. This is especially pertinent in the older population given the potential adverse effects associated with sleep aid medication, such as an increased risk of falls (see Chapter 16), and next-day sedation and confusion (Gooneratne & Vitiello 2014).

Non-pharmacological interventions include cognitive behavioral therapy. This is an effective evidence-based approach delivered by a trained professional, which aims to address negative behaviours and beliefs around sleep that may perpetuate insomnia (Gooneratne & Vitiello 2014). Other non-pharmacological interventions with mixed results include mindfulness, bright light therapy, social activities, acupuncture, acupressure and exercise regimens (MacLeod et al 2018).

If non-pharmacological interventions fail to improve the older person's sleep, pharmacological approaches can be considered. Sleep aid medications may be appropriate as a short-term measure; however, they become less effective over long periods of use. In addition, these medications produce unnatural sleep that disturbs the normal phases of NREM and REM sleep. Sedatives and hypnotics are the two common classes of sleep

Text continued on p. 164

Subject's Initials_____ID#_____Date_____Time_____ AM PM

PITTSBURGH SLEEP QUALITY INDEX

INSTRUCTIONS:
The following questions relate to your usual sleep habits during the past month only. Your answers should indicate the most accurate reply for the majority of days and nights in the past month. Please answer all questions.

1.   During the past month, what time have you usually gone to bed at night?

BED TIME _____

2.   During the past month, how long (in minutes) has it usually taken you to fall asleep each night?

NUMBER OF MINUTES _____

3.   During the past month, what time have you usually gotten up in the morning?

GETTING UP TIME _____

4.   During the past month, how many hours of actual sleep did you get at night? (This may be different than the number of hours you spent in bed.)

HOURS OF SLEEP PER NIGHT _____

For each of the remaining questions, check the one best response. Please answer all questions.

5.   During the past month, how often have you had trouble sleeping because you . . .

a)   Cannot get to sleep within 30 minutes

Not during the   Less than   Once or twice   Three or more
past month_____ once a week_____ a week_____   times a week_____

b)   Wake up in the middle of the night or early morning

Not during the   Less than   Once or twice   Three or more
past month_____ once a week_____ a week_____   times a week_____

c)   Have to get up to use the bathroom

Not during the   Less than   Once or twice   Three or more
past month_____ once a week_____ a week_____   times a week_____

FIG. 14.1 **Pittsburgh Sleep Quality Index** Buysse et al (1989).

d) Cannot breathe comfortably

Not during the   Less than   Once or twice   Three or more
past month_____   once a week_____   a week_____   times a week_____

e) Cough or snore loudly

Not during the   Less than   Once or twice   Three or more
past month_____   once a week_____   a week_____   times a week_____

f) Feel too cold

Not during the   Less than   Once or twice   Three or more
past month_____   once a week_____   a week_____   times a week_____

g) Feel too hot

Not during the   Less than   Once or twice   Three or more
past month_____   once a week_____   a week_____   times a week_____

h) Had bad dreams

Not during the   Less than   Once or twice   Three or more
past month_____   once a week_____   a week_____   times a week_____

i) Have pain

Not during the   Less than   Once or twice   Three or more
past month_____   once a week_____   a week_____   times a week_____

j) Other reason(s), please describe_____

_____

How often during the past month have you had trouble sleeping because of this?

Not during the   Less than   Once or twice   Three or more
past month_____   once a week_____   a week_____   times a week_____

6. During the past month, how would you rate your sleep quality overall?

Very good   _____

Fairly good   _____

Fairly bad   _____

Very bad   _____

FIG. 14.1, cont'd   *Continued*

7. During the past month, how often have you taken medicine to help you sleep (prescribed or "over the counter")?

Not during the   Less than   Once or twice   Three or more
past month_____ once a week_____   a week_____   times a week_____

8. During the past month, how often have you had trouble staying awake while driving, eating meals, or engaging in social activity?

Not during the   Less than   Once or twice   Three or more
past month_____ once a week_____   a week_____   times a week_____

9. During the past month, how much of a problem has it been for you to keep up enough enthusiasm to get things done?

No problem at all   _____

Only a very slight problem   _____

Somewhat of a problem   _____

A very big problem   _____

10. Do you have a bed partner or room mate?

No bed partner or room mate   _____

Partner/room mate in other room   _____

Partner in same room, but not same bed   _____

Partner in same bed   _____

If you have a room mate or bed partner, ask him/her how often in the past month you have had . . .

a) Loud snoring

Not during the   Less than   Once or twice   Three or more
past month_____ once a week_____   a week_____   times a week_____

b) Long pauses between breaths while asleep

Not during the   Less than   Once or twice   Three or more
past month_____ once a week_____   a week_____   times a week_____

c) Legs twitching or jerking while you sleep

Not during the   Less than   Once or twice   Three or more
past month_____ once a week_____   a week_____   times a week_____

FIG. 14.1, cont'd

d)   Episodes of disorientation or confusion during sleep

| Not during the past month_____ | Less than once a week_____ | Once or twice a week_____ | Three or more times a week_____ |

e)   Other restlessness while you sleep; please describe_____

_____

| Not during the past month_____ | Less than once a week_____ | Once or twice a week_____ | Three or more times a week_____ |

Buysse DJ, Reynolds CF, Monk TH, Berman SR, Kupfer DJ: *Psychiatry Research*, 28:193-213, 1989.

FIG. 14.1, cont'd

Practice Scenario

Mr Williamson is an 80-year-old man with a history of falls, obesity and cardiovascular disease. He has been admitted to hospital for further investigations of angina. On admission, Mr Williamson tells you that he does not sleep very well. He explains that he tends to have two naps during the day, approximately 1.5 hours each, but struggles to sleep at night. He often wakes early and feels unrefreshed. His wife tells you that he is a very loud snorer and is often coughing and spluttering overnight.

MULTIPLE CHOICE QUESTIONS

1. You suspect that Mr Williamson may have:
   a. insomnia
   b. narcolepsy
   c. obstructive sleep apnoea
   d. restless leg syndrome

2. Which of the following would <u>not</u> be recommended during the night to promote good sleep for an older person in residential aged care?
   a. Keep noise levels as low as possible during the night

   b. Encourage use of eye mask at night
   c. Ensure the older person is asked if they are OK during the night
   d. Keep lighting low during the night

3. Mr Williamson requests a hypnotic medication to aid his sleep. He has never had a hypnotic before. What is the best course of action for Mr Williamson?
   a. Ensure his medication is prescribed and encourage him to follow up with his GP for regular check-up
   b. Suggest beginning cognitive behavioral therapy to improve sleep
   c. Educate Mr Williamson regarding the importance of losing weight in order to control his OSA and thus improve his sleep quality
   d. Suggest he obtains over-the-counter (OTC) sleeping aid medication

---

aid medications. Sedative medications act by reducing anxiety and irritability thus indirectly promoting sleep. Hypnotic medications have a direct depressant effect on the central nervous system and directly induce sleep. Prescribing and administering medications targeting sleep disturbances requires holistic assessment and sound clinical reasoning to ensure potential adverse effects are outweighed by potential benefit. There is minimal evidence supporting the use of melatonin supplementation in older people with very modest effects observed (Reynolds & Adams 2019).

Evaluation

The nurse can play an important role in regularly assessing an older person's sleep, rest and fatigue by way of a sleep history using a sleep diary, or use of a validated tool. Improved sleep, decreased fatigue and sleepiness and improved wellbeing are all indicative of improvements in sleep quality and quantity.

SUMMARY

Sleep is essential in maintaining health and wellbeing in all populations, including older people. Normative age-related changes result in decreased quality and quantity of sleep. Older people are also more likely to

be diagnosed with a sleep disorder. Treatment of sleep disturbances should focus on sleep hygiene principles and non-pharmacological mechanisms. If unsuccessful, pharmacological interventions may be considered; however, thorough considerations must be made for the potential risks associated with sleeping medications in older people. Nurses are well placed to assess sleep disruption and provide education supporting optimal sleep opportunity.

REFERENCES

Abad VC, Guilleminault C (2018) Insomnia in elderly patients: recommendations for pharmacological management. Drugs and Aging 35(9):791–817.

Adams RJ, Appleton SL, Taylor AW et al (2017) Sleep health of Australian adults in 2016: results of the 2016 Sleep Health Foundation national survey. Sleep Health 3(1):35–42.

Australasian Sleep Association (2020a) On-the-spot management. Information for health professionals. Insomnia. Online. Available: https://sleep.org.au/Public/Resource-Centre/F-HP-Info/F-Adult/Insomnia.aspx

Australasian Sleep Association (2020b) On-the-spot management. Information for health professionals. Obstructive sleep apnoea. Online. Available: https://sleep.org.au/Public/Resource-Centre/F-HP-Info/F-Adult/Obstructive-Sleep-Apnoea.aspx

Brewster GS, Riegel B, Gehrman PR (2018) Insomnia in the older adult. Sleep Medicine Clinics 13(1):13–19.

Buysse DJ, Reynolds CF, Monk TH et al (1989) The Pittsburgh Sleep Quality Index: A new instrument for psychiatric practice and research. Psychiatry Research 28(2):193–213.

Capezuti E, Sagha Zadeh R, Woody N et al (2018) A systematic review of non-pharmacological interventions to improve nighttime sleep among residents of long-term care settings. BMC Geriatrics 18(1):143.

Chung F, Yegneswaran B, Liao P et al (2008) STOP-BANG questionnaire. Anesthesiology 108:812–821. Online. Available: https://aci.health.nsw.gov.au/__data/assets/pdf_file/0005/204728/10._STOP_BANG_Questionnaire_Safe_Procedural_Sedation_Project.PDF

Cross N, Terpening Z, Rogers NL et al (2015) Napping in older people 'at risk' of dementia: relationships with depression, cognition, medical burden and sleep quality. Journal of Sleep Research 24(5):494–502.

Delaney LJ, Currie MJ, Huang H-CC et al (2018) They can rest at home: an observational study of patients' quality of sleep in an Australian hospital. BMC Health Services Research 18(1):524.

Department of Health, Government of Western Australia (n.d.) Sleeping difficulties. Online. Available: https://healthywa.wa.gov.au/Articles/S_T/Sleeping-difficulties

Duffy JF, Zitting K-M, Chinoy ED (2015) Aging and circadian rhythms. Sleep Medicine Clinics 10(4):423–434.

During EH, Winkelman JW (2019) Drug treatment of restless legs syndrome in older adults. Drugs and Aging 36(10):939–946.

Dzierzewski JM, Dautovich N, Ravyts S (2018) Sleep and cognition in older adults. Sleep Medicine Clinics 13(1):93–106.

Elder GJ, Wetherell MA, Barclay NL (2014) The cortisol awakening response – applications and implications for sleep medicine. Sleep Medicine Reviews 18(3):215–224.

Gooneratne NS, Edwards AYZ, Zhou C et al (2012) Melatonin pharmacokinetics following two different oral surge-sustained release doses in older adults. Journal of Pineal Research 52(4):437–445.

Gooneratne NS, Vitiello MV (2014) Sleep in older adults: normative changes, sleep disorders, and treatment options. Clinics in Geriatric Medicine 30(3):591–627.

Gulia KK, Kumar VM (2018) Sleep disorders in the elderly: a growing challenge. Psychogeriatrics 18(3):155–165.

Hirshkowitz M, Whiton K, Albert SM et al (2015) National Sleep Foundation's sleep time duration recommendations: Methodology and results summary. Sleep Health 1(1):40–43.

Holth J, Patel T, Holtzman DM (2017). Sleep in Alzheimer's disease – beyond amyloid. Neurobiology of Sleep and Circadian Rhythms 2:4–14.

Johns MW (1991) A new method for measuring daytime sleepiness: The Epworth Sleepiness Scale. Sleep 14(6):540–545.

Kinnunen KM, Vikhanova A, Livingston G (2017) The management of sleep disorders in dementia: an update. Current Opinion in Psychiatry 30(6):491–497.

Lam S, Macina LO (2017) Therapy update for insomnia in the elderly. The Consultant Pharmacist 32(10):610–622.

Leng Y, Goldman SM, Cawthon PM (2018) Excessive daytime sleepiness, objective napping and 11-year risk of Parkinson's disease in older men. International Journal of Epidemiology 47(5):1679–1686.

Leng Y, Redline S, Stone KL et al (2019) Objective napping, cognitive decline, and risk of cognitive impairment in older men. Alzheimer's and Dementia 15(8):1039–1047.

MacLeod S, Musich S, Kraemer S (2018) Practical non-pharmacological intervention approaches for sleep problems among older adults. Geriatric Nursing 39(5):506–512.

Mander BA, Winer JR, Walker MP (2017) Sleep and human aging. Neuron 94(1):19–36.

Mattis J, Sehgal A (2016) Circadian rhythms, sleep, and disorders of aging. Trends in Endocrinology and Metabolism 27(4):192–203.

Nakakubo S, Makizako H, Doi T et al (2018) Long and short sleep duration and physical frailty in community-dwelling older adults. The Journal of Nutrition, Health and Aging 22(9):1066–1071.

Parliament of the Commonwealth of Australia (2019) Bedtime reading: inquiry into sleep health awareness in Australia. House of Representatives Standing Committee on Health, Aged Care and Sport. Commonwealth of Australia, Canberra.

Reynolds AC, Adams RJ (2019) Treatment of sleep disturbance in older adults. Journal of Pharmacy Practice and Research 49(3):296–304.

Schroeck JL, Ford J, Conway EL et al (2016) Review of safety and efficacy of sleep medicines in older adults. Clinical Therapeutics 38(11):2340–2372.

Schwarz JFA, Åkerstedt T, Lindberg E et al (2017) Age affects sleep microstructure more than sleep macrostructure. Journal of Sleep Research 26(3):277–287.

Shi L, Chen S-J, Ma M-Y et al (2018) Sleep disturbances increase the risk of dementia: A systematic review and meta-analysis. Sleep Medicine Reviews 40:4–16.

Walker M (2017) Why we sleep. Penguin, London.

Xu W, Tan CC, Zou J-J et al (2020) Sleep problems and risk of all-cause cognitive decline or dementia: an updated systematic review and meta-analysis. Journal of Neurology, Neurosurgery and Psychiatry 91(3):236–244.

Promoting Healthy Skin

ROBYN RAYNER

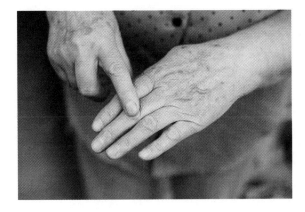

INTRODUCTION

Nurses confront a range of challenges and priorities when promoting healthy skin in older people. The older person's age, gender, genetics, skin type and lifelong exposure to environmental and lifestyle factors have an impact on the skin and influence its response to stressors. Ageing is associated with morphological and physiological skin changes that can lead to poor health outcomes

and impact on an older person's quality of life. A clear understanding of the skin's anatomy and physiology, concomitant awareness of age-related skin changes, an ability to conduct a thorough skin assessment and the capacity to apply appropriate evidence-based best practices are essential for promoting healthy skin. Table 15.1 presents a glossary of terms used within this chapter.

AGE-RELATED CHANGES

The skin is the largest and most dynamic organ of the human body. It comprises the epidermis, dermis and hypodermis. It provides a physiological buffer against harsh elements in the environment, preserves life-supporting functions, and provides an active immuno-logical barrier. Over the course of a lifetime, changes in the condition of the skin are influenced by:
- ageing
- gender
- genetics
- skin type
- environmental (exposure to ultraviolet radiation [UVR], pollutants, gravity)
- lifestyle-related factors (smoking, nutrition, alcohol, stress, exercise, medications).

TABLE 15.1
Glossary of Terms

Actinic keratosis	pre-cancerous scaly spots or patches on the top layer of skin from long-term exposure to the sun
Actinic purpura	a benign clinical condition resulting from sun-induced damage to the connective tissue of the dermis that leads to bleeding into the skin from loss of blood vessel support
Autolytic debridement	Autolysis or autolytic debridement uses the body's own enzymes and moisture to re-hydrate, soften and finally liquefy hard eschar and slough. Autolytic debridement is selective as only necrotic tissue is liquefied
Cellular senescence	characterised by the cessation of cell division
Cellulitis	an acute common and often painful bacterial infection of the dermis and hypodermis that presents as a red, swollen area that feels hot and tender to touch. The redness and swelling can spread quickly
Critical colonisation	when host defences are unable to maintain a healthy [bacterial] balance and bacteria are sufficient in number to delay healing without exhibiting signs of inflammation
Dermatomes	an area of skin in which sensory nerves derive from a single spinal nerve root
DNA telomeres	the terminal end of a chromosome involved in chromosomal replication
Exudate	any fluid that filters from the circulatory system into lesions or areas of inflammation. It can be a pus-like or clear fluid. When an injury occurs, leaving skin exposed, it leaks out of the blood vessels and into nearby tissues. The fluid is composed of serum, fibrin and white blood cells
Functional fibroblasts	these maintain the structural integrity of connective tissues by continuously secreting precursors of the extracellular matrix
Hyperkeratotic	the thickening of the outer layer of the skin
Induration	an increase in the fibrous elements in tissue commonly associated with inflammation and loss of elasticity
Intracellular environment	the internal environment of the cells
Intercellular microenvironment	the environment between cells
Intertrigo	a superficial inflammatory condition of skin folds resulting from friction and moisture
Ischaemic	restricted blood supply causing damage to tissues
Keratinocyte	an epidermal cell which produces keratin
Lentigines	or liver spots – benign lesions that occur on the sun-exposed areas of the body. Commonly found on the backs of hands and face
Lymphoedema	a chronic condition arising from the accumulation of protein-rich fluid within the hypodermis from abnormal development or impairment of a lymphatic system
Maceration	caused by exposure of the skin to excessive moisture. Skin may present as wrinkly, wet or soggy to the touch and is often associated with improper wound care
Oedema	a condition characterised by an excess of watery fluid collecting in the cavities or tissues of the body
Photoageing	premature ageing of the skin caused by repeated exposure to ultraviolet radiation (UV), primarily from the sun and other factors, including smoking and pollution
Pruritus	or itch, the unpleasant sensation of the skin that increases the urge to scratch
Reactive oxygen species (ROS)	highly reactive chemicals derived from oxygen that interact with other molecules to cause damage

TABLE 15.1
Glossary of Terms—cont'd

Revascularisation	a procedure to restore the blood flow to an area
Semmes–Weinstein monofilament	non-invasive clinical test that uses a monofilament to measure sensation
Solar elastosis	an accumulation of abnormal elastin (elastic tissue) in the dermis of the skin, which occurs as a result of the cumulative effects of prolonged and excessive sun exposure, a process known as photoageing
Stratum corneum	the outermost layer of the skin, consisting of keratinised cells
Subepidermal low echogenicity band (SLEB)	a marker of photoageing. A hypoechoic band that is visible in the papillary dermis by ultrasound and which is exacerbated by exposure to UVR and photoageing
Transepidermal water loss	the loss of water that passes from inside the body through the epidermis to the surrounding atmosphere via diffusion and evaporation processes
Transudate	watery fluid with scant cells or proteins that is squeezed through tissue or into the extracellular space
Truncal adiposity	also known as abdominal fat deposits
Ulceration	the formation of a break on the skin forming when the surface cells die
Uneven pigmentation	irregular discolouration of the skin
Xerosis	the term used for dry skin

Ageing reduces collagen and elastin synthesis, and when combined with the cumulative effects of UVR the mechanical properties of the skin progressively weaken (Garcia-Martinez et al 2020; Han et al 2014). The impact of natural (intrinsic or chronological) and external (extrinsic or photoageing) ageing processes become more pronounced over time. Skin manifestations commonly associated with intrinsic ageing include fine wrinkles and loss of elasticity. Conversely, extrinsic ageing is an accumulative process superimposed on natural ageing and characterised by solar elastosis, uneven pigmentation, actinic purpura, lentigines, actinic keratosis and yellowing (Vierkötter & Krutmann 2012).

Ageing is an individual and complex process affecting all three layers of the skin. The pH of exposed skin is normally weakly acidic. It contributes to the skin's protective function by:
- providing a barrier to water and electrolyte movement
- maintaining the integrity and cohesion of the skin surface
- activating cytokines
- forming a buffer against microorganisms and chemicals.

As the skin ages, the pH increases (becoming more alkaline) and surface lipid concentration decreases. Together, these changes impair the integrity of the epidermal barrier. Dermal collagen and elastin fibres also decline and fragment, reducing the skin's mechanical force properties. The deleterious effects of reactive oxygen species production, progressive shortening of the DNA telomeres and reduced efficiency of enzymes that repair DNA, alter the intracellular environment. Chronic low-grade inflammation and extracellular matrix disruption damage the intercellular microenvironment. The hypodermis reduces in the face, hands and feet and generally increases around the torso and thighs. Ageing decreases the functional capacity of the skin and increases the risk of non-inflammatory skin diseases (Algiert-Zielińska et al 2017; Barth et al 2019; Birch 2018; Choi 2019; Cole et al 2018).

RISK FACTORS FOR SKIN DAMAGE
Environmental Exposure
Long-term exposure to deleterious environmental agents profoundly impact on the skin's structural integrity.

Accumulative exposure to UVR is associated with DNA structural changes, inflammation and photoageing. The Fitzpatrick Skin Type Tool was developed to predict the reactivity of skin to photochemotherapy and is now commonly used to identify the clinical sensitivity of skin to UV exposure and sun protective behaviours. This system classifies skin types according to the amount of pigment and the skin's reaction to sun exposure. Skin types range from 1 (highest risk of skin damage, skin ageing from sun exposure and skin cancer) to 6 (lowest risk). Individuals with lower Fitzpatrick skin types (i.e. skin types 1 and 2) who engage in an outdoor lifestyle are at greater risk of the harmful effects of UVR (Fitzpatrick 1988; Sachdeva 2009).

Although inflammation is implicated in both intrinsic and extrinsic ageing, the effects are more pronounced in those with photoaged skin. Photoaged skin is characterised by:

- dryness
- deep wrinkles
- coarse texture
- increased thickness
- pigmentation
- microvascular changes.

Low-grade asymptomatic chronic inflammation accelerates cellular senescence, suppresses the immune system and damages the epidermis, extracellular matrix, dermal–epidermal junction (DEJ) and dermis to prematurely age skin (Amano 2016). There is also an increased susceptibility to both pre-cancerous and cancerous lesions.

Lifestyle-Related Factors

Numerous lifestyle-related choices, including smoking, alcohol intake, level of physical activity and diet, induce age-related skin changes. The effects of smoking, which are more pronounced in females than males, accelerate ageing and negatively impact on the epidermal skin barrier, degrade dermal collagen, reduce skin elasticity and impair wound healing (Ortiz & Grando 2012).

Regular consumption of alcohol tends to impair skin healing. After surgery, older people who regularly drink alcohol are at higher risk of superficial surgical site infection and wound dehiscence, which are associated with longer length of hospital stay and postoperative mortality. Moreover, alcohol contributes to weight gain and increased truncal adiposity, is a major risk factor for cancer and, among chronic users, can cause peripheral neuropathy (Julian et al 2019; Rehm et al 2019). Chronic alcohol consumption reduces the absorption of essential vitamins (A, folate, B_{12}, C), proteins, carbohydrates and lipids.

Inactivity is associated with loss of functional fibroblasts, collagen production and the skin's mechanical strength. At the other end of the spectrum, extreme activity promotes the production of inflammatory mediators that can lead to degeneration of collagen and extracellular matrix. Regular physical activity enables cells to adapt to oxidative stress and increase tissue resistance to reactive oxygen species damage (Kruk & Duchnik 2014).

Lifelong nutritional behaviour significantly influences ageing. Over time, dietary behaviours have a gradual, cumulative effect on the skin, culminating in poor health outcomes. Malnutrition is associated with increased risk of morbidity and mortality. Malnutrition accelerates ageing as insufficient macro- and micronutrients are available to protect and regenerate skin cells. Nutrient deficiencies prolong inflammation and increase the risk of infection. Fibroblast proliferation and collagen synthesis decrease to delay wound-healing and reduce the tensile strength of tissue. Malnutrition increases the risk of pressure injuries and is associated with dryness (xerosis), pruritus and purpura.

The skin of obese persons is characterised by roughness, diminished moisturising function, an impaired skin barrier and reduced intercellular lipids (Mori et al 2017). Impaired collagen and elastin production reduce the skin's mechanical strength, increasing the risk of tissue breakdown and delayed healing. Excessive hypodermal tissue folds are susceptible to intertrigo and the secondary growth of bacterial and fungal organisms. Vascular and lymphatic changes increase the susceptibility of the lower extremities to cellulitis, oedema, lymphoedema and ulcerations.

Infection

Age-related changes to the immune composition of the skin increase the skin's susceptibility to infections and malignancies (Chambers & Vukmanovic-Stejic 2019). The outermost layer or stratum corneum is marked by decreased lipids and an impaired skin barrier that leads to xerosis, fissures and increased risk for inflammation and infections (Farage et al 2017). These are normal effects seen with ageing.

Medications

Older people who take multiple prescription and non-prescription medications are at greater risk of pruritus (itching). The drug, or its preservative, can initiate or exacerbate pruritus by inducing an allergic reaction. Classes of medications most associated with the development or exacerbation of pruritus include:

- antihypertensives
- hypolipidemics

- antibiotics
- opioids
- antidiuretics (Garibyan et al 2013).

COMMON SKIN CONDITIONS IN OLDER PEOPLE

The three most common skin conditions in older age include:

- xerosis
- pruritus
- actinic purpura.

Xerosis

Xerosis, or generalised skin dryness, occurring with or without pruritus, is one of the most common and uncomfortable dermatological conditions affecting older people. The condition results from decreased epidermal lipids and a related increase in transepidermal water loss. Management of xerosis is directed at promoting the skin's natural moisture by improving hydration and restoring the skin's barrier function through regular application of topical moisturisers or lipid-replenishing agents (Augustin et al 2019). The *Tips for Best Practice* box shows the assessment and treatment of xerosis.

Tips for Best Practice
Assessment and Treatment of Xerosis

ASSESSMENT

- Observe the skin for: dryness, dull colouration, roughness, flakiness, fissures, erythema and scratch marks that indicate itching.
- Identify precipitating factors, including: heat, hot showers or bathing, the use of soaps and seasonal variation, such as winter months when the relative humidity is reduced.
- Assess effectiveness of current therapies.

TREATMENT

- Keep the skin cool by minimising duration, frequency and temperature of water when bathing.
- Use low pH lipid-replenishing cleansers.
- Apply moisturisers to the skin when still moist from bathing.
- Gently pat dry the skin using soft non-abrasive materials.
- Use humidification during winter months.

Encourage adequate fluid intake to rehydrate the skin.

Pruritus

Pruritus, or an undesirable urge to scratch, is a common and debilitating skin condition of older people that negatively impacts on quality of life. The unpleasant itch sensation results from inflammation of cutaneous nerve fibres and the skin (Mollanazar et al 2016). Pruritus in older people is associated with a multitude of factors, including:

- age-related skin changes
- systemic conditions (renal failure, liver disease)
- neuropathic disorders (herpes zoster, small-fibre polyneuropathy)
- psychogenic illnesses (psychosis, obsessive compulsive disorder)
- polypharmacy (Garibyan et al 2013).

The priority of management is to identify and eliminate the cause of the itch. While management is individualised, skincare measures recommended to treat xerosis can also address the itch. Finger nails also need to be kept short to minimise scratching, as this increases inflammation and exacerbates the condition. The *Tips for Best Practice* box presents ways to promote a healthly skin barrier.

Tips for Best Practice
Promoting a Healthy Skin Barrier

- Limit the time taken to bath or shower.
- Use tepid or warm water when bathing or showering.
- Use pH neutral non-alkaline skin cleansers.
- Apply emollients or moisturisers while the skin is still moist from bathing.
- Select an emollient or moisturiser containing urea or glycerin to prevent xerosis.

Actinic Purpura

Actinic purpura is a benign manifestation that occurs in older people from the progressive loss of dermal collagen and increased fragility of blood vessels. Dark purple macules or patches form on the forearms, hands and lower limbs from extravasation of blood on sun-exposed skin surfaces. The lesions are clearly demarcated and occur following relatively minor trauma. Despite appearing unsightly for the individual, they generally resolve within 1–3 weeks without any complications. Where purpuric lesions repeatedly occur at the same site, a residual brown pigmented skin stain can develop. Management of purpura is directed at protecting exposed skin surfaces from trauma.

SKIN ASSESSMENT

The initial skin assessment involves evaluating the person's past medical history to identify pre-existing conditions that can impact on skin health. These include:

- peripheral vascular disease
- diabetes
- lower extremity ulcers
- incontinence.

Review of the older person's use of prescription and over-the-counter (OTC) medications can identify therapies which have the potential to induce a skin reaction or impair healing. Determining the Fitzpatrick skin type will indicate the person's reaction to UVR and level of risk for sun damage, photoageing and skin cancers. It is important to evaluate recent skin changes in relation to pre-existing skin conditions, previous skin problems or application of skincare products.

As skin conditions are commonly associated with virtually every older person, a head-to-toe skin assessment should be routinely conducted to identify skin, nail or hair problems. A general list of signs and symptoms to be considered when conducting a skin assessment is provided in Table 15.2.

Findings of the skin assessment need to be documented. Any identified skin condition requires further examination and investigation to establish appropriate management and prevention strategies.

WOUND ASSESSMENT AND MANAGEMENT

Wound assessment and management are key to a successful outcome. A comprehensive and systematic approach is needed to assess the wound, identify the cause, mitigate factors that impair healing and optimise management.

Wound Assessment

A detailed wound assessment is conducted using a recognised assessment tool in conjunction with clinical judgement. Nursing assessment of a wound involves:

- taking a comprehensive history: location, duration, cause (known or presumed), management to date and any previous response to treatment
- measuring the size of the wound: length, width and depth
- evaluating characteristics of the wound:
  - tissue type – granulation, hypergranulation, epithelialisation, slough, necrotic or fibrotic
  - exudate – quantity and quality
  - margins – rolled, undermined, hyperkeratotic
  - odour

TABLE 15.2
General Skin Assessment Signs and Symptoms

	General Skin Assessment	
Signs	Temperature	Areas of warmth or heat
		Cool or cold extremities
	Colour	Normal skin hue
		Paleness
		Flushing
		Cyanosis
		Pigmentation
		Bruising
		Jaundice
		Blanchable or non-blanchable skin
	Skin integrity	• Wounds
		• Lesions
		• Fissures
		• Rashes
		• Blisters
	Skin texture	• Coarse
		• Smooth
		• Fragile
		• Moist, dry or sweaty
		• Turgor
		• Induration
		• Oedema
Symptoms	Pain can be assessed using the acronym SOCRATES (Koneti & Jones 2016)	
	Site	
	Onset	
	Character	
	Radiation	
	Association	
	Time course	
	Exacerbating/ relieving factors	
	Severity	
	Neuropathy	
	Pruritus	
	Odour	
	Bleeding	

- assessing the surrounding skin: inflammation, induration, and oedema.

Utilise a recognised wound assessment tool, such as TIME (Tissue, Infection, Moisture and Edge) framework or MEASURE (Measurement, Exudate, Appearance, Suffering, Undermining, Re-evaluate and Edge) to assess and guide clinical management (Keast et al 2004; Schultz et al 2003). Various tools are also available to assess specific types of wounds, including: skin tears, pressure injuries, venous leg ulcers and diabetic foot ulcers. The assessment generates meaningful information that better directs management and supports dressing selection to optimise healing.

Wound Management

Wound management refers to evidence-based decisions taken to treat the wound. Effective management involves identifying, treating or eliminating any factor that causes the wound, including correcting ischaemia, promoting venous return or off-loading pressure.

The choice of dressing or topical therapy is dependent on:

- assessment of the wound that indicates the cause
- type of tissue
- amount of exudate
- presence of microbes
- wound care objective
- the older person's preference.

The ideal dressing needs to provide a warm, moist and innocuous environment to promote healing. The exception is if the wound is ischaemic; then it must be kept dry to reduce the risk of infection until a vascular review and revascularisation have been completed. If an ischaemic wound is suspected, the nurse should refer back to the GP for further referral to a specialist.

Dressing products broadly address three wound characteristics and include:

- a rehydrating product to reduce desiccated, necrotic or eschar tissue
- an absorbent product to contain excessive transudate or exudate
- an antimicrobial product where there is evidence of critical colonisation or infection.

Table 15.3 lists examples of dressings products, indications for use and any contraindications or precautions.

SKIN TEARS

Skin tears are defined as trauma-induced, partial or full thickness wounds, which primarily occur on the extremities of older people who are at higher risk due to age-related changes to the skin's structural and mechanical support

properties. These wounds are commonly associated with elastosis and/or ecchymosis (Rayner, Carville & Leslie 2019). Ageing and photoageing have been implicated in the risk for skin tears (Rayner et al 2019a, 2019b).

A range of classification tools are available to assess skin tears, standardise evaluation and improve management. The Skin Tear Audit Research (STAR) classification system is widely used in Australia (Carville et al 2007). The STAR classification system comprises three categories and two sub-categories (Fig. 15.1). Fig. 15.2 shows an image of a STAR category 2b skin tear on the arm of a 90-year-old man with chronic photoageing.

The *Tips for Best Practice* box discusses the assessment, treatment and prevention of skin tears.

Tips for Best Practice
Assessment, Treatment and Prevention of Skin Tears

ASSESSMENT
- Classify the skin tear.

TREATMENT
- Control bleeding.
- Gently clean the wound with potable water or normal saline.
- Realign the skin edges or flap to the normal anatomical position.
- Apply an atraumatic low adherent dressing, such as silicone.
- On outer dressing, date and draw arrow pointing to the wound edge to indicate direction to remove.
- Document assessment and treatment.

PREVENTION
- Identify at-risk person (history of skin tears, history of falls, chronic UVR exposure, purpura/ecchymosis, elastosis, frail skin).
- Wear longsleeve shirts and long trousers to protect extremities.
- Use pH-friendly cleanser and tepid water when bathing.
- Apply moisturisers twice daily to the extremities.
- Use hoists and sliding sheets to transfer the person.
- Minimise environmental hazards (poor lighting and clutter).
- Pad hard contact surfaces (bed rails, wheelchair arms and leg support).
- Avoid adhesive skin products.
- Keep fingernails and toenails short.

TABLE 15.3
Dressing Types, Indications for Use and Contraindications or Precautions

Dressing Type	Indications for Use	Contraindications or Precautions
Semi-permeable films	Low exudating wounds Can be used to secure a primary dressing	Non-absorbing Not recommended for high exudating wounds Removal can cause skin trauma
Hydrogels	Dry–low exuding wounds Promotes moist wound healing Facilitates autolytic debridement	Not recommended for higher exudating wounds Can cause maceration
Silicone	Prevents trauma and pain Suitable for superficial and fragile wounds	Known sensitivity to silicone Primary layer not absorbent
Hydrocolloids	Low–moderate exudate wounds Facilitates autolytic debridement	Not recommended for fragile or infected wounds May cause hypergranulation or maceration
Calcium alginates	Moderate–heavy exudating wounds Promotes blood coagulation	Non-exudating wounds May adhere to and desiccate a wound
Gelling fibre dressings	Heavy exudating wounds Reduces periwound maceration Promotes moist wound healing	Non-exudating wounds
Foams	Moderate exudating wounds Protection Promotes moist wound healing	Not recommended for high exudating or infected wounds
Cadexomer iodine	Broad-spectrum antimicrobial activity Facilitates autolytic debridement	Known thyroid disease or sensitivity
Hypertonic saline	Exudating infected wounds Inhibits bacterial growth	Dry saline-impregnated gauze not recommended for dry slough, eschar or minimal exudating wounds
Medical grade honey	Broad-spectrum antimicrobial activity Infected wounds Reduces malodour Promotes moist wound healing Facilitates autolytic debridement	May cause a drawing sensation Known sensitivity
Polyhexamethylene biguanide	Broad-spectrum antimicrobial activity Topical antiseptic Reduces malodour	Dry necrotic wounds Known sensitivity
Silver	Broad-spectrum antimicrobial activity Infected wounds Reduces inflammation	May cause skin discolouration Re-evaluate after 2 weeks
Odour absorbing dressings	Malodorous wounds Malignant/fungating wounds Infected wounds	Not suitable for cutting

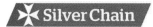 **STAR Skin Tear Classification System**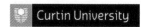

STAR Skin Tear Classification System Guidelines

1 Control bleeding and clean the wound according to protocol.
2 Realign (if possible) any skin or flap.
3 Assess degree of tissue loss and skin or flap colour using the STAR Classification System.
4 Assess the surrounding skin condition for fragility, swelling, discolouration or bruising.
5 Assess the person, their wound and their healing environment as per protocol.
6 If skin or flap colour is pale, dusky or darkened reassess in 24-48 hours or at the first dressing change.

STAR Classification System

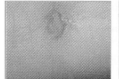 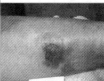 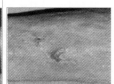 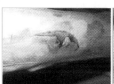 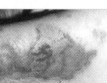

Category 1a	**Category 1b**	**Category 2a**	**Category 2b**	**Category 3**
A skin tear where the edges **can** be realigned to the normal anatomical position (without undue stretching) and the skin or flap colour **is not** pale, dusky or darkened.	A skin tear where the edges **can** be realigned to the normal anatomical position (without undue stretching) and the skin or flap colour **is** pale, dusky or darkened.	A skin tear where the edges **cannot** be realigned to the normal anatomical position and the skin or flap colour **is not** pale, dusky or darkened.	A skin tear where the edges **cannot** be realigned to the normal anatomical position and the skin or flap colour **is** pale, dusky or darkened.	A skin tear where the skin flap is completely absent.

Skin Tear Audit Research (STAR). Silver Chain Group and Curtin University, (2007), Revised 4/2/2010.

FIG. 15.1 **STAR skin tear classification system.** (Skin Tear Audit Research (STAR). Silver Chain Group and Curtin University. (2007), Revised 4/2/2010.)

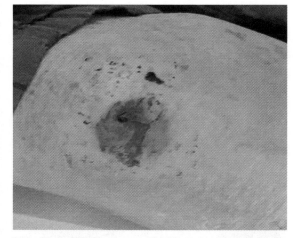

FIG. 15.2 **STAR category 2b skin tear on upper arm of 90-year-old male.**

Promoting Wellness

Australian researchers have demonstrated that twice-daily application of moisturiser can reduce the incidence of skin tears by nearly 50% (Carville et al 2014).

PRESSURE INJURIES

Pressure injuries (PIs) are defined as 'a localised injury to the skin and/or underlying tissue usually over a bony prominence, as a result of pressure, or pressure in combination with shear' (European Pressure Ulcer Advisory Panel et al 2014). PIs commonly occur at sites such as the sacrum, heels and greater trochanters (hips), where soft tissue can be compressed between a bony prominence and an external surface. The risk that an older person will develop a PI increases with higher intensities and

Research Highlights

- Australian researchers collected extensive data and used statistical modelling to identify factors that significantly predicted skin tears in older people.
- Factors that predicted the risk of skin tears included: history of skin tears, history of falls, male gender, clinical purpura and elastosis (Rayner et al 2019a).
- Four individual characteristics (age, history of skin tears, history of falls, antiplatelet therapy) and three skin properties (pH, subepidermal low echogenicity band of the forearms [indicating photoageing], skin thickness) predicted the risk of purpura (Rayner et al 2019b).
- Three individual characteristics (age, gender, smoking), three clinical skin characteristics (uneven skin pigmentation, cutis rhomboidalis nuchae [deep furrows at the nape of the neck from chronic photoaging], history of actinic keratosis) and one skin property (collagen type IV) predicted the risk of elastosis (Rayner et al 2019b).

  Research findings indicated that chronological ageing, environmental and lifestyle-related factors progressively changed the structural and mechanical properties of skin to increase the risk of skin tears.

longer duration of localised pressure and a decreased ability of soft tissue to withstand these forces. Sustained pressure compresses blood vessels, leading to ischaemia and necrosis. Characteristics of the older person which increase the risk of developing a PI include:

- increasing age
- compromised skin integrity
- impaired mobility and impaired activity
- malnutrition or obesity
- impaired sensory perception
- compromised or reduced blood supply to pressure points
- severely compromised status of health.

The consequence of a PI in an older person is significant. These injuries can take a long time to heal and cause the older person severe pain, disturbing sleep and increasing susceptibility to infection. They can also impact on mobility and rehabilitation, and lead to lower long-term quality of life (Gillespie et al 2014). Prevention is therefore important (Clinical Excellence Commission and Pressure Injury Prevention Project 2014). Strategies that reduce the risk for a PI include:

- using a validated assessment tool such as the BRADEN Score (Braden & Bergstrom 1988) to identify at-risk persons

- identifying and removing causative factors that increase localised pressure
- optimising tissue integrity and the skin's ability to withstand localised pressure (effective skincare, appropriate nutrition, mobilisation, repositioning, application of protective dressings)
- utilising pressure-relieving support surfaces (European Pressure Ulcer Advisory Panel et al 2014; Lin et al 2020).

LEG ULCERS

Leg ulcers occur in about 4% of people aged over 65 years and frequently become chronic without appropriate management. The principal causes of leg ulcers are venous disease, arterial disease or neuropathy. The most common features of these ulcers are listed in Table 15.4.

Venous Leg Ulcers (see Fig. 15.3)

Venous ulcers account for about 70% of leg ulcers reported in the older age group. The wound represents the advanced stage of long-term venous insufficiency from venous hypertension, valvular incompetence or impaired calf muscle pump. These ulcers typically occur on the medial lower leg or calf and are generally irregular in shape.

The gold standard management of venous leg ulceration is compression therapy, which acts to reduce venous hypertension. Compression bandages can only be applied by competently trained nurses. Conservative measures for reducing venous insufficiency include:

- encouraging movement and exercise to improve the calf-muscle pump
- avoiding sitting or standing for prolonged periods
- when resting, elevating legs above the heart to alleviate venous pressure and maximise venous return.

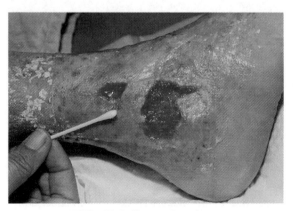

FIG. 15.3 **Venous leg ulcer.**

TABLE 15.4
Common Characteristics of Venous, Arterial and Neuropathic Lower Extremity Ulcers

	Venous	Arterial	Neuropathic
Location	Medial lower leg or calf	Lateral malleolus Toes Feet	Feet Toes

Clinical characteristics	Shallow
	Irregular shape
	Slough and/or granulating
	  wound bed
	Moderate–heavy exudate
		Deep
		Punched out appearance
		Dry, pale, fibrous or necrotic
		  wound base
		Scant exudate
			Depth variable
			Surrounding callus
			Punched out appearance
			Necrotic tissue

Surrounding skin	Oedematous
	Exudating
	May show signs of stasis
	  dermatitis (ill-defined reddish
	  patches and plaques)
	Presence of hair
	Brown pigmentation
		Pale
		Thin
		Shiny
		Absence of hair
		Pale, cyanotic or dusky red
			Warm
			Dry

Skin temperature	Warm	Cool or cold	Warm

Pain	Variable
	Dull or aching discomfort
	  exacerbated when legs
	  dependent or swollen
		Moderate to severe
		Presence of intermittent
		  claudication
		Worse at night or when legs
		  elevated
			Painless

Pedal pulses	Present	Diminished or absent	Present

The person should also be referred to a vascular surgeon for a review.

Arterial Leg Ulcers (see Fig. 15.4)

Arterial ulcers account for about 10% of leg ulcers and result from impaired arterial blood flow to the lower extremities. Factors associated with development of arterial leg ulcers include:

- ageing
- smoking
- hypertension
- diabetes
- hyperlipidaemia
- hypercholesterolaemia
- atherosclerotic disease.

Arterial ulcers are extremely painful, hard to heal and typically occur on the lower leg or over a bony prominence. Walking and exercising are encouraged to promote collateral or auxiliary circulation to the lower extremities. Local wound management is aimed at providing comfort, promoting healing and reducing any risk of infection. A referral to a vascular surgeon is necessary to assess for any treatment to restore arterial blood flow.

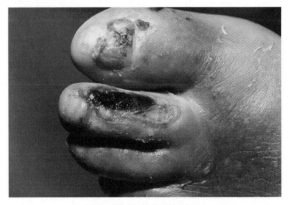

FIG. 15.4 Arterial ulcer.

Neuropathic Ulcers (see Fig. 15.5)

Neuropathic ulcers result from damage to sensory, motor and autonomic fibres. Peripheral neuropathy can be caused by diabetes, alcohol abuse, spinal cord injuries, drugs, leprosy or spina bifida. Neuropathic feet show diminished sensation to light touch when measured with the 5.07/10-gram Semmes–Weinstein monofilament.

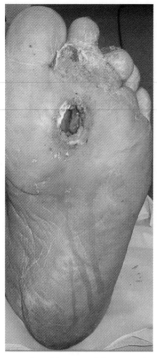

FIG. 15.5 **Neuropathic foot ulcer.**

The older person will typically report that they do not feel pain in the feet and often develop ulcers at sites of pressure or repeated trauma, such as from poorly fitted shoes or walking bare-footed. A palpable foot pulse and a warm foot generally indicates sufficient blood supply. Conversely, signs indicating impaired arterial blood flow include:

- a foot that is cool to the touch
- presence of ache at rest
- slow capillary refill time (> 2 seconds)
- diminished or absent foot pulses
- pallor in the feet when elevated.

The disrupted skin integrity and underlying poor blood supply mean that neuropathic ulcers can become infected. There is also a risk of osteomyelitis where bone is exposed.

The management of neuropathic ulcers involves removing pressure and limiting further trauma; this necessitates an interdisciplinary approach comprising of (but not limited to) a vascular surgeon, general practitioner (GP), podiatrist, orthotist, dietitian and nurse. Any calluses, hyperkeratotic skin or corns need to be expertly removed and areas of pressure need to

be off-loaded. Instructions concerning care of the feet (routine inspection, cleaning, correct technique to trim nails) need to be provided. Shoes need to be correctly fitted to avoid friction and accommodate any deformity. The toe of the shoe should be broad with sufficient room to contain the toes. Orthotic insoles may cushion the foot and prevent ulcers from forming. Active ulcers may need to be surgically debrided and benefit from therapeutic footwear that offloads pressure.

SKIN CANCERS

Skin cancers are the most common form of cancer and are broadly classified as melanoma or non-melanoma. While excessive exposure to UVR can damage all skin types, persons with lower Fitzpatrick skin types are at greater risk of skin cancers than those with more darkly pigmented skin.

Melanoma

Melanomas derive from changes to the skin pigment, forming melanocytes, and is associated with significant morbidity and mortality. The incidence of melanoma in Australia has nearly doubled since 1982 (Australian Institute of Health and Welfare [AIHW)] 2016). The risk of developing melanoma increases with age, exposure to UVR, history of sunburn, low Fitzpatrick skin types and family history. Melanomas occur on sun-exposed skin sites, including the face, upper arms, shoulders, back and legs.

Despite melanomas varying in presentation, the ABCDEFG (Woltsche et al 2016) mnemonic can aid early detection of the lesion's principal clinical features:
- Asymmetry
- Border irregularity
- Colour variation
- Diameter greater than 6 mm (smaller sizes should not be ignored)
- Elevated above skin surface
- Firm
- Growing

Early detection and complete excision of the primary lesion averts invasion and improves prognosis.

Non-Melanoma Skin Cancers
Basal cell carcinoma

Basal cell carcinoma (BCC) is the most common non-melanoma skin cancer reported in older people. These lesions are slow-growing, rarely metastasise and primarily occur in low Fitzpatrick skin types from chronic sun exposure. BCC initially appears as a small nodule with rolled edges, which can ulcerate if untreated. Early identification and surgical removal of the lesion is necessary.

Squamous Cell Carcinoma

Squamous cell carcinoma (SCC), the second most common skin cancer, is more aggressive and is at risk of metastasising without treatment. Individuals at most risk of SCC are those:

- with a history of chronic sun exposure
- with a lower Fitzpatrick skin type
- infected by the human papilloma virus
- who are immunosuppressed.

Routine screening is essential as SCC have a high risk of reoccurrence. SCCs have a firm texture despite the clinical appearance varying from wart-like to irregular, reddish, scaly patches that rapidly increase in size. Early identification and surgical removal of the lesion is necessary.

HERPES ZOSTER

Herpes zoster or shingles (see also Chapter 10) is a painful condition that causes a rash to develop along a nerve pathway or dermatome. It generally occurs in older people from reactivation of the dormant varicella-zoster virus that initially causes chicken pox and can reappear as shingles later in life when the immune system is compromised, or when the older person is experiencing stress or has a malignancy. The severity of symptoms increases with age, when it encompasses the face, or when numerous dermatomes are involved. Malaise, fever, itch or pain may be experienced between one and five days prior to the development of a rash, which develops along the nerve in which it has been residing. Contagious vesicles form along the nerve pathway to form pustules, which ultimately rupture, crust and resolve. The condition can lead to considerable morbidity, including post-herpetic neuralgia (see Chapter 19) and herpes zoster ophthalmicus (see Chapter 21). Scarring can occur when lesions are scratched or from a secondary bacterial infection. While there is no cure for herpes zoster, treatment is aimed at reducing complications and managing the symptoms, and may include:

- antiviral medication (most effective when started within 72 hours of onset of rash)
- analgesia to reduce pain
- topical therapies to relieve pruritus.

A vaccine is recommended for persons aged over 50 years to prevent or to reduce the risk and severity of this condition.

FOOT CARE

Ageing is associated with structural, functional and biomechanical foot problems that can lead to pain, deformities, disabilities and an increased risk of falling. Older people may have greater difficulty maintaining basic personal hygiene measures that increase the risk for foot problems. Proper foot care is essential to reduce infection and wounds, and for maintaining mobility. The feet should be screened to identify:

- changes in skin colour, warmth and texture
- turgor
- presence of infection
- deformities
- peripheral neuropathy
- peripheral vascular disease
- abnormalities of the toenails.

Where screening detects potential foot problems, a referral to a dermatologist, vascular surgeon or podiatrist for specialist review is indicated.

Care of the foot includes daily inspection, cleansing and measures to maintain healthy skin (see *Tips for best practice*: Promoting a healthy skin barrier on p. 171). If the older person is independent, the nurse can provide education and encouragement for the person and/or family members to undertake daily foot care. However, the nurse may need to provide this care for an older person with functional limitations in acute care or residential aged care settings. Daily foot inspection involves observing the skin for:

- redness
- fissures
- xerosis
- infection
- calluses and corns (thick, hard patches of skin developing in response to pressure or friction).

Feet should be gently cleaned with a pH neutral cleanser and tepid water, and thoroughly dried. Pay particular attention to the areas between the toes by drying thoroughly and avoiding moisturisers to reduce the risk of fungal infections. Do not soak feet, as prolonged immersion in water removes natural moisturising factors, causes fissures and increases the risk for infection. Apply low-scent skin moisturiser (other than between toes) to prevent xerosis and fissures. Discourage the use of heat packs and hot water on the feet to prevent the risk of burning, particularly with older people who cannot feel heat or communicate how they feel (see Chapter 19). Dissuade the older person from using OTC therapies to treat corns and calluses and recommend professional attention from a podiatrist. Encourage the wearing of professionally fitted

Practice Scenario

Mrs Bryant is an active 81-year-old woman who sustained a skin tear to her right forearm from an unknown cause. While assessing the wound, you observe that her skin is dry and coarse, with uneven pigmentation and isolated areas of purpura. Mrs Bryant reports her skin feels constantly uncomfortable, dry and itchy, with the symptoms exacerbated by showering.

MULTIPLE CHOICE QUESTIONS
On the basis of this scenario:

1. Which solutions would you use to clean the wound?
   a. Potable water or normal saline
   b. Chlorhexidine or potable water
   c. Povidone-iodine and normal saline
   d. Chlorhexidine and povidone-iodine
2. Which dressing product would you apply to this wound?
   a. Calcium alginate
   b. Hypertonic saline
   c. Silicone
   d. Semi-permeable film
3. Which strategies would you recommend to reduce skin tear recurrence?
   a. Apply moisturisers twice a day to the extremities
   b. Wear short-sleeve clothing
   c. Apply adhesive dressing products
   d. Avoid using hoists and slide sheets when transferring
4. What advice would you give to Mrs Bryant to improve skin hydration?
   a. Use soap when washing the skin
   b. Frequently wash the skin
   c. Use pH friendly cleanser and tepid water when bathing
   d. Dry the skin using a rubbing action

low-heeled, broad-toe shoes to provide comfort and support, and to reduce the risk of friction, pressure and deformities.

SUMMARY

The skin is the largest and most dynamic organ of the body that reacts to and physiologically reflects the effects of the exposed environment. Skin ageing is individualised and is influenced by gender, genetics, skin type and environmental and lifestyle-related factors. Ageing skin is more susceptible to infections, malignancies, xerosis, pruritus and purpura, and is at greater risk of developing wounds. A comprehensive approach is needed when assessing both the skin and skin abnormalities to help identify the cause, alleviate factors that impair healing and optimise management.

REFERENCES

Algiert-Zielińska B, Batory M, Skubalski J et al (2017) Evaluation of the relation between lipid coat, transepidermal water loss, and skin pH. International Journal of Dermatology 56(11):1192–1197.

Amano S (2016) Characterization and mechanisms of photoageing-related changes in skin. Damages of basement membrane and dermal structures. Experimental Dermatology 25(S3):14–19.

Augustin M, Wilsmann-Theis D, Körber A et al (2019) Diagnosis and treatment of xerosis cutis – a position paper. Journal der Deutschen Dermatologischen Gesellschaft 17(S7): 3–33.

Australian Institute of Health and Welfare (AIHW) (2016) Skin cancer in Australia. CAN 96. Canberra: Commonweath of Australia.

Barth E, Srivastava A, Stojiljkovic M et al (2019) Conserved aging-related signatures of senescence and inflammation in different tissues and species. Aging 11(19):8556–8572.

Birch HL (2018) Extracellular matrix and ageing. In: JR Harris & VI Korolchuk (eds) Biochemistry and cell biology of ageing: Part I biomedical science. Springer Singapore, Singapore.

Braden B, Bergstrom N (1988) Braden Score for predicting pressure sore risk. Online. Available: healthywa.wa.gov.au/~/media/Files/Corporate/general%20documents/safety/PDF/Bradenscale.pdf

Carville K, Leslie G, Osseiran-Moisson R et al (2014) The effectiveness of a twice-daily skin-moisturising regimen for reducing the incidence of skin tears. International Wound Journal 11(4):446–453.

Carville K, Lewin G, Newall N et al (2007) STAR: A consensus for skin tear classification. Primary Intention 15(1):18–28.

Chambers ES, Vukmanovic-Stejic M (2019) Skin barrier immunity and ageing. Immunology 160(2):10.1111/imm.13152

Choi EH (2019) Aging of the skin barrier. Clinics in Dermatology 37(4):336–345.

Clinical Excellence Commission & Pressure Injury Prevention Project (2014) Pressure Injury Prevention and Management Policy Implementation guide. Online. Available: www.Chealth.nsw.gov.au/__data/assets/pdf_file/0003/259257/Pressure-Injury-Prevention-and-Management-Policy-Implementation-Guide.pdf

Cole MA, Quan T, Voorhees JJ et al (2018) Extracellular matrix regulation of fibroblast function: redefining our perspective on skin aging. Journal of Cell Communication and Signaling 12(1):35–43.

European Pressure Ulcer Advisory Panel, National Pressure Ulcer Advisory Panel, & Pan Pacific Pressure Injury Alliance (2014) Prevention and treatment of pressure ulcers: Quick reference guide. In: E Haesler (ed.). Cambridge Media, Perth.

Farage MA, Miller KW, Maibach HI (2017) Degenerative changes in aging skin. In: MA Farage, KW Miller, HI Maibach (eds), Textbook of aging skin. Springer, Berlin, Heidelberg.

Fitzpatrick TB (1988) The validity and practicality of sun-reactive skin types I through VI. Archives of Dermatology 124(6):869–871.

Garcia-Martinez D, Leyva-Mendivil MF, Gefen A et al (2020) Biomechanical aspects of skin aging – the risk of skin breakdown under shear loading increases with age. In: A. Gefen (ed.), Innovations and emerging technologies in wound care. Academic Press, London.

Garibyan L, Chiou AS, Elmariah SB (2013) Advanced aging skin and itch: Addressing an unmet need. Dermatologic Therapy 26(2):92–103.

Gillespie BM, Chaboyer WP, McInnes E et al (2014) Repositioning for pressure ulcer prevention in adults. Cochrane Database of Systematic Reviews. 2014(4). Online. Available: https://doi.org/10.1002/14651858.cd009958.pub2

Han A, Chien AL, Kang S (2014) Photoaging. Dermatologic Clinics 32(3):291–299.

Julian T, Glascow N, Syeed R et al (2019). Alcohol-related peripheral neuropathy: a systematic review and meta-analysis. Journal of Neurology 266(12):2907–2919.

Keast DH, Bowering CK, Evans AW et al (2004). Measure: a proposed assessment framework for developing best practise recommendations for wound assessment. Wound Repair and Regeneration 12:S1–S17.

Koneti KK, Jones M (2016) Management of acute pain. Surgery (Oxford) 34(2):84–90.

Kruk J, Duchnik E (2014) Oxidative stress and skin diseases: Possible role of physical activity. Asian Pacific Journal of Cancer Prevention 15(2):561–568.

Lin F, Wu Z, Song B et al (2020). The effectiveness of multi-component pressure injury prevention programs in adult intensive care patients: a systematic review. International Journal of Nursing Studies 102:103483.

Mollanazar NK, Smith PK, Yosipovitch G (2016) Mediators of chronic pruritus in atopic dermatitis: Getting the itch out? Clinical Reviews in Allergy and Immunology 51(3):263–292.

Mori S, Shiraishi A, Epplen K et al (2017) Characterization of skin function associated with obesity and specific correlation to local/systemic parameters in American women. Lipids in Health and Disease 16(1):214.

Ortiz A, Grando SA (2012) Smoking and the skin. International Journal of Dermatology 51:250–262.

Rayner R, Carville K, Leslie G (2019) Defining aged-related skin tears: A review. Wound Practice & Research 27(3):135–143.

Rayner R, Carville K, Leslie G et al (2019a) A risk model for the prediction of skin tears in aged care residents: A prospective cohort study. International Wound Journal 16(1):52–63.

Rayner R, Carville K, Leslie G et al (2019b) Clinical purpura and elastosis and their correlation with skin tears in an aged population. Archives of Dermatological Research 311(3):231–247.

Rehm J, Soerjomataram I, Ferreira-Borges C et al (2019) Does alcohol use affect cancer risk? Current Nutrition Reports 8(3):222–229.

Sachdeva S (2009) Fitzpatrick skin typing: Applications in dermatology. Indian Journal of Dermatology, Venereology and Leprology 75(1):93–96.

Schultz GS, Sibbald RG, Falanga V et al (2003) Wound bed preparation: A systematic approach to wound management. Wound Repair and Regeneration 11(Supp 1):S1–S28.

Vierkötter A, Krutmann J (2012) Environmental influences on skin aging and ethnic-specific manifestations. Dermato-Endocrinology 4(3):227–231.

Woltsche N, Schwab C, Deinlein T et al (2016) Dermoscopy in the era of dermato-oncology: From bed to bench side and retour. Expert Review of Anticancer Therapy 16(5):531–541.

CHAPTER 16

Falls and Falls Prevention

KEITH HILL

LEARNING OBJECTIVES

After reading this chapter, you will be able to:

- discuss the importance of encouraging older people to have a medical review if they are increasingly unsteady or have falls
- identify risk factors for falls among older people, and understand the cumulative impact of multiple risk factors
- differentiate between falls risk screening and falls risk assessment, and be able to describe examples of these tools
- describe interventions that can reduce the risk of falling in older people.

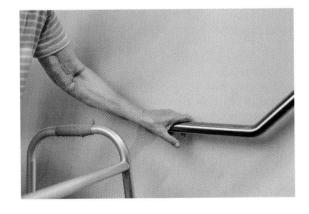

INTRODUCTION

Falls are common for older people and can have serious consequences and impacts for the older person, their family and social network, the broader community and the health and care system. While they are commonly experienced by older people, falls are not just due to age. Strategies can usually be implemented to reduce an older person's risk of falling, irrespective of the

multiple risk factors and co-morbidities that may be contributing to this risk. Acute health problems, such as those requiring hospitalisation or additional care at home, increase an older person's usual level of falls risk, which may necessitate short or longer term additional strategies to manage the increased falls risk. Effective falls prevention programs aim to maintain or improve social and physical activity participation and engagement safely in the context of the individual's level of falls risk.

Definitions

- **Fall:** It is important that a consistent definition is used, so that everyone understands what is being referred to. For the purposes of this chapter, the World Health Organisation (WHO) definition is used: a fall is any event where a person 'inadvertently comes to rest on the ground, floor or other lower level, excluding intentional change in position to rest in furniture, wall or other objects' (WHO 2007).
- **Injurious fall:** a fall where any physical harm occurred as a result of the fall.
- **Fear of falling:** a psychological concern about the risk of falling, or a psychological consequence of falling, that can often result in restriction of activities

and mobility, increasing risk of future falls (Jorstad et al 2005).

HEALTHY AGEING AND PREVENTION OF FALLS

Older people present across the health and wellbeing spectrum, from being very well through to being frail with many co-morbidities. Most of those in hospital or residential aged care, or who are receiving community care services, have multiple chronic health problems, and at times an additional acute health problem (for example, urinary tract infection, stroke, heart attack) superimposed. A healthy ageing and prevention approach aims to optimise health and wellbeing outcomes irrespective of the health status of an individual, and implement interventions to minimise the risk of future health problems.

In this way, the principles of falls reduction and falls injury prevention that are discussed throughout this chapter apply across the health and wellbeing spectrum – for those older people who are generally well through to those with many chronic health problems, poor mobility and a high risk of falling. Although the principles apply to all older people, the implementation approach should be tailored to the individual older person's needs. For example, exercise that includes balance training can reduce falls risk across the health spectrum; however, depending on the number, severity and nature of co-morbidities, different types, intensity and range of the exercises may be required.

Promoting Wellness

- Focus on the abilities of the older person.
- Incorporate joint decision-making with the older person regarding treatment priorities and goals in working to reduce the risk of future falls.
- Encourage older people to report new health problems to a health professional, to ensure early and effective interventions can be implemented before a health condition becomes more severe.

INCIDENCE OF FALLS AND FALL-RELATED INJURIES

Falls are common among older people, with approximately one-third of older people experiencing one or more falls each year. Fortunately, most falls do not cause serious injuries, although some falls do cause death, and up to 10% cause serious injuries, often requiring

hospitalisation. In Australia, there were 125,021 hospital admissions for falls in people aged 65 years and older in 2016–17 (Pointer 2019), while in New Zealand in 2016 there were 27,000 hospital admissions for falls in people aged 50 years and older (HSQCNZ 2016). Most common sites of serious injuries from falls are the head (26% of all hospital admissions) and the hip or thigh (22%) (Pointer 2019). Over 22,000 of these hospital admissions in Australia were for a hip or thigh fracture (Pointer 2019). Given the ageing populations in Australia, New Zealand and other developed parts of the world, the actual number of hospitalisations for serious injuries will continue to increase unless systematic population-level approaches to reducing falls and falls injuries can be effectively implemented.

Falls among older people are common in community, hospital and residential aged care settings. In one large Australian study across general medicine, specialist medicine, general surgical and specialist surgical wards in six hospitals, 3.6% of admitted patients fell (966 falls among 27,026 admissions) (Morello et al 2015). In residential aged care, 50% of residents have been found to experience one or more falls (Barker et al 2009; Whitney et al 2012), a proportion that increases in dementia-specific facilities.

While the majority of falls do not cause serious injuries, many cause minor injuries and/or loss of confidence (also called fear of falling). This psychological effect often makes an older person reduce their usual levels of activity (for example, making the decision to drive instead of walking to the local shops). Over time, reduced activity can result in greater muscle weakness and poorer balance, and thereby increase an older person's risk of having future falls. Staff working with older people who have fallen should ask them about a fear of falling (for example, 'Are you more afraid of falling when walking now than before the fall?'), and activity level ('Have you been doing fewer activities since you had the fall?'). Another option is to use a falls efficacy scale to evaluate an older person's confidence in performing a number of routine activities without overbalancing, such as the Falls Efficacy Scale International (FES-I) Short Form (Kempen et al 2008; University of Manchester n.d.).

Older people identified to have loss of confidence or reduced activity level should be recommended for a medical or other health professional assessment to determine causes and possible interventions (which may include exercise, use of a walking aid or cognitive behavioural training). Interventions such as cognitive behavioural therapy, multifactorial falls prevention interventions and exercise have been shown to reduce fear of falling (Papadimitriou & Perry 2020; Sjosten et al 2008).

Do Older People Report Falls?

In order for doctors or other health professionals to be able to determine a person's risk of falling and introduce appropriate interventions, they need to be aware that the older person is experiencing these problems. This is particularly important because having had a recent fall, even one that did not cause an injury, is a strong indicator that the person is likely to have a future fall. Unfortunately, only around half of older people who have a fall report it to their doctor (Lee et al 2015).

It is essential that anyone working with older people, who becomes aware about falls or increasing unsteadiness, encourages the older person to discuss the fall/s or unsteadiness with their doctor.

COSTS

Costs associated with falls can be considered as costs to the individual, and can include a broad range of elements such as costs of additional medications, services, tests and so on, as well as personal impacts such as pain, loss of independence and fear of falling. For frailer older people receiving informal care at home, falls have been shown to reduce the older person's function and to increase caregiver burden (Meyer et al 2012).

Health and care system costs associated with falls are high, though they vary depending on what is included in analyses. One Queensland report found that the costs associated with fall-related hospitalisations were on average AU$8139 per hospitalisation episode in 2007–08 (Black & Begg 2010). These cost estimates did not include non-hospitalisation costs, including short-term (transition care) or permanent residential care, when required, so are considered an underestimate of the real costs for older people who are hospitalised due to a fall. Although the costs of falls for older people who are not hospitalised due to serious injuries would not be as high, they can be a moderate cost burden if recovery is prolonged. For example, an older person injured in a fall may require long-term community care support for activities such as cleaning and gardening, which he or she was previously able to undertake.

Costs of falls are also high in hospital and residential aged care settings. One large Australian study reported that every fall occurring in an acute hospital resulted in an average increased length of stay of eight days, and an increase in costs of AU$6669 (Morello et al 2015).

In residential care, the cost of falls per person was estimated at AU$1887 (Haines et al 2013).

> **Safety Alert**
>
> It is essential that anyone working with older people, who becomes aware of falls or increasing unsteadiness, encourages the older person to discuss the fall/s or unsteadiness with their doctor.

STAFF REPORTING OF FALLS

All falls that occur in hospitals and residential care should be recorded in the institution's incident reporting systems. One study in a hospital setting compared incident reports for falls, falls documentation in nursing notes and patient reports of falls, and identified that only 75% of falls were reported on the incident reporting system (Hill et al 2010). Without accurate falls reporting, strategies are unlikely to be instituted to reduce the risk of a future fall occurring.

Falls Risk Factors and Falls Risk Screening and Assessment Tools

Falls risk factors can be grouped as intrinsic (within the body/health problems), extrinsic (e.g. environmental, footwear) or behavioural (e.g. taking unnecessary risks relative to abilities).

Falls risk *screening tools* are brief evaluations or checklists that give an indication of overall level of falls risk (often high, medium or low) that could be targeted with falls prevention interventions; however, they do not provide information about specific falls risk factors for a particular older person. One of the strongest indicators of future falls risk is having had a previous fall, so this question often forms part of a falls risk screening tool, either in isolation or with other items. Screening tools or checklists may also be useful for older people themselves to complete (for example, in a doctor's waiting room). An example of a self-check list for risk of falling (indicating the need to discuss falls risk with a doctor) has been developed by Injury Matters (Western Australia) (see Fig. 16.1).

Falls risk *assessment tools* are more in-depth and should be completed for older people with an increased risk of falling (either based on a falls risk screening tool or if the person is known to have a condition associated with high falls risk, such as stroke, Parkinson's disease or dementia). These tools assess the main intrinsic risk factors for falls (see Table 16.1), and contributory falls risk factors identified for an individual older person.

STAY ON YOUR FEET®

| Move | Improve | Remove |

Did you know....?

> Falling is not a normal part of ageing. Falls are preventable!
> Only a small proportion of falls are caused by tripping, slipping or "not being careful" – most are the result of health or lifestyle factors.
> One in four people aged 60 or over fall at least once a year.

COMPLETE THIS CHECKLIST TO DETERMINE YOUR RISK OF FALLING

Yes

☑

Have you had a fall in the last year? ☐

Having previously fallen increases your chance of falling again.

Do you do less than 30 minutes of physical activity a day? ☐
Are you unsteady on your feet, do you find it difficult to get up from a chair or do you have trouble walking? ☐

Many falls are the result of muscle weakness and/or impaired balance.

Are you taking three or more medicines? ☐
Are you taking sleeping tablets, tranquillisers or anti-depressants? ☐
Has it been more than 12 months since your GP reviewed your medicines? ☐

Some side effects and combinations of medicines can increase your risk of a fall.

Do you have diabetes, arthritis or Parkinson's Disease? ☐
Have you had a stroke or do you have problems with your heart or circulation? ☐
Has it been more than 12 months since your eyes were tested or your glasses checked? ☐
Do you experience dizziness, light headedness, unsteadiness, drowsiness, blurred or double vision or have difficulty thinking clearly? ☐

Many health conditions can increase your risk of falling.

If you answered "yes" to one or more of these questions you are at risk of falling.
The good news is that there are steps you can take now to reduce your risk.

If you answered "no" to all of these questions, but are aged 60 or over, you should still take falls seriously and take action to stay mobile and independent.

To learn how you can prevent slips, trips and falls visit www.stayonyourfeet.com.au or call 1300 30 35 40.

Partner:
Department of Health
GOVERNMENT OF WESTERN AUSTRALIA

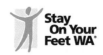
Stay On Your Feet WA®

injury matters

Stay On Your Feet® is provided by Injury Matters and funded by the Western Australian Department of Health.

FIG. 16.1 **Self-check list for risk of falling** (Stay On Your Feet®, State of Western Australia 2020, reproduced with permission.)

TABLE 16.1
Falls Risk Factors, and Possible Interventions to Reduce Falls Risk

Falls risk factors	Possible intervention approaches
Intrinsic risk factors[#]	
Previous fall	Falls risk assessment; address identified falls risk factors
Vision impairment (see Chapter 21)	Vision assessment and correction (e.g. cataract surgery) Encourage older person to wear their glasses
Reduced balance or impaired mobility (see Chapter 22)	Balance and strength training exercise or tai chi Use of walking aid
Polypharmacy or use of high falls risk medications (e.g. psychotropic medications) (see Chapter 11)	Medication review Use of non-pharmacological approaches where possible Review use of medications associated with high falls risk (e.g. psychotropic medications)
Chronic health problems such as stroke, dizziness, arthritis, Parkinson's disease	Falls risk assessment, and address identified falls risk factors
Cognitive impairment (delirium, dementia) (see Chapter 26)	Screen for delirium, and treat if present Review other falls risk factors for people with dementia, and address modifiable falls risk factors
Urinary incontinence (see Chapter 13)	Medical review and treatment of causes of urinary incontinence
Multiple risk factors/multiple falls or unexplained falls	Geriatrics review; or Multi-disciplinary falls clinic assessment
Extrinsic risk factors	
Indoors environment (poor lighting, loose carpets, slippery surfaces)	Assessment of environment in context of individual's risk (in community setting, should be undertaken by an occupational therapist or other trained health professional), and environmental modifications implemented
Poor footwear	Advice regarding good/safe footwear characteristics
Outdoors environment (in the garden/backyard at home, and away from home)	Assessment of outdoor environment at home (as for indoors environment, above) Regular reviews of outdoor environments by councils Reporting of unsafe outdoor environments for correction (e.g. levelling of uneven footpaths)
Behavioural risk factors	
Mismatch between regularly performed activities and ability and safety	Review of regularly performed activities with a health professional, and discussion about alternatives (e.g. change environment to make the activity safer, or change the method of performing the activity)

[#]Intrinsic risk factor list adapted from Deandrea et al (2010).

This information can then be used to discuss possible intervention approaches to reduce future falls risk with the older person who fell. Falls risk assessments can be undertaken by doctors, nurses or health professionals, such as physiotherapists or occupational therapists, and by assessors for services such as community care.

Cognitive impairment (including delirium) is an independent risk factor for falls. Delirium is a form of cognitive impairment that develops quickly and is especially prevalent in older people with acute illness (see Chapter 26). Delirium can be prevented in many cases, and is often treatable (McCrow & Dementia Australia 2015). However, it is often not recognised, and therefore often not treated in older hospitalised patients, contributing to an increased falls risk in these patients.

Extrinsic falls risk factors are also important to assess. These can be indoors within the home, hospital or residential care setting or outdoors. Extrinsic falls risk factors within indoor environments include:

- loose rugs
- electrical cords on floors
- poor lighting
- slippery surfaces
- glare on floor surfaces
- stairs/uneven surfaces.

Falls can also be associated with a mismatch of the older person's abilities and their environment. For example, standing on a step ladder or stool to reach objects in a high cupboard at home, rather than locating regularly used items in lower cupboards, can increase risk. In this context, a home assessment by a qualified health professional, such as an occupational therapist, is beneficial to identify not just the obvious hazards, but also how the environment can be modified to suit the abilities and safety for an individual older person. The Home-FAST tool is a useful tool for evaluating the home environment and safety needs of an older person in the context of their abilities (Mackenzie et al 2009; University of Newcastle n.d.). Environmental assessments are also important in hospital, residential care and outdoor environments.

Falls can be due to a combination of different falls risk factors, often including a combination of intrinsic and extrinsic factors. For example, an older woman with cataracts and polypharmacy (including sleeping tablets) trips on an uneven footpath near her home. Each of the following factors individually or in combination could have contributed to the fall:

- Poor vision due to cataracts, which can reduce the ability to detect tripping hazards.
- Polypharmacy, including sleeping tablets, that may slow down balance reactions.
- The presence of the uneven footpath.

Each factor should be discussed as part of a plan to reduce this older person's future falls risk.

Examples of several falls risk screening tools and falls risk assessment tools for use in the community, hospital and residential aged care setting are detailed in Table 16.2. Although risk factors can be fairly similar across settings, there can be additional elements that are of greater or lesser importance between the settings, and therefore usually different tools are used in different settings.

Falls risk assessments should be repeated whenever there is a change in function, or if the older person becomes more unsteady or nearly falls, and after any fall (do not assume that a new fall is always due to pre-existing or previously identified falls risk factors).

In particular, a common contributor to increased unsteadiness or falls can be an acute health problem (such as a urinary tract infection or a chest infection), which has an effect of increasing an individual's risk of falling. Early recognition and treatment of these acute health problems can reduce the risk of falls, so should be considered when there is an acute change in physical and/or cognitive status. When an older person experiences these type of acute health problems, staff (if the person is in hospital or residential aged care) or informal and formal caregivers (if in the home environment) and the older person, need to be aware of this increased risk of fall, and exercise greater vigilance, and possibly implement additional falls prevention strategies for the duration of the acute health problem.

> **Practice Point**
>
> A critical aspect to maximise the success of falls risk screening and assessment processes is to implement evidence-based actions that address the main identified risk factors after completion of the tool. *It is of no value to complete a screening or assessment tool, but not develop and implement an action plan to address any risk factors identified.* All staff involved in the care of the individual must be aware of the outcomes of the assessment and the interventions being implemented.

Post-fall huddles have primarily been reported in hospital settings and have been shown to reduce the risk of subsequent falls (Jones et al 2019). Post-fall huddles are an opportunity for team members to debrief after an event such as a fall, and to:

- review circumstances of the fall
- review identified falls risk factors in the context of current fall prevention actions
- determine additional or different approaches to minimise the risk of a future fall for the individual who fell.

Changes to environments, perhaps in combination with an acute health problem, can cause the older person to become confused and also increase the risk of falls. In this context, periods of acclimatisation to a new environment and the associated new routines (for example, admission to hospital, admission to respite or residential care) can be associated with an increase in the risk of falling. Bed moves (transferring patients between wards or even within a ward) have been shown to increase the risk of falling among high falls risk older patients in hospitals (Toye et al 2019).

TABLE 16.2

Examples of Falls Risk Screening and Assessment Tools, Used in Different Settings

Tool	Description	Practical issues
Community setting screening tool		
FROP-Com screen[#]	Three-item screening tool. Classifies falls risk into low (0–3) or high risk (4–9)	Two self-report questions, and one observation and rating of steadiness in walking and turning
Elderly Falls Screening Test (EFST) (Cwikel et al 1998)	Five-item screening tool. Classifies falls risk into low (0–1) or high risk (2–5)	One item requires measurement of gait speed over 5 metres
Community setting assessment tool		
FROP-Com tool[#]	28 items assessment; includes broad range of falls risk factors. High risk score ≥19	Takes approximately 20 minutes to complete
FallsScreen© (Physiological Profile assessment – PPA)	Short form and long form – involves detailed assessment of five physiological falls risk factors (balance, muscle strength, proprioception, vision and reaction time) Does not include non-physiological assessment items such as cognition, medications or impaired mobility	Takes approximately 45 minutes. Moderate cost to purchase assessment kit Provides comparison to computerised normative profile on each risk factor
Hospital setting screening and assessment tools		
STRATIFY[#] (St. Thomas's Risk Assessment Tool in Falling Elderly inpatients)	Five items screening tool. High risk if score ≥2	Quick to use, widely used
The Ontario Modified STRATIFY[#] (Sydney scoring)	Expanded version of the STRATIFY. Six items, with different weighting for each item. High risk if score ≥ 17 (although originally validated tool rated ≥ 9 as high risk)	Need to add different scores for each item, according to different weightings
Morse falls scale	Six items, with different weighting for each item. No Risk (0–24), Low Risk (25–50), High Risk (≥ 51)	Need to add different scores for each item, according to different weightings Widely used
FRHOP tool[#]	Nineteen items evaluating main falls risk factors. Scores: 0–5 = low risk; 6–20 = medium risk; 21–45 = high risk	Takes approximately 20 minutes
Residential care setting screening and assessment tools		
Peninsula Health Falls Risk Assessment Tool (FRAT)[#]	Initial four-item screen, with additional assessment tool for those identified at high falls risk – low risk (5–11), medium risk (12–15), high risk (16–20)	Developed in mixed residential care and sub-acute hospital sample Need to add different scores for each item, according to different weightings
Care Home Falls Risk Screen (CaHFRiS) (Whitney et al 2012)	Six items assessed. Identifies absolute risk of falling in next 6 months based on score	Need to add different scores for each item, according to different weightings

[#]Tools reported and copies available in Australian falls prevention best practice guidelines (ACSQHC 2009a, 2009b, 2009c).
FROP-Com = Falls Risk for Older People – Community version; FRHOP = Falls Risk for Hospitalised Older People.
ACSQHC (2009a, 2009b, 2009c).

RISK FACTORS FOR INJURIES FROM FALLS

Some older people are at greater risk of sustaining more severe injuries from falls, such as fractures. Risk factors for injuries from falls include:

- osteoporosis or osteopenia (see Chapter 22)
- vitamin D deficiency
- low calcium intake
- corticosteroid use
- smoking
- low levels of physical activity.

Assessment of bone health (such as a DEXA scan, checking vitamin D levels) can guide additional treatment to reduce the risk of fractures from falls, in combination with interventions that aim to reduce the risk of falls.

FALL RISK REDUCTION STRATEGIES ACROSS SETTINGS

There is strong research evidence that the risk of falling can be reduced in older people living in the community (Gillespie et al 2012; Hopewell et al 2018; Sherrington et al 2019), including among people with a high falls risk, such as older people presenting to emergency departments (EDs) after a fall. Types of interventions have been classified as:

- single interventions (using one single intervention approach)
- multifactorial interventions (using two or more interventions, where the interventions are targeted to an individual's needs, usually based on a falls risk assessment)
- multiple interventions (using two or more fixed interventions for all individuals, irrespective of their specific risk factor profile; for example, a service may only offer an exercise program and a home assessment/modification program and offer these to all who are referred for the intervention, irrespective of the presence of other falls risk factors).

Single interventions were shown to be effective in reducing falls in community settings in at least one randomised controlled trial (Gillespie et al 2012; Sherrington et al 2019; Spink et al 2011). Interventions include:

- exercise that includes balance and strengthening exercises. This can be done at home, or in group settings (Sherrington et al 2019). There is also growing evidence about the effectiveness of these exercise approaches in reducing the falls risk for people with dementia
- home assessment and modification – it is recommended that this is undertaken by a trained health professional, such as an occupational therapist
- vision correction – cataract surgery. The use of separate distance and reading glasses rather than using bi-focal

or multi-focal glasses is also recommended, as it reduces the risk of falls outdoors

- a medication review, including reviewing and rationalising the need for medications, as well as a targeted review of medications associated with increased risk of falls
- foot exercise, sturdy footwear and the use of orthotics to reduce foot pain.

Multiple interventions and multifactorial interventions, including falls clinics, have also been shown to be effective in reducing falls risk in community settings (Hopewell et al 2018).

The amount of research and evidence of successful interventions in residential aged care and hospital settings is substantially smaller than in the community setting. In residential care settings, the strongest research evidence includes vitamin D supplementation for vitamin D deficient residents, and multifactorial interventions (Cameron et al 2018). The SUNBEAM strength and balance exercise program has been shown to reduce falls in residential aged care settings, with nearly 50% of participating residents having a cognitive impairment (Hewitt et al 2018). A community of practice supporting falls prevention translation into practice across a number of residential care facilities has also been shown to achieve positive outcomes (Francis-Coad et al 2018).

In hospital settings, patient education about falls risk factors and strategies to minimise risk in the hospital setting have been shown to be effective for cognitively intact older patients (Haines et al 2011), and combined with staff education programs have been shown to reduce falls in sub-acute wards for both cognitively intact and cognitively impaired patients (Hill et al 2015). Multifactorial approaches (based on falls risk assessments and the targeting of individual risk factors) may reduce falls rates in hospitals, with this effect shown to be stronger in sub-acute settings (Cameron et al 2018).

There are some approaches to reducing falls risk in older people that do not have strong research evidence, but are recommended by best practice guidelines. These should be considered in a comprehensive falls risk management program. Some of these include:

- using a walking aid to reduce unsteadiness (but with correct assessment and instructions for use)
- wearing good footwear (low heels, thin, hard, non-slippery soles, firm fit and a supportive heel collar) (Menant et al 2008)
- continence management approaches (Batchelor et al 2013).

In addition, there are a number of generic falls prevention recommendations that can be applied to reduce the risk for all residents or patients (see Box 16.1).

BOX 16.1
Recommended Falls Prevention Actions for all Older People in Hospital or Residential Care Settings

- Familiarise older person with ward or unit layout and routines (regularly for people with cognitive impairment)
- Safe environments around beds (brakes on, remove clutter or possible trip hazards, call bell within reach, walking aid within reach)
- Screen eyesight, ensure use of correct glasses, ensure glasses are clean
- Measure postural blood pressure – investigate causes and treat hypotension; encourage slow and safe sit-to-stand for transfers and walking, acclimatise to each position change before moving
- Screen for urinary tract infections
- Educate patients or residents about falls and reducing falls risk
- Ensure clear communication for all staff about an individual's mobility instructions (safety, independence, walking aid use), falls risk and falls prevention strategies
- Have a policy in place and implemented to minimise the use of restraints.

ACSQHC (2009b, 2009c).

Research Highlight

The RESPOND falls prevention program recruited older people who presented to the EDs of two Australian hospitals with falls over a 15-month period. When the fallers were discharged back home, they were presented with a limited suite of evidence-based interventions (balance and strength training program, vision correction, bone health and medication management). The program used phone call follow-up with motivational interviewing to support sustained participation, and achieved a significant 35% reduction in falls, and 63% reduction in fractures (Barker et al 2019).

The ED is an important setting in which to consider falls risk management, particularly when the person is being discharged back home. Some 50% of older people that present to an ED with a fall will fall again at least once in the following 12 months. Considering the high risk of recurrent falls and potential future admissions, targeting falls risk interventions for this high-risk population can yield positive outcomes. In the busy constraints of the ED, this may involve a falls risk screen and/or assessment, and appropriate referrals or case management on and after discharge.

REVIEWING STRATEGIES FOR PREVENTING FALLS

It is important to review current practice in the context of emerging research evidence. In some cases, practices implemented to reduce falls may need to be reviewed and possibly discontinued, especially if quality new evidence indicates a particular intervention approach is not effective. A recent example is that of using bed and chair alarms as routine practice for high falls risk patients in hospitals. A large randomised controlled trial (> 27,000 patients) demonstrated that the use of bed and chair alarms in hospitals was not effective in reducing the rate of falls, number of fallers, falls injuries or the number of patients who were placed in a physical restraint (Shorr et al 2012). This outcome was reinforced in the Cochrane Review of falls prevention in hospitals (Cameron et al 2018). Many falls prevention interventions such as this are associated with substantial cost, including staff time, infrastructure and administration.

As such, it is important to intermittently review the mix of current practices in any particular setting, in the context of new research evidence. Where there is quality evidence of no effect, organisations should consider opportunities to dis-invest in those interventions, which may enable greater resources, including staff time, for those interventions with good research evidence of effect (Mitchell et al 2018). It should be noted that many intervention areas in hospitals and residential care need further research in order to make clear decisions about whether an intervention is effective or not, because in many cases large high-quality randomised controlled trials have not been conducted.

Adherence to Falls Prevention

A consistent limitation of current falls prevention research is the lack of uptake and sustained engagement in falls prevention activities over time. This includes a focus on older people remaining involved long term with recommended interventions, as well as staff remaining up to date with knowledge and skills, and consistently implementing best practice across all settings. The use of motivational interviewing has been shown to be an effective approach in falls prevention to help older people commence and sustain participation in interventions (Barker et al 2019). Sustainability of interventions needs to have a stronger focus in practice.

INTERVENTIONS TO REDUCE INJURIES FROM FALLS

While the focus of this chapter has been on reducing falls risk, it is also important to consider strategies to reduce the risk of injuries from falls, particularly for older people with poor bone health (for example, osteoporosis or osteopenia) (see Chapter 22). Resistance and weightbearing exercises or impact exercises can improve bone density and reduce the risk of injurious falls and fractures (Tricco et al 2017). Hip protectors can also reduce fracture risk (Santesso et al 2014), but have low adherence.

Falls Prevention for People With Cognitive Impairment

While the presence of cognitive impairment is an independent risk factor for falls, it does not mean that people with cognitive impairment cannot benefit from falls prevention approaches. Many falls risk factors can be addressed in the same way for people with cognitive impairment as for those without cognitive impairment (for example, cataract surgery, medication review). Some other falls prevention interventions may need some tailoring for people with cognitive impairment, e.g. exercise (Suttanon et al 2013).

Cost Effective Interventions

An important consideration for wide uptake and translation of interventions shown to be effective in reducing falls is that they need to be cost-effective. Home assessment and modification programs and medication review and adjustment programs (including vitamin supplementation in residential aged care) have been shown to be cost effective, while some exercise interventions and some multifactorial interventions have also been cost effective (Church et al 2015; Olij et al 2018). There is a need for further research investigating cost-effective interventions across all settings.

Evaluating Falls Prevention Programs

Whether a falls prevention program is implemented for an individual older person or across a unit, ward, hospital, residential care facility or program, there should be an established process to intermittently review progress, effectiveness and sustained participation in the recommended intervention/s. Evaluation outcomes should be reported back to relevant individuals (i.e. the older person) or within organisations (e.g. wards or units, executive team etc). It is common that there may need to be an ongoing review and modifications to programs over time, to respond to evaluation findings. Implementation guides which outline key steps in evaluation and continuous improvement in each of the community, hospital and residential care settings have been developed by the ACSQHC (2009a, 2009b, 2009c).

Practice Points

- Many single, multiple and multifactorial falls prevention approaches can reduce falls in older people
- Nurses, medical and allied health staff have key roles in understanding falls risk factors and interventions, identifying risk factors, developing action plans and motivating sustained engagement with interventions
- Falls prevention programs can be safely and effectively implemented for people with high levels of falls risk, including people with cognitive impairment.

There is a need for falls prevention programs to include an emphasis on engaging all older people with increased falls risk to commence and support sustained participation in recommended interventions, to maximise outcomes.

Practice Scenario (Case Study)

Geoff is an 85-year-old man who lives alone since his wife Mary died 3 years ago. Last year, Geoff was taken to hospital after falling at home. While there he was diagnosed with Parkinson's disease, high blood pressure and chronic insomnia, and commenced on several medications. His daughter Jenny is concerned that he is becoming more unsteady when walking and seems a little confused at times, often forgetting to wear his glasses. She recently helped Geoff move from the family home to a small unit, which she hoped would be easier for him to manage. She tries to keep Geoff's unit in order, but finds this difficult as he insisted on bringing most of the family furniture and all of Mary's treasured pot plants. Geoff has expressed concern that he might fall over and so avoids activities unless Jenny is nearby.

REVIEW QUESTIONS

1. What intrinsic factors might contribute to Geoff's increased falls risk?
2. What extrinsic factors may contribute to Geoff's increased falls risk?
3. What behavioural factors may contribute to Geoff's increased falls risk?
4. What falls prevention strategies could be implemented to address these risk factors?

Online. Available: www.safetyandquality.gov.au/sites/default/files/migrated/Guidelines-HOSP1.pdf.

Australian Commission on Safety and Quality in Health Care (ACSQHC) (2009c) Preventing falls and harm from falls in older people: Best practice guidelines for Australian residential aged care facilities. Online. Available: www.safetyandquality.gov.au/sites/default/files/migrated/Guidelines-RACF.pdf.

Barker A, Cameron P, Flicker L et al (2019) Evaluation of RESPOND, a patient-centred program to prevent falls in older people presenting to the emergency department with a fall: A randomised controlled trial. PLoS Medicine 16(5): e1002807.

Barker AL, Nitz JC, Low Choy NL et al (2009) Measuring fall risk and predicting who will fall: clinimetric properties of four fall risk assessment tools for residential aged care. The Journals of Gerontology Series A: Biological Sciences and Medical Science 64(8):916–924.

Batchelor FA, Dow B, Low MA (2013) Do continence management strategies reduce falls? A systematic review. Australasian Journal of Ageing 32(4):211–216.

Black A, Begg S (2010) Rate and cost of hospital admissions due to fall-related injuries among older Queenslanders, 2007–08. Health Statistics Centre, Queensland Health. Online. Available: www.health.qld.gov.au/__data/assets/pdf_file/0027/435078/0708-hosp-admissions.pdf,

Cameron ID, Dyer SM, Panagoda CE et al (2018) Interventions for preventing falls in older people in care facilities and hospitals. Cochrane Database Systematic Reviews 9:Cd005465.

Church JL, Haas MR, Goodall S (2015) Cost effectiveness of falls and injury prevention strategies for older adults living in residential aged care facilities. Pharmacoeconomics 33(12):1301–1310.

Cwikel JG, Fried AV, Biderman A et al (1998) Validation of a fall-risk screening test, the Elderly Fall Screening Test (EFST), for community-dwelling elderly. Disability and Rehabilitation 20(5):161–167.

Deandrea S, Lucenteforte E, Bravi F et al (2010) Risk factors for falls in community-dwelling older people: a systematic review and meta-analysis. Epidemiology 21(5):658–668.

Francis-Coad J, Etherton-Beer C, Bulsara C et al (2018) Evaluating the impact of a falls prevention community of practice in a residential aged care setting: a realist approach. BMC Health Services Research 18(1):21.

Gillespie LD, Robertson MC, Gillespie WJ et al (2012) Interventions for preventing falls in older people living in the community. Cochrane Database Systematic Reviews(9):Cd007146.

Government of Western Australia Department of Health (2020) Stay On Your Feet® Online. Available: https://www.stayonyourfeet.com.au/wp-content/uploads/2020/05/200506_SOYF_FallsRiskChecklist2.pdf

Haines TP, Hill AM, Hill KD et al (2011) Patient education to prevent falls among older hospital inpatients: a randomized controlled trial. Archives of Internal Medicine 171(6):516–524.

Tips for Best Practice

- Ensure all falls are reported and reviewed.
- Look for new risk factors when a fall occurs, even for those with a large number of risk factors.
- Discuss with the older person, and where appropriate, their caregivers, about their individual falls risk, and possible strategies to reduce the risk of future falls. The older person should be actively involved in discussions about their falls management plan.
- Ensure older people are informed that many falls are preventable, and of the approaches known to reduce the risk of falling.

SUMMARY

Falls are common in older people and can have serious adverse outcomes. Therefore, principles of falls prevention apply for older people across the health spectrum, from those who are generally well to those with chronic illness and poor mobility. A fall can cause an older person to develop a 'fear of falling'. This psychological effect often leads the older person to reduce their activity levels, leading to muscle weakness and poorer balance, thereby increasing the risk of future falls. Nurses who become aware that an older person has fallen or is becoming more unsteady on his or her feet must encourage the older person to discuss this with their doctor. Falls risk factors include intrinsic risks, extrinsic risks and behavioural risks. Falls risk screening and falls risk assessment tools identify an individual's falls risk factors that must then be addressed with evidence-based interventions. Falls prevention strategies include single interventions, multifactorial interventions (targeted to an individual's needs, or multiple interventions (program applied to everyone in a specific group). Falls prevention strategies, whether implemented for an individual, or for a ward or an organisation, should have a process in place to intermittently review progress. It is common to require modifications over time to sustain effectiveness and participation in the intervention.

REFERENCES

Australian Commission on Safety and Quality in Health Care (ACSQHC) (2009a) Preventing falls and harm from falls in older people: Best practice guidelines for Australian community care. Online. Available: www.safetyandquality.gov.au/sites/default/files/migrated/Guidelines-COMM.pdf.

Australian Commission on Safety and Quality in Health Care (ACSQHC) (2009b) Preventing falls and harm from falls in older people: Best practice guidelines for Australian hospitals.

Haines TP, Nitz J, Grieve J et al (2013) Cost per fall: a potentially misleading indicator of burden of disease in health and residential care settings. Journal of Evaluation in Clinical Practice 19(1):153–161.

Health Safety and Quality Commission New Zealand (HSQCNZ) (2016) Falls Atlas domain: falls in people aged 50 and over. Online. Available: www.hqsc.govt.nz/our-programmes/health-quality-evaluation/projects/atlas-of-healthcare-variation/falls/

Hewitt J, Goodall S, Clemson L et al (2018) Progressive resistance and balance training for falls prevention in long-term residential aged care: a cluster randomized trial of the Sunbeam Program. Journal of American Medical Directors Assocation 19(4):361–369.

Hill AM, Hoffmann T, Hill K et al (2010) Measuring falls events in acute hospitals – a comparison of three reporting methods to identify missing data in the hospital reporting system. Journal of the American Geriatrics Society 58(7):1347–1352.

Hill AM, McPhail SM, Waldron N et al (2015) Fall rates in hospital rehabilitation units after individualised patient and staff education programmes: a pragmatic, stepped-wedge, cluster-randomised controlled trial. Lancet 385(9987):2592–2599.

Hopewell S, Adedire O, Copsey BJ et al (2018) Multifactorial and multiple component interventions for preventing falls in older people living in the community. Cochrane Database Systematic Reviews 7:Cd012221.

Jones KJ, Crowe J, Allen JA et al (2019) The impact of post-fall huddles on repeat fall rates and perceptions of safety culture: a quasi-experimental evaluation of a patient safety demonstration project. BMC Health Services Research 19(1):650.

Jorstad EC, Hauer K, Becker C et al (2005) Measuring the psychological outcomes of falling: a systematic review. Journal of the American Geriatrics Society 53(3):501–510.

Kempen GI, Yardley L, van Haastregt JC et al (2008) The Short FES-I: a shortened version of the falls efficacy scale-international to assess fear of falling. Age & Ageing 37(1):45–50.

Lee DC, Day L, Hill K et al (2015) What factors influence older adults to discuss falls with their health-care providers? Health Expectations 18(5):1593–1609.

Mackenzie L, Byles J, D'Este C (2009) Longitudinal study of the Home Falls and Accidents Screening Tool in identifying older people at increased risk of falls. Australasian Journal of Ageing 28(2):64–69.

McCrow J, Dementia Australia (2015) Q & A sheet – Delirium and Dementia. Online. Available: www.dementia.org.au/files/helpsheets/Helpsheet-DementiaQandA21_Delirium_english.pdf.

Menant JC, Steele JR, Menz HB et al (2008) Optimizing footwear for older people at risk of falls. Journal of Rehabilitation Research and Development 45(8):1167–1181.

Meyer C, Dow B, Bilney BE et al (2012) Falls in older people receiving in-home informal care across Victoria: influence on care recipients and caregivers. Australasian Journal of Ageing 31(1):6–12.

Mitchell, D, Raymond M, Jellett J et al (2018) Where are falls prevention resources allocated by hospitals and what do they cost? A cross sectional survey using semi-structured interviews of key informants at six Australian health services. International Journal of Nursing Studies 86:52–59.

Morello RT, Barker AL, Watts JJ et al (2015) The extra resource burden of in-hospital falls: a cost of falls study. Medical Journal of Australia 203(9):367.

Olij BF, Ophuis RH, Polinder S et al (2018) Economic evaluations of falls prevention programs for older adults: a systematic review. Journal of the American Geriatrics Society 66(11):2197–2204.

Papadimitriou A, Perry M (2020) Systematic review of the effects of cognitive and behavioural interventions on fall-related psychological concerns in older adults. Journal of Aging and Physical Activity 28(1):155–168.

Pointer S (2019) Trends in hospitalised injury due to falls in older people, 2007–08 to 2016–17. Injury research and statistics series no. 126. Cat. no. INJCAT 206. AIHW, Canberra.

Santesso N, Carrasco-Labra A, Brignardello-Petersen R (2014) Hip protectors for preventing hip fractures in older people. Cochrane Database Systematic Reviews (3):Cd001255.

Sherrington C, Fairhall NJ, Wallbank GK et al (2019) Exercise for preventing falls in older people living in the community. Cochrane Database Systematic Reviews 1:Cd012424.

Shorr RI, Chandler AM, Mion LC et al (2012) Effects of an intervention to increase bed alarm use to prevent falls in hospitalized patients: a cluster randomized trial. Annals of Internal Medicine 157(10):692–699.

Sjosten N, Vaapio S, Kivela SL (2008) The effects of fall prevention trials on depressive symptoms and fear of falling among the aged: a systematic review. Aging & Mental Health 12(1):30–46.

Spink MJ, Menz HB, Fotoohabadi MR et al (2011) Effectiveness of a multifaceted podiatry intervention to prevent falls in community dwelling older people with disabling foot pain: randomised controlled trial. BMJ 342:d3411.

Suttanon P, Hill KD, Said CM et al (2013) Feasibility, safety and preliminary evidence of the effectiveness of a home-based exercise programme for older people with Alzheimer's disease: a pilot randomized controlled trial. Clinical Rehabilitation 27(5):427–438.

Toye C, Slatyer S, Kitchen S et al (2019) Bed moves, ward environment, staff perspectives and falls for older people with high falls risk in an acute hospital: a mixed methods study. Clinical Interventions in Aging 14:2223–2237.

Tricco AC, Thomas SM, Veroniki AA et al (2017) Comparisons of interventions for preventing falls in older adults: a systematic review and meta-analysis. JAMA 318(17):1687–1699.

University of Manchester (n.d.) FES-I. Online. Available: https://sites.manchester.ac.uk/fes-i/)

University of Newcastle (n.d.) Home falls and accidents screening tool (HOMEFAST). Online. Available: www.newcastle.edu.au/__data/assets/pdf_file/0007/137185/HOMEFAST-Home-Falls-Accidents-Screening-Tool.pdf

Whitney J, Close JC, Lord SR et al (2012) Identification of high risk fallers among older people living in residential care facilities: a simple screen based on easily collectable measures. Archives of Gerontology and Geriatrics 55(3):690–695.

World Health Organisation (WHO) (2007) WHO Global report on falls prevention in older age. WHO, Geneva.

CHAPTER 17

Palliative Care

RUTH WEI • SUSAN SLATYER

LEARNING OBJECTIVES

After reading this chapter, you will be able to:

- describe the elements of a *good* death
- define the six guiding principles for quality palliative care
- explain the application of a palliative approach in residential aged care settings
- describe the signs of imminent death
- discuss the elements of nursing care for the older person at the end of life
- explain the nurse's role in communication, advance care planning and decision-making to support older people who are approaching the end of life.

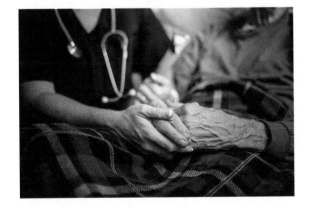

You matter because you are you, and you matter to the end of your life. We will do all we can not only to help you die peacefully but also to live until you die.

**DAME CICELY SAUNDERS, FOUNDER OF THE
MODERN HOSPICE MOVEMENT (1918–2005)**

INTRODUCTION

Death is a natural part of life. If we describe life as a journey, then birth and death are the beginning and end of that journey and we experience our life in between. Without life, there is no death. While an impending birth is prepared for and celebrated, and the new baby warmly welcomed into the world, an impending death may not be acknowledged as people shy away from the topic of dying. Philosophers, psychologists and researchers have attempted to understand and explain the fear of death, but it remains a myth. As Woody Allen remarked, 'I am not afraid of death. I just don't want to be there when it happens' (Allen 1975).

In 2018, approximately 158,000 deaths were recorded in the Australian population of 25 million, with 66% being people aged 75 years or older (Australia Institute of Health and Welfare [AIHW] 2020). The median age at death was 78 years for males and 84 years for females (AIHW 2020). In New Zealand, population 5 million, there were approximately 34,000 deaths in the year to June 2020, with two-thirds being people aged 70–94 years (Stats NZ 2020). Older people will continue to make up the majority of deaths as the population ages and the prevalence of cancer and age-related chronic diseases increases. For example, by 2066, it is projected that 25% of Australians will be aged over 65 years, with approximately 29% diagnosed with three or more co-morbid chronic conditions (Australian Government Department of Health 2018).

Older people who have irreversible and progressive conditions require quality care to help them live life as fully and comfortably as possible. This chapter will discuss the role of palliative care for older people with life-limiting conditions, recognition of the dying older person and the nursing management of terminal symptoms. The goal of palliative care is to provide comfort rather than cure and to enhance the *quality* instead of the *quantity* (length) of a person's remaining life. The evidence demonstrates that benefits for older people who receive palliative care include better quality of life, fewer hospitalisations and shorter length of hospital stay, which also bring cost-savings in healthcare expenditure (Australian Government Department of Health 2018).

Although inevitable as a natural part of life, death is not the goal for most people. Thoughts of separating from loved ones and leaving them behind, perceptions of an unfulfilled life, fear of pain and suffering during the dying process, as well as uncertainty after death can make it difficult to openly discuss dying, or even to prepare for death. The consistent and purposeful avoidance of thinking about and discussing dying only reinforces the consensus view that death is a taboo subject, with some cultures even believing that discussion on the subject brings about misfortune (Wei et al 2019). However, people expect a *good* death or *successful* dying, even though death may be unspeakable and the person unprepared.

A GOOD DEATH

There is a long historical, cultural and literary tradition that discusses the concept of a *good* death. In 1997, a good death was defined as death 'free from avoidable distress and suffering for patient, family and caregivers, in general accord with the patient's and family's wishes, and reasonably consistent with clinical, cultural and ethical standards' (Institute of Medicine 1997). Since then it has been debated in several disciplines, including medicine, sociology, theology and psychology, with the point made that whether a death is good depends on the perspective of the dying person.

Perceptions of a good death are influenced by culture, customs, social norms, religion and previous experiences of death and dying. For most people, this means dying without pain or suffering, and with respect and dignity. One review by Meier and colleagues (2016) of the literature articulated 11 core themes thought to define a good death:

- Preferences for the dying process: where, when and how, e.g. dying during sleep

- Pain-free status: both pain and symptoms under control and no suffering
- Emotional wellbeing
- Family and relatives present (and prepared for their loved one's death)
- Dignity
- A sense of completion of life (saying goodbye, a life well lived)
- Religiosity and spirituality
- Preferences for treatment (not prolonging life, control over treatment decisions)
- Quality of life
- Relationship with healthcare providers (support from care team, experience in end-of-life care)
- Other (cultural aspects, comfort through physical touch, being with pets).

With these principles in mind, a good death is most often achieved when the person dies in a calm, peaceful and private environment, without pain or suffering, and under the care of a team that is familiar to the dying person and their family (Marie Curie Cancer Care 2014). Dying and death are not merely biomedical events, but rather the finishing of a life. Therefore, care for a person approaching the end of life is holistic, with the physical, psychological, social and spiritual needs and preferences of both the dying person and their family at the centre of the experience (Cherny et al 2015).

PALLIATIVE CARE

Palliative care emerged from the hospice movement in the United Kingdom. In 1967, Dame Cicely Saunders, who trained as a nurse, then a medical social worker, and finally as a doctor, founded the St Christopher's Hospice in London to care for terminally ill people (St Christopher's Hospice 2020). She had recognised the inadequacy of end-of-life care provided in busy acute care hospitals and sought to create an environment that emphasised the dying person and their family as the unit of care, and included bereavement services to support families after death. In doing so, she brought together medical and nursing care with holistic support to meet the physical, emotional, social and spiritual needs of the dying persons and their families.

In the early 1970s, William Lamers in the United States pioneered a homecare model of hospice care, allowing terminally ill people to live out their lives at home (Woo 2012). In 1975, a Canadian urologic cancer specialist named Balfour Mount coined the term 'palliative care' and established a hospital-based model which delivered hospice care in a dedicated palliative care ward at the Royal Victoria Hospital (Williams &

Wheeler 2001). These three care models (hospice care, home-based palliative care and hospital-based palliative care) are the foundation for contemporary end-of-life care service delivery.

Definition of Palliative Care

The definition of palliative care was first provided by the World Health Organisation (WHO) in 1990. It was revised in 2012 to incorporate new developments and concepts, and currently states:

> *Palliative care is an approach that improves the quality of life for patients and their families facing the problem/s associated with life-threatening illness through the prevention and relief of suffering by means of early identification and impeccable assessment and treatment of pain and other problems, physical, psychosocial and spiritual (WHO 2020b).*

Similarly, palliative care has been defined for the contemporary Australian and New Zealand contexts as:

> *… person and family-centred care provided for a person with an active, progressive, advanced disease, who has little or no prospect of cure and who is expected to die, and for whom the primary goal is to optimise the quality of life (Palliative Care Australia n.d.)*

> *Palliative care is the provision of caring and dignified support and services for people of all ages facing a life-limiting condition. It is provided wherever the person is, whether that is in the home, hospital, community clinic or hospice (Health Navigator New Zealand 2020).*

As these definitions emphasise, palliative care takes a person and family-centred approach, recognising that dying is an inevitable part of life and ensuring access to palliative care services for all. In Australia, six guiding principles fundamental to quality palliative care have been identified and are expected to be demonstrated in all service delivery at the end of life (Australian Government Department of Health 2018). These are:

- palliative care is person-centred care
- death is recognised as part of life
- carers are valued and receive the support and information they need
- care is accessible
- everyone has a role to play in palliative care
- care is high quality and evidence-based.

PALLIATIVE CARE SERVICES

There are two main types of palliative care provided to people with a life-limiting illness according to the level and complexity of care needed. *Primary palliative care* is provided by healthcare professionals, such as general practitioners (GPs), nurses, personal care workers and other allied health professionals who have primary responsibility for the health needs of a person diagnosed with a life-limiting illness. *Specialist palliative care* is provided by a dedicated multidisciplinary team with specialised skills, competencies, experience and training in palliative care, when the person's complex needs exceed the expertise of primary palliative care providers (Australian Government Department of Health 2018). The primary goals of specialist palliative care services are to:

- assess and treat complex physical symptoms
- provide information and advice on complex issues, such as ethical issues and family issues, through effective communication
- manage psychosocial care needs (Australian Government Department of Health 2018).

Primary and specialist palliative care can be delivered in a variety of settings, including community, home, hospitals, hospices, special palliative care units or residential aged care facilities. Older people receiving palliative care may transition between these settings depending on their, and their family's, needs, preferences and values. In general, palliative care services provide:

- pain relief
- symptom management: dyspnoea, nausea, vomiting, terminal restlessness
- equipment and other resources to enable home-based care
- support for families to talk about sensitive issues
- links to other services such as home help and financial support
- support for people to meet cultural obligations
- emotional, social and spiritual support
- counselling and bereavement support
- referral to respite care (Palliative Care Australia n.d.)

STANDARDS FOR PALLIATIVE CARE

A variety of standards, guidelines and policies have been developed to guide specialist palliative care for people with a life-limiting illness and their families. In Australia, the first National Standards were established in 1994 and have been regularly updated since then to reflect developing knowledge, with the 5th edition released in 2018 (Palliative Care Australia 2018). The most recent version of Hospice New Zealand Standards for Palliative Care was launched in 2019 after an extensive consultation and review process (Hospice New Zealand 2019). Both versions of standards are divided into two categories:

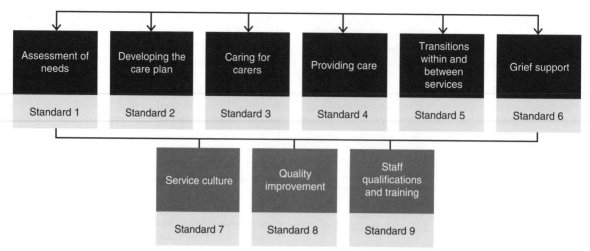

FIG. 17.1 **Overview of Palliative Care Standards, Australia.** (Source: Palliative Care Australia 2018, p. 9.)

Care Standards and Governance Standards, with nine specific Standards. These are depicted in Fig. 17.1, with Care Standards in blue, and Governance Standards in red. While not mandatory, these Standards articulate the person-centred approach to end-of-life care for all and apply to every service providing palliative care.

PALLIATIVE CARE FOR OLDER PEOPLE

Most people now die at an older age, commonly with frailty and co-morbidities. In Australia, around 25% of Australians will be aged over 65 years by 2066, with approximately 29% having three or more co-morbid chronic conditions (Australian Government Department of Health 2018). Three distinct trajectories of decline towards death in people with chronic progressive disease, most common in older people, have been described (Murray et al 2005). Fig. 17.2 provides the three trajectories in three graphs, each of which plots level of function (*y*-axis) over time (*x*-axis). Graph A demonstrates a trajectory where the person maintains a reasonable functional ability for a period of time and then declines quickly in the last few (usually) months before death. With a clear terminal phase that often includes specialist palliative care input, this trajectory is usually seen in people with cancer. Graph B describes a gradual decline during which the person has episodes of acute deterioration, from which they never fully recover. Despite the continual decline, death often seems to come suddenly when an acute episode cannot be reversed. This trajectory usually continues over a period of 2–5 years and is seen

in older people with heart or respiratory disease. The last trajectory, shown in Graph C, describes a prolonged, ongoing and gradual decline towards death. This dwindling is typically seen in frail older people or people with dementia.

Fig. 17.3 shows that the most common recipients of palliative services globally in 2018 were diagnosed with cardiovascular disease (38.5%), followed by cancer (34%), and then chronic respiratory diseases (10.3%) (WHO 2020a). These three conditions are delineated in the first two illness trajectories in Fig. 17.2. Additionally, dementia, most commonly associated with a long, slow, dwindling decline, was the second leading cause of death in New Zealand in 2017 (Institute for Health Metrics and Evaluation 2020) and is the current leading cause of death for women and the third leading cause of death for men in Australia (Dementia Australia 2020).

A PALLIATIVE APPROACH IN RESIDENTIAL AGED CARE

Many older people experiencing chronic illness, functional decline, dementia and/or frailty will move into a residential aged care facility when they are no longer able to live independently at home (see Chapter 6). Despite the support, residents with progressive disease, including dementia, will continue on a declining illness trajectory (see Fig. 17.3). There may be no distinctive delineation as to when curative treatment becomes futile and palliative care becomes the more appropriate goal as the person nears the end of life.

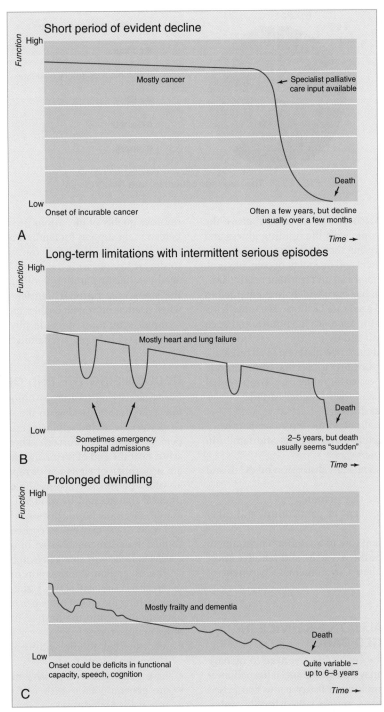

FIG. 17.2. Typical illness trajectories for people with progressive chronic illness. A. Short evident decline (mostly cancer). B. Progressive decline with episodes of acute deterioration (mostly cardiovascular disease or respiratory disease). C. Long, slow dwindling (mostly frailty or dementia). (RAND Corporation, Santa Monica, California 2005.)

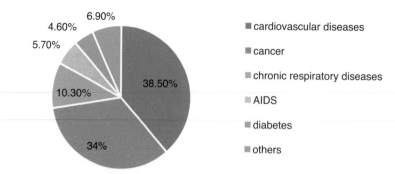

6.90%
4.60%
5.70%

38.50%

10.30%

34%

- cardiovascular diseases
- cancer
- chronic respiratory diseases
- AIDS
- diabetes
- others

FIG. 17.3 **The need for palliative care** (WHO 2020a)

A palliative approach to care aims to improve the quality of life for people with life-limiting illness and their families, by reducing their suffering through early identification, assessment and treatment of pain, physical, cultural, psychological, social and spiritual needs (AMA 2015). This approach has been widely implemented in Australian residential aged care facilities. The underlying philosophy of a palliative approach is a positive and open attitude towards death and dying. This is evidenced by the introduction of advance care planning to all residents, offering them an opportunity to discuss, communicate and document their wishes for future care. The potential benefits to residents and their families include:

- reducing potential distress
- reducing non-beneficial admission to acute care
- increasing involvement by residents and family in decisions about their care
- encouraging open and early discussion on death and dying
- facilitating advance care planning
- improving management of pain control and other symptoms
- providing consistent care in a familiar environment from the staff that the residents and families know and trust (Australian Government Department of Health 2018).

SPECIALISED PALLIATIVE SERVICE IN RESIDENTIAL AGED CARE

As a resident nears the end of life, the need to manage complex symptoms may necessitate specialist palliative care provided by a multidisciplinary team, comprised of medical practitioners, nurses, allied health professionals and volunteers with expertise in palliative support. Working with the facility staff and families, specialised palliative services can provide intermittent or ongoing care to address the resident's holistic care needs to improve quality of life, minimise suffering and facilitate bereavement support for family and friends (Toye 2012). In doing so, the care team can fulfil a resident's wish to die 'at home', with the home being the residential aged care facility, among familiar people and without the stress of a hospital transfer. Identifying early on when death is imminent enables the care team to manage terminal symptoms, provide physical and emotional comfort and help prepare family members.

RECOGNISING THE END OF LIFE

Everyone's dying journey is unique. An older person may take months or days to die. The nurse's role is to work with the multidisciplinary team to ensure the older person remains comfortable whether the condition is acute, near the end of life or anywhere in between. There are a number of signs and symptoms indicating that an older person is reaching the end of life. However, physical changes may be confused with frailty and acute exacerbations of chronic disease, while agitation, anxiety and restlessness may be categorised as manifestations of confusion or dementia. Nurses must be familiar with the common indicators that a person may be nearing death.

The Australian Commission on Safety and Quality in Health Care (ACSQHC) states that a person is 'approaching the end of life' when he or she is considered likely to die within the next 12 months. This includes older people who:

- are expected to die within a few hours or days (imminent death)
- have an advanced, progressive and incurable condition
- are generally frail, with one or more co-existing progressive conditions
- have a chronic condition that puts them at risk of dying from a sudden acute health crisis
- experience a life-threatening acute condition caused by a sudden catastrophic event.

Source: ACSQHC (2015).

The Supportive and Palliative Care Indicators Tool (SPICT™)

The SPICT™ is a useful instrument to help determine that an older person's health is deteriorating, putting them at risk of dying within 12 months (SPICT 2020). Developed in the UK, SPICT™ is widely used to indicate when a person with advancing chronic disease or multimorbidity may have unmet holistic needs requiring support and would benefit from a palliative approach. SPICT™ is not a structured assessment tool, but rather indicates when someone requires further assessment to gauge the urgency of their needs and to structure care planning. The SPICT™ tool is available at https://www.spict.org.uk/. It has six general indicators of deteriorating health, each of which could by itself prompt an assessment or be combined with the SPICT™ indicators of chronic advancing conditions, which include:

- cancer
- dementia/frailty (see Chapter 26)
- heart/vascular disease (see Chapter 23)
- neurological disease (see Chapter 26)
- respiratory disease (see Chapter 24)
- liver disease
- kidney disease.

The older person should be reviewed regularly using SPICT™, including at key transition points in his or her trajectory, for example:

- if there has been a significant functional or medical decline
- if there is a sudden acute event
- if discussions around goals of care are required, particularly around futile treatment
- following hospitalisation.

Signs of Imminent Death

As a person nears the end of life, bodily functions slow and certain signs and symptoms will occur. As a general guide, one to three months before death an older person may start to eat less, show a decreased desire for food, increasing sleep and a tendency to withdraw. As the person draws closer to death (one to two weeks before dying), he or she may demonstrate:

- increased sleepiness
- confusion
- changes in temperature and vital signs (pulse, respiration, blood pressure)
- respiratory congestion
- lack of appetite, and/or
- restlessness.

Indicators that a person is nearing the last days or hours of life provided in *Tips for best practice: Recognising the dying person*.

Nursing Care for the Older Person at the End of Life

Care for the older person at the end of life is focused upon comfort (PalliAGED 2020). As death approaches, he or she will become less responsive and the nurse will need to rely on changes in the person's body language, facial expression, respiratory rate and vocalisations to assess comfort. The multidisciplinary team may consider stopping therapies, such as blood glucose monitoring, nasogastric feeding, unnecessary medications (e.g. hypoglycaemics, antihypotensives, anticoagulants). Oxygen may be ceased unless it helps to relieve agitation and dyspnoea (see below). The nurse can encourage family members to be with the dying person, reassuring them that hearing is the last sense to be lost, so their loved one will probably be able to hear them. Invite the family to assist with care if they wish. The components of essential nursing care for the dying older person are provided in *Promoting wellness: Essential components of end-of-life care*. Care also needs to incorporate effective management of terminal symptoms to facilitate a comfortable and peaceful death. Resources are available that provide detailed information about the use of medications in end-of-life care. See *Tips for best practice: Further resources to guide medication use in end-of-life care*. The most common include pain, dyspnoea, nausea and vomiting, constipation and terminal restlessness.

Pain

Pain is a common symptom in older people dying of incurable conditions, particularly cancer, and can be a source of considerable distress for them and their families (Kehl & Kowalkowski 2013). However, pain at the end

Tips for Best Practice
Recognising the Dying Person

Identifying when the older person is approaching death enables the nurse to ensure family members are notified and given the opportunity to be with the person during the last moments of their life. If family is not available, the nurse or another staff member must stay with the dying person, so that he or she is not alone. Even if apparently unresponsive, the dying person should be touched and spoken to.

In the last days or hours of life, the dying person is likely to exhibit:

- dyspnoea and periods of apnoea (no breathing)
- pain
- noisy respiratory secretions
- confusion
- sleepiness, unresponsive
- reduced (or no) food and fluid intake
- loss of swallow and gag reflexes
- weak, rapid pulse
- declining blood pressure
- cool extremities
- pale, mottled skin
- slow or no pupil reactions
- restlessness
- little or no urine output
- bowel and bladder incontinence (Kehl & Kowalkowski 2013).

At the point of death, the older person may exhibit gasping breaths that gradually slow and stop. Signs that the older person has died include:

- no pulse
- not breathing
- no muscle tension
- eyes partially shut and pupils fixed
- bowel and bladder releasing.

Family members may wish to stay for a time with their loved one who has died. The next step will be to make contact with a funeral provider. See Chapter 29 for information on supporting bereaved family members.

Tips for Best Practice
Further Resources to Guide Medication Use in End-of Life-Care

Two useful resources are:
Australian Medicines Handbook Aged Care Companion Online
https://agedcare.amh.net.au/auth

Havard's Nursing Guide to Drugs
www.elsevierhealth.com.au/havards-nursing-guide-to-drugs-9780729542548.html

Promoting Wellness
Components of Essential Terminal Care

Essential care for the person in the last days or hours of life include:

- *Oral care*: apply products to keep the mouth clean and moist at least four times per day. Use oral hygiene sponges or swabs soaked with normal saline 0.9% (avoid products with glycerin, sodium bicarbonate, lemon, pineapple or other juices)
- *Lip care*: apply lip balm or paraffin (avoid petroleum-based products)
- *Moisten mouth*: encourage sips of water or ice chips to keep the mouth moist
- *Skin care*: apply emollient twice daily (avoid products with lanolin or fragrance). Relieve pressure and promote comfort with sheepskin products, a pressure mattress and gentle repositioning as tolerated. Consider skin cooling measures using regular sponging with cool water and fans.
- *Eye care*: use normal saline 0.9% to remove exudate several times per day. Artificial tears may relieve dryness. Provide soft, indirect lighting.
- *Bladder care*: urinary output will decrease as death approaches, urinary retention is common and may cause restlessness (see below), manage incontinence with absorbent pads, indwelling catheters or uridome draining (in men).
- *Bowel care*: constipation may cause restlessness and require rectal laxatives, position incontinence pads to minimise disruption during changes.
- *Maintain hygiene*: provide sponge baths in bed and change sheets as the person can tolerate and as required.

Note: Nurses must use clinical judgement to determine when the person requires assistance as routine care may not always be appropriate as the person deteriorates.
Queensland Health (2019); Therapeutic Guidelines Limited (2020).

of life can be managed effectively and nurses have a central role in the prevention, assessment and relief of any pain or discomfort. Older people may express their pain differently due to biological, emotional and psychosocial factors (see Chapter 19). Common indicators that a person at the end of life is experiencing pain include:

- complaints of pain or discomfort
- agitation
- refusing food
- reluctance to move (Marie Curie Cancer Care 2014).

Effective pain management depends on regular nursing assessment of pain using validated tools (see Chapter 19). Following assessment, treatment comprises analgesic medication to relieve or reduce pain symptoms in combination with non-pharmacological comfort measures. See Chapter 19 (pages 234–237) for a discussion of pharmacological approaches to pain management. Non-pharmacological comfort measures used in end-of-life care are provided in the *Tips for best practice* box.

Tips for Best Practice

Non-pharmacological measures to supplement analgesic medications to promote comfort in older people at end of life include:

- repositioning
- pressure relieving aids – appropriate mattress, positioning, pillow supports
- treating reversible causes such as urinary retention
- heat and cold packs. Note: not appropriate for people who cannot feel temperature or communicate – see Chapter 19 Safety Alert
- diversion therapy – music or reminiscence
- complementary therapies – massage, aromatherapy, relaxation, acupuncture/acupressure
- TENS (Transcutaneous Electrical Nerve Stimulation)

Queensland Health (2019); Therapeutic Guidelines (2020).

Dyspnoea

Dyspnoea, or breathlessness, is a common and distressing problem for people who are at the end of life, which becomes more frequent in the terminal stages of most conditions. The shortness of breath can cause the older person to feel:

- panic
- a sense of being suffocated
- a sense of drowning
- claustrophobia
- anxiety
- fear (Therapeutic Guidelines 2020).

Family members may become distressed watching their loved one struggle for breath and may reflect the older person's panic. It is essential to be proactive and address symptoms early. Non-pharmacological strategies to alleviate breathlessness include:

- reassurance – they are *not* going to die gasping for breath
- drug treatment for symptoms
- sitting the person upright
- providing air movement in the room – ventilation (open windows), a fan, moving visitors away from the person

- providing a cool, calm environment
- relaxation (Therapeutic Guidelines 2020).

Regular oral care to relieve mouth dryness (see *Promoting wellness: Components of essential terminal care*). Oxygen is not recommended in terminal care, unless the person with dyspnoea is hypoxic, as breathlessness is usually due to metabolic changes (PalliAGED 2020). If not relieved by non-pharmacological measures, opioid medication may be used; however, the older person needs to be monitored closely for adverse effects (Therapeutic Guidelines 2020). Careful adjustment of the dose of opioid to the level of dyspnoea can minimise the risk of causing respiratory depression (Therapeutic Guidelines 2020). Morphine, administered orally or subcutaneously, is the drug of choice. Small doses are usually effective.

Nausea and Vomiting

Many older people nearing the end of life experience nausea and vomiting, which can be intermittent or persistent, but become less common as death approaches (Therapeutic Guidelines 2020). It can be difficult to determine the cause, which is often multifactorial, and treatment is often aimed at relieving symptoms. Nursing strategies include:

- regular doses of antiemetic medication (more effective than 'as required'; reassess regularly need for treatment)
- small, frequent, appetising meals
- providing a clean and pleasant environment
- providing oral hygiene
- positioning the person on their left side, which is likely to be more comfortable (lying on the right side may increase vomiting)

Constipation

Constipation at the end of life is characterised by slowed transit of gastrointestinal contents and rectal evacuation (e.g. straining), and can cause significant discomfort and embarrassment (Therapeutic Guidelines 2020). Constipation is the most common side effect of opioid medication. Other causes include decreased oral intake of fluids and dietary fibre, dehydration, reduced mobility and electrolyte imbalances (e.g. uraemia, hypothyroidism, hypokalaemia). Addressing constipation is important to promote comfort and maintain appetite. Nursing assessment and monitoring are essential, along with a proactive approach that addresses the multifactorial causes. Prevention strategies include:

- all persons receiving opioid medication require regular laxatives
- encourage the person to use the toilet at the same time each day, and take advantage of gastrocolic reflex that occurs after eating
- increase fluid intake

- increase fibre intake if possible (e.g. fruit, prune and pear juice)
- increase exercise if tolerated (control pain and dyspnoea)
- provide privacy
- assist the person with positioning when attempting a bowel movement (e.g. sitting upright).

There are several types of laxative medication, classified according to the mechanism of action. Selection of the appropriate laxative is informed by the underlying cause of the constipation (Therapeutic Guidelines 2020). First-line treatments for opioid-induced constipation are stool softeners and stimulant laxatives. Some laxatives, particularly the fibre-based 'bulk forming' type, require a sufficient fluid intake and therefore have a limited role in end-of-life care.

Terminal Restlessness

Delirium (see Chapter 26) is common in older people who are approaching end of life. Terminal restlessness is a specific form of delirium, very prevalent in the last days of life, which commonly presents with physical restlessness or agitation, confusion and hallucinations (Therapeutic Guidelines 2020). This can be distressing for family to watch and may contribute to complicated grief (see Chapter 29). Causes include:

- uncontrolled pain
- urinary retention (common in the last days of life)
- faecal impaction
- decreasing renal and hepatic function and inability to clear toxins from the body
- fluid and electrolyte imbalances
- metabolic disorders
- low perfusion status
- effects of medications
- withdrawal from medications
- low blood glucose level.

Management is aimed at reducing harm to the dying person and the family, such as physical injury to the person from agitated movements or emotional distress in family members. It may be possible to address reversible causes to promote comfort, but an older person in the last days of life may not respond. Strategies include:

- assess and manage pain
- consider urinary catheterisation to relieve urinary retention
- rectally administered laxative to address faecal impaction
- consider de-prescribing and/or tapering dosages to wean the person off medications
- consider oxygen therapy if the person is hypoxic, for comfort only

- provide a calm, quiet environment
- provide gentle music
- differentiate between night and day
- limit people attending and visiting the dying person to familiar faces.

If these measures are ineffective and the agitation persists, the dying person may benefit from very small doses of a benzodiazepine (e.g. clonazepam or midazolam) or haloperidol as required. Monitor patient response and adjust or give an additional dose as needed. The doctor may consider regular medication therapy if agitation persists or the dying person requires more than three intermittent doses within 24 hours (Therapeutic Guidelines 2020).

COMMUNICATION AND DECISION-MAKING IN PALLIATIVE CARE

The effective provision of palliative care for an older person who is approaching the end of life depends on timely communication that facilitates decision-making about the goals of care. This communication will include the older person, their family members and the multi-disciplinary team. Discussions are focused on the older person's physical, emotional, social and spiritual needs, along with his or her preferences on how these needs are met. Ideally, this communication should occur when the older person has decision-making capacity and the ability to think about future care options, well before the older person is declining towards death.

Advance care planning (see below) enables older people to have these discussions and document their wishes for end-of-life care well before they become too ill to make and communicate their decisions. While not legally binding, advance care plans provide guidance for medical and nursing staff as to the extent and type of treatment the older person would prefer should he or she not be able to tell them. More enforceable is an advance care directive (ACD), a legal document that enables a person to direct in writing exactly which treatments he or she would want – or not want – should they become incapacitated. The ACD is an important component of the hierarchy of decision-making also discussed below.

Nurses have an ethical and legal obligation and responsibility to understand the legal requirements, policies and relevant skills to promote an older person's informed decision-making about end-of-life care. Clayton and colleagues (2007) developed clinical practice guidelines, encapsulated in the acronym PREPARED, to guide health professionals to discuss issues of prognosis, likely illness trajectory and future care needs with older people and their family (see Table 17.1).

TABLE 17.1 Prepare: Steps for Communicating Prognosis and End-of-Life Issues	
P	**Prepare** for the discussion, where possible
R	**Relate** to the person
E	**Elicit** patient and caregiver preferences
P	**Provide** information, tailored to the individual needs of both the patient and the family
A	**Acknowledge** emotions and concerns
R	**Realistic** hope (e.g. foster realistic expectations for the potential for peaceful death, support)
E	**Encourage** questions and further discussions
D	**Document**

Adapted from Clayton et al (2007).

Advance Care Planning

An advance care plan can provide an older person with peace of mind that their wishes will be known, should they come to the point of no longer being able to make and communicate their decisions. Advance care planning is defined as 'a process that supports adults at any age or stage of health in understanding and sharing their personal values, life goals and preferences regarding future medical care' (Sudore et al 2017:821). Advance care plans are developed through a collaborative process, where health professionals work with the older person and his or her family to understand the person's preferences, forecast potential future care needs and construct a plan to be implemented if and when the person becomes seriously ill and unable to communicate for themselves (Advance Care Planning Australia 2020). This is a routine part of health and personal care for older people with chronic progressive conditions which, ideally, results in a formally documented and legally binding advance care directive.

While advance care planning should be part of routine care, certain situations can prompt a conversation with the older person to initiate planning or revisit a plan already in place. These include:

- if you answer 'No' to the 'surprise' question: 'Would you be surprised if this older person died in the next 12 months?' (see *Tips for best practice: The surprise question*).
- the older person or family member raises the issue of future care
- if there is a diagnosis of dementia, meaning that the older person's decision-making capacity is likely to decline (see Chapter 26)

Promoting Wellness
Benefits of Advance Care Planning

- Enables older people to receive care that is consistent with their values and preferences
- Improves the quality of end-of-life care provided to the older person
- Helps the older person and their family to feel more satisfied with care
- Families of people who have prepared an advance care plan tend to feel less stress, anxiety and depression
- Knowing the older person's wishes tends to reduce transfers to acute care that are unlikely to benefit the person, thereby improving outcomes and care for the person and reducing demand on the healthcare system.

There are better outcomes for older people and their families when advance care planning is part of ongoing, routine care, rather than a reaction to the older person becoming acutely ill or experiencing a health crisis.

Advance care planning discussions should be conducted when the older person is feeling comfortable and medically stable, and accompanied by a family member or substitute decision-maker (see below) if required (see Chapter 7).

Advance Care Planning Australia (2018b); Brinkman-Stoppelenburg et al (2014); Detering et al (2010).

- if the older person:
  - has an advanced chronic illness, such as heart failure (Chapter 23), chronic obstructive respiratory disease (Chapter 24) or end-stage renal failure
  - has advanced cancer
  - receives a new diagnosis of a significant disease, such as metastatic cancer
  - is aged 75 years or older, or 55 years or older if an Aboriginal or Torres Strait Islander person
  - indicates that progressive disease is advancing e.g. repeated hospitalisation
  - is a resident of or moving to a residential aged care facility
  - does not have a family member or friend who can act as substitute decision-maker (see below)
- if there is the possibility of future decision-making conflict (Advance Care Planning Australia 2020).

Advance care planning may involve a number of conversations. The nurse has an important role in helping the older person to prepare by encouraging them to think and talk about their beliefs, values and wishes for current and future care. The *Tips for best practice: Starting the conversation* box provides suggestions for gentle prompts that the nurse might use to start this conversation. When the older person is ready, he or she can then take part in discussions that include the multidisciplinary care team, family and, perhaps, friends to talk about their preferences. Advance care planning can also include the older person choosing a 'substitute decision-maker(s)' to make decisions on their behalf if they become unable to communicate (see below). Ideally, advance care planning results in a formal, written, legally binding advance Care Directive that ensures the older person's wishes are respected should he or she lose decision-making capacity.

Tips for Best Practice
Starting the Conversation

Nurses can find it difficult to know how to start a conversation with an older person about his or her wishes for future treatment and care. Suggestions include:

'I try to talk to all the older people that I care for about what they would like if they became more unwell. Have you ever thought about this?'

'I am pleased that you are feeling better after your recent illness. If you became very sick again, have you thought about what treatment you would want or not want?'

'Do you have any thoughts or feelings about where things are going with your illness/health?'

Advance Care Planning Australia (2018).

Advance Care Directive

An advance care directive (ACD) is a legally binding, written document that details a person's wishes for what treatment and care they want – or do not want – should they become seriously ill. It can only be written by the person themselves and is often called a 'living will' (Advance Care Planning Australia 2020). This directive only comes into effect if and when the person loses decision-making capacity. In Australia, ACDs may also be called an advance health directive (Western Australia, Queensland), advance personal plan (Northern Territory) or health direction (Australian Capital Territory). Being constituted in state law, statutory ACDs may also differ in how they are required to be written between states and territories. In general, an ACD which is valid in one state will apply in other places in Australia, although a few further requirements or limitations may be needed. Information about advance care planning and the law

in each state is available from Advance Care Planning Australia. In New Zealand, the ACD is called an advance directive and available under the Code of Health and Disability Services Consumers' Rights (see Health and Disability Commissioner 2020).

In both countries, any person over 18 years of age, who has decision-making capacity can make an ACD. However, an audit of older Australians ($n = 2285$) receiving health services and residential aged care from September 2017 to January 2018 revealed that only about 30% had an accessible ACD, with a further 20% having some form of advance care plan (Detering et al 2019).

Substitute Decision-Makers

Advance care planning may involve an older person choosing to appoint a substitute decision-maker (see Chapter 7), who has the legal authority to make a health-care decision on their behalf in the event that they lose capacity. Anyone who is aged 18 years and above with full legal capacity and who is willing to make decisions on the older person's behalf can be a substitute decision-maker. In New Zealand, a substitute decision-maker will be either an individual with the enduring power of attorney (EPA) or a court-appointed welfare guardian (Ministry of Justice 2020). In Australia, more than one substitute decision-maker can be appointed in some states. Some family members or persons designated as next of kin mistakenly believe they hold the right to make a decision on behalf of the dying person, should there be no legally authorised substitute decision-maker. Rather, state regulations set out a hierarchy of who has the power to make healthcare decisions when the person loses capacity. An example from Western Australia is provided by the Office of the Public Advocate (Government of Western Australia Department of Justice, 2020). It can be can be viewed online at https://www.publicadvocate.wa.gov.au/M/making_treatment_decisions.aspx?uid =4727-3795-2343-5639. In this state, an ACD is known as an advance health directive, which supersedes all other legally appointed guardian or family relationships.

VOLUNTARY ASSISTED DYING

Advance care planning is not the same as voluntary assisted dying (VAD), which has now been legislated in two Australian states: in Victoria under the *Voluntary Assisted Dying Act 2017* (Vic), and Western Australia, with the passing of the *Voluntary Assisted Dying Act 2019* (WA). VAD is defined as a medical practitioner assisting a competent individual who voluntarily requests help to end his/her life with self-administered drugs. First legalised in Switzerland in 1942, VAD is now legal in five states in the USA, Canada, the Netherlands, Belgium, Luxembourg and Columbia (Munday & Poon 2019). In New Zealand the *End of Life Choice Act 2019* legalising assisted dying is set to come into effect in November 2021 after 65% of voters supported the Act in a public referendum in 2020 (New Zealand Herald 2020).

Peak medical bodies in Australia and New Zealand generally oppose the legalisation of VAD and euthanasia. For example, a recent cross-sectional online survey by Munday and Poon (2019) researched attitudes of Australian and New Zealand Society for Geriatric Medicine (ANZSGM) members. Findings showed that only 24% supported legislation on VAD and even fewer (12%) were willing to prescribe the life-ending medications, although 61% would refer the person to a third party for VAD if it was legalised. The greatest concern of these medical practitioners was a risk to vulnerable patients. This study highlights a gap between community expectations for assistance to die in order to end suffering and those in the medical profession responsible for its implementation (Munday & Poon 2019).

SUMMARY

This chapter has discussed the role of palliative care for older people with life-limiting conditions, recognition of the dying older person, symptom management and the nurse's role in communication and decision-making in end-of-life care. For most older people, a good death is achieved when the person dies in a calm, peaceful and private environment, without pain or suffering, and under the care of a team familiar to them and their family. As older people with life-limiting conditions approach the end of life, palliative care that recognises death as part of life is person-centred, accessible, inclusive and values carers is appropriate. For those living in residential aged care, a palliative approach guides the nurse-led multidisciplinary care team in regularly reviewing care planning and symptom management. Nurses are well placed to recognise when an older person is imminently dying and implementing care that includes families where possible, while focusing on comfort and symptom management. The nurse also has an important role in facilitating the process of advance care planning to ensure an older person's choices for end of life care are known and documented. Ideally, this process results in a written, legally binding advance care directive that ensures the older person's wishes are respected, and may include the older person choosing a substitute decision-maker, should they lose decision-making capacity.

Research Highlight

A recent prospective, multi-centre, cross-sectional study explored the associations between the country of birth and advance care planning (ACP) in Australia. This study audited the ACP documentation in the health records of people aged 65 years or older who had accessed GP clinics, hospitals and long-term care facilities at 100 participating study sites across eight Australian jurisdictions. The health records were randomly selected to collect information about any ACDs or ACP documentation, including advance care directives (ACDs) completed by the person and ACP documents completed by a health professional or other person, with demographic data.

The results show that 3839 out of 4187 audited health records in total reported the country of birth, in which 30% ($n = 1152$) were born outside Australia. People who were born outside Australia were less likely to complete ACDs, compared to those born in Australia (21.9% vs 28.9%, X^2 (1, $n = 3840$) = 20.3, $p < 0.001$). However, the prevalence of the ACP documents completed on their behalf by a health professional or other person was higher among people who were born outside Australia (46.4% vs 34.8%, X^2 (1, $n = 3840$) = 45.5, $p < 0.001$). This dichotomy could be interpreted as cultural values influencing communication styles between patients, health professionals and family members. People who received palliative care were more likely to have ACDs in place, even though there was no statistical significance. The study also shows those who speak English proficiently may be more able to engage in completing their ACD forms directly to make their values and preferences known, compared to migrants. The study also reported that people who received palliative care and had poorer functional status were more likely to have an ACP completed on their behalf by a health professional or someone else.

Promoting advance care planning in a culturally and linguistically diverse community is challenging to all health professionals. Personal views, beliefs, values and practices of death and dying are heavily influenced by cultures, traditions, customs and religions. More studies are required to explore how culture, language and specific diseases impact on people's capacity to complete ACDs.

REFERENCE

Sinclair C, Sellars M, Buck K et al (2020) Association between region of birth and advance care planning documentation among older Australian migrant communities: A multi-center audit study. The Journals of Gerontology Series B:gbaa127.

Practice Scenario

Mrs Kelly Lee is a 70-year-old woman who has been admitted to your medical ward with a diagnosis of liver cancer. Kelly has a long history of diabetes mellitus type 2, which has been well managed with medications, diet and exercise. One year ago, she was diagnosed with liver cancer and recently noticed lumps under the ribs. She was admitted to the medical ward for a procedure to biopsy the lumps.

Kelly migrated to Australia from China in 2009. Her husband died two years ago and she now lives with her son Mark and his family. She knows she has liver cancer, but has been receiving treatment and believes her health condition is generally good. Mark teaches maths at the local high school and is married with three young children. He has recently changed his work hours so that he can care for his mother.

After the biopsy procedure, the surgeon visits Kelly and Mark on the ward. He gives them the biopsy results which reveal that the lumps are cancerous, meaning that Kelly's liver cancer has metastasised. He has organised for Kelly to stay on the ward for further tests to determine the spread and treatment options.

QUESTIONS:

1. What are the benefits of advance care planning for Kelly and her family?
2. Who should be involved in discussions about advance care planning for Kelly?
3. How could the nurse start a conversation with Kelly about her preferences for future care?
4. How could the nurse apply the PREPARED communication process in discussions with Kelly about her end-of-life care?
5. Kelly asks the nurse about options for euthanasia. How could the nurse respond?

REFERENCES

Advance Care Planning Australia (2020) Advance care planning Australia. Online. Available: www.advancecareplanning.org.au

Advance Care Planning Australia (2018) Advance care planning in Western Australia. Frequently asked questions. Online Available: www.advancecareplanning.org.au/resources/advance-care-planning-for-your-state-territory/wa

Allen W (1975) Without feathers. Warner Books, London.

Australian Commission on Safety and Quality in Health Care (ACSQHC) (2015) National consensus statement: essential elements for safe and high-quality end-of-life care. Sydney. Online. Available: www.safetyandquality.gov.au/sites/default/files/migrated/National-Consensus-Statement-Essential-Elements-forsafe-high-quality-end-of-life-care.pdf

Australian Government Department of Health (2018) National palliative care strategy 2018. Canberra. Online. Available: www.health.gov.au/resources/publications/the-national-palliative-care-strategy-2018

Australian Institute of Health and Welfare (AIHW) (2020) Deaths in Australia. Online. Available: www.aihw.gov.au/reports/life-expectancy-death/deaths-in-australia/contents/summary

Australian Medical Association (2015) Palliative approach in residential aged care – 2015. Online. Available: https://ama.com.au/position-statement/palliative-approach-residential-aged-care-2015

Brinkman-Stoppelenburg A, Rietjens JA, van der Heide A (2014) The effects of advance care planning on end-of-life care: a systematic review. Palliative Medicine 28: 1000–1025.

Cherny NI, Fallon MT, Kassa S et al (2015) Oxford textbook of palliative medicine. Oxford University Press, Oxford.

Clayton JM, Hancock KM, Butow PN et al (2007) Clinical practice guidelines for communicating prognosis and end-of-life issues with adults in the advanced stages of a life-limiting illness, and their caregivers. Medical Journal of Australia 186(S12):S77–S105.

Dementia Australia (2020) Dementia statistics: Key facts and statistics. Online. Available: www.dementia.org.au/statistics

Detering KM, Buck K, Ruseckaite R et al (2019) Prevalence and correlates of advance care directives among older Australians accessing health and residential aged care services: multicentre audit study. British Medical Journal Open 9(1):e025255.

Detering KM, Hancock AD, Reade MC et al (2010) The impact of advance care planning on end of life care in elderly patients: randomised controlled trial. British Medical Journal 340:c1345.

Government of Western Australia Department of Justice. (2020). Making treatment decisions. Online. Available: www.publicadvocate.wa.gov.au/M/making_treatment_decisions.aspx?uid=4727-3795-2343-5639

Health and Disability Commissioner (2020) Advance directives and enduring powers of attorney. Online. Available: www.hdc.org.nz/your-rights/about-the-code/advance-directives-enduring-powers-of-attorney/

Health Navigator New Zealand (2020) Palliative care overview. Online. Available: www.healthnavigator.org.nz/health-a-z/p/palliative-care/palliative-care-overview/

Hospice New Zealand (2019) Hospice New Zealand Standards for palliative care. Wellington.

Institute for Health Metrics and Evaluation (2017) New Zealand. Online. Available: www.healthdata.org/new-zealand

Institute of Medicine (US) Committee on Care at the End of Life (1997) In: Field MJ & Cassel CK (eds) Approaching death: improving care at the end of life. National Academies Press, Washington.

Kehl KA, Kowalkowski JA (2013) A systematic review of the prevalence of signs of impending death and symptoms in the last 2 weeks of life. American Journal of Hospice and Palliative Medicine 30(6):601–616.

Marie Curie Cancer Care (2014) Difficult conversations with dying people and their family. Online. Available: www.mariecurie.org.uk/globalassets/media/documents/policy/policy-publications/march-2014/difficult-conversations-with-dying-people-and-their-families—executive-summary.pdf

Meier EA, Gallegos JV, Thomas LPM et al (2016) Defining a good death (successful dying) literature review and a call for research and public dialogue. The American Journal of Geriatric Psychiatry 24(4):261–271.

Ministry of Justice (2020) Powers to make decisions for others. Online. Available: www.justice.govt.nz/family/powers-to-make-decisions/

Munday T, Poon P (2019) Geriatricians' attitudes towards voluntary assisted dying: A survey of Australian and New Zealand Society for Geriatric Medicine members. Australasian Journal on Ageing 39(1):e40–e48.

Murray SA, Kendall M, Boyd K et al (2005). Illness trajectories and palliative care. British Medical Journal 330(7498):1007–1011.

New Zealand Herald (2020) Euthanasia referendum: Doctors prepare to put law into action. 2 November. Online. Available: www.nzherald.co.nz/nz/euthanasia-referendum-doctors-prepare-to-put-law-into-action/H5DB2FWNU6Y7OJUKRVKTMXRQVI/

PalliAGED (2020) Terminal care. Online. Available: www.palliaged.com.au/tabid/4470/Default.aspx

Palliative Care Australia (2018) National Palliative Care Standards, 5th edn. http://palliativecare.org.au/standards

Palliative Care Australia (n.d.) What is palliative care? Online. Available: https://palliativecare.org.au/what-is-palliative-care

Queensland Health (2019) Care plan for the dying person: health professional guidelines. Online. Available: https://clinicalexcellence.qld.gov.au/resources/clinical-pathways/care-plan-dying-person

St Christopher's Hospice (2020) Dame Cicely Saunders: Her life and work. Online. Available: www.stchristophers.org.uk/about/damecicelysaunders.

Stats NZ (2020) Births and deaths: Year ended June 2020. Online. Available: www.stats.govt.nz/information-releases/births-and-deaths-year-ended-june-2020

Sudore RL, Lum HD, You JJ et al (2017) Defining advance care planning for adults: a consensus definition from a multi-disciplinary Delphi panel. Journal of Pain and Symptom Management 53(5):821–832.e1.

Supportive and Palliative Care Indicators Tool (SPICT) (2020) The Supportive and Palliative Care Indicators Tool (SPICT™). Online. Available at: www.spict.org.uk/

Therapeutic Guidelines (2020) eTG complete: Terminal care: care in the last days of life. Online. Available: https://tgldcdp.tg.org.au/index#toc_d1e258

Toye C, Blackwell S, Maher S et al (2012) Guidelines for a palliative approach for aged care in the community setting: A suite of resources. Australasian Medical Journal 5(11):569–574.

Wei L, Walters J, Guo Q et al (2019) Meaningful and culturally appropriate palliative care for Chinese immigrants with a terminal condition: A qualitative systematic review protocol. JBI Database of Systematic Reviews and Implementation Reports 17(12):2499–2505.

Williams MA, Wheeler MS (2001) Palliative care: what is it? Home Healthcare Nurse 19(9):550–557.

Woo E (2012) Dr William Lamers Jr dies at 80; championed modern hospice care. Los Angeles Times. Online. Available: www.latimes.com/local/obituaries/la-xpm-2012-feb-19-la-me-william-lamers-20120219-story.html

World Health Organisation (WHO) (2020a) Palliative care: key facts. Online. Available: www.who.int/news-room/fact-sheets/detail/palliative-care

World Health Organisation (WHO) (2020b) WHO definition of palliative care. Online. Available: www.who.int/cancer/palliative/definition/en/

CHAPTER 18

Safety and Security

DANA DERMODY

LEARNING OBJECTIVES

After reading this chapter, you will be able to:

- discuss common safety and security issues of concern to older people
- describe types of natural disasters and implications for the safety of older people
- identify the risk factors and implications of homelessness in older adults
- understand the challenges in balancing road safety in older drivers with independence and quality of life
- describe innovative technologies used to facilitate ageing in place and quality of life.

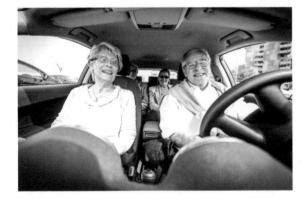

INTRODUCTION

Ageing brings with it a myriad of physiological changes that increase an older person's vulnerability to certain situations. Cognitive impairment, which can have an impact on decision-making and critical thinking, places some older people at risk of becoming victims of crimes,

including scams and fraud. Older people are also more vulnerable to extremes in climate, as they have less physiological ability to regulate temperature and declining muscle mass, muscle strength, total body water and intracellular water, which increase the risk of dehydration. Age-related vision and hearing impairment can reduce the older person's ability to detect hazards or to react to sudden environmental changes. This can be of particular concern when an older person is undertaking an activity in rapidly changing conditions, such as driving a car or facing an unpredictable natural hazard such as bushfire. Age-related decline in immune function and higher prevalence of co-morbidities in older age also tend to increase an older person's chance of succumbing during an infection epidemic or pandemic.

SAFETY AND SECURITY CONCERNS IN OLDER PEOPLE

Older people may be targets of crimes including scams, fraud and identify theft. 'Elder abuse' is the term generally used to describe 'a single, or repeated act, or lack of appropriate action, occurring within any relationship where there is an expectation of trust which causes harm or distress to an older person' (World Health Organisation [WHO] n.d.:3). Elder abuse can include physical, psychological or emotional, sexual and financial abuse (see Chapter 27). Crimes may be perpetrated by third parties unknown to the victim, or by family, friends or carers.

Evidence shows that Australians aged 55 years and older were significantly less likely than all other age groups to experience physical assault in the past 12 months (Australian Bureau of Statistics [ABS] 2019). Furthermore, older Australians were less likely than any other age group to have experienced face-to-face threatened assault (ABS 2019). However, the Royal Commission into Aged Care Safety and Quality (2019) recently acknowledged that many older people living in the aged care environment are experiencing physical harm and neglect. Older Australians are also increasingly vulnerable to perpetrators of dishonest schemes, often referred to as scams, and in 2018 submitted over 26,400 reports to Scamwatch amounting to losses of over AU$21.4 million (Australian Competition and Consumer Commission [ACCC] 2019). Estimates show that financial abuse affects 1.1% of older people in Australia, while consumer fraud is estimated to affect 5% of older Australians (Gardiner et al 2015). In New Zealand, the number of scams targeting older adults continues to rise; however, the direct financial loss associated with these scams is decreasing (Computer Emergency Response Team New Zealand [CERT NZ] 2019). This indicates an increasing ability among older people to identify scams and take appropriate action to protect themselves and their finances (CERT NZ 2019).

According to the ACCC, older Australians are often targeted by scams because they are more likely to have accumulated wealth and may be less familiar with technology (ACCC 2019). Older people with cognitive impairment may have compromised decision-making, placing them at greater risk of falling victim to fraudsters (Duke Han et al 2016; Wood & Lichtenberg 2017). Common scams targeting older Australians include schemes focusing on dating and romance, investments, unexpected prizes/lottery wins, inheritance and financial rebates (ACCC 2019). These dishonest schemes generally use deceptive tactics to obtain money or to gain access to personal information or financial information (ACCC 2019). In addition to financial loss, such fraud may place older people at risk of poor health outcomes (Sullivan-Wilson & Jackson 2014). Older victims may feel embarrassed or ashamed to have been duped and reluctant to report the incident (Sullivan-Wilson & Jackson 2014). Nurses can play a role in encouraging older people to report incidents to appropriate authorities.

Nurses and other health professionals are well placed to identify elder abuse (see Chapter 27), and signs of diminished financial and decision-making capacity that may leave an older person vulnerable to scams and fraud (Gardiner et al 2015). Nurses can provide education to older people in how to recognise signs of potentially deceptive schemes and the importance of financial planning (Gardiner et al 2015). In some cases it may be appropriate to refer the older person for a formal assessment, such as, depending on the concern, by a general practitioner (GP) or allied health professional (Gardiner et al 2015), or the Aged Care Assessment Team (ACAT), which is required for the older adult to access government-funded services and support. Nurses can also educate the older adult, family and carers about the signs of elder abuse (see Chapter 27), including financial exploitation and fraud (Sullivan-Wilson & Jackson 2014).

Tips for Best Practice
Elder Abuse

Be familiar with elder abuse assessment tools and protocols for the geographic location in which you work.

EXAMPLES OF TOOLS AND PROTOCOLS
Elder Abuse Prevention Unit (2012) A guide for elder abuse protocols. Queensland Government. Available: www.eapu.com.au/uploads/EAPU_general_resources/EA_Protocols_FEB_2012-EAPU.pdf
Alliance for the Prevention of Elder Abuse: Western Australia (2018) Elder abuse protocol: guidelines for action. Government of Western Australia, Department of Communities, Perth. Available: https://publicadvocate.wa.gov.au/_files/Elder-Abuse-Protocols-2018.pdf

---

NATURAL DISASTERS: IMPLICATIONS FOR OLDER PEOPLE

As well as what some describe as 'the silver tsunami' of an ageing population, Australia and New Zealand are facing an increase in the frequency and severity of natural hazards (Fountain et al 2019; Tuohy & Stephens 2016). Natural hazards in Australia include heatwaves, bushfires, droughts, floods, severe storms and tropical cyclones (Fountain et al 2019; Verity et al 2020), while New Zealand commonly experiences earthquakes and volcanic events. Both countries are at risk of pandemic infections (Verity 2020). Older people are especially at risk of harm from these events, which may also present a challenge for the growing 'ageing in place' movement (Astill & Miller 2017; Tuohy & Stephens 2016). In 2020, the COVID-19 pandemic proved far more hazardous for older people, with mortality rates estimated to be higher in people aged 60 years or older, and up to 13.4% in those aged 80 years and over (Verity et al 2020) (see Chapter 10, New and Emerging Diseases section).

Natural hazards have the potential to cause significant harm to the individual and the community. In addition to injury and fatality, natural hazards may disrupt telecommunications, transport, health, energy utilities, access to food and water, agriculture and employment (Astill & Miller 2017; Gilmartin et al 2019). Older people who are highly dependent on these services may be displaced for long periods of time, including being left homeless (Holle et al 2019). The impact on health services may extend beyond the initial disaster period, with research from the United States indicating higher rates of all-cause hospital admission up to 30 days after one natural hazard event which entailed a superstorm bearing multiple tornadoes (Bell et al 2018). As this evidence suggests, the vulnerable, such as those in older age groups, may remain at risk of harm despite the immediate threat having passed (Bell et al 2018).

Natural hazards are not necessarily experienced equally across the community. Some groups, particularly those who are physically, culturally, politically or otherwise disadvantaged, may be disproportionately impacted by natural hazards (O'Donnell & Forbes 2016). In the initial phase, older people may be less able to escape the hazard as they frequently lack the transportation, financial resources and family support required during an evacuation (Kim & Zakour 2017). Older people may be particularly at risk of poor outcomes when a natural disaster exacerbates physical and mental health issues, reduces access to health services, disrupts services and in-home care and restricts public transport (Gilmartin et al 2019). Furthermore, trauma from a natural hazard event, and possible displacement, may cause a significant decrease in cognitive abilities for older people with dementia or may lead to delirium (see Chapter 26) (Holle et al 2019). Older people with dementia are at particular risk in a natural hazard event due to the potential for increased confusion, anxiety and behavioural changes (Schnitker et al 2019).

PREPARING FOR THE UNEXPECTED TO KEEP OLDER PEOPLE SAFE

Older people are more vulnerable to harm from extreme temperatures, such as heat waves or cold snaps, due to physiological changes that impair thermoregulation (Balmain et al 2018). Health professionals are well placed to identify older people at most risk and initiate discussions about management strategies (Fountain et al 2019). These strategies may include increasing fluid intake, the use of emergency buttons and using available resources such as air-conditioning or heaters (Fountain et al 2019).

Preparedness to cope with unforeseen events, such as natural hazards, is linked to an older person's general health and wellbeing. Levels of informal social support and community membership have been identified as predictors of disaster preparedness (Kim & Zakour 2017), while spirituality and a positive attitude significantly predict survivor resilience (Almazan et al 2018). On this basis, nurses and other health professionals can help prepare older people for the unexpected through provision of holistic healthcare that fosters social engagement and support to maintain spiritual strength.

Nurses working with older people in the community can promote their preparedness for natural disaster (Fountain et al 2019), the key challenge of which is the lack of warning (Schnitker et al 2019). Planning is crucial. The Australian Red Cross provides free resources to assist with natural hazard preparedness, including *Emergencies happen: protect what matters most guide* (known as the RediPlan), designed for use by all age groups (Australian Red Cross 2016). The RediPlan provides a step-by-step template to assist people to prepare for an emergency. The template considers not only healthcare needs, mobility and important contacts, but also the individual's social connections and having local relationships in place (Australian Red Cross 2016).

Technology can play an important part in both preparing for and recovering from a natural disaster. Electronic warning systems and alerts, social media, general information and communication technology can all support information sharing (Fountain et al 2019). However, older people, who may be less digitally literate, can miss out on critical information (Fountain et al 2019). Depending on the context, nurses have a role in encouraging older people to 'upskill' in digital communication, or facilitate access to information and communication through other less technical modes of communication. From another perspective, increasing use of digital health is improving the ability for people to access healthcare during and after a natural hazard event. In 2019, the use of the Australian 'My Health Record' system, which holds an online summary of individuals' health information, demonstrated the value of being able to access electronically stored health information during severe floods (Australian Digital Health Agency [ADHA] 2019). Anecdotal reports indicated how the system was used by pharmacies to ensure that people who were displaced or unable to contact usual health providers were still able to obtain required medications (ADHA 2019). Nurses have a role in explaining this digital health record system to older people and its implication in both routine healthcare and times of disruption.

Promoting Wellness
Emergency Preparedness for Older Adults

- Create an emergency plan with the older person and their family members that will fit their needs, so that they are prepared for potential natural disasters.
- Create a care plan and keep a copy in the emergency supply kit.
- Work with the older person, their family members and neighbours, to create an emergency supply kit, as well as a list of elderly neighbours to check on and provide special assistance, if needed.

BASIC DISASTER SUPPLIES MAY INCLUDE THE FOLLOWING:*

- Water (about 4 litres per person per day for at least 3 days for drinking and sanitation)
- Food (at least a three-day supply of non-perishable food considering medical/allergy needs (gluten free, sugar free, etc.))
- Battery-powered or hand-crank radio and battery-powered radio tuned to the local radio station to listen for weather and warning updates
- Torch
- Extra batteries
- Whistle (to signal for help)
- Mask to filter contaminated air
- Manual can opener
- Mobile phone with chargers and backup battery
- Blankets
- Complete change of clothing appropriate to the geographic location
- Fire extinguisher
- Matches/lighter in waterproof container
- Paper and pencils/pens
- Moist towelettes, alcohol hand sanitiser

*Note this will depend on the geographic location and the unique needs of the older person; for example, rurally dwelling older adults' supplies may need to be increased for longer durations. Family Caregiver Alliance (2012).

Promoting Wellness
Emergency Preparedness for Older Adults

BASIC MEDICAL SUPPLIES MAY INCLUDE THE FOLLOWING:*

- A 3-day supply of medicine, at a minimum. If medications need to be kept cold, have a cooler and ice packs available.
- ID band: Full name, contact number for family member/caregiver, and allergies
- Hearing aids and extra batteries
- Glasses and/or contact lenses and contact solution
- Medical supplies such as syringes or extra batteries for devices, e.g. blood glucose monitor
- Information about medical devices, such as wheelchairs, walkers and oxygen, including model numbers and vendors
- Important documents should be kept in a waterproof bag; photo of each document should be taken for backup:
  - the care plan
  - contact information for family members, doctors, pharmacies and/or caregivers
  - list of all medications, including the exact name of the medicine and the dosage, and contact information for pharmacy and doctor who prescribed medicine
  - list of allergies to foods or medicines
  - copies of medical insurance cards
  - copies of a photo ID
  - copies of medical living will/enduring or durable power of attorney for health

*Note this will depend on the geographic location and the unique needs of the older person; for example, rurally dwelling older adults' supplies may need to be increased for longer durations. Family Caregiver Alliance (2012).

VULNERABLE OLDER PEOPLE AND HOMELESSNESS

Homelessness is a significant problem in Australia for people of all ages, but it is emerging as an increasing concern for older Australians (Australian Institute of Health and Welfare [AIHW] 2018). Importantly, homelessness does not just include situations where someone does not have a place to stay; it also includes inadequate living conditions. Homelessness is defined by the ABS as 'when a person does not have suitable accommodation … their current living arrangement is in a dwelling that is inadequate, has no tenure, or if their initial tenure is short or not extendable, or does not allow them to have control of, and access to, space for social relations' (ABS 2016).

With an ageing population and declining rates of home ownership in Australia and New Zealand, it is expected that homelessness will continue to increase (AIHW 2018; Johnson et al 2018). According to the AIHW, one in six homeless people in Australia were aged 55 years or over in 2016 (AIHW 2018). Homelessness among older people tends to present differently compared to younger people. While younger homeless people commonly live in overcrowded conditions, older people experiencing homelessness are more likely to report living in boarding houses, or staying temporarily with other households (AIHW 2020).

Causes of homelessness among older people are varied. For some, a relationship breakdown, trauma or having experienced child abuse may contribute to an individual becoming homeless (Bower et al 2017; Davies & Wood 2018). Other contributing factors include poor mental and physical health, and the use of alcohol and other drugs (Davies & Wood 2018). Importantly, homelessness further compounds these issues and places the individual at increased risk of poor physical and mental health outcomes, poor dental health, blood-borne viruses and a range of other health problems (Davies & Wood 2018).

It is difficult to ascertain data on specific older population groups experiencing homelessness. However, Culturally and Linguistically Diverse (CALD) older adults, older women, veterans and Aboriginal and Torres Strait Islander older adults may be at particular risk of homelessness. In New Zealand, Māori and Pacific people are at greater risk of homelessness because of a reduction in available state housing and increasing rental prices (Johnson et al 2018).

In 2018–19 in Australia, more women presented as homeless (58,700) than men (53,300) (AIHW 2020). Moreover, some researchers suggest that data used to determine rates of female homelessness are underestimated, as women are more likely to be living with friends or family, or in an unsafe environment (Petersen 2015). Risk factors for homelessness among older women include domestic violence, relationship breakdown and financial difficulty (AIHW 2018). Women are also more likely to experience poverty and financial hardship in older age due to the current superannuation system compounding the impact of the gender pay gap and the influence of family responsibilities on employment. In Australia, it is estimated that women retire with 47% less superannuation than men (Hetherington & Smith 2017). New Zealand shows similar trends, with the average woman retiring with NZ$80,000 less than a male (Groom 2018).

Older adults from CALD backgrounds face additional barriers to housing, such as language barriers, a lack of information in languages other than English and discrimination (White 2018). Aboriginal and Torres Strait Islander people are at risk of homelessness across their lifetime and older Aboriginal and Torres Strait Islander people are increasingly seeking support from specialist homelessness services, with an annual growth of 15.4% each year (AIHW 2018). Veterans may be at increased risk of homelessness due to distress, alcohol and other drug use, post-service relationship breakdown and unemployment (Hilferty et al 2019).

ROAD SAFETY IN OLDER DRIVERS

With an ageing population in Australia, it is no surprise that the number of people aged 65 years and older with a driver's licence is growing (Bureau of Infrastructure, Transport & Regional Economics [BITRE] 2017). Despite a decrease in road fatalities over the past decade, the rate of fatalities in older people has increased (BITRE 2017). In addition, older people involved in a road crash require longer periods in hospital, with people over 75 years spending an average of three days longer in hospital compared to people aged 25–54 years (BITRE 2017).

Older age alone is not a barrier to driving and chronological age should not be used as the sole criterion for driving ability (Austroads 2016; Kirk Wiese & Wolff 2016). It must be acknowledged that not all drivers over 65 years have reduced or impaired driving ability. The stereotype of older people as 'bad drivers' can be detrimental to driver ability (Lambert et al 2016). This supports the importance of focusing on functional ability, rather than generalising the ability of all older people based on chronological age.

Nevertheless, older age may bring changes that affect an older person's capacity to drive safety. These changes may include sensory, cognitive and musculoskeletal impairments, reduced motor function and a risk of sudden incapacitation (Austroads 2016). In some cases, the older person may have a progressive condition that will inevitably reduce driving ability as he or she deteriorates (Austroads 2016).

In Australia, there is no nationally consistent approach to assessing safety to drive in older people. In some states, drivers must undergo a medical assessment at 75 years, while other states have no mandatory driving assessments (Austroads 2016). The publication titled *Assessing Fitness to Drive 2016* sets out agreed standards for assessing medical fitness to drive for use by health professionals and licensing authorities (Austroads 2016). The standards establish assessment principles, which include consideration of driving task, as well as a clinical examination of various body systems, including physical and cognitive functioning (Austroads 2016).

Nurses can support older adults to maintain safe driving ability by promoting the importance of regular health checks, including eye examinations and regular exercise (Kirk Wiese & Wolff 2016). Changes in driver behaviour to maintain safe driving include:

- avoiding driving in bad weather and at night
- driving a familiar route
- avoiding distractions in the car (Kirk Wiese & Wolff 2016).

Some research also indicates that older people may self-regulate their own driving by:

- adjusting the frequency of driving
- avoiding certain driving situations (Bergen et al 2017).

In this way, older drivers can match their skills to the driving environment, enabling them to continue driving safely for longer (Conlon et al 2017). Nurses can promote and encourage driver self-regulation to support safe driving and maintain driving ability.

Nurses can also play an important role in identifying signs that an older person may be unsafe to drive. Indicators include:

- a change in medical condition
- a new diagnosis
- a history of previous road accidents (Somes & Donatelli 2017).

In some cases, presentation at an emergency department (ED) following a road accident triggers discussion about driving ability (Somes & Donatelli 2017), or family, friends or carers voice concerns about the older person's driving ability. In these instances, nurses can recommend the use of a driving self-assessment, such as that developed by the National Institute of Ageing (Kirk Wiese & Wolff 2016). The nurse is then well placed to facilitate communication between the older person and concerned family and friends (Kirk Wiese & Wolff 2016).

The loss of driving ability can have a significant impact on an older person's life. Consequences can include:

- reduced social interaction
- loss of independence
- social isolation
- depression
- reduced access to services (Stav 2014).

In contrast, however, some older people find that losing driving ability becomes an opportunity for better physical mobility. Research indicates that pedestrian travel is the preferred method of transport for older people, second only to driving (Stav 2014). For some older people, walking (with or without aids) is a viable option to maintain independence with the by-product of improving overall health and wellbeing.

The rise of innovative technologies may also help to overcome some of the challenges that arise when an older person's driving ability is becoming compromised. Firstly, new driver assistive technologies can take over some driving functions. Secondly, when the person ceases to drive, in-home technologies can promote social connectedness that might otherwise be lost. Advanced systems embedded in vehicles are increasingly commonplace. These systems include monitoring software that documents driving performance, warning systems that detect potential risks, such as blind spots or driver fatigue, and assistive technologies, such as adaptive cruise control, automated parking and emergency braking (Albert et al 2018). However, these innovations can present a paradox. While they aim to support driving ability, the new functionality in the car may create uncertainty for the driver and act as a distraction. It is therefore important that older drivers are trained and familiar with the technology to experience the safety benefits (Albert et al 2018). In addition to driving, smart home technologies, robotics, general information, communication technology and personal mobility devices offer opportunities to promote social engagement and independence once the older person is no longer able to drive (Khosravi et al 2016).

Tips for Best Practice

As many older adults prefer to age in place at home, family members will need to support the healthcare of their older family member. Nurses need to assess the knowledge, skills and capacity of the caregiver to provide care. In addition, the caregiver's wellbeing and health should be assessed to detect and prevent burnout and prevent more serious health problems for families in the long term (see Chapter 28).

Family Caregiver Alliance (2012).

TECHNOLOGIES TO SUPPORT OLDER PEOPLE AS THEY AGE

There has been explosive growth in digital technologies geared to empowering older people to facilitate a good quality of life and enable ageing in place. The concept of ageing in place refers to an older person's ability to live in his or her own home and community safely, independently and comfortably, regardless of age, income or ability level (Age in Place 2019). Gerontechnology is a term that was coined in the 1990s in Europe to describe a new, interdisciplinary field of scientific research focusing on developing technologies to support the holistic health goals of people as they age (Bouma & Graafmans 1992). Scientists working in this field develop and design products and services to promote good health and independence for as long as possible (Harrington & Harrington 2000).

There are many disruptive technologies that are being developed and integrated into the healthcare system. The idea that drones could be delivering urgent medications or blood to rural hospitals or individuals is not so far-fetched (Rosser et al 2018). Surgical procedures using robots are common in many hospitals (Cresswell et al 2018), and social companion robots, such as the animated seal PARO, have been studied in use with older people (Hung et al 2019). Virtual reality using head-mounted displays for older people is used to improve postural control to prevent falls, reduce pain and help with memory in those with cognitive changes (Dermody et al 2020). While no one can predict the future, reports have made it clear that the healthcare workforce, including nurses, must be prepared to use technologies in care delivery across the care continuum (Schwartz 2019; The Topol Review 2018).

Ageing in place gives older adults choice as to how and where they would like to age. Technological advances are the future of Health Smart Homes that could facilitate the desire of older people to remain at home for as long as possible. 'Smart Home' is a general term that is used when referring to in-home sensor technology. For example, products such as Amazon's Echo® and Alexa®, as well as Google Home® and Geeni™ support consumer comfort and also provide a level of security via interconnected devices such as motion-activated lights, sounds and security cameras. For example, Geeni™ provides cameras for the Google Home® device with an emphasis on safety and security within the home. Features include:

- both visual and audio live-streaming
- night vision technology, enabling the viewer to see clearly who may be outside at night
- two-way audio communication
- automatic recording in case of a security breach.

While a plethora of devices and software applications are available to enhance comfort and security, the emerging science creating smart-home sensor technology specifically designed for older people and persons with disabilities has the potential to take ageing in place to new levels.

The Health Smart Home is designed to remotely recognise changes in an older person's health status to facilitate early intervention (Dermody & Fritz 2019). Sensors placed strategically inside a person's home (usually ceilings and walls) collect a variety of data, including, but not limited to, the older person's:

- sleep
- general activity level
- walking speed
- interest in food via monitoring of the person's stove temperature and opening of the fridge door
- grooming
- toileting frequency.

Every person has a usual daily routine that may change with fluctuations in their health; for example, if a person is getting up later or spending more time in bed or in a chair. Alternatively, someone with a urinary tract infection is likely to use the toilet more frequently throughout the day. The Health Smart Home uses artificially intelligent (AI) algorithms to monitor behaviours of activities of daily living (ADLs) and detect these changes. The Smart Home can send nurses an alert that an unusual change has occurred. Remote monitoring is also available to enable health professionals to visually inspect data from motion sensors, picking up an older person's movement in order to make inferences about potential health problems and intervene if necessary (Fritz & Dermody 2019). Early intervention is important to reducing unnecessary hospital visits (Pollina et al 2017). The ability to intervene early and to provide integrated care in the home not only improves the quality of life of older adults, but also potentially reduces healthcare costs (Rantz et al 2015).

A variety of other health-related technologies are used, including telehealth and wearables. Telehealth is a concept that has gained popularity, especially to support isolated healthcare services and people living remotely, who may require access to specialist services. Bluetooth-enabled blood pressure cuffs, weight scales, glucose monitors, pulse oximeters and other similar devices are part of telehealth technology which older people can currently use in their home to monitor their health. Direct upload of these patient-collected assessment data to the Cloud (software and services that run on the internet instead of a local computer) means that information is readily accessible to a nurse or healthcare team remotely. This allows the healthcare team to monitor a patient's medical condition and wellbeing between in-person visits at the clinic or at

Research Highlight

A study evaluated a collaborative home fire safety program provided by three emergency services in New South Wales to vulnerable and isolated older people living at home. The Home Fire Resilience Project (HFRP) was an extension of a community-based program that installed and checked smoke alarms. The aim of the HFRP was to strengthen older people's preparedness for home fire emergencies. The HFRP involved a home visit by a firefighter to develop a fire emergency escape plan that included: having a working smoke alarm and knowing how to maintain it; finding out what to do if there was a fire at home and how to escape the home in an emergency; and making a plan to escape the home in the event of a fire.

The HFRP was offered to 1713 older people via the Australian Red Cross's Telecross program and 370 registered and completed a baseline survey. During the study period, 253 older people received a home visit, of which 156 completed a post-visit survey. Most participants were female (76%) and lived in private housing (88%). Although 58% were born outside of Australia, the vast majority (97%) spoke English at home. The mean age was 81 years (range 48–97 years).

Results indicated that after the home visit participants were significantly more likely to find out what to do if there was a fire in their home, make an escape plan, find out how to escape their home in an emergency, and how to maintain their smoke alarm. However, female participants were found to be less likely to have an escape plan than male participants. Additionally, people who spoke languages other than English at home were less likely to have a working smoke alarm. The authors concluded that home visit programs can increase the fire safety of vulnerable and isolated older people.

Tannous & Agho (2019).

home. Many older people and their family members express concern about whether the older person remains safe living alone at home. Remote health monitoring and telehealth offer an opportunity for older people who desire to age in place, particularly those in rural areas, to remain connected to and monitored by their healthcare team (Bradford et al 2016; Grant et al 2015).

A variety of wearable devices have been available and used by older people for quite some time. An example of one such technology is a pendant containing an alert button that can contact emergency services in the event of a fall, as well as alerting family members as to which hospital the older person has been taken. Another rapidly expanding market is that of wearable activity tracking devices, such as FitBit® and smart watches. These devices have enabled older people to monitor their physical activity (steps or distance ambulated), heart rate and calories burned. The next generation of wearable technologies has brought together health monitoring and emergency response features by connecting to the wearer's smart phone. Additionally, these devices will connect to the older person's Smart Home, enabling adjustments to be made to the living environment as required. The uptake of wearables, or any technology, can depend on a variety of factors such as perceived need, cost, user-friendliness and user experience with the technology (Alharbi et al 2019; Li et al 2019).

The ability to interconnect with other devices is a useful feature. For example, devices like the Apple™ Series 5 smart watch and the Garmin® wearable provide real-time heart monitoring and are compatible with the Cardiogram Heart Health application which interprets cardiac data, enabling the wearer to decide what action to take. Similarly, older people with diabetes can synchronise continuous glucose monitoring devices with a smart phone or other wearable device, providing rapid information about their blood glucose levels.

Innovations in hearing aid devices include smarter hearing technology coupled with artificial intelligence, termed 'hearables' (see also Chapter 20). These augmented hearing aids can assist older adults with age-related hearing loss to hear in very noisy environments, which is often difficult to achieve with conventional hearing aids. Using smart technology, the Oticon Opn™ hearable will connect to a person's smart home, enabling it to adjust according to the changes in the ambient noise level. There is also potential for new technologies to assist older people experiencing age-related vision changes (see Chapter 21). One company is developing specialised contact lenses that can correct conditions such as far-sightedness.

Overall, wearables provide a fairly inexpensive and reliable source of health data, which are particularly useful for older people, with potentially life-saving ramifications as several health conditions can be monitored. Features that allow the various wearables to be interconnected, along with remote health monitoring coupled with telehealth, can maximise the independence of older people living in the community. For those who desire to age in place, the sense of security and connection to a healthcare team can enhance wellbeing and quality of life, and enable early intervention to address health problems, potentially reducing the need for hospital care or the financial burden of entering residential aged care.

Practice Scenario

John is a 72-year-old farmer living in remote Western Australia. His wife died 3 years ago, and his two children live overseas. John is very attached to his home, especially as his wife is buried nearby. He mobilises well, loves his farm animals and still does some farming. He says it keeps him going and makes his life more enjoyable. Lately, his blood pressure has been high and he has complained of puffiness in both ankles. While he still drives a tractor on the farm, John does not have a driver's licence any more, making it difficult for him to get to a GP appointment in town. John is the son of immigrant parents who were also farmers. He worked on the farm from a very young age and did not attend school. John has one of his friends read him his mail, and while he has recently invested in a smart phone for safety reasons, John struggles to use it as he can't read. One of his neighbours informed him that he could access his aged care package to obtain support to manage at home. John was unaware of this but agreed that some aged care services could be helpful.

REVIEW QUESTIONS

1. Identify John's safety and security vulnerabilities.
2. Describe the technological approaches that could be used to support John's desire to remain living on the farm.
3. Develop an interdisciplinary care plan for John, including the technological approaches that could help to facilitate healthy ageing in place for John.

SUMMARY

Many older people are at increased risk of harm due to age-related changes in the body. Cognitive limitations can impact on an older person's decision-making, while physiological changes can leave an older person more vulnerable to extreme weather. Reduced mobility and vision can decrease the ability to detect and avoid hazards. Elder abuse can occur in relationships where there is an expectation of trust, but instead it causes harm or distress. Older people may be reluctant to report distressing incidents due to embarrassment or shame. Therefore, nurses are well placed to identify older people who may be vulnerable to or experiencing elder abuse, and to provide them with education or referral for a formal assessment. Nurses also have a role in supporting older people who experience homelessness, which disproportionately affects older women, veterans, culturally and linguistically diverse (CALD) and Indigenous people. While chronological age alone does not determine an older person's safety on the road, older age brings changes

that can affect driving ability. It is important that nurses identify signs that an older person may be unsafe to drive and promote regular health and vision checks and changes in driver behaviour to limit driving to safer times of the day and routes. New technologies, such as 'driver assistive' technology, 'smart homes', telehealth, 'wearables' and 'hearables' are empowering older people to remain independent and will facilitate ageing in place into the future, giving older people choice about where and how they live regardless of age, income or ability.

REFERENCES

Age in Place (2019) What is aging in place? Online. Available. https://ageinplace.com/aging-in-place-basics/what-is-aging-in-place/aa

Albert G, Lotan T, Weiss P et al (2018) The challenge of safe driving among elderly drivers. Healthcare Technology Letters 5:45–48.

Alharbi M, Straiton N, Smith S (2019) Data management and wearables in older adults: A systematic review. Maturitas 124:100–110.

Almazan JU, Cruz JP, Alamri MS et al (2018) Predicting patterns of disaster-related resiliency among older adult Typhoon Haiyan survivors. Geriatric Nursing 39:629–634.

Astill S, Miller E (2017) 'We expect seniors to be able to prepare and recover from a cyclone as well as younger members of this community': emergency management's expectations of older adults residing in ageing, remote hamlets on Australia's cyclone-prone coastline. Disaster Medicine and Public Health Preparedness 12(1):14–18.

Australian Bureau of Statistics (ABS) (2019) Crime Victimisation, Australia 2017–18. Online. Available: www.abs.gov.au/australia

Australian Bureau of Statistics (ABS) (2016) Census of population and housing: estimating homelessness 2016. Online. Available: www.abs.gov.au/Ausstats/abs@.nsf/Latestproducts/2049.0Appendix12016?opendocument&tabname=Notes&prodno=2049.0&issue=2016&num=&view

Australian Competition and Consumer Commission (ACCC) (2019) Targeting scams – Report of the ACCC on scams activity 2018. Online. Available: www.asial.com.au/documents/item/1838

Australian Digital Health Agency (ADHA) (2019) Annual Report 2018–19. Online. Available: www.digitalhealth.gov.au/about-the-agency/publications/reports/annual-report/Annual_Report_Australian_Digital_Health_Agency_2018–2019_Online.pdf.

Australian Institute of Health and Welfare (AIHW) (2020) Specialist homelessness services annual report 2018–19. Online. Available: www.aihw.gov.au/reports/homelessness-services/shs-annual-report-18-19/contents/summary

Australian Institute of Health and Welfare (AIHW) (2018) Older Australia at a glance. Online. Available: www.aihw.gov.au/reports/older-people/older-australia-at-a-glance/contents/diversity/people-at-risk-of-homelessness

Australian Red Cross (2016) Emergencies happen: protect what matters most. Your Emergency RediPlan. Red Cross, Carlton. Online Available: www.redcross.org.au/getmedia/b896b60f-5b6c-49b2-a114-57be2073a1c2/red-cross-rediplan-disaster-preparedness-guide.pdf.aspx

Austroads (2016) Assessing fitness to drive 2016. Online. Available: https://austroads.com.au/drivers-and-vehicles/assessing-fitness-to-drive

Balmain B, Sabapathy S, Louis M et al (2018) Aging and thermoregulatory control: the clinical implications of exercising under heat stress in older individuals. BioMed Research International 2018: 8306154.

Bell SA, Abir M, Choi H et al (2018) All-cause hospital admissions among older adults after a natural disaster. Annals of Emergency Medicine 71(6):746–754.

Bergen G, West BA, Luo F et al (2017) How do older adult drivers self-regulate? Characteristics of self-regulation classes defined by latent class analysis. Journal of Safety Research 61:205–210.

Bouma H, Graafmans J (1992) Gerontechnology. Amsterdam: IOS Press.

Bower M, Conroy E, Perz J (2017) Australian homeless persons' experiences of social connectedness, isolation and loneliness. Health and Social Care in the Community 26(2):241–248.

Bradford NK, Caffery LJ, Smith AC (2016) Telehealth services in rural and remote Australia: a systematic review of models of care and factors influencing success and sustainability. Rural and Remote Health 16(4):3808.

Bureau of Infrastructure, Transport and Regional Economics (BITRE) (2017) Drivers Licences in Australia. Commonwealth of Australia, Canberra. Online. Available: www.bitre.gov.au/sites/default/files/is_084.pdf

Computer Emergency Response Team New Zealand (2019) Quarter Three Report 2019. Online. Available: www.cert.govt.nz/assets/Uploads/Quarterly-report/2019-Q3/cert-nz-highlights-report-q3-2019.pdf

Conlon EG, Rahaley N, Davis J (2017) The influence of age-related health difficulties and attitudes toward driving on driving self-regulation in the baby boomer and older adult generations. Accident Analysis and Prevention 102:12–22.

Cresswell K, Cunningham-Burley S, Sheikh A (2018) Health care robotics: qualitative exploration of key challenges and future directions. Journal of Medical Internet Research 20(7):e10410.

Davies A, Wood LJ (2018) Homeless health care: meeting the challenges of providing primary care. Medical Journal of Australia 209(5):230–234.

Dermody G, Whitehead L, Wilson G et al (2020) The role of virtual reality in improving health outcomes for community-dwelling older adults: systematicreview. Journal of Medical Internet Research 22(6):e17331.

Dermody G, Fritz R (2018) A conceptual framework for clinicians working with artificial intelligence and health-assistive Smart Homes. Nursing Inquiry 26(1):e12267.

Duke Han S, Boyle PA, Yu L et al (2016) Grey matter correlates of susceptibility to scams in community-dwelling older adults. Brain Imaging and Behavior 10(2):524–532.

Family Caregiver Alliance (2012) Selected caregiver assessment measures: A resource inventory for practitioners. 2nd edn. FCA. Available: www.caregiver.org/selected-caregiver-assessment-measures-resource-inventory-practitioners-2012

Fountain L, Tofa M, Haynes K et al (2019) Older adults in disaster and emergency management: What are the priority research areas in Australia? International Journal of Disaster Risk Reduction 39:1–11.

Fritz RL, Dermody G (2019) A nurse-driven method for developing artificial intelligence in "smart" homes for aging-in-place. Nursing Outlook 67(2):140–153.

Gardiner PA, Byrne GJ, Mitchell LK et al (2015) Financial capacity in older adults: a growing concern for clinicians. Medical Journal of Australia 202(2):82–85.

Gilmartin MJ, Spurlock WR, Sinha SK (2019) Improving disaster preparedness, response and recovery for older adults. Geriatric Nursing 20:445–447.

Grant LA, Rockwood T, Stennes L (2015) Client satisfaction with telehealth in assisted living and homecare. Telemedicine Journal and e-Health 21(12):987–991.

Groom M (2018) Beyond the pay gap: the retirement disadvantage of being female. Policy Quarterly 14(1):doi.org/10.26686/pq.v14i1.4755

Harrington TL, Harrington MK (2000) Gerontechnology why and how. Shaker Publishing BV: Mastricht.

Hetherington D, Smith W (2017) Not so super, for women: superannuation and women's retirement outcomes. Per Capita & Australian Services Union. Available: asu-percapita-repoert--not-so-super-for-woment-v2-08-2017.pdf

Hilferty F, Katz I, Zmudzki F et al (2019) Homelessness amongst Australian veterans: summary of project findings. Australian Government Department of Veteren's Affairs. Online. Available: www.ahuri.edu.au/__data/assets/pdf_file/0019/46540/AHURI-Report_Homelessness-Amongst-Australian-contemporary-veterans_Final-Report.pdf

Holle CL, Turnquist MA, Rudolph JL (2019) Safeguarding older adults with dementia, depression, and delirium in a temporary disaster shelter. Nursing Forum 54:157–164.

Hung L, Liu C, Woldum E et al (2019) The benefits of and barriers to using a social robot PARO in care settings: a scoping review. BMC Geriatrics 19(1):232.

Johnson A, Howden-Chapman P, Eaqub S (2018) A Stocktake of New Zealand's Housing. Online. Available: www.beehive.govt.nz/sites/default/files/2018–02/A%20Stocktake%20Of%20New%20Zealand%27s%20Housing.pdf

Khosravi P, Rezvani A, Wiewiora A (2016) The impact of technology on older adults' social isolation. Computers in Human Behavior 63:594–603.

Kim H, Zakour M (2017) Disaster preparedness among older adults: social support, community participation, and demographic characteristics. Journal of Social Service Research 43(4):498–509.

Kirk Wiese L, Wolff L (2016) Supporting safety in the older adult driver: a public health nursing opportunity. Public Health Nursing 33(5):460–471.

Lambert AE, Watson JM, Stefanucci JK et al (2016) Stereotype threat impairs older adult driving. Applied Cognitive Psychology 30(1):22–28.

Li J, Ma Q, Chan AH et al (2019) Health monitoring through wearable technologies for older adults: Smart wearables acceptance model. Applied Ergonomics 75:162–169.

O'Donnell M, Forbes D (2016) Natural disaster, older adults, and mental health – a dangerous combination. International Psychogeriatrics 28(1):9–10.

Petersen M (2016) Addressing older women's homelessness: service and housing models. Australian Journal of Social Issues 50(4):419–438.

Pollina L, Guessous I, Petoud V et al (2017) Integrated care at home reduces unnecessary hospitalizations of community-dwelling frail older adults: a prospective controlled trial. BMC Geriatrics 17(1):53.

Rantz M, Lane K, Phillips LJ et al (2015) Enhanced registered nurse care coordination with sensor technology: Impact on length of stay and cost in aging in place housing. Nursing Outlook 63(6):650–655.

Rosser JC Jr, Vignesh V, Terwilliger BA et al (2018) Surgical and medical applications of drones: a comprehensive review. Journal of the Society of Laparoendoscopic Surgeons 22(3):e2018.00018.

Royal Commission into Aged Care Safety and Quality (2019) Interim report: neglect. Commonweath of Australia, Canberra. https://agedcare.royalcommission.gov.au/publications/Documents/interim-report/interim-report-volume-1.pdf

Schnitker L, Fielding E, MacAndrew M et al (2019) A national survey of aged care facility managers' views of preparedness for natural disasters relevant to residents with dementia. Australian Journal of Ageing 38:182–189.

Schwartz S (2019) Educating the nurse of the future report of the independent review of nursing education. Commonwealth of Australia. Online. Available: www.health.gov.au/sites/default/files/documents/2019/12/educating-the-nurse-of-the-future.pdf

Somes J, Donatelli NS (2017) Giving up the keys – the older adult driving in a rural setting. Journal of Emergency Nursing 43(1):74–77.

Stav W (2014) Updated systematic review on older adult community mobility and driver licensing policies. American Journal of Occupational Therapy 68(6):681–689.

Sullivan-Wilson J, Jackson KL (2014) Keeping older adults safe, protected, and healthy by preventing financial exploitation. Nursing Clinics of North America 49(2):201–212.

Tannous WK, Agho K (2019) Domestic fire emergency escape plans among the aged in NSW, Australia: the impact of a fire safety home visit program. BMC Public Health 19: 872.

The Topol Review (2018) Preparing the healthcare workforce to deliver the digital future. Interim report, June 2018. Online. Available: www.hee.nhs.uk

Tuohy R, Stephens C (2016) Older adults' meanings of preparedness: A New Zealand perspective. Ageing and Society 36(3):613–630.

Verity R, Okell LC, Dorigatti I et al (2020) Estimates of the severity of coronavirus disease 2019: a model-based analysis. The Lancet 20(6):669–677.

White G (2018) Housing related challenges for culturally and linguistically diverse communities. Parity 31(4):23–25.

Wood S, Lichtenberg PA (2017) Financial capacity and financial exploitation of older adults: research findings, policy recommendations and clinical implications. Clinical Gerontologist 40(1):3–13.

World Health Organisation (WHO) (n.d.). Ageing and life course: Elder abuse. Online. Available: www.who.int/ageing/projects/elder_abuse/en/

CHAPTER 19

Pain Assessment and Management

ROGER GOUCKE • SUSAN SLATYER

LEARNING OBJECTIVES

After reading this chapter, you will be able to:

- explain the differences between acute and chronic pain
- describe the biopsychosocial model of pain in older people
- explain the differences between nociceptive and neuropathic pain
- describe the components of a comprehensive pain assessment
- outline common non-pharmacological and pharmacological pain relief measures
- discuss considerations of pain in older people with cognitive and communicative impairments.

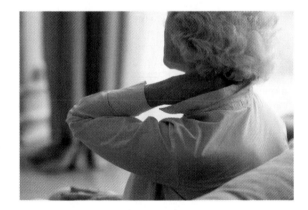

INTRODUCTION

In 2018, just over one million people aged 65 and over in Australia were living with chronic pain, which represented rates almost double that of the working population (Painaustralia 2019). In New Zealand, in 2018–19, an estimated 28% of people aged 65–74 years and 33.5% of those aged 75 years or older experienced chronic pain (Ministry of Health NZ 2020).

Pain can be defined as '… a distressing experience associated with actual or potential tissue damage with sensory, emotional, cognitive and social components' (Williams & Craig 2016:2420). Pain is classified as either acute or chronic. *Acute pain* usually has a sudden onset that coincides with tissue damage from an injury, surgery or other procedure, and which resolves as the tissue heals. *Chronic pain* is pain that persists after an injury has healed and is often defined as pain that persists for 3 months or longer. Older people tend to experience chronic pain due to pain-producing pathologies that are more common in later life. Pain can build gradually with the worsening of a chronic condition, such as arthritis, or the older person can be left with chronic pain after the acute pain of a condition such as shingles. Additionally, older people are at increased risk of injury and can experience acute pain related to tissue trauma on top of pre-existing chronic pain.

Acute Pain

Acute pain has an important function as a warning system to protect the body from mechanical, thermal and chemical injury. The experience of pain is unpleasant and as it becomes more intense will prompt the person to move away from the painful stimulus or seek treatment. Should injury occur, pain will then guide the person to avoid activities that might exacerbate the tissue damage (e.g. walking on a fractured ankle) and to undertake activities to promote healing (e.g. rest).

Chronic Pain

While acute pain has a vital protective role, many older people live with chronic pain that diminishes quality of life and increases disability. Pain is not a natural part of growing older, but rather is related to the increasing pathologies as people age (Australian & New Zealand Society of Geriatric Medicine 2016). Older people are more prone to developing conditions that impair function and many live with long-term, pain-producing diseases. Evidence has shown that older people tend to experience more complex pain problems, which often involve multiple sites in the body and multiple types of pain (Miaskowski et al 2019). Pain can fluctuate, but while it may vary in intensity, it will often be there to a certain degree. Common conditions that cause chronic pain in older people include:

- undertreated acute pain
- osteoarthritis (see Chapter 22)
- vertebral compression fractures
- chronic neuropathic pain (post-herpetic pain; diabetes)
- cancer and cancer treatments
- other chronic illnesses (Miaskowski et al 2019).

THE BIOPSYCHOSOCIAL MODEL OF PAIN

Pain is a personal experience built over a lifetime and influenced by the person's psychological, emotional and cognitive processes (Williams & Craig 2016). The biopsychosocial model of pain (Fig. 19.1) explains the subjectivity of the pain experience and why multimodal approaches are best to treat pain (Scherer 2019; Turk et al 2016). This understanding of pain brings together physical (biological) causes with the ways people think about pain and how they interact with others (psychosocial). While there is always some form of physiological change in the skin or muscles, the resulting sensory input is transmitted to the brain, where it is perceived, processed and given meaning (Turk et al 2016). Fig. 19.1 shows the three dimensions of factors that shape how a person feels pain (Scherer 2019). Importantly, these dimensions overlap.

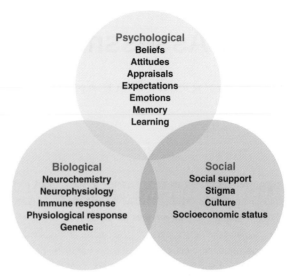

FIG. 19.1 **The biopsychosocial model of chronic pain.** (Goucke 2019:21.)

Biological aspects relate to physical changes in nerves, muscles and joints affecting neurological pathways that conduct pain signals. These changes can be due to:

- genetics
- the function of the immune system
- physiological responses to the unpleasantness of pain, such as activation of the sympathetic nervous system
- a number of co-morbid conditions
- behaviours (Miaskowski et al 2019; Seth & de Gray 2019).

In one systematic review of international studies, being female and of an older age were associated with higher rates of chronic pain (Mansfield et al 2016). An earlier population study conducted in New Zealand found that the presence of two or more co-morbid conditions not related to pain increased the likelihood of self-reported chronic pain (Dominick et al 2012). Fatigue and sleep disturbance (see Chapter 14) are associated with chronic pain, and linked to anxiety, depression, lower levels of physical activity and poorer physical wellbeing (Miaskowski et al 2019). Behaviours affecting physical function which are associated with chronic pain include smoking, with smokers reporting more chronic pain and more intense pain. Alcohol and substance misuse (see Chapter 25) are often seen in combination with chronic pain and add to the complexity of pain management (Miaskowski et al 2019). A relationship between chronic pain and obesity has also been demonstrated (Dong et al 2018).

Psychological aspects refer to the way an older person is thinking and feeling. These thoughts and feelings affect how the brain processes and interprets pain signals (Seth & de Gray 2019; Turk et al 2016). A person's beliefs about pain and what it means for their health is important in shaping their pain experiences. For example, an otherwise healthy person who has surgery to remove their appendix is likely to see the postoperative pain as 'normal' and manageable while the tissues heal. In contrast, a person with a history of cancer may view the onset of a new pain as a sign that the cancer has spread and become fearful, stressed and focused on the pain. Additionally, an older person's belief about how well they cope with pain can determine whether they adjust emotionally and engage in therapeutic interventions, or lose confidence and avoid activity that would help manage pain.

People with pain often experience emotional distress, because of both the meaning it may hold for them and the stress of ongoing physical discomfort. There is a body of evidence showing that stress, anxiety and depression in older people are associated with higher rates of chronic pain, more intense pain and increased disability (Miaskowski et al 2019; Turk et al 2016).

'Catastrophising' is a cognitive process whereby a person assumes the worst possible outcome in a situation and interprets even minor issues as major catastrophes (Turk et al 2016). This negative appraisal can influence how the person remembers events and expects things to happen in the future. It can lead the person to concentrate on the pain and feel helpless. The tendency to catastrophise about pain has been shown to define how people go on to experience pain episodes. Catastrophising is associated with more emotional distress in people with pain, more intense chronic pain in older people and more pain-related disability (Miaskowski et al 2019; Seth & de Gray 2019; Turk et al 2016). Examples of the types of things an older person who is catastrophising might say are:

- 'I can't go on like this.'
- 'I feel that my spine has collapsed.'
- 'I feel completely helpless.'

The *Tips for best practice* box on this page provides some examples of the language nurses can use to gently challenge these thoughts to promote the older person's coping and confidence.

Other psychological factors that influence an older person's experience of chronic pain include:

- *Pain-related coping* – how a person adjusts to their pain. How a person copes with pain can determine how much pain they report, their level of emotional distress, how well they adapt and how much disability

> **Tips for Best Practice**
> *Suggested Statements a Nurse Can Use to Gently Challenge an Older Person's Negative Thoughts About Pain*
>
> 'These tablets might not get rid of all your pain, but they should reduce it. Then we can try a small walk together.'
>
> 'You managed very well walking yesterday. Let's try another small walk today.'
>
> 'You have dealt with this pain before, and you can do it again.'
>
> 'If you plan your activities, you will find that you can usually avoid increasing your pain.'
>
> 'You have options to cope better with pain.'

they experience (Turk et al 2016). Evidence indicates that older people use a wider range of coping strategies when living with chronic pain than younger people and that their attitudes and beliefs can determine changes in daily activities (Miaskowski et al 2019).

- *Pain-related fear of movement* (also known as fear-avoidance) – when a person with chronic pain avoids undertaking a movement that he or she believes will trigger more pain (Miaskowski et al 2019; Turk et al 2016). This begins a cycle where the older person is constantly vigilant about pain and limits their physical activity, causing deconditioning of joints and muscles (see Chapter 22) that exacerbates pain and leads to decreased function and confidence and, ultimately, more disability (Seth & de Gray 2019).
- *Self-efficacy* – the personal belief that one can successfully perform certain activities to accomplish a particular task or deal with a specific situation (Turk et al 2016). When related to pain, self-efficacy is a person's expectation that he or she can undertake an activity and feel confident despite having pain. Lower self-efficacy has been associated with higher chronic pain ratings, and is a predictor for disability in older people with chronic pain (Miaskowski et al 2019; Turk et al 2016).

Social aspects relate to the influence the environment has on an older person's functioning and health, including the society in which they live, cultural factors and the built environment. These include:

- social supports (family and friends)
- quality of relationships
- work issues
- cultural issues

- financial security
- stigma
- level of isolation (de Ruddere & Craig 2016; Seth & de Gray 2019).

The level and quality of support available through family, friends and co-workers can influence how an older person responds to pain and engages with healthy coping strategies (Turk et al 2016). The supportive behaviours of others are generally beneficial and associated with older people reporting less pain, less distress and better adjustment to living with chronic pain. In contrast, social isolation and loneliness are both risk factors for and consequences of chronic pain in older people (Emerson et al 2018). Older people with less income and education have been shown to report more pain (Grol-Propopczyk 2017).

The influence of ethnicity on rates of chronic pain in older people is unclear (Miaskowski et al 2019). However, cultural factors can determine an older person's willingness to report pain and seek pain relief. Some cultures, such as Hispanic, Mediterranean and Middle Eastern, value the expression of pain and encourage people to communicate their pain verbally and non-verbally. In contrast, other cultures, such as those from Asia and Northeastern Europe, value a stoic attitude to pain, preferring that people keep their pain to themselves. The experiences of Australian Indigenous people living in two rural communities revealed a 'cultural preference for bravery' that influenced decisions not to communicate pain (Strong et al 2015:182). The Australian Indigenous people in the study also described past experiences of not feeling listened to and a resulting reluctance to talk about pain (Strong et al 2015). Older people from cultural minorities have also been shown to receive fewer prescription analgesics and use more complementary approaches to manage their pain (Lavin & Park 2014).

'Stigma' is an attribute or behaviour that causes a person to be socially discredited by others and classified as different to the social majority. People with chronic pain often experience stigmatising responses from others. This is because they usually do not have evident tissue damage to explain their pain and therefore deviate from the widely held belief that a clear pathology underlies the pain (de Ruddere & Craig 2016). The lack of clarity about an observable cause for the older person's pain report can cause others to react with confusion and uncertainty. There is ample evidence that people with chronic pain feel the effects of stigma. Many do not feel believed by family and friends or believe that health professionals think they are exaggerating or imagining their experiences of pain. In turn, health professionals, including nurses, doctors and physiotherapists, have reported a tendency to attribute lower pain scores to people who lack a physical reason for their pain or have chronic pain (de Ruddere & Craig 2016). Stigma is detrimental to a person's wellbeing and associated with poorer physical and psychological outcomes. This could be because the lack of acceptance from others causes a person with chronic pain to question themselves and the reality of their pain symptoms. Additionally, the person may feel a sense of injustice and the stigmatising responses of others may translate to fewer prescriptions of pain relief (de Ruddere & Craig 2016).

The biopsychosocial model of chronic pain explains why a person's report of pain is always subjective. In this model, aspects overlap to shape how an older person experiences chronic pain. For example, the physical discomfort of unrelieved pain causes stress and anxiety. In turn, this emotional upset and worry for what the pain might mean for their health leads the older person to focus on it, intensifying the physical sensation of pain. If the older person feels isolated by stigma and unwilling to seek help for fear of not being believed or because their cultural traditions value bravery, then without adequate treatment the physical pain may be prolonged. Psychosocial and behavioural variables that affect physical symptoms of chronic pain and that are also affected by the experience of chronic pain include:

- emotional state (affect)
- beliefs and expectations of pain
- coping resources
- sleep quality
- physical function
- interference with daily activities (Seth & Gray 2019; Turk et al 2016).

CONSEQUENCES OF CHRONIC PAIN

Chronic pain is detrimental to an older person's physical and emotional wellbeing, as well as their ability to function and to socially connect (Emerson et al 2018). Musculoskeletal pain is most common in older people and a major contributor to disability across the world (see Chapter 22). Unrelieved pain has been associated with more rapid memory decline and increased risk of dementia (Whitlock et al 2017), increased risk of falls (Stubbs et al 2014) and the development of frailty (Saraiva et al 2018; Sodhi et al 2020). Additionally, older people with persistent knee pain related to osteoarthritis have been shown to be twice as likely to develop depression as those with no knee pain (Sugai et al 2018). In summary, impacts of chronic pain on older people include:

- fear and loss of confidence to move and undertake daily tasks
- loss of physical function and fitness

- limited mobility
- development of frailty
- increased risk of falls
- increased risk of dementia
- poor sleep
- loneliness
- anxiety and depression
- disability
- potential for drug/alcohol misuse (Dominick et al 2012; Emerson et al 2018; Saraiva et al 2018; Sodhi et al 2020; Sugai et al 2018; Whitlock et al 2017).

TYPES OF PAIN

Pain can be classified as nociceptive or neuropathic. This differentiation is based on how the pain signal is generated, which has implications for treatment options.

Nociceptive pain arises from stimulation of pain receptors known as nociceptors. It is usually caused by some form of tissue damage in the skin, muscle, bone or mucosa. Common stimuli include:

- inflammation
- fracture
- ischaemia (inadequate blood supply to tissue)
- infection
- ulceration
- distension or obstruction of visceral (internal) organs.

Treatment consists of non-pharmacological approaches and pharmacological treatments that act on pain receptors in the peripheral and central nervous systems.

Neuropathic pain arises from damage to the neural pathways that carry or process pain signals. It is caused by a lesion or disease in the central or peripheral nervous system as a consequence of conditions such as diabetes, shingles, peripheral vascular disease or stroke. An older person will often describe neuropathic pain as:

- burning
- shooting
- tingling
- stabbing
- pricking.

See *Tips for best practice: Different characteristics of nociceptive pain and neuropathic pain* for more information on p. 230. Treatment can be very difficult and usually consists of pharmacological measures that modify nerve transmission and psychological approaches that promote coping abilities (Brooks & Kessler 2017).

AGE-RELATED CHANGES AND PAIN

As a person ages, there are widespread changes in the peripheral and central nervous systems that tend to increase the older person's pain threshold (Gibson & Farrell 2004). This means that sensations need to be stronger to be felt as pain. Additionally, the older person's tolerance of pain is reduced. This changed sensitivity to pain coupled with slower reaction times may place the older person at greater risk of injury. There is also evidence that the body's natural analgesic systems weaken and post-injury pain resolves more slowly with age, making it more difficult for the older adult to cope once injury occurs (Rajan & Behrends 2019).

PAIN IN OLDER PEOPLE WITH COGNITIVE IMPAIRMENT

It is not precisely known how people with cognitive impairment experience pain. There is a suggestion that degeneration of the nervous system associated with dementia (see Chapter 26) reduces some elements of the pain experience, although this has not been definitively established (Cravello et al 2019; Savvas 2019). Nevertheless, the high prevalence of persistent pain reported by older people generally would suggest that many people with dementia and other forms of cognitive impairment experience some degree of pain. It cannot be assumed that this pain is less bothersome than for people who are cognitively intact. Evidence has shown that older people with cognitive impairment receive less pain relief than their cognitively intact peers (Liu & Leung 2017). Additionally, unrelieved pain can commonly cause a person with dementia to display responsive behaviours (see Chapter 26), such as agitation, aggression or restlessness, driven by distress associated with significant discomfort (Savvas & Gibson 2015).

PAIN ASSESSMENT

Nurses have a responsibility to address pain. The nurse needs to understand the high prevalence of pain in the older population and be alert to verbal and non-verbal cues that an older person may be in pain. As part of the multidisciplinary team, nurses have a role in a 'pain vigilant' culture that prioritises the timely identification and management of pain (Scherer 2019). However, as described previously, older people can adopt a stoic attitude, preferring to 'grin and bear' pain and assume (wrongly) that it is part of growing old. Nurses who work with older people are well placed to identify and respond to verbal and non-verbal cues that the person is in pain.

A comprehensive assessment is the first step towards effective pain management. This assessment must always include the older person's experience of pain at rest and when moving. The nurse gathers information about the nature of the pain, the physical and psychosocial influences and the impact of the pain experience. This is important because different types of pain respond to different treatments. Additionally, understanding the complexities of the pain experience enable the nurse to use a holistic and collaborative approach to address the pain, ease distress and promote functional ability.

The most reliable indicator of the presence and severity of pain is the person's self-report of what he or she is experiencing. If the older person can talk about their pain, it is important to ask direct questions and listen to the answers. Some older people require more time and support to be able to express how they are feeling through words or movements. It may be useful to re-phrase questions to make it easier for the older person to answer, such as by asking 'Do you hurt anywhere?' or 'What is stopping you from doing what you want to do?' (Schofield & Abdulla 2018:325). The nurse may need to ask more often, using simple language and alternative words for pain.

The biopsychosocial model explains how each person's experience of pain is subjective and highly personal. How people express pain is similarly individual. An older person may describe their pain using words such as:

- sore
- ache
- hurt
- a niggle
- a nuisance.

Some older people may be reluctant to talk about their pain because:

- they think pain is a natural part of ageing
- they think pain is a sign that they are becoming more dependent
- they worry about becoming addicted to pain medication (Savvas & Gibson 2015).

The nurse has a role to gently challenge these beliefs. If the older person cannot or prefers not to talk about their pain, the nurse needs to observe closely for signs of discomfort. This means being highly attentive to non-verbal cues, such as pain on movement or facial expression (see *Tips for best practice: Non-verbal pain cues in older people*).

A comprehensive pain assessment is the first step to effective pain management. Pain should be assessed at rest and during movement, and at different times of the day and night (Scherer 2019). The 'PQRST' acronym (see *Promoting wellness: Pain assessment*) provides a useful set of questions to structure the pain assessment (Harris 2007). Using this acronym, the 'Q' component refers

---

Tips for Best Practice
Non-Verbal Pain Cues in Older People

Facial: grimacing; pleading expression; clenching teeth

Vocalisation: groaning; moaning; saying 'ouch'; crying without clear reason; vocalising more or less than usual

Physical changes: pallor; flushing; sweating; increased pulse and/or respiration and/or blood pressure

Protective behaviours: Limping; holding; rubbing; guarding (trying to reduce pain in a part of the body by keeping it still or not letting others move it)

Other behaviours: restlessness or agitation; clenching hands; changes in movement, such as unsteady walking; movements that cause facial grimacing or vocalisations

Activities of daily living: decreased appetite; decreased sleep; suddenly resistant to anyone trying to help

---

Promoting Wellness
Pain Assessment – PQRST Approach

These questions are worded to prompt the older person to give descriptive answers, not 'yes/no' answers. This will provide more insight into the person's pain.

P: Provokes or Palliates – What makes your pain worse? What makes your pain better?

Q: Quality – Please describe the pain (e.g. burning, shooting or tingling, indicating neuropathic pain, or sharp, indicating nociceptive pain)

R: Radiate – Where is the pain? Does it radiate (to other parts of the body)?

S: Severity – How intense is your pain? (can use simple numerical rating scale or a verbal descriptor scale) (see Figs 19.2 and 19.3)

T: Time – How long have you had the pain? Does it change over time?

Harris (2007).

---

to the quality of pain being experienced. The descriptive words an older person uses are particularly useful to indicate the type of pain (nociceptive or neuropathic), which will inform the appropriate treatment. Nurses need to understand the differences between nociceptive pain and neuropathic pain, as provided in *Tips for best practice: Different characteristics of nociceptive pain and neuropathic pain* on p. 230. Nursing assessment and documentation of the older person's description of their pain will assist diagnosis and treatment decisions.

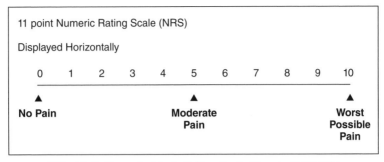

FIG. 19.2 **Numerical Pain Rating Scale** (Goucke 2019:153.)

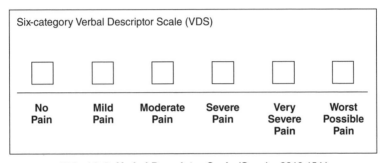

FIG. 19.3 **Verbal Descriptor Scale** (Goucke 2019:154.)

In the acronym, 'S' refers to the severity of pain the older person is feeling. Some older people may find it useful to self-report the severity of their pain using a numerical rating scale (Wood et al 2010) (see Fig. 19.2) or verbal descriptor scale (see Fig. 19.3) (Rajan & Behrends 2019).

The nurse should also ask what pain relief the person has received; if it was medication, when it was given; if it was a non-pharmacological treatment, did they use it and how effective had it been? It is also useful to know how the older person has managed their pain in the past. Other important questions relate to the older person's medical history, in particular pain-producing conditions, such as:

- arthritis
- cancer
- diabetes
- vascular or neurological diseases
- recent falls.

The nurse then supplements these questions with a physical examination. Body areas indicated as painful should be inspected for swelling, bruising, redness, heat and other signs of injury or inflammation. General observation of the person's movement and activities can yield information about the source and effect of pain. Observation of the older person's emotional responses, affect (level of emotional expression), sleep and family dynamics can reveal psychosocial influences on and impacts of the pain experience. The general principles for managing pain in older people are provided in the *Promoting wellness* box on p. 232.

Assessment and Cognitive Impairment

Pain assessment is particularly challenging when the older person has cognitive impairment. Many cognitively impaired older people have limited, or no, ability to communicate their pain experiences. In this group, pain often goes unrecognised, resulting in poor pain management (Nowak et al 2019; Schofield & Abdulla 2018). Therefore, the nurse needs to be extra vigilant and consider the following:

- Is the older person capable of self-reporting?
- Does this self-reporting seem reliable?

Tips for Best Practice
Different Characteristics of Nociceptive Pain and Neuropathic Pain

NOCICEPTIVE PAIN

- Tissue damage stimulates the nociceptors in the peripheral nervous system to send a pain signal along the spinal cord to the brain
- Tissue damage caused by:
  - mechanical injury
  - thermal damage
  - chemical release
- Examples: sprains, burns, headache, bumps, bruises, inflammation, obstruction
- Usually time-limited, resolves when the tissue heals (except for arthritis pain)
- Usually constant and easy to locate (except for internal visceral pain, which can be dull and episodic)
- Can radiate along a nerve root (e.g. sciatic pain radiates down a leg; gall bladder pain radiates to right shoulder tip)
- Words used to describe:
  - sharp
  - aching
  - throbbing

NEUROPATHIC PAIN

- Damage to peripheral or central nervous system that results in nerves sending aberrant pain signals
- Often caused by injury that has healed leaving scarred or compressed nerves that continue to generate pain signals
- Examples: post-herpetic neuropathy, diabetic neuropathy, peripheral vascular disease (ischaemic neuropathy), phantom limb pain
- Not time-limited. Can persist for months or years
- Usually presents as altered sensation or discomfort
- Can also cause 'allodynia' defined as non-painful stimulus such as a light touch being experienced as painful
- Words used to describe:
  - burning
  - shooting
  - tingling
  - stabbing
  - pricking

- Can the older person describe the impact pain is having, e.g. on their sleep?
- What does the older person's family think is the impact of pain on their loved one?

Many older people with cognitive impairment can report their pain when prompted (Cravello et al 2019; Schofield & Abdulla 2018). Knowing the prevalence of pain-producing conditions in older people can highlight 'red flags' (see *Tips for best practice: Red flags that indicate a person with cognitive impairment may be experiencing pain pain* on p. 232) that alert the nurse to the likelihood that the older person living with a cognitive impairment has pain, even though they may be unable to tell anyone (Savvas 2019).

Some older people with a mild to moderate cognitive impairment may be able to use a verbal descriptor scale to rate their pain (Cravello et al 2019) (see Fig. 19.3). However, assessment using an observational pain scale is warranted if:

- the older person cannot communicate verbally
- the nurse is unsure or suspects pain upon noting the older person's behaviour
- a 'red flag' condition (see *Tips for best practice: Red flags ...*) is present.

The Abbey Pain Scale (Abbey et al 2004) was developed in Australia, is quick to administer and assesses non-verbal pain cues including behaviour along with physical and physiological changes (see Fig. 19.4). It does not discriminate between pain and distress from other causes. Therefore, it is important to administer the scale again one hour after analgesia to see if the pain score improves, and then again regularly until the older person's pain indicators diminish.

INTERVENTIONS TO ADDRESS PAIN

The nurse may need to support the older person to report and address their pain. The aim of pain management is to promote comfort, maintain function and balance risks and benefits of pharmacological treatment options. The goals of pain therapy should be:

- developed collaboratively with the older person, family carer and multidisciplinary team
- to promote comfort, function and independence
- to balance treatment risks and benefits.

Acute pain is usually well managed with timely analgesic medication. However, complete relief of chronic pain, particularly neuropathic pain, may not be possible. Nevertheless, treatment can yield benefits for the older person, in terms of less discomfort and improved sleep and mobility.

A multimodal approach to treating pain in older people recognises the complex biopsychosocial factors

Abbey Pain Scale

For measurement of pain in people with dementia who cannot verbalise.

How to use scale: While observing the resident, score questions 1 to 6

Name of resident: ....

Name and designation of person completing the scale: ....

Date: .... **Time:**...................................

Latest pain relief given was...**at** ....**hrs.**

Q1. Vocalisation
eg. whimpering, groaning, crying **Q1** ☐
Absent 0   Mild 1   Moderate 2   Severe 3

Q2. Facial expression
eg: looking, tense, frowning grimacing, looking frighten **Q2** ☐
Absent 0   Mild 1   Moderate 2   Severe 3

Q3. Change In body language
eg: fidgeting, rocking, guarding part of body, withdrawn **Q3** ☐
Absent 0   Mild 1   Moderate 2   Severe 3

Q4. Behavioural Change
eg: increased confusion, refusing to eat, alteration in usual **Q4** ☐
patterns
Absent 0   Mild 1   Moderate 2   Severe 3

Q5. Physiological change
eg: temperature, pulse or blood pressure outside normal **Q5** ☐
limits, perspiring, flushing or pallor
Absent 0   Mild 1   Moderate 2   Severe 3

Q6. Physical changes
eg: skin tears, pressure areas, arthritis. contractures, **Q6** ☐
previous injuries.
Absent 0   Mild 1   Moderate 2   Severe 3

Add scores for 1 – 6 and record here ⟹ Total Pain Score ☐

Now tick the box that matches the
Total Pain Score ⟹

0 – 2	3 – 7	8 – 13	14+
No pain	Mild	Moderate	Severe

Finally, tick the box which matches
the type of pain ⟹

Chronic	Acute	Acute on Chronic

Dementia Care Australia Pty Ltd
Website: www.dementiacareaustralia.com

Abbey, J; Piller, N; De Bellis, A; N; Esterman, A; Giles, L; Parker, D and Lowcay, B.
Funded by the JH & JD Gunn Medical Research Foundation 1998 – 2002
(This document may be reproduced with this acknowledgment retained)

FIG. 19.4 **Abbey Pain Scale** (Source: Abbey et al 2004 CC 2.0. Funded by the JH & JD Gunn Medical Research Foundation 1998–2002.)

- Every older person deserves adequate pain management. Maintain a 'pain vigilant' culture that prioritises and addresses older people's pain.
- Pain management requires a multidisciplinary and multimodal approach.
- Pain is a subjective experience, shaped by the older person's biological, psychological and social factors.
- The older person's self-report is the best measure of their pain.
- Older people with mild to moderate cognitive impairment may be able to self-report pain when prompted. Use of a simple verbal descriptor scale may be helpful.
- Older people who cannot communicate should be regularly assessed for indications of pain using an observational pain assessment tool, e.g. Abbey Pain Scale.
- A blend of non-pharmacological and pharmacological approaches is most effective to treat pain, and may allow use of lower, and therefore safer, analgesic doses.
- Always start pain medications with a low dose, monitor closely, and slowly titrate doses upwards to achieve best possible pain relief with fewest side effects. **'Start low, go slow, but go'**
- Acute pain is usually well managed with timely analgesic medication.
- Complete relief of chronic pain, particularly neuropathic pain, may not be possible. Nevertheless, treatment can yield benefits for the older person, including less discomfort with better sleep and improved mobility.
- Consider age-related changes in medication effectiveness and metabolism and the potential for side effects (see also Chapter 11).
- Observe for and manage side effects of medication (may be more troublesome than the pain).
- Perform regular and frequent reassessment to identify treatment effectiveness and emergence of side effects.

Goucke (2019).

The following diseases, conditions, circumstances and environments potentially cause pain. Each warrants a rigorous pain assessment.

- Pain-related diseases, e.g. musculoskeletal conditions (see Chapter 22), diabetes, recent stroke, cancer
- Impairments in gait, e.g. speed, variability, unable to walk and talk
- Immobility, e.g. cannot weight bear, has contractures
- High friction factors, e.g chafing from clothing
- Obesity
- Poor nutrition or weight loss
- Skin breakdown, e.g. pressure injuries, wounds
- Recent surgery or medical procedure
- Responsive behaviours in older people with dementia (see Chapter 26)
- Concerns about pain from family
- Falls (see Chapter 16)

Savvas (2019).

A blend of non-pharmacological and pharmacological therapies is most effective, and may allow lower, and therefore safer, analgesic drug doses to be used (Cravello et al 2019; Stitzlein Davies 2017). Psychological approaches to calm emotional distress, which can make the pain worse, are important in any pain management plan. Physical treatments that change physiological processes in the body tissues, including superficial heat and cold, can reduce pain intensity, but are generally not recommended for regular pain relief and therefore are of limited use for treating chronic pain in older people. Tailored exercise programs and complementary therapies, such as tai chi and yoga, can help to manage chronic pain. When adding pharmacological treatment, the type and severity of pain guides the choice of analgesic medication.

Non-Pharmacological Approaches

Non-pharmacological strategies can be used alone or in combination with pharmacological treatments to reduce pain and provide comfort for an older person experiencing acute or chronic pain. The biopsychosocial model of pain explains how non-pharmacological strategies can target biological pain processes, psychological distress and/or social factors. As the overlapping nature of the

that interact to shape the pain experience. The prevalence of chronic pain in the older population requires an holistic approach that addresses pain processes in the central nervous system along with the various sources and impacts of pain.

model explains, non-pharmacological strategies often address several factors contributing to the older person's pain. For example, using gentle massage can:

- produce muscle relaxation that reduces pain signals
- calm emotional distress
- provide another sensation to distract the older person's attention away from the pain
- communicate a therapeutic presence that reduces isolation.

A brief summary of commonly used non-pharmacological comfort measures is provided.

Physical Treatments
Superficial heat and cold therapy

The application of heat or cold can modify pain signals to the brain. However, the effect is temporary and there are safety considerations when using with older people, particularly those who cannot feel heat or communicate their experiences (see *Safety Alert: Precautions when using physical treatments*). Application of heat to the skin causes vasodilation. It is best suited to the short-term use for acute pain that is expected to resolve quickly (Moore 2019). Older people with sensory loss, such as those with diabetes-related neurological damage, may sustain burns if they are unable to feel excessive levels of heat.

Cold packs act by cooling the skin and underlying tissues to temporarily reduce swelling and inflammation that can cause pain, and to reduce nerve conduction of pain signals. Cold therapy is best used within the first 48 hours after a traumatic injury, particularly muscle strain/sprain, which is common in older people, and applied intermittently. As with heat, cold should not be used with older people who cannot feel low temperatures or cannot communicate how they are feeling (see *Safety Alert*: *Precautions when using physical treatments*).

Transcutaneous Electrical Nerve Stimulation (TENS)

TENS works by applying a weak electrical charge to the skin with the aim of modulating transmission of pain signals in the peripheral nerves. It may be of use to relieve pain related to post-herpetic neuralgia (see Chapters 10, 15 and 21) and osteoarthritis of the knee. The TENS machine is small and portable and worn in a pocket or on a belt as the older person goes about his or her daily activities. While it can be left in place for long periods, it should not be used with older people who cannot communicate what they are feeling (see *Safety Alert: Precautions when using physical treatments*).

Mind and Body Approaches
Relaxation, meditation and guided imagery

- *Relaxation* involves quietening the mind and body and should be added to all pharmacological pain relief measures for all types of pain. Relaxation calms emotional distress and causes muscles to release tension, potentially reducing aches and pains. Deep controlled breathing and progressive muscle relaxation (tensing and releasing various muscle groups) can promote relaxation. Meditation and guided imagery are also useful.
- *Meditation* encourages the older person to 'detach from their pain by focusing on what is going on around them rather than what is going on inside' (Twigg & Wallace 2019:42). The older person needs to be able to follow simple instructions. Older people with mild to moderate cognitive impairment may be able to use meditation, but may require an individual session and the use of non-verbal gestures and visual cues.
- *Guided imagery* involves the older person listening to a gentle voice that evokes objects or activities that promote wellbeing. The older person visualises and imagines these images focusing their attention away from the pain and promoting muscle relaxation. Guided imagery can be done face-to-face with a trained facilitator or via an app, CD or online. Evidence suggests it reduces discomfort, stress, anxiety and depression (Mantopoulos 2019).

Massage

Gentle massage is widely used to promote comfort and relaxation. It involves manipulating the skin and soft tissues using various movements, such as kneading, rolling, tapping and pressing. Similarly, back rubs and hand and foot massages are relaxing and communicate care and a therapeutic presence that reduces stress and anxiety.

Tai chi

Tai chi is a gentle mind and body exercise that involves a sequence of slow controlled movements, breathing and concentration. When done regularly, it can help older people to build muscle strength and flexibility, and to improve balance. Studies suggest that tai chi in addition to medication can improve arthritic pain. It is also effective in reducing falls risk in older people (see Chapter 16).

Other Approaches
Distraction

Distraction involves diverting the older person's mental focus away to something other than the pain experience

Safety Alert
Precautions When Using Physical Treatments

Physical treatments for pain work by stimulating tissue in or below the skin. They include:

- superficial heat: hot packs
- superficial cold: ice pack, cold packs
- Transcutaneous Electrical Nerve Stimulation (TENS).

These treatments carry a risk of tissue damage. To minimise the risk of harm:

- use only with older people who can communicate to give feedback on the experience
- conduct regular pain assessment to determine any benefit
- use with caution on sensitive skin.

Note: skin sensitivity can increase with painful conditions such as diabetic neuropathy, post-herpetic neuralgia (Moore 2019).

SUPERFICIAL HEAT

- Do not use within 48 hours of pain onset to avoid increasing swelling
- Only use if the older person can feel heat
- Only use if the older person can communicate how much warmth they can feel
- Best for short-term relief of acute pain
- May be useful prior to stretching to relax muscle and nervous tissue.

SUPERFICIAL COLD

- Do not use for regular pain relief:
  - Cooling the skin over a long period can cause tissue damage

- Superficial cooling does not give long enough pain relief
- Cold therapy is not well tolerated
- Only use if the older person can feel cold
- Only use if the older person can communicate their discomfort
- Can help when applied within 48 hours of pain onset, but significant cooling required and not recommended for older people
- Older people report less pain relief from superficial cold.

TRANSCUTANEOUS ELECTRICAL NERVE STIMULATION (TENS)

May relieve some pain in certain conditions such as post-herpetic nerve pain and knee osteoarthritis.

- Only use if the older person can communicate how they are feeling
- Titrate level of stimulation by level of change in pain (measured by regular pain assessments)
- Excessive stimulation is uncomfortable.

Note: The brain will adjust and filter out TENS stimulation. Recommended use is: apply for 20 minutes, then turn off for up to 1 hour, then use with a 'pulsed' or 'ramped' setting that applies a constantly changing stimulation to the skin (Moore 2019).

---

and associated stress and worry. Distraction works by slowing transmission of pain messages to the brain (Jett 2018). When absorbed in another activity, the older person may become completely unaware of the physical pain or at least experience less intense pain. Common behaviours that provide distraction include:

- rhythmic tapping
- rhythmic singing
- listening to music
- rhythmic massage and breathing
- humour
- creative pursuits such as art, craft, playing music, gardening.

Acupuncture and acupressure

Acupuncture is an ancient Chinese practice that involves inserting fine needles into the skin at various points in the body. Acupressure involves using the thumbs or finger tips to apply pressure at the same locations. It is thought that acupuncture and acupressure stimulate nerves to block pain signals and/or stimulate the release of endorphins that act on opiate receptors reducing pain and promoting comfort. Evidence suggests that acupuncture is effective in reducing pain that arises in the back, neck and shoulder, and in osteoarthritis and headache (National Center for Complementary and Integrative Health 2016).

Pharmacological approaches

Analgesic medication is prescribed to relieve or reduce pain symptoms. These medications aim to alter the transit of sensory pain signals in the nervous system. They do not address the underlying condition causing the pain. In older people, individual responses to medication vary, with some reporting much improved comfort while others achieve only minimal pain relief with significant side effects. The goal of pharmacological management is to provide medication that achieves the best possible pain relief with the least possible side effects (Rajan & Behrends 2019).

A number of age-related changes in the body modify the way in which analgesic medication is absorbed, metabolised, distributed and excreted. Chapter 11 provides details on the safe use of analgesic medications in older people. These changes may mean that the medication's action is increased or decreased, or that the side effects are more pronounced.

The nurse must be alert to the older person's responses when giving analgesic medication, regularly reassessing pain levels and looking for signs or symptoms that indicate an adverse reaction.

The nurse must also be prepared to titrate dosages or change analgesics depending on response. With the older person, it is essential to begin with the lowest dose possible and build up gradually while not delaying dosage increases and prolonging the pain, particularly in those patients with cancer pain. In gerontological nursing, the adage holds true: 'Start low, go slow, but go!' (Jett 2018:243). It must also be remembered, however, that when treating many types of chronic non-cancer pain, the goal should be less pain rather than no pain.

Following a comprehensive assessment, the nurse will be aware of which type of pain and its severity is being treated: whether acute or chronic, nociceptive or neuropathic, cancer (or palliative) or non-cancer. This will dictate which medication, in addition to non-pharmacological approaches, should be used.

For acute nociceptive pain, for example, osteoarthritis, back pain or gout where inflammation may be a component, paracetamol and a low-dose non-steroidal anti-inflammatory drug (NSAID) can be used with caution. These options may also be useful in bone metastases from cancer. While pain persists, regular around-the-clock medications are preferred.

For acute *severe* nociceptive pain, a short-acting opioid can be added to paracetamol and the NSAID. Pre-emptive analgesia can promote comfort when given before the older person undertakes a painful activity (e.g. wound dressing), timing the activity for when the medication reaches maximum effect.

For acute or chronic, severe, nociceptive cancer pain, the recommendation is to start with a short-acting opioid, monitor the older person for effectiveness and any side effects, and then titrate doses to achieve the best pain relief possible with the fewest adverse effects. Initial doses should always be at the lower end with small incremental dose increases. Once adequate pain relief is achieved, the short-acting formulation is converted to a more convenient long-acting preparation and given regularly to achieve the required amount of medication over 24 hours.

> ### Safety Alert
> #### *Changing Opioid Formulations*
>
> Different formulations of opioid medications have different strengths. When converting formulations, the doctor will calculate equianalgesic doses and make a new prescription. The doctor will consider starting the new opioid medication at a lower dose, because people vary in the way they respond to opioids, particularly frail and older people.
>
> **The nurse has an essential role to carefully and regularly reassess the older person when analgesic medications are changed:**
>
> - **Are the older person's pain symptoms being controlled?**
> - **Is the older person experiencing any side effects?**
>
> More information is available at: PalliAGED (2019) Opioids: Switching between formulations. Online. Available: www.palliaged.com.au/tabid/5536/Default.aspx

For chronic nociceptive non-cancer pain, non-pharmacological strategies are preferred. Regular use of paracetamol may be helpful. Opioids are less effective and should be carefully managed. Side effects are common and worsening pain from hyperalgesia may occur. Keeping the opioid dose below a morphine equivalent of 50 mg per day has been recommended (Hogg 2019).

For chronic neuropathic pain, non-pharmacological treatments are recommended with consideration of low-dose antidepressant or anti-epileptic adjuvant medications (see below).

Non-opioid analgesics

The most common non-opioid analgesic medications used with older people are paracetamol and NSAIDs. Paracetamol is often used to relieve pain related to musculoskeletal conditions, including osteoarthritis (see Chapter 22). In general, older people can use paracetamol at the same doses as younger people (see Chapter 11), although lower doses may be required if the older person has frailty, low body weight (< 50 kg), or renal/hepatic impairment. Regular dosing (around the clock) is most effective; however, do not exceed the maximum of 4 g paracetamol in 24 hours (i.e. 8×500 mg tablets).

NSAIDs are used to relieve acute and chronic pain caused by inflammatory conditions.

NSAIDs can cause adverse effects, which include gastrointestinal, cardiovascular and renal problems (see Chapter 11). In general, they should be used in the lowest dose and for the shortest duration possible. The Australian Pain Society recommends that a 'review or stop order should be routine after two weeks of treatment' (Hogg 2019:81). It may be appropriate for the older person on NSAID therapy to also be prescribed a gastro-protective medication, such as a proton pump inhibitor. Topical NSAIDS, applied as a cream or gel, have been found to effectively relieve pain from osteoarthritis in peripheral joints (hand, knee) and the side effect profile is safer, as much less medication is absorbed systemically.

Opioid analgesics

Opioid analgesics are first-line treatment for older people with moderate-to-severe acute pain from trauma (e.g. fractured hip), cancer and those nearing the end of life. They are not recommended for chronic non-cancer conditions (such as osteoarthritis or neuropathic pain). In older people, opioid analgesics have a longer duration of effect, a higher peak effect, and a greater analgesic effect compared to younger people. However, older people are also more sensitive to the side effects of opioids, including:

- constipation
- sedation
- respiratory depression
- cognitive impairment
- falls
- nausea
- pruritis (itch) (Hogg 2019; Stitzlein 2017).

Opioids are not effective when treating neuropathic pain. *The Safety Alert: Education for older people who are taking opioid medication* box provides information that should be given to an older person on opioid therapy and their caregivers. Opioid medications can be classified as 'atypical', 'weak opioids' or 'strong opioids'.

Atypical opioids

- *Tapentadol* has a weak action on the *mu*-opioid receptors in the brain and spinal cord, and also blocks noradrenaline reuptake in the nervous system. This combination makes it useful to treat both nociceptive and neuropathic pain. Tapentadol has a potency of about one-third that of morphine and causes less constipation than other opioids and fewer interactions with other drugs. It is given orally and is available in immediate and modified release formulations (Hogg 2019).

Safety Alert
Education Topics for Older People Who Are Taking Opioid Medication

- Do not combine opioid medication with alcohol or other sedating medications. This combination increases risk of:
  - oversedation
  - respiratory depression
  - accidental overdose
  - death.

  Sedating medications include benzodiazepines (e.g. diazepam, temazepam); benzodiazepine receptor agonists (e.g zolpidem); muscle relaxants (e.g. baclofen); and sedating antihistamines (e.g. diphenhydramine)

- Fall prevention
- Driving safety: opioids increase reaction time and increase the risk of motor vehicle accidents
- Safe storage to prevent accidental overdose by child or pet or intentional theft
- Alert caregivers to signs of over-sedation and instruct to call an ambulance if older person becomes deeply sedated or unarousable (dial 000 in Australia; dial 111 in New Zealand)

Hogg (2019); Stitzlein Davies (2017).

- *Tramadol*, in addition to weak opioid receptor action, inhibits both noradrenaline and serotonin reuptake, leading to a combined analgesic effect. Tramadol's effects on the serotonin and noradrenaline systems produce a different side effect profile compared with typical opioids, including increased nausea, dizziness, tremors and headaches, although with comparatively less constipation and lower risk of respiratory depression. Due to its complex pharmacology and potential for serious adverse effects, *tramadol is no longer preferred as an early use analgesic in older people*.
- *Buprenorphine* is a semi-synthetic partial *mu*-opioid atypical opioid that works on several types of pain receptors in the central nervous system. In higher doses, it has similar analgesic effects to strong opioids. It is given sub-lingually or via a transdermal patch and tends to have fewer adverse effects, particularly less constipation and sedation. The ease of administration and low risk of constipation make it suitable for use in older people.

Weak opioid

- *Codeine* is a relatively weak opioid that is short-acting and often used in combination with paracetamol or

NSAIDS. It is given orally but has a direct effect on the gastrointestinal system, with significant potential to cause constipation. This is often a limiting factor against using codeine in older people (Hogg 2019).

Strong opioids

- *Morphine* works on the *mu*-opioid receptors in the brain and spinal cord, and is considered the 'gold standard' preparation against which other *mu*-opioid agonist medications are measured. It comes in various formulations, is widely available, and is usually first-line treatment in palliative care settings. Morphine has a number of side effects, most commonly constipation, and the potential for toxicity and sedation.
- *Fentanyl* is a synthetic opioid that is 100 times more potent than morphine and shorter acting. It can be given sub-lingually (under the tongue) or via the skin. Fentanyl has an affinity for lipids (fats) and is ideal for use as a transdermal patch, where it is absorbed slowly and steadily. However, **the transdermal patch must only be used with people who are already taking opioids**. Also, older people with a higher ratio of fat to lean body mass can be at risk of absorbing too much of the drug, leading to potential overdose. Fentanyl should be reserved for older people with cancer or receiving palliative care, who:
  - require high doses of opioids to manage their pain, or
  - cannot take oral analgesia, or
  - cannot tolerate side effects from other medications.
- *Oxycodone* is a full-strength opioid that works on the *mu*-opioid receptors. It is equivalent to around 1.5 times the strength of morphine. Oxycodone is given orally and available in immediate release and in slow-release formulations. Slow-release tablets must not be crushed or chewed (Hogg 2019).

Adjuvant analgesics

Adjuvant analgesics are medications developed to manage other conditions, which are also useful in treating pain. Primarily, they work by modifying nerve transmission and are of particular value for neuropathic pain (Finnerup et al 2015). Adjuvant medications can help to reduce pain caused by sensitisation of the central nervous system (e.g. non-specific low back pain) (Hogg 2019). While adjuvant analgesics rarely achieve complete pain relief, the reduction of pain severity is usually valued by the older person. Adjuvant analgesics used with older people include:

- tricyclic antidepressants: amitriptyline, nortripyline
- serotonin-noradrenaline reuptake inhibitors: venlafaxine, duloxetine

- antiepileptics: gabapentin, pregabalin
- antihypertensive: clonidine.

Some types of adjuvant medications are formulated as a cream or gel and applied to the skin (topical). These analgesics work on the peripheral nerves and are useful for localised neuropathic pain, including post-herpetic neuralgia and diabetic neuropathy. Adjuvant analgesics available for topical use include:

- lidocaine
- capsaicin
- amitriptyline
- ketamine (Hogg 2019).

When using topical agents, the skin must be intact and the area observed regularly for signs of irritation.

Research Highlight
Biopsychosocial Factors and Risk of Developing Pain in Older Adults

A longitudinal study conducted in Ireland surveyed 4458 adults, who were aged 50 years or over and not bothered by pain, at baseline and at a two-year follow-up. Participants provided data on their pain, and 11 personal variables: depressive symptoms, anxiety, loneliness, self-rated physical health, number of chronic conditions, physical disability, sleep, amount of physical activity, alcoholism, smoking and body mass index. The researchers classified participants into four classes based on the prevalence of each variable and postulated each group's risk of developing bothersome pain over the two-year period.

Results showed that people in the 'high-risk' class, who more frequently reported depression, loneliness, sleep problems, co-morbidities, disability, obesity and lower physical activity, were over three times more likely to develop pain than those in the 'low-risk' class, who self-reported good physical and mental health. Additionally, 22.9% of participants who fell into the 'high-risk' class reported multi-site pain or pain that limited their usual activities compared to 5.6% of those in the 'low-risk' class. The risk classes, which grouped biopsychosocial factors, were also more strongly associated with development of pain than the factors by themselves.

O'Neill et al (2018).

SUMMARY

Pain is a common problem for many older people, which can lead to immobility, disability and diminished quality of life. The biopsychosocial model of pain explains how pain is a subjective experience and why multimodal approaches are best to treat pain. An older person's physical condition, thoughts and feelings, cultural traditions and social environment influence how they experience, express and cope with pain. Acute pain usually occurs suddenly with the onset of tissue damage and resolves as tissue heal. Chronic pain persists after an injury has healed. Many older people experience chronic pain due to pain-producing pathologies that are more common in later life.

The older person's self-report is the best measure of their pain. Older people with mild to moderate cognitive impairment can provide a self-report of pain with prompting and the help of a simple verbal descriptor scale. Older people who cannot communicate may express pain through facial expression, vocalising and changes in activity, and should be regularly assessed using an observational pain assessment tool.

A blend of non-pharmacological and pharmacological approaches is most effective to treat pain in older people. Always start pain medications at a low dose, then monitor closely and slowly titrate doses upwards to achieve the best possible pain relief with the fewest side effects. Complete relief of chronic pain, particularly neuropathic pain, may not be possible. Nevertheless, treatment can yield benefits for the older person in terms of less discomfort, leading to better sleep and mobility. Regular and frequent reassessment of the older person are required to identify treatment effectiveness and emergence of side effects, which may be more troublesome than the pain.

Practice Scenario

Mr K is a 70-year-old man who sustained a back injury at work 10 years ago. At the time, he took sick leave for 6 weeks and then resumed work part-time until he retired 4 years ago. He reports being left with constant pain in his lower back, which gets worse when he bends down or stretches forward to pick something up. He also describes 'shooting' pains in his legs that come and go, and numbness across the balls of his feet. Mr K states that he tries not to do too much and says that he is frightened that 'the movement will set the pain off'. He has been able to position pillows on his favourite chair to support his back and legs and spends a lot of time resting in it by the window. He used to enjoy his daily walk to the shops until the pain became too much. Mr K feels sad that his wife left him 2 years ago, but says he understands why she would not want to live with someone 'who will probably end up in a wheelchair'. Still he misses her and their friends, and doesn't sleep well. Mr K says that the pain medication he takes doesn't seem to work, but he doesn't like to complain to the doctor and hasn't had the energy to visit the physiotherapist for an exercise program as the doctor advised. Mr K says, 'Nothing will change this pain, so why should I bother?'

MULTIPLE CHOICE QUESTIONS

1. Chronic pain is:
   a. Pain from an injury that hasn't healed
   b. An imaginary feeling of pain often experienced by older people with depression
   c. Pain that persists after an injury has healed and is experienced for 3 months or longer.
   d. Pain experienced by older people in the last year of life.

2. What is meant by 'catastrophising'?
   a. A psychological response when a person has an unrealistic expectation of a good outcome in a bad situation
   b. A psychological response when a person assumes the worst possible outcome in a situation
   c. A psychological response when the older person exaggerates their pain to receive sympathy from others
   d. A social response where the older person describes their situation is a catastrophe to encourage others to stay away and not bother them

3. What is the recommended approach to managing pain in older people:
   a. To get pain under control as quickly as possible with regular large doses of oral morphine and a transdermal patch of fentanyl to ease pain and calm distress
   b. Limit pain management to non-pharmacological strategies for older people aged over 80 years to avoid dangerous side effects of medication
   c. Use a blend of non-pharmacological and pharmacological strategies, with regular and frequent reassessment to achieve the best possible pain relief with minimal side effects
   d. Use the WHO analgesic ladder beginning at the 'step' appropriate to the older person's level of pain

REVIEW QUESTIONS

1. What biological (physical) aspects are influencing Mr K's pain?
2. What psychological aspects are influencing Mr K's pain?
3. What social aspects are influencing Mr K's pain?
4. What statements could the nurse use to gently challenge Mr K's thoughts about his pain?
5. What non-pharmacological and pharmacological pain management strategies might help Mr K?

REFERENCES

Abbey J, De Bellis A, Piller N et al (2004) The Abbey pain scale: a 1-minute numerical indicator for people with end-stage dementia.

Abbey J, Piller N, De Bellis AD et al (2004) The Abbey pain scale: a 1-minute numerical indicator for people with end-stage dementia. International Journal of Palliative Nursing 10(1):6–13.

Australian & New Zealand Society for Geriatric Medicine (2016) Australian & New Zealand Society for Geriatric Medicine Position Statement Abstract: Pain in older people. Australasian Journal on Ageing 35(4):293.

Brooks KG, Kessler TL (2017) Treatments for neuropathic pain, Clinical Pharmacist. Online. Available: www.pharmaceutical-journal.com/research/review-article/treatments-for-neuropathic-pain/20203641.article?firstPass=false

Cravello L, Di Santo S, Varrassi G et al (2019) Chronic pain in the elderly with cognitive decline: A narrative review. Pain and Therapy 8(1):53–65.

de Ruddere L, Craig KD (2016) Understanding stigma and chronic pain: A state of the art review. Pain 157:1607–1610.

Dominick CH, Blyth FM, Nicholas MK (2012) Unpacking the burden: Understanding the relationships between chronic pain and comorbidity in the general population. Pain 153(2):295–304.

Dong H-J, Larsson B, Levin L-A et al (2018) Is excess weight a burden for older adults who suffer chronic pain? BMC Geriatrics 18:270.

Emerson K, Boggero I, Ostir G et al (2018) Pain as a risk factor for loneliness among older adults. Journal of Ageing Health 30(9):1450–1461.

Finnerup NB, Attal N, Haroutounian S et al (2015) Pharmacotherapy for neuropathic pain in adults: a systematic review and meta-analysis. The Lancet Neurology 14(2):162–173.

Gibson S, Farrell M (2004) A review of age differences in the neurophysiology of nociception and the perceptual experience of pain. The Clinical Journal of Pain 20(4):227–239.

Goucke CR (ed.) (2019) Pain in residential aged care facilities: Management strategies, 2nd edn. Australian Pain Society, North Sydney.

Grol-Propopczyk H (2017) Sociodemographic disparities in chronic pain, based on 12-year longitudinal data. Pain 158(2):313–322.

Harris D (2007) Pain management in older people. Geriatric Medicine: Midlife and beyond Pain. July:23–25. Online. Available: www.gmjournal.co.uk/media/21438/jul07p23.pdf

Hogg M (2019) Pharmacological treatments. In: CR Goucke (ed) Pain in residential aged care facilities: Management strategies, 2nd edn. Australian Pain Society, North Sydney.

Jett K (2018) Pain and comfort. In: Touhy TA & Jett K (eds) Ebersol and Hess' gerontological nursing and healthy aging, 5th edn. Elsevier, St Louis Missouri.

Lavin R, Park J (2014) A characterization of pain in racially and ethnically older adults: A review of the literature. Journal of Applied Gerontology 33(3):258–290.

Liu J, Leung D (2017) Pain treatments for nursing home residents with advanced dementia and substantial impaired

communication: a cross-sectional analysis at baseline of a cluster randomized controlled trial. Pain medicine (Malden, Mass.) 18(9):1649–1657.

Mansfield K, Sim J, Jordan JL et al (2016) A systematic review and meta-analysis of the prevalence of chronic widespread pain in the general population. Pain 157(1):55–64.

Mantopoulos S (2019) Complementary approaches to pain. In: CR Goucke (ed.) Pain in residential aged care facilities: management strategies, 2nd edn. Australian Pain Society, North Sydney.

Miaskowski C, Blyth F, Nicosia F et al (2019) A biopsychosocial model of chronic pain for older adults. Pain Medicine, December 2019; pnz329. doi:10.1093/pm/pnz329

Ministry of Health NZ (2020) New Zealand health survey, indicator chronic pain 2018/2019. Online 25 May 2020. Available: https://minhealthnz.shinyapps.io/nz-health-survey-2018-19-annual-data-explorer/_w_fdeeaa4e/#!/explore-indicators

Moore N (2019) Movement and physical activity. In: CR Goucke (ed.) Pain in residential aged care facilities: management strategies, 2nd edn. Australian Pain Society, North Sydney.

National Center for Complementary and Integrative Health (2016) Acupuncture in depth. Online 13 July 2020. Available: www.nccih.nih.gov/health/acupuncture-in-depth

Nowak T, Neumann-Podczaska A, Tobis S et al (2019) Characteristics of pharmacological pain treatment in older nursing home residents. Journal of Pain Research 12, 1083–1089.

O'Neill A, O'Sullivan K, O'Keeffe M et al (2018) Development of pain in older adults: a latent class analysis of biopsychosocial risk factors. Pain 159(8):1631–1640.

Painaustralia Limited (2019) Painful facts. Online 25 May 2020. Available: www.painaustralia.org.au/about-pain/painful-facts

Rajan J, Behrends M (2019) Acute pain in older adults. Anaesthesiology Clinics 37:507–520.

Saraiva MD, Suzuki GS, Lin SM et al (2018) Persistent pain is a risk factor for frailty: a systematic review and meta-analysis from prospective longitudinal studies. Age and Ageing 47(6):785–793.

Savvas S (2019) Dementia and cognitive impairment: Special considerations. In: CR Goucke (ed.) Pain in residential aged care facilities: management strategies, 2nd edn. Australian Pain Society, North Sydney.

Savvas S, Gibson S (2015) Pain management in residential aged care facilities. Australian Family Physician 44:198–203.

Scherer S (2019) About pain. In: CR Goucke (ed.), Pain in residential aged care facilities: management strategies, 2nd edn. Australian Pain Society, North Sydney.

Schofield P, Abdulla A (2018) Pain assessment in the older population: what the literature says. Age & Ageing, 47(3):324–327.

Seth B, de Gray L (2019) The genesis of chronic pain. Anaesthesia and Intensive Care Medicine 20(8):410–414.

Sodhi JK, Karmarkar A, Raji M et al (2020) Pain as a predictor of frailty over time among older Mexican Americans. Pain 161(1):109–113.

Stitzlein Davies P (2017) Opioids for pain management in older adults: Strategies for safe prescribing. The Nurse Practitioner 42(2):20–26.

Strong J, Nielson M, Williams M et al (2015) Quiet about pain: Experiences of Aboriginal people in two rural communities. Australian Journal of Rural Health 23:181–184.

Stubbs B, Schofield P, Binnekade T et al (2014) Pain is associated with recurrent falls in community-dwelling older adults: evidence from a systematic review and meta-analysis. Pain Medicine 15(7):1115–1128.

Sugai K, Takeda-Imai F, Michikawa T et al (2018) Association between knee pain, impaired function, and development of depressive symptoms. JAGS 66(3):570–576.

Turk DC, Fillingim RB, Ohrbach R et al (2016) Assessment of psychosocial and functional impact of chronic pain. The Journal of Pain 17(9), Supplement 2:T21–T49.

Twigg O, Wallace M (2019) Beyond medication: Psychological and educational approaches to pain management. In: CR Goucke (ed.) Pain in residential aged care facilities: management strategies, 2nd edn. Australian Pain Society, North Sydney.

Whitlock EL, Diaz-Ramirez LG, Glymour MM et al (2017) Association between persistent pain and memory decline and dementia in a longitudinal cohort of elders. JAMA Internal Medicine 177(8):1146–1153.

Williams AC, Craig KD (2016) Updating the definition of pain. Pain 157(11):2420–2423.

Wood BM, Nicholas MK, Blyth F et al (2010) Assessing pain in older people with persistent pain: The NRS is valid but only provides part of the picture. The Journal of Pain 11(12):1259–1266.

World Health Organisation (n.d.) WHO guidelines for the management of cancer pain. Online. Available: www.who.int/ncds/management/palliative-care/Infographic-cancer-pain-lowres.pdf

CHAPTER 20

Hearing

EMMA CHAFFEY • SUSAN SLATYER

LEARNING OBJECTIVES

After reading this chapter, you will be able to:

- describe rates of hearing loss in the Australian and New Zealand gerontological population, and the associated risk factors
- explain the three types of hearing loss and their implications for communication in older people
- describe the nursing assessment of hearing and the ear in older people
- describe strategies to promote older persons' hearing and communication
- define the roles and referrals pathways within the hearing healthcare industry in Australia and New Zealand.

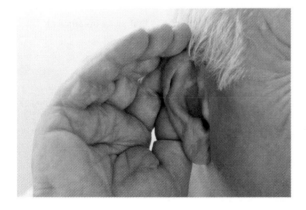

INTRODUCTION

Hearing loss is the most common disability in adult populations and poses a particular challenge for older adults. Not only are older people with hearing loss more likely to report communication difficulties, they are also reluctant to seek rehabilitation services and remediation devices. Once accessed, rehabilitation programs can be challenging for older people, who commonly present with co-morbid vision impairment, poor dexterity, cognitive decline, limited mobility and frailty (Wilson et al 1999). Nurses have a role in identifying potential hearing deficits in older people, and implementing strategies to enhance hearing, overcome communication difficulties and minimise further hearing loss to maintain the person's quality of life and social connectedness. This chapter will outline types of hearing loss, strategies to determine how well an older person can hear and interventions to promote hearing and communication. A glossary of terms is provided in Table 20.1.

Rates of Hearing Impairment in Older People in Australia and New Zealand

Hearing loss refers to the reduced sensitivity of the auditory system to sound. It is expected that most older people in Australia and New Zealand experience some degree of hearing loss. In Australia, for adults over 70 years, 87% of men and 63% of women will have at least a mild hearing loss (Hearing Care Industry Association [HCIA] 2017). Moreover, it is estimated that the prevalence of hearing loss across the whole

TABLE 20.1
Glossary

Word	Meaning
Atresia	Absence or abnormal narrowing of the ear canal
Acoustic neuroma	A benign tumour originating in the vestibulocochlear nerve
Audiogram	A graph that shows the audible threshold for standardised frequencies as measured by an audiometer
Auditory deprivation	Decline in the brain's ability to process auditory information due to continued lack of auditory stimulation
Basal turn	(of the cochlear): the anterior two and a half turns of the shell-shaped cochlear (inner ear): responsible for hearing high frequency sounds
Cerumen	Ear wax
Cholesteatoma	A non-cancerous cystic mass of skin cells arising in the middle ear
Cognitive loading	The used amount of working memory resources
Ear mould	Moulded plastic fitting that sits in the ear canal to couple the ear with a hearing aid
Epithelial regeneration	Renewal of skin cells
Hearing dog	A specifically-trained dog that will respond to environmental sounds as an alert and/or guide for a hearing impaired or deaf owner
Linguistic redundancy	The nature of acoustic information in spoken language that allows a normal listener to recognise speech, even when parts of the speech signal are missing
Mastoid surgery	Surgery on the bony portion of the skull-base behind the ear to remove diseased regions of the mastoid
Microtia	Congenital deformity where the pinna (external ear) is underdeveloped or absent
Perforation	Hole in the eardrum caused by infection or trauma
Personal amplifier	Set of headphones connected to an adjustable microphone that picks up ambient sound from a distance of 1–4 metres
Pinna	The external part of the ear
Presbycusis	Loss of hearing that gradually occurs in most individuals as they grow older
Otitis externa	Inflammation of the passage of the outer ear (ear canal)
Otitis media	Inflammation of the middle ear
Otosclerosis	A hereditary disorder causing progressive deafness due to overgrowth of bone in the inner ear
Spatial auditory processing	Auditory perception to a location in space
Temporal auditory processing	Perception of time differences or changes of an audible acoustic event(s)
Tinnitus	Perceived ringing or buzzing heard in one or both ears or heard centrally
Working memory	The cognitive system with a limited capacity that is responsible for temporarily holding information available for processing

population will increase, with 7.8 million Australians (18.9%) reporting hearing impairment by 2060 (HCIA 2017). In New Zealand, rates of hearing loss are expected to be similar (Exeter et al 2015; Williams 2019). Some older adults may manage or mask the degree of their hearing loss using additional communication strategies, but most would benefit from additional intervention such as hearing aids, assistive listening devices or medical treatment (Exeter et al 2015; HCIA 2017).

TYPES OF HEARING LOSS

There are three main types of hearing loss: sensorineural, conductive and mixed. Determining the cause of hearing loss is important because some conditions, such as wax build-up or ear infection, can be treated. Other types of hearing loss are less amenable to treatment. Once hearing loss is permanent, knowing the underlying cause is unlikely to alter the strategies or management plan to enhance hearing and communication. Nevertheless, it can be useful to understand the diagnosis because some pathologies result in fluctuating levels of hearing ability. Being able to anticipate the rate at which an older person's hearing is likely to deteriorate is also useful when planning clinical care.

Sensorineural Hearing Loss

Sensorineural hearing loss is caused by defects in the cochlear (inner ear) or the neural pathways that send and process sound. Sensorineural hearing loss is usually permanent and is the most common type of hearing loss. The three main causes of sensorineural hearing loss are age-related changes, accumulated exposure to excessive noise and genetic variations.

Presbycusis, also called age-related hearing impairment, has been linked to a breakdown of hair cells within the cochlear, most commonly in the basal turn, which is sensitive to high frequency sounds. This primarily affects an individual's ability to understand speech and to hear in the presence of background noise. Presbycusis generally has many contributing factors that have compiled over a person's lifetime.

Noise-induced hearing loss is the second most common form of sensorineural hearing loss. Continuous exposure to loud noise is more damaging than intermittent exposure, and once it occurs hearing loss becomes permanent. Noise-induced hearing loss is entirely preventable; however, rates of hearing protection have historically been very low. As such, older people who worked in industries such as farming, manufacturing, trades, transportation, music, entertainment or the armed services are very likely to have had exposure to damaging levels of noise that have caused or contributed to a hearing loss (Sliwinska-Kowalska & Davis 2012; Thorne et al 2008). While previous exposure cannot be reversed, hearing protection is critical for older people who still participate in noisy activities (Davis et al 2016; Sułkowski et al 2017).

Medication-induced hearing loss arises when a person ingests particular drugs that have 'ototoxic' (ear damaging) side effects. An ototoxic medication can cause degeneration of the cochlear, the auditory nerve and/or the vestibular system (Ganesan et al 2018).

Over 600 categories of medications can potentially cause ototoxicity. The most commonly used ototoxic medications are:
- aminoglycoside antibiotics (gentamycin, tobramycin, amikacin, kanamycin)
- platinum-based chemotherapy agents (cisplatin, carboplatin)
- loop diuretics (furosemide (frusemide) at doses above 240 mg/hour)
- macrolide antibiotics (erythromycin, roxithromycin, azithromycin, clarithromycin)
- antimalarials (quinines) (Ganesan et al 2018; Hammill & Campbell 2018).

Older people, along with the very young, are at higher risk of side effects from ototoxic drugs. Other factors that can increase the risk of ototoxicity include renal failure or transplant, hepatic dysfunction, and use of two or more ototoxic medications. Symptoms are variable, can present gradually or rapidly, and, depending on the duration and dose of the medication treatment, can be temporary or permanent. Symptoms include:
- tinnitus
- high-frequency hearing loss
- complete deafness
- dizziness
- vertigo.

At present, there are no treatments to reverse medication-induced hearing loss, other than ceasing the medication. However, these medications have significant therapeutic effects, which are in some cases life-saving. Prevention and management, therefore, is focused on early detection through prospective ototoxicity monitoring to enable treatment modification to minimise or prevent permanent hearing and balance impairment (Ganesan et al 2018).

Conductive Hearing Loss

Conductive hearing loss describes decreased hearing sensitivity due to disruption in the transmission of sound waves to the cochlear. This can occur when there is a mechanical obstruction in the outer ear, or structural damage to the middle ear. Conductive hearing loss can be temporary if properly treated, such as in the case of wax build-up and infections of the ear canal (otitis externa) or middle ear (otitis media).

Other types of conductive hearing loss, however, may persist or become permanent. These include long-term perforation of the eardrum or disruption of the structures of the middle ear, such as in otosclerosis, cholesteatoma or mastoid surgery. Some pathologies that cause conductive hearing loss may prohibit a person from wearing a conventional hearing aid, including deformities of the outer ear such as microtia and atresia, or an actively discharging ear infection.

Cerumen (ear wax) build-up is common among older adults. As people age, the glands that produce cerumen lose some of their secretory function, the skin is dryer and there is reduced epithelial regeneration. Cerumen therefore becomes hard and dry, leading to impaction and reduced hearing when sound waves are prevented from reaching the eardrum (Roland et al 2008).

Mixed Hearing Loss

Mixed hearing loss is simply when an individual has a hearing loss that is both conductive and sensorineural in nature. It is expected most older people will have sensorineural or mixed hearing loss. The conductive portion of a mixed hearing loss may be fluctuating or treatable, as already described.

Tinnitus

Tinnitus is the experience of hearing sounds that are not there. It is most commonly described as a ringing, buzzing or roaring heard in one or both ears (Pienkowski 2019). While not a type of hearing loss, tinnitus is often a consequence of damage to the auditory system. It is most commonly associated with noise-induced hearing loss or any other form of sensorineural hearing loss (Mazurek 2018). While many people report tinnitus as a temporary, sporadic and non-bothersome phenomenon, between 11% and 30% of adults report distressing or debilitating tinnitus (Esmaili & Renton 2018; McCormack et al 2016). These forms of tinnitus are most often associated with additional stress, mental health issues or undesirable experiences, with the tinnitus being the focus of many negative thoughts or reactions. There are successful interventions for distressing or bothersome tinnitus which are summarised in *Tips for best practice: Strategies to reduce distressing or bothersome tinnitus*.

ADDITIONAL RISK FACTORS FOR HEARING LOSS IN OLDER ADULTS

Dementia

Dementia is often associated with hearing loss, in that an older person living with dementia is more likely to have poorer hearing than the general older population. There is a growing body of research about the risk of hearing loss contributing to dementia. Moreover, hearing loss potentially accelerates cognitive decline (Ford et al 2018; Gurgel et al 2014). While there is no causal link identified between hearing loss and dementia, there is a suggestion that auditory deprivation, social isolation

---

Tips for Best Practice
Strategies to Reduce Distressing or Bothersome Tinnitus

- Referral to a specialist audiologist, who can offer:
  - assessment of the underlying hearing loss and prescription of hearing aids or other listening devices
  - structured sound therapy to partially mask the tinnitus and promote acclimatisation and filtering.
- Referral to a psychologist, who can offer:
  - cognitive behavioural therapy to disrupt the distressing reaction to tinnitus
  - counselling and other psychological support to address additional mental and emotional stressors contributing to the overall distress.

Beukes et al (2018); Pienkowski (2019).

---

and increased cognitive loading may contribute to a dementia disease pathway (Amieva et al 2015; Lin et al 2013; Pichora-Fuller et al 2015).

Indigenous Population

Rates of hearing loss are significantly higher among Māori, Aboriginal and Torres Strait Islander populations. This is attributed to both genetic and environmental factors. Many Aboriginal and Torres Strait Islander people are left with poor hearing as a result of untreated otitis media in childhood (Australian Medical Association [AMA] 2017). Otitis media develops when fluid builds up in the middle ear. While this condition is readily treatable, evidence shows that between the ages of 2 and 20 years, an Indigenous child will experience hearing loss due to middle ear infections for at least 32 months, compared to a total of 3 months for non-Indigenous children (AMA 2017). Chronic otitis media is linked to poorer social determinants of health (see Chapter 3), including poverty and absence of health services. The impacts are life-long and include a higher risk of adult social problems, poor physical health and disability (AMA 2017). Indigenous peoples are also less likely to receive early intervention for hearing loss (Closing the Gap Clearinghouse 2014; Digby et al 2014; Williams 2019). As such, older Indigenous people are much more likely to have had a long-term hearing loss and may continue to have ongoing or chronic middle ear problems.

FUNCTIONAL IMPACTS OF HEARING LOSS

Hearing loss is not an inevitable symptom of ageing. Nevertheless, as current rates of hearing loss indicate, a significant number of older people, including the majority living in residential aged care, have a degree of hearing impairment. The inability to hear properly has a significant impact on quality of life and reduces an older person's opportunities for meaningful interactions (Wittich et al 2016). Even a mild hearing loss can result in breakdowns in conversation, leading to:

- frustration or mistrust
- difficulty using the telephone
- misunderstanding of medical or clinical advice
- medication errors
- increased falls risk
- social isolation
- less awareness of common environmental sounds in the home and elsewhere (Bainbridge & Wallhagen 2014).

Speech Discrimination

Being able to hear the voices of other people and our own is essential to communication. It is also critical to understand what is being said in a particular environment. Speech discrimination refers to the ability to identify and understand specific spoken words. Generally, this ability deteriorates in older people when they are in more complex listening situations, such as when there is background noise, unfamiliar speakers or subjects, or conversations involving multiple speakers.

The nurse may notice an older person's poor 'hearing' when talking in a busy or noisy place, particularly when earlier conversations have been conducted in ideal listening conditions and seemed relatively easy. These changes can be attributed to sensorineural hearing loss or processing abnormalities in higher-level regions of the brain. In addition, age-related cognitive decline may affect complex auditory functions crucial to speech, which include temporal and spatial auditory processing, working memory and linguistic redundancy.

ASSESSMENT

Ascertaining how well an older person can hear and communicate is critical to the success of care. In the early stages, older people are often not aware that their hearing is gradually diminishing. Additionally, the older person's poor hearing and consequent difficulty communicating may not be evident to others. It is not unusual for older people to feign understanding of a conversation or instruction they have not heard in order

Research Highlight

Researchers in the United States sought to determine whether dietary patterns influence the development of hearing loss over time. A cohort of 81,818 women in the Nurses' Health Study II, aged 27–44 years when they entered the study in 1991, completed questionnaires about their diet every 4 years and then self-reported levels of hearing loss in 2009 and 2013. The dietary questionnaires assessed how much participants, over the previous year, followed any of three healthy diets: the Alternate Mediterranean diet (AMED), the Dietary Approaches to Stop Hypertension (DASH) diet and the 2010 USDA Dietary Guidelines for Americans as measured by the Alternative Healthy Eating Index-2010 (AHEI2010).

The AMED consists of nine food types: higher quantities of vegetables (except potatoes), fruits, nuts, legumes, fish, monounsaturated fats, whole grains and lower quantities of red or processed meats and alcohol. This diet has been consistently associated with lower risk of chronic disease.

The DASH diet comprises higher quantities of fruits, vegetables, nuts, legumes, low-fat dairy, whole grains, and lower intake of sodium, red/processed meat and sugar sweetened beverages. This diet is linked to lower rates of hypertension, diabetes, cardiovascular disease and dementia.

The 2010 USDA Dietary Guidelines recommend higher intake of fruit, vegetables, whole grains, nuts, legumes, and lower intake of red/processed meat, trans fat, sodium, sugar sweetened beverages and fruit juice, along with moderate alcohol consumption.

The study controlled for the presence of a number of confounding variables including: age, race, smoking, body mass index, waist circumference, physical activity, total energy intake, hypertension, diabetes, use of paracetamol or ibuprofen, and tinnitus.

Results showed that women who adhered more closely to the healthy diets tended to be slightly older, leaner, more physically active and less likely to smoke. During the follow-up (which equated to >1 million person-years of follow-up), 2306 cases of moderate or worse hearing loss were reported. Higher cumulative average AMED and DASH scores were significantly associated with lower rates of hearing loss. A higher recent AHEI2010 score was also associated with lower risk.

The authors concluded that adhering to a healthy diet is linked to lower risk of hearing loss in women and, therefore, may be helpful in reducing acquired hearing loss.

Curhan et al (2018).

to avoid looking uninterested, stupid or confused. In a clinical setting, it can be problematic to gauge how much the older person has understood.

Hearing Assessment

There are several ways to assess how well an older person can hear and understand. The *Promoting wellness* box details strategies the nurse can use during routine interactions with the older person. A further simple test of hearing acuity uses a ticking wristwatch (Pich & Govind 2018). The older person covers one ear and the nurse moves out of sight and holds the ticking watch 2–3 cm away from the person's other ear. The nurse then asks the older person whether he or she can hear the ticking, repeats the test with the other ear and documents the outcome. The Shortened Hearing Handicap Inventory For Elderly (HHIE-S), a validated functional screening tool, may also be helpful (Sindhusake et al 2001; Ventry & Weinstein 1983).

Promoting Wellness
Assessing Hearing and Understanding

- Ask the older person if he or she has ever been fitted with hearing aids.
- If so, ask the older person if he or she is using these devices now or has them available to use. *Note*: There is little correlation between self-reported hearing loss and a diagnosable hearing loss. The older person may not be able to describe their hearing loss (Haanes et al 2014).
- Move 2 metres away from the older person and ensure that he or she cannot see your face. Ask simple closed-ended questions (i.e. a question requiring only one specific and unique answer).
- If the person is unable to answer correctly or asks you to repeat the question, move to face the person while remaining at the same distance. This will indicate whether the person is able to use visual cues to assist communication (e.g. potentially indicating presence of poor vision or other impairments).
- Administer the Shortened Hearing Handicap Inventory For Elderly (HHIE-S), a functional questionnaire validated as a useful screening tool for hearing loss (Sindhusake et al 2001; Ventry & Weinstein 1983). Available: www.audiology.org/sites/default/files/PracticeManagement/Medicare_HHI.pdf.

Ear Assessment

Nursing assessment of the ear involves questioning to determine the older person's history of ear and hearing problems, followed by physical observation and palpation of the external ear (Pich & Govind 2018). Only a doctor or nurse trained in the procedure should visualise the ear canal and eardrum using an otoscope. Ear assessments should be conducted in a quiet environment, with the older person sitting or standing at the same level as the nurse.

Assessment questions to obtain and document the older person's ear or hearing problems should ask about:
- hearing problems or loss (onset, contributing factors)
- family history
- current or past use of hearing aids
- difficulty hearing in noisy environments
- ear pain
- medication use (particularly if the older person has ringing in the ears)
- interference with daily life from hearing loss, and
- if the person uses a hearing device, when and how obtained (Pich & Govind 2018).

When observing the external ear (pinna), look for:
- redness that may indicate infection
- lesions (e.g. cysts)
- flaky, scaly skin, especially behind the pinna, which may indicate seborrhoea (Pich & Govind 2018).

Gentle palpation of the external ear can identify areas of tenderness, swelling, texture and elasticity:
- Slightly pull pinna downwards and backwards.
- Push on the tragus.
- Fold pinna forward and release (normal finding is that it recoils).
- Apply pressure behind the pinna to assess the bony mastoid process (Pich & Govind 2018).

INTERVENTIONS

Nursing actions in response to an indication that the older person has diminished hearing include referral for medical review or to an audiologist for specialist assessment and, often, prescription of assistive devices. Nurses are also well placed to educate older people about the risks associated with hearing loss and how to minimise these, the benefits of regular hearing checks and strategies to manage communication difficulties and distress related to tinnitus.

If the hearing loss is caused or exacerbated by a medical condition, referral for further investigation and treatment can have a big impact. Treatment of simple infective ear disease requires review by a general practitioner (GP) and generally responds to antibiotic treatment. In more complex cases, including chronic otitis media, otosclerosis, cholesteatoma and acoustic neuroma, management by an ear, nose and throat (ENT) specialist is required. If cerumen build-up or impaction is identified, then gentle cerumen removal by a GP, ENT specialist or qualified nursing staff under medical supervision may be indicated.

Referral to a Hearing Health Professional

Audiologists are allied health professionals who provide a specialist comprehensive hearing assessment and develop tailored hearing interventions. A medical referral is not needed to see an audiologist, unless the consultation is required during hospital inpatient care. The most common hearing assessment used by audiologists is 'puretone' audiometry, which records the sensitivity of the auditory system to sounds. While this does not measure real world listening function, it gives frequency-specific thresholds of an individual's hearing that the audiologist can use to diagnose the type and severity of hearing loss and program hearing devices. You may see results of puretone audiometry represented in an audiogram (Lasak et al 2014).

In Australia, for people over 65 years of age, funding for hearing services and some devices may be available via the Hearing Services Program. The first step to determining an older person's eligibility for funding support is to contact an audiology practice. In New Zealand, government funding for hearing services is available for holders of the SuperGold Card and through the Ministry of Health. Having ascertained funding options, the older person can be assessed and provided with a hearing management plan. This service is available via community audiology clinics, aged-care facilities, in some tertiary hospitals or in a private residence where the person has extreme mobility challenges, as confirmed by a medical practitioner.

Strategies to Promote Hearing and Communication

Given the high rates of hearing loss in older people, in the absence of specific information about a patient's hearing or communication ability, the nurse should assume the older person has at least a mild hearing loss. This means interacting with the older person as though they, even if wearing hearing aids, may not be able to understand when standing more than 2 metres away or with any competing background noise (Dementia Australia 2020). Strategies to optimise communication with an older person who has poor hearing are outlined in *Tips for best practice: Communication strategies*.

Devices

There are two main types of device used in Australia and New Zealand to rehabilitate permanent hearing loss: hearing aids and assistive listening devices (ALDs).

Tips for Best Practice
Communication Strategies

- Change the physical environment:
  - Ensure you are 1–2 metres away from the older person whenever speaking to them
  - Make sure the person can see your face clearly, while ensuring the room has good lighting
  - Turn off or move away from background noise
  - If unable to reduce background noise, position yourself away from the source of the noise. This directs the noise to the older person's back while you speak to the person from the opposite direction.
- Adjust your speaking style:
  - Do not speak loudly or shout. Use slow, clear speech
  - Avoid obstructing the view of your face with your hands or other objects
  - In extreme cases use short sentences consisting only of 'key' words, such as 'Point to where the pain is' might become 'Pain? Point'
  - Use gestures
  - Ask the older person to repeat key information to check understanding rather than asking for yes or no responses.
- Using technologies:
  - Check if the older person uses any hearing technology. If so, check whether they have it with them and whether it is working
  - If available, a generic personal amplifier with headphones can be used and easily adjusted to the older person's preferred volume
  - Explore whether the older person can use phone technology that incorporates captioning or video technology.

Hearing aids

The most commonly prescribed rehabilitation strategy for hearing loss is a hearing aid. These devices are battery-powered personal amplifying instruments worn in the ear to improve the audibility of sounds. Hearing technology has changed dramatically over the last 30 years and now digital signal processing is more advanced. Most hearing aids now come with features that aim to improve speech signal quality when there is background noise, which is the most common communication challenge for someone with a hearing loss (Davis et al 2016; Dawes et al 2015).

There are many styles of hearing aid devices. Those classified as 'behind-the-ear' or 'receiver-in-the-ear' devices have components that sit behind the pinna, with tubing or wire fitted to a component (such as an ear mould) that sits inside the ear canal (Fig. 20.1).

A third style, the 'in-the-ear' hearing aid, is custom-fitted to sit inside the ear canal and surrounding areas with no components required behind the ear.

Advancing technology has enabled the development of hearing aids that are very small, an attractive feature that has improved hearing aid adoption (Fig 20.2). However, the smaller size can present challenges for older people, who can find them difficult to see and

handle. Those with vision loss, poor dexterity or impaired cognition can find the daily maintenance tasks required to use a hearing aid particularly difficult. It is, therefore, important that nurses are familiar with the different devices in order to optimise the older person's use of their hearing technology as a critical step in promoting healthy hearing and communication.

The nurse is well placed to ensure the older person removes their hearing aids at night. If left in place overnight, the hearing aids will amplify any noise and disrupt the older person's sleep, particularly if they are in hospital. Additionally, the continuous use will run the device batteries down quickly, necessitating frequent replacement. *Tips for best practice: Ensuring hearing aids (and most bone-conduction devices) are working effectively* provides strategies for troubleshooting device-related problems (Hickson et al 2014; Ng & Loke 2015; Pichora-Fuller et al 2015; Wittich et al 2016).

Some types of conductive hearing loss warrant the use of a bone-conduction device. This is typically worn on a headband and makes direct contact with the skin around the ear to provide the sound via vibrations rather than through the ear canal. These devices can also be partially implanted and attach to the individual's head via a magnet or abutment protruding from the skull (Fig 20.3) (Reinfeldt et al 2015).

Assistive listening devices (ALDs)

This category covers a range of devices that can assist with hearing and communication in specific situations, often in conjunction with hearing aids. The more common types of ALDs recommended for older adults with a hearing loss include:

- amplified headphones for the TV
- visual or tactile alerting systems for a smoke alarm, doorbell, bedside alarm or telephone

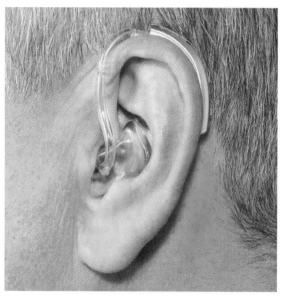

FIG. 20.1 **Behind-the-ear hearing aid** (© Starkey Hearing Technologies)

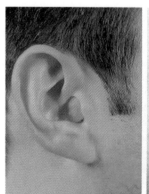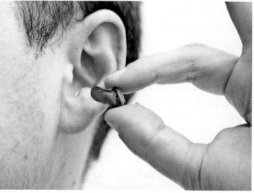

FIG. 20.2 **In-the-ear hearing aid**

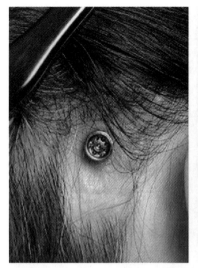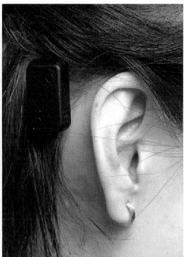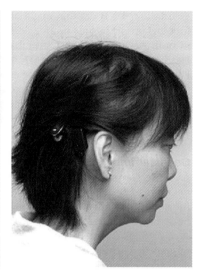

FIG. 20.3 **Bone conduction implant with abutment**

Tips for Best Practice
Ensuring Hearing Aids (and Most Bone-Conduction Devices) Are Working Effectively

- When a hearing aid is working, there should be squeaking or whistling noises coming from the device when it is loosely cupped in your hand. If you cannot hear these sounds, here are some tips for troubleshooting:
  - Ensure the areas that collect sound (microphone ports) and emit sound (speaker) are clear of wax and debris. Clean with a brush and/or alcohol wipe if needed
  - Ensure any tubing is free of moisture and wax. You may need to rinse an ear mould in warm water, drying the tubing well before use
  - Check and replace the battery, remembering each hearing aid takes a specific sized battery and will have a correct orientation when inserting the battery
  - Check for loose or damaged components
  - If you are still unable to her the sound from the hearing aid, most audiology clinics have onsite

technicians who can repair the devices or provide advice.
- If there is a clear sound heard when the hearing aid is cupped in your hand but the older person still reports they cannot hear properly (or you suspect they are not hearing well with the device), you can also try the following:
  - Check the person's ears for excessive wax and refer them to a medical practitioner for wax removal if necessary
  - Ascertain when the older person last had a hearing test and specialist audiology review
- **Cochlear implants** are not able to be tested and repaired in the same way as hearing aids. If an older person with a cochlear implant is reporting issues with their devices, replacing the batteries is one troubleshooting option available. If this does not resolve the issue, the device will require review by a specialist implant audiologist.

- enhanced telephones that amplify and slow speech
- wireless communication devices (WCDs) that most often link in with someone's hearing aids and allow a hearing aid user to hear a speaker's voice over a distance or with a clearer signal in background noise. Other common technologies such text messaging, email, captioning and computers are also beneficial for a person

with a hearing loss. However, older people are often less familiar with these newer electronic modes of communication. The nurse can provide direction to learning resources that enable older people access to these non-sound-based technologies and offer a means to connect with people and activities that are important in their lives (Aberdeen & Fereiro 2014).

Additional services that might also provide benefit for older people include hearing dogs, which are trained in both New Zealand and Australia (Australian Lions Hearing Dogs 2020; Hearing Dogs NZ 2020); the National Relay Service, which allows phone calls to be translated from verbal speech to text; and interpreting services for people who are profoundly deaf and communicate via a visual language such as Signed English, AUSLAN or New Zealand Sign Language (NZSL).

Cochlear implants

As medical technology has evolved, the cochlear implant or 'bionic ear' has emerged as a successful solution for some individuals with hearing loss that cannot be remedied by use of a hearing aid. The criteria for cochlear implantation have expanded, meaning more and more people would benefit from a cochlear implant as technology improves (Fig. 20.4) (Friedmann et al 2016; Sorkin & Buchman 2016). The success and performance has also improved (Mosnier et al 2015; Tang et al 2017).

The cochlear implant has two components. One is implanted under the skin to turn sound into electrical stimulation of the cochlear nerve. The other component is the sound processor which detects sound via microphones and transmits it to the implant under the skin via a coil. The sound processor will often sit behind the ear with a cord connecting it to a magnet that couples it to the implant underneath (Yawn et al 2015). Using a cochlear implant is very different to a hearing aid and the troubleshooting tips are also different (see *Tips for best practice: Ensuring hearing aids (and most bone- conduction devices) are working effectively*).

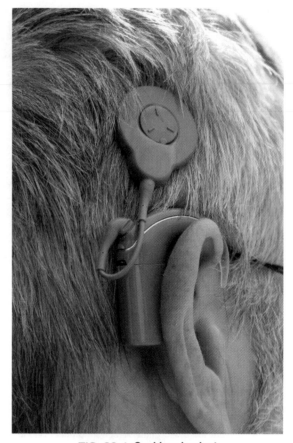

FIG. 20.4 **Cochlear implant**

Practice Scenario

Mrs Jackson is 72 years of age and has recently been admitted to residential aged care. She has mild cognitive impairment, but manages her activities of daily living with assistance. As the registered nurse, you have been dressing a wound on her lower leg and find her cheerful. In answer to your questions she has described her nine grandchildren and how much she enjoyed her 30 years working as a seamstress and factory supervisor for a large fashion label. You are therefore surprised that Mrs Jackson does not seem to interact with other residents over meals or when mixing in the activities areas. She smiles and nods but doesn't talk much and certainly doesn't initiate conversation. You are concerned that Mrs Jackson is becoming isolated. When asked, she denies any problems with her ears or hearing, but you remain concerned, particularly when she trips over an electrical cord, not realising the cleaner is vacuuming nearby.

REVIEW QUESTIONS

1. What factors indicate that Mrs Jackson may have hearing loss?

2. Why might Mrs Jackson deny any problems with her hearing?

3. What are the impacts on Mrs Jackson of a potential hearing loss?

4. How could the nurse assess how well Mrs Jackson can hear and understand?

5. What nursing interventions are appropriate if an assessment indicates that Mrs Jackson has a potential hearing loss?

6. What strategies could the nurse use to promote effective communication with Mrs Jackson?

SUMMARY

It is expected that most older people in Australia and New Zealand will experience some degree of hearing loss. Indigenous populations are at increased risk of hearing loss in older age due to social determinants of health. Additionally, evidence suggests an association between hearing loss and dementia, although no causal link has been established. The three types of hearing loss are sensorineural hearing loss, conductive hearing loss and mixed hearing loss. Tinnitus is the experience of hearing sounds that are not there, most commonly described as a ringing or buzzing in one or both ears, which can be distressing. Nursing assessment of the ear involves questioning to determine the older person's history of ear and hearing problems; physical observation; and gentle palpation of the external ear. Only a doctor or nurse trained in the procedure should visualise the ear canal and eardrum using an otoscope. Given the high rates of hearing loss, the nurse should assume that the older person has at least a mild hearing loss and modify interactions (face-to-face within 2 metres), adjust the physical environment (good lighting, little background noise), speak slowly, clearly use gestures and access technologies if available. Some older adults may manage or mask the degree of their hearing loss using additional communication strategies, but most would benefit from additional intervention. Devices to rehabilitate hearing loss include hearing aids, assistive listening devices and cochlear implants.

REFERENCES

Aberdeen L, Fereiro D (2014) Communicating with assistive listening devices and age-related hearing loss: Perceptions of older Australians. Contemporary Nurse 47(1–2):119–131.

Amieva H, Ouvrard C, Giulioli C et al (2015) Self-reported hearing loss, hearing aids, and cognitive decline in elderly adults: A 25-year study. Journal of the American Geriatrics Society 63(10):2099–2104.

Australian Lions Hearing Dogs (2020) Available: https://hearingdogs.asn.au/

Australian Medical Association (AMA) (2017) AMA Report card on Indigenous health: A national strategic approach to ending chronic otitis media and its life long impacts in Indigenous communities. Available: https://ama.com.au/system/tdf/documents/2017%20Report%20Card%20on%20Indigenous%20Health.pdf?file=1&type=node&id=47575

Bainbridge KE, Wallhagen MI (2014) Hearing loss in an aging American population: extent, impact, and management. Annual Review of Public Health 35(1):139–152.

Beukes EW, Andersson G, Allen PM et al (2018) Effectiveness of guided internet-based cognitive behavioral therapy vs face-to-face clinical care for treatment of tinnitus: a randomized clinical trial. JAMA Otolaryngology Head & Neck Surgery 144(12):1126–1133.

Closing the Gap Clearinghouse (2014) Ear disease in Aboriginal and Torres Strait Islander children. Resource sheet no. 35. Closing the Gap Clearinghouse. Australian Institute of Health and Welfare, Canberra & Australian Institute of Family Studies, Melbourne. Available: www.aihw.gov.au/getmedia/c68e6d27-05ea-4039-9d0b-a11eb609bacc/ctgc-rs35.pdf.aspx?inline=true

Curhan SG, Wang M, Eavey RD et al (2018) Adherence to healthful dietary patterns is associated with lower risk of hearing loss in women. Journal of Nutrition 148(6):944–951.

Davis A, McMahon CM, Pichora-Fuller KM et al (2016) Aging and hearing health: the life-course approach. The Gerontologist 56(Suppl_2):S256–S267.

Dawes P, Cruickshanks KJ, Fischer ME et al (2015) Hearing-aid use and long-term health outcomes: Hearing handicap, mental health, social engagement, cognitive function, physical health, and mortality. International Journal of Audiology 54(11):838–844.

Dementia Australia (2020) Managing changes in communication. Online. Available: www.dementia.org.au/national/support-and-services/carers/managing-changes-in-communication

Digby JE, Purdy SC, Kelly AS et al (2014) Are hearing losses among young Māori different to those found in the young NZ European population? The New Zealand Medical Journal (Online) 127(1398):98–110.

Esmaili AA, Renton J (2018) A review of tinnitus. Australian Journal of General Practice 47(4):205.

Exeter DJ, Wu B, Lee AC et al (2015) The projected burden of hearing loss in New Zealand (2011–2061) and the implications for the hearing health workforce. The New Zealand Medical Journal 128(1418):12.

Ford AH, Hankey GJ, Yeap BB et al (2018) Hearing loss and the risk of dementia in later life. Maturitas 112:1–11.

Friedmann DR, Ahmed OH, McMenomey SO et al (2016) Single-sided deafness cochlear implantation: candidacy, evaluation, and outcomes in children and adults. Otology & Neurotology 37(2):e154–e160.

Ganesan P, Schmiedge J, Manchaiah V et al (2018) Ototoxicity: A challenge in diagnosis and treatment. Journal of Audiology & Otology 22(2):59–68.

Gurgel RK, Ward PD, Schwartz ST et al (2014) Relationship of hearing loss and dementia: a prospective, population-based study. Otology & Neurotology 35(5):775.

Haanes GG, Kirkevold M, Horgen G et al (2014) Sensory impairments in community health care: A descriptive study of hearing and vision among elderly Norwegians living at home. Journal of Multidisciplinary Healthcare 7:217–225.

Hammill TL, Campbell KC (2018) Protection for medication-induced hearing loss: The state of the science. International Journal of Audiology, 57:S87–S95.

Hearing Dogs NZ (2020) Available: https://hearingdogs.org.nz/

Hearing Care Industry Association (HCIA) (2017) The social and economic cost of hearing loss in Australia. Available: www.hcia.com.au/about-hearing-loss/#.XlsbQ_lua71

Hickson L, Meyer C, Lovelock K et al (2014) Factors associated with success with hearing aids in older adults. International Journal of Audiology 53(sup1):S18–S27.

Lasak JM, Allen P, McVay T et al (2014) Hearing loss: diagnosis and management. Primary Care: Clinics in Office Practice 41(1):19–31.

Lin FR, Yaffe, K, Xia J et al, Health ABC Study Group (2013) Hearing loss and cognitive decline in older adults. JAMA Internal Medicine 173(4):293–299.

Mazurek B (2018) Tinnitus – New challenge and therapeutic approaches. HNO 66(2):47–48.

McCormack A, Edmondson-Jones M, Somerset S et al (2016) A systematic review of the reporting of tinnitus prevalence and severity. Hearing Research 337:70–79.

Mosnier I, Bebear J-P, Marx M et al (2015) Improvement of cognitive function after cochlear implantation in elderly patients. JAMA Otolaryngology – Head & Neck Surgery 141(5): 442–450.

Ng JH-Y, Loke AY (2015) Determinants of hearing-aid adoption and use among the elderly: A systematic review. International Journal of Audiology 54(5):291–300.

Pich J, Govind N (2018) Health assessment. In A Bermen et al (Eds), Kozier and Erb's fundamentals of nursing: concepts, process and practice, 4th Australian edition. Pearson Australia, Melbourne.

Pichora-Fuller MK, Mick P, Reed M (2015) Hearing, cognition, and healthy aging: Social and public health implications of the links between age-related declines in hearing and cognition. Seminars in Hearing 36(3):122–139.

Pienkowski M (2019) Sound therapies for tinnitus and hyperacusis. The Hearing Journal 72(1):22–23.

Reinfeldt S, Håkansson B, Taghavi H et al (2015) New developments in bone-conduction hearing implants: a review. Medical Devices (Auckland, NZ) 8:79.

Roland PS, Smith TL, Schwartz SR et al (2008) Clinical practice guideline: cerumen impaction. Otolaryngology – Head and Neck Surgery, 139(3_suppl_1):S1–S21.

Sindhusake D, Mitchell P, Smith W et al (2001) Validation of self-reported hearing loss. The Blue Mountains Hearing Study. International Journal of Epidemiology 30(6):1371–1378.

Sliwinska-Kowalska M, Davis A (2012) Noise-induced hearing loss. Noise and Health 14(61):274–280.

Sorkin DL, Buchman CA (2016) Cochlear implant access in six developed countries. Otology & Neurotology 37(2): e161–e164.

Sułkowski W, Owczarek K, Olszewski J (2017) Contemporary noise-induced hearing loss (NIHL) prevention. Otolaryngologia polska = The Polish Otolaryngology 71(4):1–7.

Tang L, Thompson CB, Clark JH et al (2017) Rehabilitation and psychosocial determinants of cochlear implant outcomes in older adults. Ear and Hearing 38(6):663–671.

Thorne PR, Ameratunga SN, Stewart J et al (2008) Epidemiology of noise-induced hearing loss in New Zealand. New Zealand Medical Journal 121(1280):33–44.

Ventry I, Weinstein B (1983). Identification of elderly people with hearing problems. American Speech-Language-Hearing Association 25(7):37–42.

Williams L (2019) Untreated severe-to-profound hearing loss and the cochlear implant situation: how policy and practice are disabling New Zealand society. The New Zealand Medical Journal 132(1505):73–78.

Wilson DH, Walsh PG, Sanchez L et al (1999) The epidemiology of hearing impairment in an Australian adult population. International Journal of Epidemiology 28(2):247–252.

Wittich W, Southall K, Johnson A (2016) Usability of assistive listening devices by older adults with low vision. Disability and Rehabilitation: Assistive Technology 11(7):564–571.

Yawn R, Hunter JB, Sweeney AD et al (2015) Cochlear implantation: a biomechanical prosthesis for hearing loss. F1000prime Reports 7.

CHAPTER 21

Vision

LAUREN ENTWISTLE

LEARNING OBJECTIVES

After reading this chapter, you will be able to:
- describe age-related changes to the eye
- identify the most common eye conditions affecting older people
- implement appropriate nursing interventions for older people with vision impairment
- reflect on the challenges of vision impairment in later life
- discuss the nature of eye health within an Australian and New Zealand context.

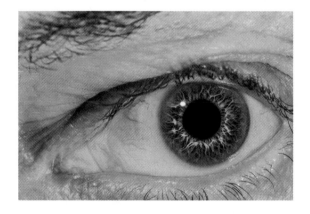

INTRODUCTION

There are currently over 600,000 people living with vision impairment or blindness in Australia and New Zealand combined (Centre for Eye Research Australia [CERA] & VISION 2020 Australia 2016; Statistics New Zealand [Stats NZ] 2013). In both countries, the prevalence of vision impairment has been shown to increase with advanced age or Indigenous descent.

As the body ages, the eye undergoes a number of physiological changes, many of which may impact on vision. Over and above normal age-related changes, older people are at greater risk for ocular pathologies that can dramatically decrease visual acuity and subsequently affect quality of life.

Nursing older people with eye conditions requires a holistic approach to health and flexibility to accommodate the changing needs of the person. Poor vision may necessitate increased assistance with the activities of daily living (ADLs) and new strategies to improve communication. The older person's physical environment may need to be adapted to ensure their safety and promote independence. Those with eye conditions may require increased psychological and emotional support as their visual acuity fluctuates or deteriorates.

This chapter will focus on the most common eye conditions affecting older people in Australia and New Zealand today, the impact of vision impairment and blindness in later life, the disparity in eye health between Indigenous and non-Indigenous populations, relevant nursing interventions and health promotion strategies.

AGE-RELATED CHANGES
(see Table 21.1 and Fig. 21.1)

The Orbit and Eyelids

Bone loss throughout the body occurs with ageing. The orbit is no different and, as bone recedes, it enlarges with advancing years. The skin of the eyelids decreases in elasticity, as the muscles of the eyelid begin to atrophy and muscle fibres separate from each other. This can cause an age-related *ptosis*, the drooping of the upper lid.

The Tear Film and Cornea

As the body ages, the production of tears decreases. This is due to an age-related loss of conjunctival goblet cells and a decrease in sexual hormones, affecting the meibomian and lacrimal glands. These three structures produce the mucus, oils and lipids that make up tear film.

Every year that a person ages, the density of endothelial cells in the cornea decreases. Usually these cells pump fluid out of the cornea, keeping it in the relatively dehydrated state necessary for refraction. It is common for older adults to develop a hazy white ring around the cornea, called *arcus senilis*, caused by an accumulation of lipids. While this may indicate high cholesterol, it is usually of no concern when present in an older eye.

TABLE 21.1
Glossary

Word	Meaning
Arcus senilis	a hazy white ring around the cornea caused by an accumulation of lipids
Blepharitis	inflammation of the eyelids
Cataract	the clouding, or *opacification*, of the intraocular lens
Conjunctival goblet cells	cells in the conjunctiva that produce the mucus component of the tear film
Drusen	deposits of yellow or white lipid material
Ectropion	the outward turning of the eyelids
Entropion	the inward turning of the eyelids
Floaters	clumps of collagen drifting across the vitreous humour, appearing as moving specks across one's vision
Globe	the overall eyeball structure, apart from its extraocular muscles
Halos	circles of bright light surrounding true light sources
Lacrimal glands	a gland located above the eye that produces the aqueous component of the tear film
Meibomian glands	a gland located in the eyelids that produces the oil component of the tear film
Optic neuritis	inflammation of the optic nerve, causing a temporary but painful loss of vision
Optometrist	an eye health specialist in vision testing and the provision of glasses or contact lenses
Orthoptist	an eye health specialist in eye assessment and the non-surgical management of eye disorders
Presbyopia	the age-related decrease in the elasticity of the lens affecting accommodation
Ptosis	drooping of the upper eyelid
Puncta	the openings of the tear ducts
Punctal plugs	a small plug inserted into the tear ducts to decrease tear drainage and treat dry eye
Rhodopsin	a protein present in rod photoreceptors that assists vision in low light
Senile miosis	an age-related decrease in pupil size
Trichiasis	the inward turning of the eyelashes, causing harmful contact with the cornea
Uveitis	inflammation of the uveal structures of the eye: the choroid, ciliary bodies and iris

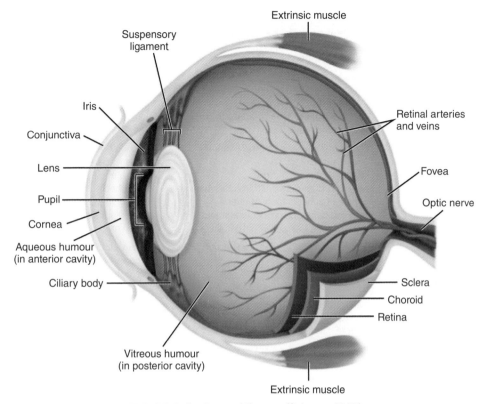

Suspensory
ligament

Extrinsic muscle

Iris

Conjunctiva

Lens

Pupil

Cornea

Aqueous humour
(in anterior cavity)

Ciliary body

Retinal arteries
and veins

Fovea

Optic nerve

Sclera

Choroid

Retina

Vitreous humour
(in posterior cavity)

Extrinsic muscle

FIG. 21.1 **Anatomy of the eye** (Solomon 2016.)

The Iris and Lens

The sphincter and dilator muscles of the iris contract to change the size of the pupil and allow light to enter the eye. Age-related atrophy of the dilator muscles leads to smaller pupils (*senile miosis*) and increased light adaptation time.

When focusing on a close object the ciliary muscle contracts, forcing the lens into a shorter, rounder shape. This increases the refractive power of the lens and enables light to focus on the retina. As a person ages, the lens enlarges, increasing in density, and becomes less elastic. This is termed *presbyopia* and affects the eye's ability to accommodate to shorter focal lengths, with a resulting decrease in near vision. Older people may find they need to hold text further away to read it.

With ageing, the transparent crystalline proteins present in the lens degenerate and become opaque. The cortex of the lens thickens and this change in shape affects the strength at which the lens can refract light rays and causes glare. A larger lens also affects the depth of the *anterior chamber*, the space between the cornea and iris. A narrower anterior chamber has the potential to detrimentally raise intraocular pressure. The lens gradually yellows, imperceptibly changing the individual's perception of colour and contrast.

The Vitreous and Retina

As a person ages, the gel-like vitreous humour, situated behind the lens in the posterior segment of the eye, condenses and become less viscous. As this occurs, the collagen fibres in the vitreous thicken, clump together and separate out from the thinner vitreous humour. The presence of floaters, tiny specks in a person's vision, may increase. Pockets of space, or *lacunae*, develop and fill with fluid. These *lacunae* join and may cause the vitreous to detach from the retina.

Photoreceptors, the key sensory receptor cells within the retina, decrease with age. Two kinds of photoreceptor cells exist: rods and cones. Rods make it possible to see in low light, whereas cones enable colour vision in bright light. The protein *rhodopsin*, present in rods, decreases with age, altering the older person's ability to adapt to the dark.

TABLE 21.2
Promoting Vision and Safety in Older People

Age-Related Change	Impact on the Older Person	Nursing Interventions
Longer dark adaptation time and light adaptation time	Increased risk of falls or other injuries when moving between areas that are lit differently May need more time to adapt to new surroundings	Support and/or supervise the older person when transitioning between differently lit areas
Decreased colour sensitivity	Different experience of the general environment Colours may appear dull May find it harder to differentiate between pills of similar size and shape May make confusing choices about wardrobe, hair colour and make-up	Provide education and clear labelling of prescribed medications Promote independence by supporting aesthetic choices Use bright, contrasting colours to highlight key items in the older person's surroundings
Decreased near vision (presbyopia)	Will require glasses for reading and fine work	Enlarge labelling of medications and other key items Promote regular evaluations by an optometrist
Smaller, less reactive pupils; reduction in number of photoreceptors	Will require more light to see compared to a younger individual	Ensure well-lit areas of activity (e.g. dinner table, bedside, bathroom sink)
Increased glare	Difficulty driving at night	Encourage regular visual acuity testing and compliance with licensing laws

Ageing impedes the retina's ability to properly eliminate cellular waste products. As a result, deposits of yellow or white lipid material accumulate within the retinal layers. These *drusen* may be hard or soft. Hard drusen are discrete entities with clearly defined edges, which often cause no impact on visual acuity and are considered a normal finding in older people. Soft drusen, however, may clump together and can lead to the development of wet age-related macular degeneration (AMD). Table 21.2 summarises the impact of age-related changes on vision and nursing interventions to promote an older person's safety, independence and emotional wellbeing.

COMMON EYE CONDITIONS
Uncorrected Refractive Error

Refractive error occurs when the eye is not able to focus light on the retina due to its size and shape. This is the result of anatomical variation between individuals or an age-related change and can be corrected with the right glasses. Despite having a simple solution, uncorrected refractive error accounts for two-thirds of cases of vision impairment in Australia and half of those in New Zealand (Access Economics 2010; CERA & Vision 2020 Australia 2016).

This is a global issue affecting people of all ages – however, it is more prevalent among the elderly (Nael et al 2019; Ye et al 2018). Uncorrected refractive error may lead to:
- falls and fractures
- worsening depression
- increased reliance on assistance with ADLs
- nutritional compromise
- medication compliance errors
- general decreased quality of life.

Investing in the development of eye health services and the training of ophthalmic health professionals are two ways to address this problem (Naidoo & Jaggemath 2012). In Australia, Indigenous people have lower rates of treatment with appropriate corrective aids. Increasing access to optometry services in remote regional communities has been a strong recommendation of researchers in this area (Foreman et al 2017).

Cataract (see Fig. 21.2)

A cataract is the clouding, or *opacification*, of the intraocular lens. This clouding limits the transmission of light

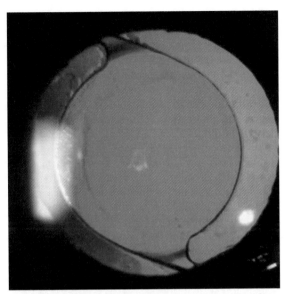

FIG. 21.2 **An artificial intraocular lens after cataract surgery** (Thomson & Lakhani 2015.)

through the lens, resulting in vision loss. Cataracts are considered an advanced stage of the process begun in presbyopia.

Cataracts are a pressing issue in gerontological health in both Australia and New Zealand. It has been estimated that in 2020 the number of New Zealanders with cataract-related vision loss was close to 23,000 people (Access Economics 2010). In New Zealand, rates of cataract are relatively similar between Māori and non-Māori people groups. However, in Australia statistics show that Indigenous Australians are not accessing cataract surgery at the same rate as non-Indigenous Australians (61% versus 88%), despite cataracts being the leading cause of blindness in this population (Access Economics 2010; CERA & Vision 2020 Australia 2016).

Age-related cataracts are the most common form of cataract. Pathogenesis is multifactorial, with oxidative stress recognised as a significant, if not the major, contributing factor (Liu et al 2017). Severe dehydration, hypertension, smoking and lipid metabolism are also thought to play a role in damage to the lens. Additionally, some medications commonly used by older people probably contribute to cataract formation, such as:

- allopurinol
- simvastatin
- potassium-sparing diuretics
- chlorpromazine
- carbamazepine.

Hormone replacement therapy has also been linked to a higher risk of cataracts (Gupta et al 2014).

Cataracts cause blurred vision, glare, halos and reduced sensitivity to contrast (the visual ability to discern an object from its background). Clinical management consists of surgical replacement of the cataractous lens with a new, artificial implant. The aim of surgery is to achieve excellent mid- to long-distance vision, after which the older person will require prescription glasses for reading and close work.

Glaucoma

Glaucoma is a group of conditions causing irreversible cell death in the optic nerve. It is a global problem responsible for 12% of blindness (WHO 2020). Advancing age is a major risk factor for any kind of glaucoma, as well as family history. It is largely associated with raised intraocular pressure (IOP), but can occur in the presence of normal IOP. Gradually, the nerve fibre layer in the retina thins out due to cell loss, causing a corresponding reduction in peripheral vision.

Individuals can be affected by glaucoma without being conscious of it. Poetically dubbed 'the thief of sight', glaucoma initially leaves central vision intact while decreasing peripheral vision. People over 65 years should have an IOP check and clinical examination of the optic nerve by an eye health professional each year (International Council of Ophthalmology [ICO] 2015).

Safety Alert
Acute Angle Closure Glaucoma

Nausea, vomiting, headaches, painful, irritated eyes, blurred vision and a cloudy cornea are signs of a dangerously high IOP, signalling a vision-threatening emergency called acute angle closure glaucoma. When accompanied by a sudden decrease in vision, warning signs include:

- nausea
- vomiting
- headaches
- halos
- a painful, irritated eye (most often occurs in one eye, but can be bilateral)
- a cloudy cornea.

Decreased vision with any combination of these signs warrants referral to the hospital's emergency department as soon as possible, as permanent damage can occur within hours. General nursing interventions include the administration of antiemetics, analgesia and ensuring the head is elevated to at least 30 degrees.

The most common form of glaucoma is primary open angle glaucoma (POAG). In POAG, the IOP increases due to the build-up of aqueous humour, the fluid that fills the anterior chamber. Aqueous is produced by the ciliary bodies and flows continually out of the eye into the systemic circulation. Resistance to the major drainage pathway causes congestion and a resulting increase of pressure in the globe. This increase of pressure is highly linked to damage of the optic nerve, although the exact mechanism of this damage is still undetermined. Medical treatment consists of eye drops to lower IOP. Surgical interventions attempt to create new aqueous drainage pathways.

While different estimates exist for the prevalence of glaucoma in Australia and New Zealand, it appears that roughly 3% of the population over 50 years old are affected by glaucoma, creating a substantial burden on the healthcare system (Keel et al 2019; Ministry of Health NZ 2020).

Age-Related Macular Degeneration
(Fig. 21.3)

Age-related macular degeneration (AMD) is a degenerative retinal condition that affects central vision. Age and genetic predisposition are key factors contributing to development of AMD. Individuals older than 75 years are three times more likely to have AMD than those between the ages of 65 and 74 (Al-Zamil & Yassin 2017). Caucasians are most affected by AMD compared to other ethnicities, and in Australia the prevalence among non-Indigenous people is eight times that of Indigenous people (CERA & Vision 2020 Australia 2016).

The macula is an area of the retina responsible for acute central vision due to its high volume of photoreceptors. The presence of drusen has a significant impact on their arrangement and subsequently on visual acuity. AMD has two different late stages – dry and wet. Most AMD sufferers have the dry form. This is characterised by atrophy of the retinal pigment epithelium, the cell layer responsible for supporting the health of the photoreceptors. There is no current treatment regimen for dry AMD, and management focuses on monitoring and health promotion. In the wet form of AMD, drusen forms in *Bruch's membrane*, a layer of the retina that separates it from its blood supply, causing it to break. Newly formed, fragile blood vessels grow through these breaks. When the vessels leak, fluid impedes the transmission of light and dramatically reduces vision. If left untreated, scarring occurs and vision loss is irreversible.

Individuals may experience blurring, areas of lost vision (*scotomas*) and distorted patches in their central line of vision; straight lines may appear wavy and deformed. The Amsler grid (Fig. 21.4) is a simple but effective screening tool for AMD. A nurse, optometrist, GP or ophthalmologist may supply the older person with a grid for their home environment, along with education on its use. The person can monitor themselves every day by standing 30 cm away and looking at the grid with one eye at a time to assess whether the lines appear straight or wavy. If lines appear wavy, the older person should seek review by their optometrist, GP or ophthalmologist.

There is no way to completely reverse scarring caused by wet AMD. However, in recent years treatment strategies have evolved to stall deterioration and preserve existing vision. These include regular injections of anti-vascular endothelial growth factor (anti-VEGF) into the vitreous chamber of the eye and laser photocoagulation to destroy ischaemic areas of the peripheral retina.

> **Research Highlight**
> *Potential New Therapy for AMD*
>
> While effective, repeated intravitreal injections are costly and put the older person at risk of injection-related complications such as infection and retinal detachment. Lately, research in this area has investigated gene therapy with adeno-associated virus vectors. This exciting innovation would require just one injection, potentially saving older people money and reducing risk (Bahadorani & Singer 2017).

Diabetic Retinopathy

Diabetic retinopathy is a condition in which high blood glucose levels caused by diabetes mellitus damage the vasculature of the retina. It has two clinical stages: non-proliferative and proliferative. In the first non-proliferative stage, asymptomatic damage begins. Glucose at high concentrations interacts with protein in vessel walls, increasing permeability and causing microaneurysms to develop and burst, filling the retina and vitreous with blood and fluid. In the second proliferative stage, this damage leads to ischaemic areas in the retina, which prompt production of vascular endothelial growth factor (VEGF) as a compensatory effort to produce more blood vessels. These new blood vessels can break, exacerbating the fluid build-up (*macular oedema*). Left untreated, this will result in irreversible vision loss. Diabetic retinopathy is currently managed with regular injections of anti-VEGF drugs. Advanced diabetic retinopathy may lead to unresolving vitreous haemorrhages and/or retinal detachments, in which case surgical intervention may be necessary.

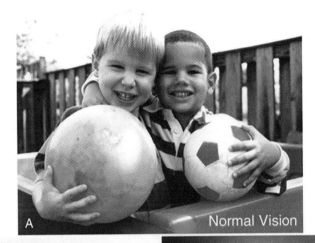

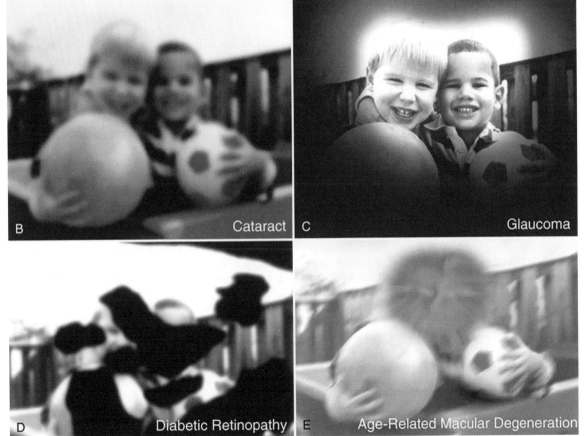

FIG. 21.3 **Vision affected by different eye conditions** A, Normal vision. B, Simulated vision with cataracts. C, Simulated vision with glaucoma. D, Simulated vision with diabetic retinopathy. E, Simulated vision with age-related macular degeneration (AMD). (Touhy 2018.)

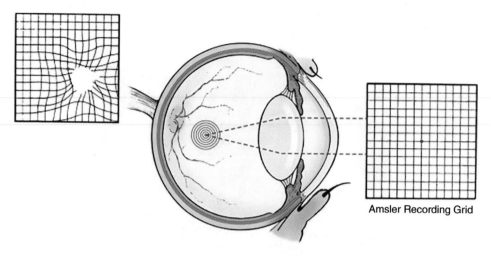

Amsler Recording Grid

FIG. 21.4 **An Amsler grid** (Touhy 2018.)

With growing rates of diabetes and an ageing population worldwide, there are increasing numbers of individuals who have had diabetes for decades. Sixty per cent of people will suffer from diabetic retinopathy 20 years after the onset of diabetes (Purbrick et al 2013). Effective measures to slow progression of diabetic retinopathy include:

- controlling blood glucose levels
- lowering cholesterol levels
- maintaining a healthy weight
- avoiding tobacco smoking
- regulation of blood pressure (Li & Wang 2013; Purbrick et al 2013).

In New Zealand, diabetes is believed to affect Māori and Pacific populations at three times the rate of other New Zealanders (Access Economics 2010). Similarly, diabetic retinopathy affects Indigenous Australians five times more than non-Indigenous people (CERA & Vision 2020 Australia 2016). On top of decreased visual acuity, diabetic retinopathy has been linked to an increase in falls and higher mortality rates in older people (Gupta et al 2017; Fisher et al 2016). This is a significant issue that is contributing to the gap in health outcomes experienced by Indigenous populations.

Posterior Vitreous Detachments and Retinal Detachments

Posterior vitreous detachments (PVDs) affect the majority of individuals over 80 years old (Bond-Taylor et al 2017). Age-related changes cause liquefaction and contraction of the vitreous humour, which may detach from the retina and collapse inwards. The uneven vitreous creates sites of traction that can lead to macular holes, retinal tears, vitreous haemorrhages and retinal detachments. Posterior vitreous detachments and their complications may present with:

- decreased vision
- flashes of light
- new or cascades of floaters, and/or
- a 'curtain' of darkness obscuring a section of the visual field.

However 20% of posterior vitreous detachments are asymptomatic. If a posterior vitreous detachment occurs without any complicating factors, such as a retinal tear, no active management is necessary. Complications may necessitate surgery. Retinal events can be diagnosed by clinical examination by an ophthalmologist at the slit lamp, by using ultrasound, and by using optical coherence tomography (OCT), a form of imaging that provides a cross-sectional view of the retinal layers.

Entropion, Ectropion, Blepharitis and Dry Eye

The production and distribution of tears over the surface of the eye are essential for its health and proper functioning. The film of tears nourishes the non-vascular cornea, helping to maintain the pristine clarity essential for the refraction of light. A number of mechanisms and structures are at work in the healthy eye to maintain this hydrated state. Tear production and drainage must both be intact. Eyelids must be properly positioned against the eye to control the amount of tear evaporation, and to effectively spread tear film with blinking. This also relies on a functioning blink mechanism, and the nervous regulation of tear production.

Glandular dysfunction leads to a decreased volume of tears. While the blink reflex is itself reduced, eyelid dysfunction, as seen in entropion and ectropion, reduces the extent to which blinking spreads tear film, allowing excess evaporation. This also disposes the older person to *blepharitis* (inflammation of the eyelids). Certain medications may also lead to dry eye, such as diuretics, anti-depressants, and medications used to treat Parkinson's disease and rheumatoid arthritis (Sharma & Hindman 2014).

Dry eye is associated with redness, irritation, pain, foreign body sensation and, paradoxically, excessive tearing. Basic interventions to alleviate dryness may include:
- instilling artificial tears
- avoiding air-conditioning
- using a humidifier
- applying warm compresses
- eyelid hygiene to promote adequate tear secretion and decrease bacterial load.

Punctal plugs may be required to block the drainage of tears, increasing their time on the eye's surface. It may also be necessary to treat underlying systemic conditions that exacerbate dry eye, such as autoimmune disorders. Many sufferers look to traditional Chinese medicine to manage dry eye symptoms. Recently, a meta-analysis of several studies showed that acupuncture may assist tear secretion (Yang et al 2015). Nutritional supplements, such as omega-3 fatty acids, are also thought to improve dry eye symptoms through managing inflammation (Ngo et al 2016).

Entropion and ectropion are eyelid malpositions where the lid margins turn inwards or outwards respectively. These malpositions can lead to irritation, sensitivity to the elements, and tearing. Corneal exposure from this kind of lid dysfunction can potentially lead to corneal ulceration and severe vision loss. Entropion has the added factor of involving the eyelashes, which turn inwards with the lid and can cause damage to the globe (*trichiasis*). Management for these conditions is surgical correction, dependent on the severity of the effects on the health of the globe.

Blepharitis is the inflammation of the lid margins. It may be acute or chronic and is considered multifactorial, involving:
- bacterial overload
- impaired immune response
- increased sensitivity to toxins
- general dermatological condition.

Lid hygiene is the mainstay of blepharitis treatment, and patients with chronic blepharitis should continue with their regimen even after their symptoms have resolved. Topical antibiotic ointment may also be prescribed in cases of staphylococcal blepharitis.

Herpes Zoster Ophthalmicus

Herpes zoster ophthalmicus (HZO) is a reactivation of the varicella zoster virus (shingles) within the ophthalmic division of the fifth cranial nerve. It produces a painful, vesicular rash in a striking distribution over just one side of the forehead and periocular skin. HZO commonly affects older people and those who are immunocompromised.

In many cases, HZO affects the eye itself, as well as the skin. This is due to the spread of inflammation as the virus moves along ciliary nerves innervating the sclera, cornea, iris, retina and the optic nerve. This can cause corneal ulcers, uveitis, retinal necrosis and detachment and optic neuritis; conditions that have the potential to cause blindness. Review by an ophthalmologist is essential, and some older people may require a hospital admission. The mainstay of treatment involves systemic antivirals and oral corticosteroids, but each case may necessitate additional management according to the severity of the potential complications (Vrcek et al 2016).

A consideration for the nurse caring for an older person with a history of HZO is post-herpetic neuralgia (see Chapter 19). This nerve pain can last for months following a bout of HZO, and places strain on the emotional health of the older person, as well as their functionality (Mallick-Searle et al 2016). Treatment for this neuropathic pain condition is pharmacological, which may exacerbate polypharmacy in older people, who may be on a number of medications.

Trachoma in Australia

Trachoma is an eye infection by *Chlamydia trachomatis*. Recurrent infections can cause the eyelids to become scarred and malformed, causing *trichiasis* and consequent irreversible scarring to the cornea. Trachoma predominantly affects children, but healthcare professionals must bear in mind that older Indigenous adults grew up during years of much higher infection rates and could be suffering the persistent effects of trichiasis from decades past.

Trachoma is highly contagious and is transmitted through close contact with an infected individual, shared fabric items such as towels and via flies. A dry, dusty environment, crowded living conditions and limited sanitation increase the transmission of trachoma. It is usually only found in developing countries, but persists today in remote Australia, contributing to socioeconomic disadvantage in Indigenous communities. Treatment follows the SAFE strategy promoted by the World Health Organisation (WHO):

- Surgery for trichiasis
- Antibiotics
- Face washing
- Environmental improvement (Harding-Esch et al 2018).

Australia has made great strides in reducing the prevalence of trachoma. In at-risk communities, rates of childhood infection have dropped from 14% in 2009 to 3.8% in 2017 (Australian Institute of Health and Welfare [AIHW] 2019). The number of identified at-risk communities has dropped from 244 in 2010 to 120 in 2018 (Kirby Institute 2018). It is now estimated that less than 1% of adults in these communities are suffering from trichiasis. However, trichiasis screening is opportunistic, and reporting is limited (AIHW 2019).

HEALTHY AGEING AND PREVENTION
General Principles

Most blindness and vision impairment are preventable or treatable (CERA & Vision 2020 Australia 2016). Providing health promotion and education may effect great change in an older person's life. The key wellness factors for eye health correspond to those for overall systemic health.

Promoting Wellness
Healthy Living for Best Vision

The following all contribute to a lower incidence of AMD, cataracts, dry eye, glaucoma and diabetic retinopathy:

- Smoking cessation and low alcohol intake
- A body mass index (BMI) in the normal range
- Good control of blood glucose, cholesterol and blood pressure
- Reduced UV exposure
- A healthy diet with a high intake of fruit, vegetables and legumes

Al-Zamil & Yassin (2017); Gupta et al (2014); Hernandez-Zimbron et al (2017); Owaifeer & Taisan (2018); Rasmussen & Johnson (2013).

Early Detection

Self-monitoring and regular check-ups with an optometrist are essential for the early recognition and management of glaucoma, AMD and diabetic retinopathy. All three conditions have asymptomatic stages where critical damage occurs. Early recognition of AMD, in particular, is key to preserving visual acuity in the ageing population. OCT (described earlier) is an imaging modality that can assess fluid build-up in the retina. It can be accessed by an optometrist or ophthalmologist. Older people can initiate their own appointment for a vision assessment. In Australia, Medicare subsidises eye health screens by optometrists annually for people aged 65 years and over. The nurse has a role to educate and encourage older people to undertake these regular vision checks.

Older people with diabetes should attend an annual diabetic eye health check with their optometrist, ophthalmologist or virtual outpatient diabetic retinal clinic to monitor for signs of diabetic retinopathy (CERA & Vision 2020 Australia 2016). Intraocular pressure can be monitored opportunistically at any eye health appointment, and individuals with a family history of glaucoma should regularly check their pressure with their optometrist or ophthalmologist. Promoting self-monitoring strategies, including regular use of an Amsler grid (Fig. 21.4) and eye health checks with OCT imaging, could make a considerable difference to an older person's life.

Smoking Cessation

Tobacco smoking damages the eye inside and out. The cornea is at risk of injury from exposure to heat, smoke and ash, while the retinal vasculature suffers from excessive inflammation and vasoconstriction. Nicotine triggers vasoconstriction in the eye, decreasing blood flow to the optic nerve, impacting cell metabolism and increasing the risk of vessel occlusion by a thrombus. Smoking particularly impacts cataract formation, AMD, diabetic retinopathy and dry eye. Nurses are well placed to:

- identify smokers
- initiate conversations about cessation
- provide education
- request intervention and assistance from medical staff
- refer patients to support groups and other assistive strategies.

Nutrition

The eye is highly susceptible to damage from oxidative stress and inflammation. Nutritional approaches to eye health focus on employing antioxidants and anti-inflammatory foods to combat these two forces. Vitamin C, vitamin E, zinc oxide, cupric oxide and lutein/zeaxanthin have been shown to have protective roles in staving off macular degeneration (Chew et al 2012; Al-Zamil & Yassin 2017). There are many commercially sold supplements that contain these nutrients. As previously noted, omega-3 fatty acids are thought to improve dry eye (Ngo et al 2016; Rasmussen & Johnson 2013). Tea, ginkgo biloba extract, fruits and vegetables and, in one study, saffron have all been shown to have protective potential against glaucoma (Owaifeer & Taisan 2018). Good nutrition will have a positive impact on the overall health of the older person and complement medical treatment of ocular diseases.

NURSING OLDER PEOPLE WITH VISION IMPAIRMENT

Communication

Adapting communication to the needs of the older person with vision loss is critical to clinical management. Communication affects the success of all aspects of care, including repositioning, mobilisation, pain assessment, health assessment, medication compliance and allied health therapy. Vision impaired or blind patients will not perceive non-verbal cues (gestures, facial expression) and body language that are obvious to those with normal vision. *Tips for Best Practice: Communicating with patients with vision loss* contains key tips for communicating with an older person who has vision loss.

Tips for Best Practice
Communicating With Patients With Vision Loss

- Identify yourself and others when approaching, before touching the older person
- Notify the person when you are leaving, and inform them who is remaining with them
- Speak in a normal volume, always facing the older person
- Reduce unnecessary background noise
- Use the analogy of an anatomical clock to alert the older person to an item's location, e.g. 'Your glass of water is on your right, at two o'clock.'

Touhy (2018); Vision Australia (2020).

Health Education

Health education provided to the older person should consist of both verbal and written communication. In written materials, use an enlarged font and a bold contrast between the colour of the paper and the text. Paper with a high gloss may be difficult to read in certain lights. Provide opportunities for the older person to ask questions and ensure that he or she knows how to contact the nurse with any further questions.

Adapting the Healthcare or Home Environment

Appropriate lighting is essential for older people with vision loss. Poor lighting can result in:
- medication errors
- miscommunication
- anxiety
- falls.

Provide bright, warm, incandescent lighting to promote the older person's safety and independence. Important items, such as cutlery or handtowels, should be brightly coloured. In the healthcare environment, strategies to assist the older person include:
- placing respectful 'low vision' signage by the bedside to alert staff to the older person's needs
- accommodation in a corner bed, which may be easier to locate
- remaining present while the older person takes medication to ensure all pills are taken with none unknowingly dropped
- assisting the older person to mobilise by standing by his or her side and extending an arm out with elbow bent so that he or she can place a hand on the arm above the elbow
- when approaching a change in the environment (e.g. a step), stopping the older person and notifying him or her before continuing
- highlighting light-coloured crockery by placing it on a coloured background, such as a coloured serviette, tray or piece of paper (Vision Australia 2020).

Corrective Aids and Assistants

Older people who have corrective aids may not be wearing them. When meeting the person for the first time, it is helpful to enquire as to whether they use glasses, contact lenses or a magnifying glass for reading. Making these items accessible empowers the older person to read health information, complete forms, identify faces of family, friends and healthcare professionals and enjoy recreational reading or television. It is also vitally important that these aids are kept clean and safe.

Assistive devices may be available to the older person in the healthcare or home environment. A nurse's diligence may be a key factor in initiating the use of an assistive device. For example, mobile phones and smart watches may have features that enhance contrast, enlarge fonts and read text out aloud. Liaising with other disciplines, such as occupational therapists, orthoptists, optometrists and specialised ophthalmic nurses, may assist staff in accessing all the aids and services available to the older person.

Available Services in Australia and New Zealand

Older people with vision loss can access free services to preserve their independence and promote their health and wellbeing. Vision Australia and Blind Low Vision New Zealand are not-for-profit organisations that provide practical and emotional support for individuals with vision impairment and blindness. Among other actions, Vision Australia can help older clients navigate the Department of Health's My Aged Care system and access a broad range of services, such as help in the home and help with assistive technology, meals and modifications such as shower rails. Blind Low Vision NZ teaches individuals how to reclaim everyday tasks such as using public transport, cooking at home or enjoying multimedia.

Practice Scenario

John, a 79-year-old man, has been admitted to your orthopaedic unit after a fall left him with a fractured neck of femur. He's upset because he can't mobilise and wants to go downstairs for a smoke. When you offer him a newspaper he sighs and explains he's struggling to see his TV, let alone the newspaper these days, even with his reading glasses. He shares that he's not been able to do his woodworking lately either, remarking that he 'hasn't got much going for him at the moment'.

MULTIPLE CHOICE QUESTIONS

1. Based on the information provided, which of the following eye conditions could John be at risk for? More than one answer may be appropriate.
   a. macular degeneration
   b. dry eye
   c. uncorrected refractive error
   d. conjunctivitis

2. Based on the information provided, which systemic conditions could John be at risk for? More than one answer may be appropriate.
   a. depression
   b. hearing loss
   c. ketoacidosis
   d. nicotine withdrawal

3. Which of the following nursing interventions would be appropriate in promoting John's health and wellbeing? More than one answer may be appropriate.
   a. referral to a diabetes nurse educator
   b. referral to a low vision service
   c. smoking cessation intervention
   d. referral to ophthalmology

Summary

An awareness of eye conditions and their effects on the lives of older people will help inform nursing care and thereby improve the quality of life of those with vision loss. This chapter has examined relevant statistics relating to vision impairment in Australia and New Zealand, detailed age-related changes in the eye and orbit, discussed the major eye conditions affecting older people and outlined nursing interventions to promote a patient's safety, health and wellbeing.

REFERENCES

Access Economics Pty Limited. (2010) Clear focus – the economic impact of vision loss in New Zealand in 2009. Online. Available: https://blindlowvision.org.nz/information/statistic-and-research/#sta

Al-Zamil WM, Yassin SA 2017 Recent developments in age-related macular degeneration: a review. Clinical Interventions in Aging 12:1313–1330.

Australian Institute of Health and Welfare (AIHW) (2019) Indigenous eye health measures 2018. Online. Available: www.aihw.gov.au/

Bahadorani S, Singer M (2017) Recent advances in the management and understanding of macular degeneration. F1000 Research 6:519.

Bond-Taylor M, Jakobsson G, Zetterberg M (2017) Posterior vitreous detachment – prevalence of and risk factors for retinal tears. Clinical Ophthalmology 11:1689–1695.

Centre for Eye Research Australia and Vision 2020 Australia (2016) National eye health survey. Online. Available: www.vision2020australia.org.au/resources/national-eye-health-survey-report/

Chew E, Clemons T, SanGiovanni J et al (2012) The age-related eye disease study 2 (AREDS2): study design and baseline characteristics (AREDS2 report number 1). Ophthalmology 119(11):2282–2289.

Fisher D, Jonasson F, Klein R et al (2016) Mortality in older persons with retinopathy and concomitant health conditions. Ophthalmology 123(7):1570–1580.

Foreman J, Xie J, Keel S et al (2017) Treatment coverage rates for refractive error in the National Eye Health survey. PLoS ONE 12(4):e0175353.

Gupta P, Aravindhan A, Gan A et al (2017) Association between the severity of diabetic retinopathy and falls in an Asian population with diabetes: the Singapore epidemiology of eye diseases study. JAMA Ophthalmology 135(12):1410–1416.

Gupta V, Rajagopala M, Ravishankar B (2014) Etiopathogenesis of cataract: an appraisal. Indian Journal of Ophthalmology 62(2):103–110.

Harding-Esch E, Kadimpeul J, Sarr B et al (2018) Population-based prevalence survey of follicular trachoma and trachomatous trichiasis in the Casamance region of Senegal. BMC Public Health 18:62.

Hernandez-Zimbron L, Gulias-Cañizo R, Golzarri M et al (2017) Molecular age-related changes in the anterior segment of the eye. Hindawi Journal of Ophthalmology 2017:1295132.

International Council of Ophthalmology (2015) ICO guidelines for glaucoma eye care. ICO, San Francisco. Online. Available: www.icoph.org/enhancing_eyecare/glaucoma.html

Keel S, Xie J, Foreman J et al (2019) Prevalence of glaucoma in the Australian National Eye Health Survey. British Journal of Ophthalmology 103:191–195.

Kirby Institute (2018) Australian trachoma surveillance report 2018. Online. Available: www1.health.gov.au/

Li X, Wang Z (2013) Prevalence and incidence of retinopathy in elderly diabetic patients receiving early diagnosis and treatment. Experimental and Therapeutic Medicine 5(5): 1393–1396.

Liu YC, Wilkins M, Kim T et al (2017) Cataracts. Lancet (London) 390(10094):600–612.

Mallick-Searle T, Snodgrass B, Brant J (2016) Postherpetic neuralgia: epidemiology, pathophysiology, and pain management pharmacology. Journal of Multidisciplinary Healthcare 9:447–454.

Ministry of Health (2020). Glaucoma. MOH, Wellington. Online. Available: www.health.govt.nz/your-health/conditions-and-treatments/diseases-and-illnesses/eye-and-vision-problems/glaucoma

Nael V, Moreau G, Monferme S (2019) Prevalence and associated factors of uncorrected refractive error in older adults in a population-based study in France. JAMA Ophthalmology 137(1):3–11.

Naidoo K, Jaggemath J (2012) Uncorrected refractive error. Indian Journal of Ophthalmology 60(5):432–437.

Ngo W, Srinivasan S, Houtman D et al (2016) The relief of dry eye signs and symptoms using a combination of lubricants, lid hygiene and ocular nutraceuticals. Journal of Optometry 10:26–33.

Owaifeer A, Taisan A (2018) The role of diet in glaucoma: a review of the current evidence. Ophthalmology and Therapy 7(1):19–31.

Purbrick R, Ah-Chan J, Downes S (2013) Eye disease in older people. Reviews in Clinical Gerontology 23:234–250.

Rasmussen H, Johnson E (2013) Nutrients for the ageing eye. Clinical Interventions in Aging 8:741–748.

Sharma A, Hindman HB (2014) Aging: a predisposition to dry eyes. J Ophthalmol 2014:781683.

Solomon E (2016) Introduction to human anatomy and physiology, 4th edn. Elsevier, Maryland Heights, Missouri.

Statistics New Zealand (2013) Disability survey: 2013. Online. Available: www.stats.govt.nz/topics/disability

Thomson J, Lakhani N (2015) Cataracts. Primary Care 42(3): 409–423.

Touhy T (2018) Diseases affecting vision and hearing. In T Touhy & K Jett (eds), Ebersole and Hess' gerontological nursing & health aging, 5th edn. Elsevier, St Louis, Missouri.

Vision Australia (2020) Communicating effectively. Online. Available: www.visionaustralia.org/information/family-friends-carers/communicating-effectively

Vrcek I, Choudhury E, Durairaj V (2016) Herpes zoster ophthalmicus: a review for the internist. The American Journal of Medicine 130(1):21–26.

World Health Organisation (2020) Priority eye diseases: glaucoma. Online. Available: www.who.int/blindness/causes/priority/en/index6.html

Yang L, Yang Z, Yu H et al (2015) Acupuncture therapy is more effective than artificial tears for dry eye syndrome: evidence based on meta-analysis. Evidence Based Complementary Alternative Medicine 2015:143858.

Ye H, Qian Y, Zhang Q et al (2018) Prevalence and risk factors of uncorrected refractive error among an elderly Chinese population in urban China: a cross-sectional study. BMJ Open 8(3):bmjopen-2017-021325.

CHAPTER 22

Musculoskeletal Health

HELENE METCALFE

LEARNING OBJECTIVES

After reading this chapter, you will be able to:

* examine current trends in musculoskeletal disorders in older people
* identify age-related changes that occur in bones, muscles and connective tissues
* highlight the physical changes that occur in inflammatory conditions, including osteoarthritis, rheumatoid arthritis and gout
* analyse the consequences associated with traumatic injury and limited mobility in older people
* discuss current nursing assessment, interventions and management of bone and joint disorders to minimise disability.

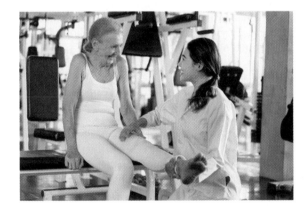

INTRODUCTION

This chapter will explore the common age-related musculoskeletal disorders seen in older people, as well as the impact of traumatic injury. The role of the nurse in assessing musculoskeletal health, providing interventions and subsequent management of common musculoskeletal disorders will be identified, along with strategies to minimise immobility. The impact a musculoskeletal disorder has on an older person's quality of life and wellbeing, resulting in withdrawal from social, community and occupational activities, will be highlighted.

MUSCULOSKELETAL HEALTH

Musculoskeletal conditions are attributed to over 150 different disorders of the bones, muscles, ligaments and connective tissues. In Australia, 29% of the population, around 7 million people, had a chronic musculoskeletal condition in 2017–18 (Australian Institute of Health and Welfare [AIHW] 2019). Arthritis was the third most common chronic condition overall, reported by one in seven Australians (15% of the population, 3.6 million people), with the highest proportion in people aged 65 years and older (57.3% of all females; and 39.9% of all males). Additionally, one in five Australians aged 75 years and over reported having osteoporosis or osteopenia (low bone density). Three out of four people with arthritis aged 45 and over reported the presence of at least one other co-morbidity, with the most common being back problems (37%), mental and behavioural conditions (31%) and asthma (19%) (AIHW 2019).

In New Zealand it was estimated that more than 45% of people aged over 65 years had some form of arthritis in 2018, with the economic and wellbeing costs calculated at $NZ12.2 billion (Arthritis New Zealand 2019). By 2040, there are projected to be 1 million cases of arthritis in New Zealand. As in Australia, osteoarthritis is the most common form; however, this is followed by gout arthritis, which is disproportionately more common in Māori and Pacific Islander peoples (Arthritis New Zealand 2019). Preventable factors associated with chronic musculoskeletal disorders include dietary factors, overweight and obesity, lack of physical activity, smoking, alcohol and occupational exposure (AIHW 2019).

AGE-RELATED CHANGES

As individuals age, key changes occur in the bone, muscles, joints and connective tissue. All these issues can contribute to decreased mobility and independence.

Bone Strength

Bone strength is essential for body structure, shape and movement. The human body consists of 206 bones divided into the axial skeleton, which contains 80 bones: skull, vertebral column and thorax; and the appendicular skeleton, comprising 126 bones (Craft et al 2019). Ageing, in combination with intrinsic and extrinsic factors, accelerates the decline in bone mass (the amount of bone tissue in the body) in both males and females, contributing to fractures, morbidities, disability and social costs (Heidari et al 2017).

Intrinsic factors include:
- genetics
- hormonal
- biochemical
- vascular changes.

Extrinsic factors include:
- nutrition
- physical activity
- comorbidities
- medications.

Typically, bone loss is accelerated in women due to oestrogen deficiency following menopause. Males are similarly affected, with oestrogen deficiency more important than testosterone deficiency in the loss of bone in ageing men. In addition to bone loss, a reduction in collagen decreases bone flexibility in response to pressure, increasing susceptibility to fracture. Other effects include the spinal column becoming curved and compressed and the foot arches becoming less pronounced, contributing

to a slight loss of height. Bone spurs (bony projections that develop along bone edges) may also form on the vertebrae due to ageing and overall wear and tear.

A bone mineral density (BMD) test can provide a snapshot of bone health (Osteoporosis Australia). This test generates a 'T-score' by comparing the person's BMD with the mean BMD of young healthy adults of the same sex. To interpret the T-score:

1 to −1 suggests normal bone density

−1 to −2.5 suggests osteopenia (low bone density)

−2.5 and lower suggests osteoporosis (low bone mass and deterioration of bone tissue).

Muscle Mass

Declining muscle tissue in older people is often caused by age-related sarcopenia, defined as 'progressive and generalised loss of skeletal muscle mass and strength' (Santilli et al 2014:177). Contributing factors include decreased physical activity, lower hormone excretion, nutritional deficits and, possibly, chronic inflammatory disease. As muscle fibres shrink, the tissue is regenerated more slowly and may be replaced with a tough fibrous tissue. This is most noticeable in the hands, which may look thin and bony. Currently, there is no definitive biological marker of sarcopenia, with dual-energy X-ray absorptiometry (DXA) often used to assist diagnosis. Management includes resistance training to improve muscle strength (Osteoporosis Australia). Additionally, muscle changes can be due to diseases, such as cancer-related anorexia and cachexia syndrome, a multifactorial condition defined by ongoing muscle loss (Fearon et al 2011).

Joints

As individuals age, joint movement becomes less flexible due to reduced lubricating fluid inside the joint, as well as a decrease and thinning of cartilage. In addition, ligaments tend to shorten and lose flexibility causing joints to become stiff (Craft et al 2019). This can lead to a decrease in range of motion (ROM) and changes in posture and gait. All these factors can contribute to the older person experiencing pain, impaired mobility, self-care deficits and an increased risk of falls (see Chapter 16).

MUSCULOSKELETAL ASSESSMENT

When undertaking a musculoskeletal assessment, it is essential to observe the older person's appearance and gait, noting indications of pain at rest or triggered by movement. Observe for any obvious structural deformities, muscle tone hypotonicity (flaccidity), as well as signs of spasticity. Ask the older person to move each joint through its various ROMs, noting any pain or crepitus (a grating sound or sensation) (Estes et al 2015). Assess the joints for changes in function and signs of inflammation using the following *Tips for best practice*.

Tips for Best Practice

Assess the joints for limitations in function and signs of inflammation:

- Ask the older person to move each joint through its ROM, noting:
  - any indicators of pain (see Chapter 19)
  - any crepitus (a grating sound or sensation) (Estes et al 2015).
- If the older person is unable to actively move any joint on their own, then the nurse passively (and gently) moves the joint through its ROM, again noting any pain or crepitus.
- Palpate each joint by applying light pressure from the periphery inwards to the centre of the joint. Note any:
  - swelling
  - indicators of pain (see Chapter 19)
  - tenderness
  - warmth
  - presence of nodules.

Always stop if the older person complains of pain. Never force a joint into a position beyond its anatomic angle.

Balance and mobility diminish as people age (Clinical Excellence Commission [CEC] 2016). With impairment of balance a key predictor of falls risk (see Chapter 16), a variety of simple tools can be used by the nurse to indicate an issue with balance, coordination or strength that affects mobility. These are explained in *A guide to understanding balance and mobility for health staff*, produced by the New South Wales Government (CEC 2016).

OSTEOPOROSIS

Osteoporosis is a common disease where the bones weaken to the point at which they easily break; most commonly affecting the hip, spine and wrist (National Institute on Aging [NIA] 2017). It affects approximately 1 million Australians (Osteoporosis Australia 2020) and occurs due to a loss of minerals such as calcium, which leads to declining bone density or mass. Osteopenia is the condition where bone mass is lowered, but not as severely as in osteoporosis. Osteopenia indicates that

bone loss has begun and can be considered a warning sign that the person is at risk for developing osteoporosis and accompanying risk for fractures (NIA 2017). Contributing factors seen in older people include:

- decreased levels of oestrogen and testosterone
- inadequate vitamin D, calcium, magnesium
- decreased activity level or sedentary lifestyle
- alcoholism
- use of corticosteroids
- cigarette smoking (Craft et al 2019).

Some of these factors may be modified with lifestyle changes. Osteopenia is diagnosed via a bone mineral density test. The goal of treatment is to prevent progression to osteoporosis with a diet that includes sufficient calcium and vitamin D (see *Promoting Wellness* box) and regular weight-bearing exercise, e.g. walking, running or jumping, ideally 30 minutes per day. Neither osteopenia nor osteoporosis produce symptoms, as losing bone mass does not cause pain. Frequently, osteoporosis is not diagnosed until a fracture occurs. Current guidelines recommend that any person over 50 years of age who experiences a broken bone from a minor fall should be investigated for osteoporosis (Royal Australian College of General Practitioners [RACGP] 2019).

Patient education is critical for the management and prevention of traumatic injury. Recommended strategies for managing osteoporosis, and its precursor osteopenia, are provided in *Tips for best practice: Recommended strategies for the management of osteoporosis and osteopenia*.

Tips for Best Practice
Recommended Strategies for the Management of Osteoporosis and Osteopenia

- nutritional and pharmacological management
- attention to diet, especially intake of vitamin D and calcium
- calcium supplementation
- weight-bearing and resistance exercise (RACGP 2019)
- smoking cessation
- avoidance of heavy alcohol use
- assessing risk factors and contributing conditions
- reducing the risk of falls (see Chapter 16)
- monitoring bone density by densitometry techniques.

Elemental calcium (1.0–1.5 g/day to maintain bone minerals) should be adjunctive therapy for all people with osteoporosis, unless contraindicated, such as in hypercalcaemia.

TABLE 22.1   Medications Affecting Bone

Therapeutic Group	Pharmacological Group	Examples
Drugs to treat hypocalcaemia	Calcium salts	calcium carbonate calcium gluconate
	Vitamin D analogues	calcitriol ergocalciferol paricalcitol
Drugs to treat hypercalcaemia	Calcitonin analogues	salcatonin
Drugs to treat osteoporosis	Bisphosphonates	alendronate, clodronate, ibandronic acid, pamidronate, risedronate, tiludronate
	Parathyroid hormone analogues	teriparatide
	Calcium uptake promoters	strontium ranelate
	Selective Estrogen Receptor Modulators (SERMs)	raloxifene
	RANKL antibody denosumab	RANKL antibody denosumab

Bryant et al (2018).

Promoting Wellness
Osteopenia Diet to Prevent Bone Loss

Dietary choices to ensure sufficient calcium and vitamin D:

- non-fat and low-fat dairy products:
  - cheese
  - milk
  - yoghurt
- Other foods with calcium include:
- dried beans
- broccoli
- wild fresh water salmon
- spinach

  Some types of orange juice, breads and cereals are fortified with calcium and vitamin D.

Patient education is critical for the management and prevention of traumatic injury. Recommended management of this condition includes:

- nutritional and pharmacological management
- attention to diet, especially intake of vitamin D and calcium (see *Promoting Wellness: Osteopenia diet to prevent bone loss*)
- calcium supplementation
- weight-bearing and resistance exercise (RACGP 2019)
- assessing risk factors and contributing conditions
- reducing the risk of falls (see Chapter 16)
- monitoring bone density by densitometry techniques.

Elemental calcium (1.0–1.5 g/day to maintain bone minerals) should be adjunctive therapy for all people with osteoporosis, unless contraindicated, such as in hypercalcaemia. The drugs used to treat osteoporosis either inhibit bone resorption (antiresorptive) or have anabolic (building up) actions (Bryant et al 2018). Table 22.1 summarises medications that affect the bone.

Safety Alert

The medication class bisphosphonates, used to treat osteoporosis, increase the risk of oesophageal erosion. It is important that the older person follows dosing instructions:

- Take tablets with a full glass of plain water.
- Stay upright for at least 30 minutes.
- Do not chew or crush tablets.
- Some formulations must be taken on an empty stomach.
- Consult the doctor if symptoms of oesophageal disease (i.e. heartburn, retrosternal pain, difficulty swallowing) develop or worsen.

These medications are not appropriate for older people with memory loss or those who cannot be relied upon to follow these instructions. Bisphosphonates are also contraindicated for people with oesophageal problems.

OSTEOMALACIA

Osteomalacia is a bone disorder in adults in which osteoid, the newly formed bone matrix, does not mineralise within the bone, resulting in soft bones (BMJ Best Practice 2020). Current research suggests this condition affects about 1 in 1000 individuals in Australia. Contributing factors include:

- deficiency in vitamin D

Research Highlight

A study conducted in Western Australia evaluated the impact of a newly created role of orthopaedic nurse practitioner in one large tertiary hospital (Coventry et al 2017). A nurse practitioner is a registered nurse with extensive clinical experience, Masters level qualification and endorsement from the Nursing and Midwifery Board of Australia, or registration with the Nursing Council of New Zealand Aotearoa. Nurse practitioners hold advanced nursing knowledge and work autonomously to improve access to healthcare and provide a wide range of assessment and treatment options in collaboration with healthcare teams. Nurse practitioners have legal authority to practise beyond the scope of a registered nurse, and can prescribe medication and order diagnostic tests. The orthopaedic nurse practitioner role provides clinical support to all hospital patients receiving treatment for bone and muscle injuries. This study assessed outcomes for patients who were treated for a 'minimal trauma' hip fracture before and after the orthopaedic nurse practitioner role was implemented. A 'minimal trauma hip fracture' results from a simple fall from no more than standing height.

The study used a retrospective cohort design. Data were extracted from electronic medical records for two cohorts of patients aged 65 years or over treated for hip fracture. The comparison cohort (354 patients) was treated in 2010, before the orthopaedic nurse practitioner role. The intervention cohort (301 patients) was treated in 2013, after the orthopaedic nurse practitioner commenced. Both cohorts had the same average age (84 years) and over 70% were female. Statistical comparison between the cohorts found that patients had a shorter length of stay in hospital after the orthopaedic nurse practitioner role came into being (4.4 days in 2013 versus 5.3 days in 2010) with a cost saving to the hospital of AU\$354,483 over one year and net annual cost saving per patient of AU\$1,178.

Coventry et al (2017).

- reduction in calcium intake
- chronic kidney disease
- limited sunlight exposure.

Clinical symptoms include bone pain, muscular weakness (particularly proximal muscle weakness) and difficultly walking. Older people with this condition may develop bone fractures, vertebral collapse and bone malformation. Management includes vitamin D supplements (see Table 22.1) and increased levels of dietary calcium (See *Promoting Wellness: Osteopenia diet to prevent bone loss*).

PAGET'S DISEASE

Paget's disease of the bone (also known as osteitis deformans) is a chronic condition causing abnormal enlargement and weakening of the skeleton. It is associated with ageing and may have a genetic origin. It tends to affect people over the age of 50 and affects slightly more men than women. Risk factors include ethnicity – it's more common in people from England, Scotland, Central Europe and Greece. The most commonly affected sites include the:

- skull
- spine
- pelvis
- femur
- tibia
- humerus.

Individuals may present with pain and aching in the bones (affected bones may become deformed or misshapen), and affected bones can feel warmer than the rest of the body. If the skull is affected, individuals may experience problems with hearing, headaches, vertigo or tinnitus (Craft et al 2019). Thickened bones can cause abnormal bone curvatures, brain compression and impaired motor function.

Nursing assessment includes:

- observing areas over long bones for warmth, deformity, pain and erythema
- observing joints for reduced ROM
- evaluating the presence of any weakness, ataxia or hearing loss
- consideration of safety and mobility issues.

Pharmacological treatment is aimed at managing pain and calcium levels. Medications used to treat Paget's disease of bone include bisphosphonates (see Table 22.1), non-steroidal anti-inflammatory drugs (NSAIDs) for temporary pain relief, calcium and vitamin D.

INFLAMMATORY JOINT DISEASE

Arthritis is a term used for a range of inflammatory conditions that affect the bones, muscles and joints. It includes rheumatoid arthritis, osteoarthritis and gout. The AIHW (2019) suggests that one in seven Australians have some form of arthritis, and it is particularly prevalent among older Australians. These inflammatory diseases result in pain and disability, restricting an individual's ability to perform activities of daily living (ADLs) with subsequent loss of independence.

Osteoarthritis

Osteoarthritis is a degenerative joint disease and the most common form of arthritis in Australia and New Zealand. An estimated 2.2 million (9.3%) Australians have this condition, according to the Australian Bureau of Statistics (ABS) 2017–18 National Health Survey. Osteoarthritis is estimated to affect 10% of adults in New Zealand (Arthritis New Zealand 2019). The conditions is characterised by:

- local damage and loss of articular cartilage
- new bone formation at joint margins
- subchondral bone changes
- variable degrees of mild synovitis
- thickening of the joint capsule (Craft et al 2019).

When joint cartilage is lost, the two bone surfaces come into contact resulting in joint pain (see Fig. 22.1). The individual may also present with stiffness, enlargement of the joint, tenderness, limited motion and deformity. The areas most commonly affected include the:

- distal interphalangeal joints
- carpometacarpal joints
- first metatarsophalangeal joints
- proximal interphalangeal joints
- knees
- hips
- spine.

Predisposing factors for development of osteoarthritis include:

- increasing age
- female gender
- joint injuries
- lifestyle (inactivity, stress)
- obesity
- genetics.

On assessment of an affected joint, crepitus (a grating sound or sensation) may be heard and felt, along with reduced ROM. In addition, there may be pain, tenderness, swelling and redness. Bony enlargements known as Heberden nodes may be seen on the distal interphalangeal joints, and Bouchard nodes may be seen on the proximal joints. Fig. 22.1 demonstrates the progressive pathological changes in joints affected by osteoarthritis.

Management includes heat and cold therapy, NSAIDs, topical gels and occasionally steroid injections (Bryant et al 2018).

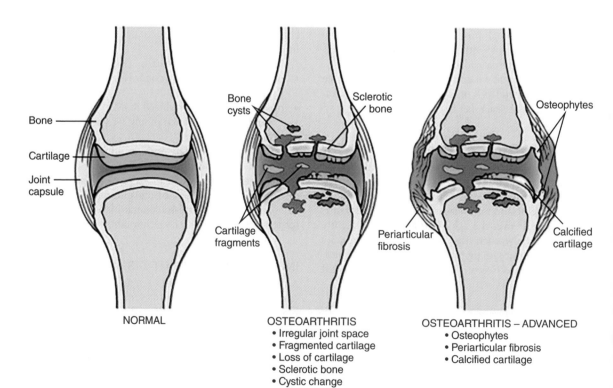

FIG. 22.1 **Progressive pathological changes underlying osteoarthritis** (Craft et al 2019.)

Rheumatoid Arthritis

Rheumatoid arthritis is a systemic autoimmune disease characterised by inflammatory damage or destruction to the synovial membrane or articular cartilage (see Fig. 22.3). It is estimated to affect approximately 2% of the Australian population (AIHW 2019). The presence of the rheumatoid factor (RF) in the blood is often used to diagnose rheumatoid arthritis. The majority of adults with rheumatoid arthritis test positive for RF, although healthy people without any autoimmune disorders can also test positive for RF (Arthritis Australia 2020a).

Other blood indicators include the erythrocyte sedimentation rate (ESR), tumour necrosis factor-alpha or c-reactive protein (CRP) levels, as all of these may indicate the presence and level of inflammation in the body. Further diagnostic tests include X-rays, ultrasounds and magnetic resonance imaging (MRI) scans to examine the joints and determine if rheumatoid arthritis is the cause of joint erosion.

As rheumatoid arthritis is a systemic disease, organs such as the heart and lungs may be affected. In the early stages, a person with rheumatoid arthritis may not exhibit the characteristic joint redness or swelling, but may experience tenderness and pain. Often more than one joint is involved and small joints (wrists, certain joints in the hands and feet) are typically affected first. The same joints on both sides of the body are affected. Many people with rheumatoid arthritis also experience fatigue and some may have a low-grade fever. Symptoms tend to come and go in flare-ups which can last from days to months (Craft et al 2019).

Monocyclic progression (sometimes called remissive) is an episode of rheumatoid arthritis in which symptoms last only 2–5 years. Monocyclic progression is usually the result of an early diagnosis and immediate aggressive treatment to ensure that the symptoms do not return. *Polycyclic progression* (sometimes called intermittent) is the constant recurrence of rheumatoid arthritis symptoms and flares, but in fluctuating stages. A person with polycyclic progression can go for long periods of time without experiencing any symptoms at all, but flare-ups usually return. The goal of treatment for rheumatoid arthritis is to:

* inhibit inflammation
* relieve symptoms
* prevent joint and organ damage
* reduce complications
* improve physical function.

Fig. 22.2 demonstrates the pathways of joint damage caused by stimulation of macrophages and fibroblasts as well as B lymphocytes. This autoimmune response ultimately leads to pannus formation, joint destruction and cartilage fibrosis.

Pharmacological management of rheumatoid arthritis begins with first-line medicines, such as paracetamol, codeine and NSAIDs. When there is insufficient symptom control, treatment progresses to include corticosteroids, disease-modifying anti-rheumatic drugs (DMARDs) and biologic disease-modifying anti-rheumatic drugs (bDMARDs). Maintaining a healthy and active lifestyle, including low-impact physical activity, can maintain mobility and strengthen muscles around the affected joints (AIHW 2019). Physiotherapy may be recommended for some people. Joint replacement surgery may also be necessary to relieve pain and restore function to severely damaged joints. Fig. 22.3 demonstrates joint deformities associated with damage from rheumatoid arthritis.

Gout

Gout is a metabolic disorder that disrupts the body's control of uric acid production or excretion. As the level of uric acid rises, it crystallises within connective tissues. When these crystals occur in the synovial fluid, the inflammation is known as 'gouty arthritis' (Craft et al 2019). Affected individuals can have accelerated purine synthesis and breakdown (with uric acid as the end product of purine metabolism), or poor uric acid secretion in the kidneys. Fig. 22.4 provides an overview of the processes of purine synthesis, metabolism and excretion.

Typically, people with gout develop three stages of the disease:

1. asymptomatic hyperuricaemia
2. acute gouty arthritis
3. tophaceous gout

The most commonly affected joint appears to be the great toe. Affected joints become hot, reddened and tender (Arthritis Australia 2020b). The pain can be severe and associated with fever and chills. It may affect a person's mobility, self-care and functional abilities. Nursing assessment involves observing the affected joint for:

* warmth
* swelling
* tophi (visible small white or yellow lumps)
* cutaneous erythema
* severe pain.

Management is aimed at pain relief, including the use of NSAIDs, colchicine and corticosteroids. Allopurinol is an effective treatment for reducing concentrations of uric acid (Bryant et al 2018). It is also essential to educate the older person regarding dietary intake of purine (see *Promoting Wellness: Dietary management of gout*) and encourage fluid intake to prevent kidney stones.

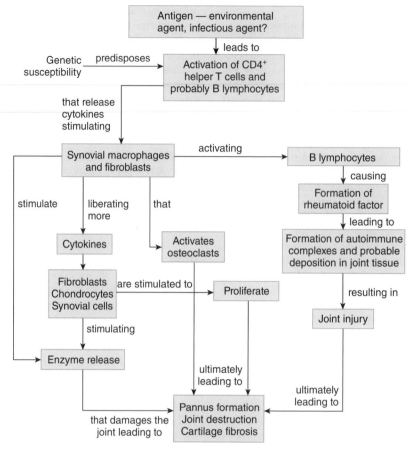

FIG. 22.2 Rheumatoid arthritis progression leading to joint damage (Craft et al 2019.)

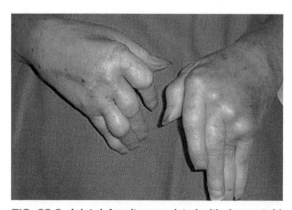

FIG. 22.3 Joint deformity associated with rheumatoid arthritis (Craft et al 2019.)

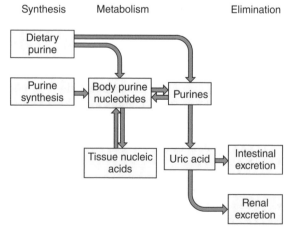

FIG. 22.4 The processes of purine synthesis, metabolism and excretion (Craft et al 2019.)

Promoting Wellness
Dietary Management of Gout

Dietary management primarily consists of reducing levels of uric acid in the body and maintaining a healthy weight. The recommended dietary modification is a low-purine diet. While it is impossible to avoid purines completely, the goal is to limit intake.

AVOID HIGH-PURINE FOODS:
- Alcoholic beverages (all types)
- Some fish, seafood and shellfish, including:
  - anchovies
  - sardines
  - herring
  - mussels
  - codfish
  - scallops
  - trout
  - haddock.
- Some meats, including:
  - bacon
  - turkey
  - veal
  - venison
  - offal, e.g. liver

LIMIT MODERATE-PURINE FOODS:
- Meats, such as:
  - beef
  - chicken
  - duck
  - pork
  - ham.
- Shellfish, such as:
  - crab
  - lobster
  - oysters
  - shrimps and prawns.

than in women. The disease causes a bony overgrowth of the facet joints of the vertebrae, leading to narrowing of the spinal canal and possible compression of the nerve roots (Craft et al 2019). The joints of the neck, back and pelvis, particularly the sacroiliac joints, become inflamed, causing pain and stiffness. It is mostly seen in the lumbar region at levels L3 and L4 and can present as progressive back pain and possible weakness of the lower extremities. Other joints, such as the hips and shoulders, can also be involved. Osteoporosis and fracture are also common. Fig. 22.5 shows the underlying bony changes in the spinal column and resulting characteristic change in posture seen in ankylosing spondylitis.

While the specific cause of ankylosing spondylitis is not known, genetic factors seem to be involved. A variation of the HLA-B27 gene is associated with an increased risk of ankylosing spondylitis, with almost nine out of ten people with the disease testing positive for this gene. However, HLA-B27 is present in 8% of the general population, including healthy people who do not have ankylosing spondylitis. Recently, two new genes (IL23R and ARTS1) were also found to be associated with ankylosing spondylitis (Arthritis Western Australia 2020).

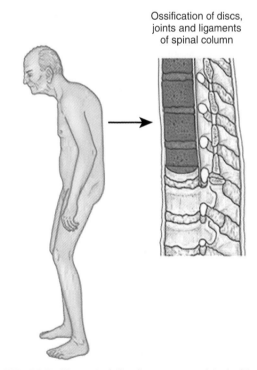

Ossification of discs, joints and ligaments of spinal column

FIG. 22.5 Characteristic changes associated with ankylosing spondylitis (Craft et al 2019.)

ANKYLOSING SPONDYLITIS

Ankylosing spondylitis is a chronic inflammatory disorder that primarily affects the axial skeleton and is present in 1–2% of Australians (Arthritis Australia 2020c). The disease usually appears between the ages of 15 and 40 years and is about three times more common in men

Management of ankylosing spondylitis includes physiotherapy (including hydrotherapy), use of NSAIDs, corticosteroids and oral bisphosphonates. In common with other inflammatory rheumatic conditions, ankylosing spondylitis is associated with increased rates of cardiovascular morbidity and mortality, and with an increased risk of falls in older people.

FRACTURES

A fracture is defined as a break in the continuity of a bone and may occur because of trauma to a bone or joint, or as the result of pathological processes. Falls are a common cause of fractures in older people (see Chapter 16). Fractures can be classified into the following categories (see Fig 22.6):
- Complete or incomplete
- Closed or open
- Oblique
- Occult
- Pathological
- Spiral
- Comminuted
- Transverse
- Greenstick
- Impacted

In older people, the most common fracture sites are:
- the hip
- the proximal femur
- the wrist (Colles fracture)
- the vertebrae
- the clavicle.

The AIHW (2019) suggests that the incidence of hip fractures is rising and is projected to increase due to the ageing population. This will present a heavy burden on the community, in terms of both acute care and

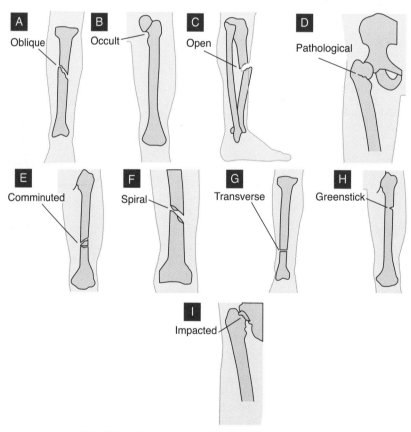

FIG. 22.6 **Fracture classification** (Craft et al 2019.)

rehabilitation. A fracture can cause damage to surrounding tissue, the periosteum and blood vessels in the bone cortex and marrow. Complications may include the presence of haematoma, compartment syndrome, loss of function and disability.

Clinical presentation of a fracture includes:
- pain
- tenderness
- swelling
- oedema
- ecchymosis (bruising)
- loss of alignment or displacement of bone
- shortening of the extremity
- internal or external rotation of the bone.

Initial assessment, when an older person has a suspected or confirmed fracture, includes observation of:
- vital signs
- level of consciousness
- limitations in ROM
- neurovascular status
- time of capillary refill
- a self-reported pain score.

Immediate management includes immobilisation and, if possible, application of a splint. For many older people, surgical intervention may be required in the form of open reduction internal fixation (ORIF). Older patients with hip fracture have a 20% to 30% mortality rate in the year following surgery. Non-operative care has higher one-year mortality rates and is generally only pursued in those with an extraordinarily high surgical risk (Sullivan et al 2019). The AIHW (2019) notes the increase in falls in older adults, with 22% resulting in injuries to the hip and thigh (see also Chapter 16).

CONSEQUENCES ASSOCIATED WITH TRAUMATIC INJURY AND LIMITED MOBILITY IN OLDER PEOPLE

Following any period of immobility, older people face the possibility of losing function and, consequently, independence. Older people are more likely to lose some capacity to perform routine ADLs during a hospital admission than those who are not hospitalised (Lafrenière et al 2017). For example, Walker and colleagues (2018) noted that 17% of older medical patients who were independently ambulating 2 weeks prior to admission needed assistance to walk following discharge. They also found that 65% of older patients became deconditioned after 2 days of hospitalisation and 67% failed to improve before discharge (Walker et al 2018).

During acute hospitalisation, it has been identified that older people spend approximately 83% of their hospital stay in bed and 12% in a chair. Prolonged immobility in the hospital is associated with a number of impairments in older people, including declines in:
- muscle strength
- muscle mass
- cognitive function
- muscle protein synthesis
- physical function.

From a musculoskeletal perspective, during a period of immobility those who cannot undertake weightbearing exercises are at significant risk of developing osteoporosis. It has been suggested that 12 weeks of bed rest reduces bone density by 50%. While all bones are affected, those most at risk are the long bones (Kramer et al 2017). It is therefore imperative that all members of the healthcare team are involved in strategies to reduce the risk of functional and cognitive decline in older people admitted to hospital.

Walker and colleagues (2018) identified the occurrence of 'deconditioning syndrome' in older people, which affects the ability to undertake everyday activities following a period of inactivity. Deconditioning can affect an older person in a very short time frame and in any environment, particularly acute care hospitals and residential aged care facilities. This deconditioning syndrome can lead to:
- reduced mobility
- falls
- functional incontinence
- low self-esteem
- longer term physiological and psychological dependence.

Re-conditioning (regaining lost abilities) can often take twice as long as deconditioning. There is, therefore, a need to commence early mobilisation in those who have experienced a traumatic injury or fracture. However, the AIHW (2019) noted that when older people are hospitalised, there is an inherent tension between preventing falls and promoting mobility. In response to this, the 'Sit Up, Get Dressed, Keep Moving' campaign has been developed (British Geriatrics Society 2017). This campaign encourages older hospital patients to wear day clothes and shoes, sit out of bed whenever possible and stay mobile during admission. Based on the principle that hospitalised people should restart normal life as soon as possible, the initiative began on a small scale and was taken up by other UK hospitals to prevent deconditioning and the resulting immobility and frailty in their older patients.

Practice Scenario

Mr David Lewis is a 71-year-old man admitted to your ward with an exacerbation of gout. He has recently returned from a month-long cruise with his wife around New Zealand. Since his return a week ago he has noticed his right great toe has become very painful, inflamed and swollen. This is now preventing him from mobilising, and he is unable to leave the house or attend his weekly bowling game. He has noticed that he has also put on some weight following his trip, as he was making the most of the daily buffets and unlimited alcohol.

MULTIPLE CHOICE QUESTIONS

1. What is the cause of gout?
   a. A chronic autoimmune disorder of the joints exacerbated by immobility.
   b. A metabolic disorder that disrupts the body's control of uric acid production or excretion.
   c. An acute disorder of the weight-bearing joints caused by increased pressure due to weight gain.
   d. A rare genetic disorder occurring in older men.
2. Nursing assessment of Mr Lewis includes:
   a. Daily weight monitoring and food intake diary
   b. Regular assessment of gait speed, balance and ankle strength
   c. Observation of affected joints for warmth, swelling, tophi, and erythema
   d. Both B and C

3. Management of Mr Lewis's condition is aimed at:
   a. Pain relief, low purine diet and adequate fluid intake to prevent kidney stones
   b. Vitamin D and calcium supplementation, adequate sunlight, pain relief
   c. Elevation of affected joints, rest, pain relief, calorie restriction
   d. All of the above
4. What dietary advice would the nurse recommend for Mr Lewis?
   a. Limit intake to 5000 kilojoules and increase fluids intake to prevent formation of kidney stones
   b. Avoid alcohol, avoid purine-containing foods, such as asparagus, scallops and oily fish (herring, sardines, anchovies)
   c. Limit alcohol and increase intake of green vegetables, nuts and low-fat meats
   d. Limit protein intake to decrease purine production
5. Strategies to prevent Mr Lewis's deconditioning while in hospital include:
   a. Early mobilisation, sitting out of bed and wearing day clothes whenever possible
   b. Intensive physiotherapy
   c. Enrolment into post-discharge community rehabilitation plan
   d. All of the above

SUMMARY

Musculoskeletal conditions are a common cause of pain and disability in older people. As individuals age, there are key changes in bones, muscles, joints and connective tissue that contribute to decreased mobility, independence and increased risk of falls and injury. Osteoporosis, in which bones weaken to the point of breaking easily, puts the older person at risk of fracture. Osteopenia, where bone mass is lowered, is a precursor to osteoporosis and a warning that bone loss has begun. Interventions to minimise ongoing bone loss include vitamin D and calcium supplementation, and regular weight-bearing exercise. Osteoarthritis is a degenerative joint disease and the most common form of arthritis in Australia and New Zealand. Management of osteoarthritis includes heat and cold therapy, NSAIDs, topical gel and occasionally steroid injections. Rheumatoid arthritis is a systemic autoimmune disease that causes inflammatory damage to the joints, resulting in joint tenderness, redness, pain and deformity. Treatment consists of symptom management and anti-rheumatic medication as the disease progresses.

In both forms of arthritis, maintaining a healthy and active lifestyle can promote mobility and function. Gout is a metabolic condition that causes chronic inflammation in joints, which can flare up acutely, causing hot, red, tender joints. Management is aimed at pain relief, medication to reduce concentrations of uric acid in the blood and dietary modification to reduce purine intake. Bone fractures are a major cause of pain, immobility and disability. Older people are at high risk of deconditioning after any period of inactivity, which can leave them less able to perform some ADLs. Early mobilisation and support to restart normal life as soon as possible after fracture or other traumatic injury can help to minimise loss of strength and flexibility and maintain function and independence.

REFERENCES

Arthritis Australia (2020a) Blood and pathology tests for arthritis. Online. Available: www.arthritisaustralia.com.au/managing-arthritis/medical-management/blood-test-for-arthritis/

Arthritis Australia (2020b) Gout. Online. Available: https://arthritisaustralia.com.au/types-of-arthritis/gout

Arthritis Australia (2020c) Ankylosing spondylitis. Online. Available: https://arthritisaustralia.com.au/types-of-arthritis/ankylosing-spondylitis/

Arthritis New Zealand (2020) Osteoarthritis. Online. Available: www.arthritis.org.nz/oesteoarthritis

Arthritis Western Australia (2020) Ankylosing spondylitis. Online. Available: www.arthritiswa.org.au/condition/ankylosing-spondylitis/

Australian Institute of Health and Welfare [AIHW] (2019) Chronic musculoskeletal conditions. Online. Available: www.aihw.gov.au/reports-data/health-conditions-disability-deaths/chronic-musculoskeletal-conditions/overview

BMJ Best Practice (2020) Osteomalacia. Online. Available: https://bestpractice.bmj.com/topics/en-us/517

British Geriatrics Society (2017) Sit up, Get Dressed, Keep Moving: Deconditioning syndrome awareness and prevention campaign: why is everyone talking about it? Online. Available: www.bgs.org.uk/blog/sit-up-get-dressed-keep-moving-the-campaign-everyone-is-talking-about

Bryant B, Knights K, Rowland A (2018) Pharmacology for health professionals, 5th edn. Elsevier, Philadelphia.

Clinical Excellence Commission (CEC) (2016) A guide to understanding balance and mobility for health staff. Online. Available: http://cec.health.nsw.gov.au/__data/assets/pdf_file/0003/327711/A-Guide-to-Understanding-Balance-and-Mobility-for-Health-Staff.pdf

Coventry L, Pickles S, Sin M et al (2017) Impact of the orthopaedic nurse practitioner role on acute hospital length of stay and cost-savings for patients with hip fracture: A retrospective cohort study. Journal of Advanced Nursing 73:2652–2663.

Craft J, Gordon C, Huether S et al (2019) Understanding pathophysiology, 3rd edn. Australian and New Zealand edn. Elsevier, St. Louis.

Estes M, Calleja P, Theobald K et al (2015) Health assessment and physical examination, 2nd edn, Cengage, South Melbourne.

Fearon K, Strasser F, Anker SD et al (2011) Definition and classification of cancer cachexia: An international consensus. The Lancet Oncology 12(5):489–495.

Heidari B, Muhammadi A, Javadian Y et al (2017) Associated factors of bone mineral density and osteoporosis in elderly males. International Journal of Endocrinology and Metabolism 15(1):e39662.

Kramer A, Gollhofer A, Armbrecht G et al (2017) How to prevent the detrimental effects of two months of bed rest on muscle, bone and cardiovascular system: an RCT. Scientific reports 7(1):1–10.

Lafrenière S, Folch N, Dubois S et al (2017) Strategies used by older patients to prevent functional decline during hospitalization. Clinical Nursing Research 26(1):6–26.

National Institute on Aging (NIA) (2017) Osteoporosis. Online. Available: www.nia.nih.gov/health/osteoporosis

Osteoporosis Australia (2020). What is it? Accessed 17 July 2020. Available: www.osteoporosis.org.au/what-it

Royal Australian College of General Practitioners (RACGP) (2019) Supporting clinical judgements for osteoporosis. Online. Available: www.racgp.org.au/clinical-resources/clinical-guidelines/key-racgp-guidelines/view-all-racgp-guidelines/osteoporosis

Santilli V, Bernetti A, Mangone M et al (2014) Clinical definition of sarcopenia. Clinical Cases in Mineral and Bone Metabolism 11(3):177–180.

Sullivan NM, Blake LE, George M et al (2019) Palliative care in the hip fracture patient. Geriatric Orthopaedic Surgery & Rehabilitation 10:2151459319849801.

Walker J, Povey J, Lai J (2018) Reducing the effects of immobility during hospital admissions. Nursing Times 114(6):18.

CHAPTER 23

Cardiovascular Health

CAROLINE VAFEAS • DEBORAH SUNDIN

LEARNING OBJECTIVES

After reading this chapter, you will be able to:

- outline the age-related changes of the cardiovascular system associated with normal ageing
- discuss common conditions of the cardiovascular system associated with older people
- briefly outline the assessment of the cardiovascular system in older people
- discuss interventions for maximising health relating to the cardiovascular system in older people.

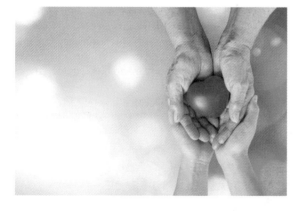

INTRODUCTION

Cardiac conditions are prominent in the health of older people with cardiovascular disease (heart disease) currently the top cause of mortality in Australia and New Zealand (see Chapter 2). Cardiovascular disease includes all disease processes of the heart and blood vessels. In 2015, 45,613 Australians died from cardiovascular disease, accounting for nearly one-third (29%) of all deaths in

one year. Cardiovascular disease is also the second largest contributor to the burden of disease in Australia, following cancer (Australian Institute of Health and Welfare [AIHW] 2019). Indigenous Australians are more likely than non-Indigenous Australians to face premature death due to chronic diseases, such as heart disease (Commonwealth of Australia 2020). In New Zealand, ischaemic heart disease and cerebrovascular disease were the highest-ranking causes of death in 2016–17. For older Māori males and females, ischaemic heart disease was the leading cause of death in 2018 (Ministry of Health NZ 2019).

This chapter will discuss the age-related changes experienced by older people in relation to cardiac health and wellbeing. Nurses caring for older people will encounter common cardiovascular conditions, therefore assessment and interventions need to be planned and implemented to ensure the best outcomes possible. The nurse is ideally placed to offer health promotion to reduce the incidence of cardiovascular disease and subsequent co-morbidities.

THE CARDIOVASCULAR SYSTEM

The cardiovascular system is comprised of the heart (the system's pump), the vasculature or blood vessels (a network of arteries, capillaries and veins) and the haematological system (the blood and blood products). The healthy heart beats an average of 70 times a minute to move blood through the body, nourishing cells and removing waste. Deficits in, or damage to, the cardiovascular system affect every other system in the body (Intensive Care NSW 2020).

In the healthy older person, several age-related changes occur. These factors on their own need not necessarily affect the individual due to the resilience and adaptive ability of the cardiovascular system (Casey 2017). Concurrent problems with other systems, particularly the respiratory system (see Chapter 24), and the presence of risk factors may leave the older person with a potential for challenges with cardiovascular health. Improved early diagnostic skills, together with enhanced public awareness of the importance of managing risk factors, such as diet and smoking, has seen a decline in the incidence of heart disease among the general population. The aged population, however, has not had the benefit of current diagnostic, prevention and treatment strategies. It is therefore vital that strategies to promote cardiovascular health in the older person are promoted and implemented when necessary.

THE AGEING CARDIOVASCULAR SYSTEM

Older age may result in a decrease in bone marrow function, reducing the ability to produce sufficient red and white blood cells, as well as platelets, which may result in anaemia and a diminished immune response (Craft et al 2017). Anaemia requires the heart to work harder to supply essential nutrients to the tissues, which may lead to heart failure. Additionally, the development of plaque within cardiac vessels narrows their diameter, reducing and potentially obstructing, blood supply to cardiac muscles. This narrowing may also result in hypertension, increasing vascular resistance against which the heart must pump to move the blood. A decrease in elasticity of the blood vessels also leads to vascular changes in the heart, kidneys and pituitary gland and reduced baroreceptor function. The decreased baroreceptor function and increased peripheral resistance leads to inefficient vasoconstriction and decreased cardiac output, often resulting in postural hypotension.

Reductions in muscle mass and subcutaneous tissue that accompany ageing may cause blood vessels in the head, neck and extremities to appear more prominent. These changes may also impair the body's ability to respond to a drop in temperature. A decrease

in blood pressure and changes in blood vessel walls compromise tissue perfusion and may lead to oedema, inflammation, pressure injury and changes in the effects of some medications (National Institute on Aging 2018). However, despite the multitude of age-related changes, physical performance is generally not affected.

Age-Related Changes

Changes in the cardiovascular system may occur with age or may be due to other factors. Those seen in later life may include:

- decreased cardiac output, compromising oxygen and nutrient supply to the tissues
- reduced heart muscle contractility and efficiency with left ventricle hypertrophy leading to decreased cardiac output
- thickening of tissue around the sinoatrial node leading to a decrease in pacemaker cells and thus rhythm disturbances (typically tachycardia and atrial fibrillation)
- decreased cardiac output during exertion or stress reducing exercise tolerance
- slight left ventricular hypertrophy, prolonged isometric contraction phase and relaxation time leading to increased diastolic filling and systolic emptying
- increased stroke volume to compensate for tachycardia, resulting in hypertension
- valves and blood vessels – the aorta may become elongated and stressed/dilated, valves become thicker and more rigid, thus resistance to blood flow increases (1% per year)
- increased blood pressure to compensate for resistance to flow and decreased cardiac output (Strait & Lakatta 2012).

RISK FACTORS AND CARDIOVASCULAR DISEASE

Risk factors can be described as those that are non-modifiable and those that are modifiable, meaning that they can be prevented or improved through interventions.

Non-modifiable risk factors include:

- genetics/family history
- age
- gender
- ethnicity.

  Modifiable risk factors include:
- smoking
- sedentary lifestyle
- poor diet high in saturated fats

- overweight and obesity
- hypertension
- hyperlipidaemia (raised blood lipids, such as cholesterol and triglycerides).
- alcohol intake
- stress.

COMMON CONDITIONS ASSOCIATED WITH CARDIOVASCULAR DISEASE

Coronary heart disease (CHD), also called coronary artery disease, is the result of reduced or impaired blood flow and thus nutrient supply to the myocardium. The most common cause is accumulation of fatty plaques within the walls of the coronary arteries due to atherosclerosis. This condition may be asymptomatic or lead to angina pectoris (chest pain), myocardial infarction, cardiac dysrhythmias, acute coronary syndrome, heart failure or even death. Despite steady advancements over the last three decades, with improvement in public health education, assessment and treatment modalities, cardiovascular disease remains one of the biggest causes of death in Australia, placing a considerable burden on the population in terms of illness and disability. The treatment options for CHD prolong life, but as people develop more risk factors such as obesity, hypertension and diabetes, the economic burden on the healthcare system increases (AIHW 2016).

Cardiovascular disease is any disease of the heart and/or blood vessels and includes conditions such as:
- myocardial infarction
- hypertension
- heart failure
- atrial fibrillation
- stroke.

Myocardial Infarction

Myocardial infarction (MI) or heart attack is caused by artherosclertic plaque formation in the cardiac arteries. The plaque may rupture or cause a clot to form within the coronary arteries reducing, and potentially obstructing, blood flow causing death of myocardial tissue (Tabloski 2019). The usual symptoms include chest pain, shortness of breath, nausea and sweating, although some people experience no pain. The development of an MI is often a consequence of an unhealthy lifestyle and/or poor healthcare. Measures to address modifiable risk factors can usually prevent MI, and include healthy diet, regular physical exercise, no smoking and regular heart health check-ups. In the event of an MI, immediate action to transfer the older person to hospital within the first few hours of symptom onset can facilitate administration of medication that can be given to dissolve clots. Aspirin is often recommended as a first aid treatment while waiting for an ambulance (Tabloski 2019).

Hypertension

Primary hypertension is a persistent elevated systemic blood pressure. Hypertension is defined as systolic blood pressure of 140 mmHg or higher or diastolic blood pressure of 90 mmHg or higher, taken over an average of three measurements on three separate occasions (AIHW 2018). People who are currently normotensive, but who take antihypertensive medications, are considered hypertensive for the sake of statistics. Despite rarely causing symptoms or noticeably limiting a person's functional ability, hypertension is a major risk factor for coronary artery disease, heart failure, stroke and renal failure. For this reason, hypertension has been called 'the silent killer'.

Heart Failure

Heart failure is a complex syndrome caused by any condition that has impaired the ability of the ventricles of the heart to fill with blood at normal pressure or efficiently eject blood into the cardiac system (Heart Foundation 2020a). Without the ability to pump sufficient oxygen and nutrient-rich blood into the cardiac system, the body's metabolic needs cannot be fulfilled (Heart Foundation 2020a). This problem is often the long-term result of a previous MI which has left extensive damage to the left ventricle, reducing cardiac output. Heart failure may also be the result of structural, inflammatory and rhythm disorders in the heart, or may be induced by excessive demand on the normal heart. Heart failure can be acute or chronic and is considered in terms of left- and right-sided heart failure. Left-sided heart failure involves the left ventricle, causing fluid to build up in the lungs and related dyspnoea (shortness of breath). Right-sided heart failure involves the right ventricle, causing fluid to build up in the abdomen, legs and feet (appearing as swelling). Generally, heart failure begins with the left side and if not effectively treated, progresses to involve the right side as well.

The cardinal symptom of heart failure is dyspnoea, with other important symptoms being palpitations and fatigue (National Heart Foundation of Australia 2018). To begin with, symptoms will manifest upon physical (and sometimes emotional) exertion, but as the heart failure progresses, symptoms occur at lower levels of physical activity and then even at rest.

Atrial Fibrillation

Atrial fibrillation is a common arrhythmia characterised by disorganised electrical activity within both atria of the heart. The arrhythmia is the result of multiple re-entry circuits within the atria, essentially developing a multitude of pacemakers. Extremely rapid electric stimulation bombards the atrioventricular node, resulting in a fast, irregular ventricular response of greater than 100 beats per minute. Atrial fibrillation may be the result of genetic or structural disorders, but is commonly associated with rheumatic heart disease, heart failure, coronary artery disease, hypertension and hyperthyroidism (National Heart, Lung and Blood Institute 2019). Atrial fibrillation increases the risk of thrombus formation and organ infarction (stroke).

Stroke

Stroke or cerebral vascular accident is a condition that causes enormous burden for older people and their families. It is often sudden, but leaves longer term difficulties for the individual involved. The causes can usually be traced back to the non-modifiable and modifiable risk factors for cardiovascular disease discussed earlier in the chapter. The 2012 Australian data show that over 40,000 people present with stroke each year, of whom over 11,000 die (AIHW 2006). Stroke can present in two distinct ways: a blockage in a cerebral blood vessel that deprives brain tissue of oxygen (ischaemic), or bleeding from a ruptured cerebral vessel or vascular malformation bleed (haemorrhagic) which affects the cerebral vascular blood flow for more than 24 hours (Sacco et al 2013). The ischaemic type accounts for 80% of all presentations. While less common than ischaemic stroke, the haemorrhagic sub-type is associated with higher mortality and morbidity (Sacco et al 2013). Immediate action can often prevent further complications. Fig. 23.1 shows how to recognise a stroke.

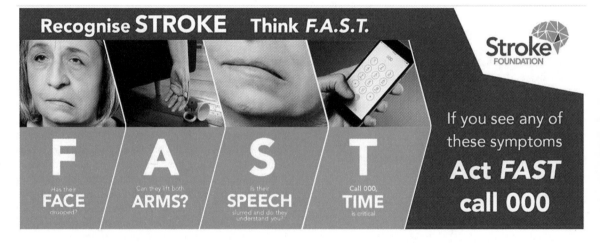

How do you know if someone is having a stroke? Think... F.A.S.T.

The Stroke Foundation recommends the F.A.S.T. test as an easy way to remember the most common signs of stroke. Using the F.A.S.T. test involves asking these simple questions:

Face Check their face. Has their mouth drooped?

Arms Can they lift both arms?

Speech Is their speech slurred? Do they understand you?

Time Is critical. If you see any of these signs call 000 straight away.

FIG. 23.1 **Recognising a Stroke** (Stroke Foundation 2020.)

Assessment

Assessment of the cardiovascular system is important for older people, who are at greater risk of developing cardiovascular complications that can diminish quality of life and independence. Assessment should include:

- clinical history
- family history
- identification of any risk factors (non-modifiable and modifiable)
- top-to-toe physical assessment (see Chapter 8)
- vital signs: temperature, pulse, respirations, oxygen saturation and blood pressure
- signs of stress or anxiety
- assessment of activities of daily living (ADLs) and instrumental activities of daily living IADLs (see Chapter 8).

DIAGNOSING CARDIOVASCULAR DISEASE

The following tests and procedures may be required to diagnose cardiovascular disease:

- blood tests
- electrocardiogram (ECG)
- stress test
- echocardiogram (ECHO)
- coronary angiogram or coronary computed tomography angiogram (CCTA)
- myocardial perfusion study (MPS)
- computerised tomography scan (CT scan) (Heart Foundation 2020b).

INTERVENTIONS

Prevention is better than cure, therefore the best intervention is to prevent cardiovascular disease in the first place. *Primary* prevention includes identification of potential risk factors which can be addressed prior to onset of signs or symptoms of any chronic health condition. This approach can be achieved through community health promotion, school education programs and media advertising to increase public awareness. *Secondary* prevention includes the early detection of any health condition, providing treatment to achieve a cure and addressing risk factors to reverse symptoms and prevent the progression of any condition. *Tertiary* prevention is aimed more at modifying any determinants of healthy ageing to improve wellbeing, reduce symptoms and delay progression of existing chronic conditions (Daly et al 2019) (see also Chapter 4).

Self-Care as an Intervention

One ideal strategy for promoting wellness is to prompt the older person to take back care and responsibility for themselves. With this approach, the nurse provides the older person with information to increase knowledge and understanding, collaborates with the older person to prepare an action plan and then supports the older person to implement the plan and monitor outcomes. This strategy needs to be assessed on an individual basis and may not suit everyone. It is important to remember that a plan without a goal or support is likely to fail.

The basic self-care activities important in cardiovascular disease and stroke prevention and management have been captured by the American Heart Association (AHA) and clearly identify the seven most important strategies to promote cardiovascular health. These are called 'Life's Simple 7' (see *Tips for best practice*).

> **Tips for Best Practice**
> *Life's Simple 7*
>
> 1. Manage blood pressure
> 2. Control cholesterol
> 3. Reduce blood sugar
> 4. Get active
> 5. Eat better
> 6. Lose weight
> 7. Stop smoking
>
> Adopting these seven behaviours can reduce the incidence of stroke and heart failure.

American Heart Association (2018).

Common Medications Prescribed to Control Symptoms of Coronary Heart Disease

- Angiotensin-converting enzyme (ACE) inhibitors – lower blood pressure and reduce the strain on the heart (e.g. captopril, enalapril).
- Anticoagulants reduce the risk of blood clots forming (warfarin, apixaban, dabigatran).
- Antiplatelet agents reduce the risk of clots forming and limit damage (clopidogrel)
- Beta blockers lower blood pressure and regulate the heart rate and rhythm (atenolol, metoprolol).
- Calcium channel blockers lower blood pressure and slow heart rate (amlodipine, verapamil).
- Nitrate medications (glyceryl trinitrate) can increase blood flow to the heart. Available in a spray or dissolvable tablet form.
- Statins can lower cholesterol and triglycerides (atorvastatin, simvastatin) (Heart Foundation 2020b).

MAXIMISING CARDIOVASCULAR HEALTH

Cardiovascular health, similar to respiratory health (see Chapter 24), can be maintained and improved through lifestyle modification. Modifications include stopping smoking, regular exercise and healthy eating (see *Tips for Best Practice: Life's Simple 7*); (Riegel et al 2009).

Smoking

Smoking is a major cause of cardiovascular disease, so must be ceased to ensure maximum improvement in health. Nicotine replacement patches can be prescribed by a doctor to assist. The older person must see the benefit of cessation of smoking or any effort is likely to fail. See the Transtheoretical model of health promotion in Chapter 4 to understand the change cycle for effective health promotion.

Exercise

Exercise is one of the most important activities for maintaining and improving cardiovascular health (Charbek et al 2018). Regular cardiovascular exercise is also important in maintaining respiratory muscle strength and mass. An exercise program may need review and clearance by a doctor. A slow build-up to a regular plan of sustained activity will be required for full benefit. It is estimated that 84% of those over 75 years do not participate in sufficient physical activity. This inactivity is also higher in women than in men (AIHW 2020).

HEALTHY DIET

Adequate nutrition is required to maintain muscle mass. A diet that is high in protein, fruits and vegetables is recommended for assisting muscle development and to maintain health (see Chapter 12). Replacing saturated fat with polyunsaturated fat in the diet reduces cardiovascular risk by 24% (Lloyd-Jones et al 2009). Being overweight or obese has been found to be a strong indicator of CHD without any other risk factors (Carbone et al 2019). Including a dietitian in the healthcare team can ensure the best recommendations are provided regarding healthy food choices, reducing obesity and improving quality of life.

Other essential factors when implementing a plan to improve cardiac health include education for the older person to ensure their knowledge on the condition, reasons for the need to stop smoking, the purpose of eating a healthy diet and stress reduction to ensure a good quality of life. Blood pressure monitoring and cholesterol testing may also be included in a health promotion plan and supported by the general practitioner (GP) and primary healthcare team.

Promoting Wellness
Key Points to Promoting Cardiovascular Wellness

- **A**wareness of family history
- **B**lood pressure monitoring
- **C**ardiovascular exercise plan
- **D**evelop and maintaining a positive attitude
- **E**at healthy, nutritious food

Safety Alert

Avoid a sudden transfer from bed on rising due to the risk of postural hypotension and subsequent fall (see Chapter 16).

Research Highlight
Influenza Vaccination as a Novel Means of Preventing Coronary Heart Disease: Effectiveness in Older Adults

- Evidence shows that infection is an independent risk factor for cardiovascular disease.
- Preliminary data also indicates that vaccination can prevent cardiovascular disease.
- This study examined the association mentioned above in a review focused on older persons.
- Influenza vaccination gives promising results that are still not completely understood.
- Given the innovative perspectives, this review points to a need to intensify research on vaccine.

Aidoud et al (2020).

SUMMARY

Many changes can occur in the cardiovascular system as people age. These changes may be due to age, as well as other factors. Although physiological changes can happen, many older people lead a normal healthy life free from cardiovascular disease. Age-related changes and modifiable risk factors need to be considered during assessment to inform an effective health promotion plan. Cardiovascular care for older people needs to be implemented on an individual basis, but generally includes a holistic assessment, stopping smoking, increasing exercise if and as able, promoting a healthy diet and encouraging a positive mental attitude.

Promoting Wellness
Heart Foundation Heart Health Basics

The Heart Foundation recommends that heart health is something everyone can work on every day.

KEY POINTS
A heart healthy diet is a pattern of food intake over days, weeks and months.

- Eat more fruit and vegetables
- Swap to wholegrains: Wholegrain cereals have more dietary fibre, B vitamins, vitamin E and healthy fats
- Include more monounsaturated and polyunsaturated fats: avocados, nuts, fish, sunflower seeds.
- Replace salt with herbs and spices.

Regular physical exercise reduces the risk of heart attack (MI) and heart disease.

- Move more: any physical activity is better than none.
- Set realistic goals: start with small goals and work up to 30 to 60 minutes of moderate exercise (e.g. brisk walking).
- Choose enjoyable activities
- Get social: do things with a group of friends, family or even the dog.
- Sit less: adults of all ages who sit less throughout the day have a lower risk of early death, including from heart attack.

Quitting smoking always decreases the risk of heart attack and stroke almost immediately.

- Understand the risks of smoking.
- Keep trying: quitting smoking may take multiple efforts and needs planning, practice and help.
- Reach out for support: call Quitline (Australia) 137 848 or Quitline (New Zealand) 0800 778 778.
- Quit for loved ones: Don't smoke in the home or other enclosed spaces.

Understanding and controlling blood pressure and cholesterol is key to heart health.

- Cholesterol is essential for normal body function. However, there are two main types: High-density cholesterol ('good cholesterol') and low-density cholesterol ('bad cholesterol'). Low-density cholesterol sticks to the walls of the arteries causing plaque that can rupture or obstruct blood flow to heart muscle (see above).
- Eating too much saturated or 'trans' fats can raise cholesterol levels. These fats are found in pizza, cakes, biscuits and deep-fried foods. Choose a heart healthy diet instead.
- Know your own cholesterol levels: anyone 45 years or older (30 years for Aboriginal and Torres Strait Islander people) should have a regular heart health check with a GP.
- Take medication as prescribed: cholesterol-lowering medications are effective and should be taken exactly as prescribed.

Adapted from Heart Foundation (2020c).

Practice Scenario

Jane Simpson is a 74-year-old lady who has been admitted to the ward with chest pain. Jane has a family history of MI and stroke. Jane weighs 92 kg and is 160 cm in height. Her blood pressure on admission is 176/95. Jane lives with her husband George, aged 75. The couple live in a retirement village and perform their ADLs and IADLs independently. The chest pain was diagnosed as an MI and Jane is now preparing for discharge home.

MULTIPLE CHOICE QUESTIONS
Which of the following answers is most appropriate?

1. One modifiable risk factor that Jane could address would be:
   a. family history
   b. being a non-smoker
   c. too much exercise
   d. overweight and obesity

2. Referral to the following would be required prior to discharge:
   a. dietitian
   b. chaplain
   c. Aged Care Assessment Team (ACAT)
   d. Occupational Therapist

3. Jane has:
   a. normotension
   b. hypertension
   c. hypotension
   d. all of the above

4. During her admission, Jane was required to have lying and standing BP monitoring:
   a. to assess for postural hypotension
   b. to reduce blood pressure
   c. to reduce chest pain
   d. to assess for postural hypertension

REFERENCES

Aidoud A, Marlet J, Angoulvant D et al (2020) Influenza vaccination as a novel means of preventing coronary heart disease: Effectiveness in older adults. Vaccine 38(32): 4944–4955.

American Heart Association (2018) Life's simple 7. Online. Available: www.heart.org/en/healthy-living/healthy-lifestyle/my-life-check–lifes-simple-7

Australian Institute of Health and Welfare (AIHW) (2020) Insufficient physical activity. Online. Available: www.aihw.gov.au/reports/risk-factors/insufficient-physical-activity/contents/physical-inactivity

Australian Institute of Health and Welfare (AIHW) (2019) Australian Burden of Disease Study: Impact and causes of illness and death in Australia 2015 – Summary. Online. Available: https://www.aihw.gov.au/reports/burden-of-disease/burden-disease-study-illness-death-2015-summary/contents/table-of-contents

Australian Institute of Health and Welfare (AIHW) (2018) High blood pressure. Online. Available: www.aihw.gov.au/reports/risk-factors/high-blood-pressure/data

Australian Institute of Health and Welfare (AIHW) (2016) Australia's health 2016. Cat no AUS 199. Online. Available: www.aihw.gov.au/getmedia/2a44d779-bff1-4302-b129-f515e7b07842/ah16-3-5-coronary-heart-disease.pdf.aspx

Australian Institute of Health and Welfare (AIHW), Senes, S (2006) How we manage stroke. AIHW cat. no. CVD 31. AIHW, Canberra.

Carbone S, Canada JM, Billingsley HE et al (2019) Obesity paradox in cardiovascular disease: where do we stand? Vascular Health and Risk Management 15:89–100.

Casey G (2017) The biology of ageing. Kia Tiaki Nursing New Zealand 23(10):20–24.

Charbek E, Espiritu JR, Nayak R et al. Frailty, comorbidity and COPD. Journal of Nutritional Health and Aging (2018) 22:876–879.

Craft JA, Gordon CJ, Huether SE et al (2017) Understanding pathophysiology, Australia and New Zealand Edition, 3rd edn. Elsevier, Chatswood.

Commonwealth of Australia, Department of the Prime Minister and Cabinet (2020) Closing the Gap Report 2020. Commonwealth of Australia, Canberra.

Daly L, Byrne G, Keogh B (2019) Contemporary considerations relating to health promotion and older people. British Journal of Nursing 28(21):1414–1419.

Heart Foundation (2020a) What is heart failure? Online. Available: www.heartfoundation.org.au/conditions/heart-failure

Heart Foundation (2020b) What is coronary heart disease? Online. Available: www.heartfoundation.org.au/conditions/coronary-heart-disease

Heart Foundation (2020c) Online. Available: Keeping your heart healthy. Online. Available: www.heartfoundation.org.au/heart-health-education/keeping-your-heart-healthy

Intensive Care NSW (2020) Cardiovascular system. Online. Available: www.aci.health.nsw.gov.au/networks/icnsw/patients-and-families/patient-conditions/cardiovascular-system

Lloyd-Jones D, Adams R, Carnethon M, et al, American Heart Association Statistics Committee and Stroke Statistics Subcommittee (2009) Heart disease and stroke statistics – 2009 update: a report from the American Heart Association Statistics Committee and Stroke Statistics Subcommittee. Circulation 119(3):e21–e181.

Ministry of Health NZ (2019) Annual update of key results 2018/2019: New Zealand Health Survey. MOH, Wellington.

National Heart Lung and Blood Foundation (2019) Atrial fibrillation. Online. Available: www.nhlbi.nih.gov/health-topics/atrial-fibrillation

National Institute on Aging (2018) Heart health and aging. Online. Available: www.nia.nih.gov/health/heart-health-and-aging

National Vascular Disease Prevention Alliance (2012) Guidelines for the management of absolute cardiovascular disease risk. Online. Available: www.heartfoundation.org.au/getmedia/4342a70f-4487-496e-bbb0-dae33a47fcb2/Absolute-CVD-Risk-Full-Guidelines_2.pdf

Riegel B, Driscoll A, Suwanno J et al (2009) Heart failure self-care in developed and developing countries. Journal of Cardiac Failure 15(6):508–516.

Sacco RL, Kasner SE, Broderick JP et al (2013) An updated definition of stroke for the 21st century. Stroke 44:2046–2089.

Strait B, Lakatta EG (2012) Aging-associated cardiovascular changes and their relationship to heart failure. Heart Failure Clinics 8(1):143–164.

Stroke Foundation (2020) Learn the F.A.S.T. signs of a stroke. Online. Available: FAST https://strokefoundation.org.au/

Tabloski P 2019 Gerontological nursing, 4th edn. eText Pearson.

CHAPTER 24

Respiratory Health

ELISABETH JACOB

LEARNING OBJECTIVES

After reading this chapter, you will be able to:

- outline the age-related changes of the respiratory system associated with normal ageing
- discuss common conditions of the respiratory system associated with older people
- consider common interventions such as inhalation therapy and continuous positive airway pressure
- briefly outline the assessment of the respiratory system in older people
- discuss methods for maximising health of the respiratory system in older people.

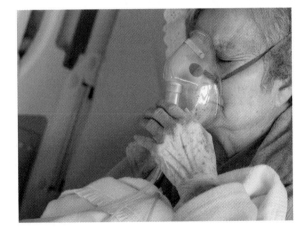

INTRODUCTION

As people age, changes occur to the respiratory system due to physiological, structural and immunological changes occurring in the body. This chapter will outline the common changes to the respiratory system experienced by older people and briefly discuss some of the respiratory health conditions often experienced in older

age. Interventions of inhalation therapy and continuous positive airway pressure (CPAP), often used for these conditions, will be discussed. This will be followed by a brief outline of respiratory assessment for older people and ways of maintaining and improving respiratory health.

AGE-RELATED CHANGES

There are several structural and functional changes that occur to the respiratory system as a person ages. Physiological changes due to ageing include a decrease in muscle mass and strength (Craft et al 2017). Chest expansion and compliance may be restricted due to a decrease in vertebral height, increased risk of osteoporosis and advancing kyphosis (Ennis 2013). This results in decreased respiratory capacity, strength and volume, meaning that less air is expelled during exhalation, causing an increased work of breathing and increased risk of ventilatory failure (Casey 2017; Craft et al 2017; Ennis 2013; Sanches et al 2014). This loss of aerobic capacity in older people is mainly impacted by the loss of muscle function and leads to a decrease in exercise tolerance and physical functioning (Casey 2017). Despite the physical changes that occur, endurance athletes in their 80s are able to maintain the aerobic function of 40-year-olds (Casey 2017).

Changes to lung tissue as a person ages cause loss of elasticity, decreasing the ability of the lungs to expand (Casey 2017). This may be seen on examination as decreased air entry in the lungs. Additionally, older people have a decreased capillary network and pulmonary atrial blood flow that reduce the ability for diffusion gas exchange in the lungs (Craft et al 2017). Small airways in the base of the lungs collapse during inspiration, redistributing air to the apex of the lungs where there is decreased blood flow, resulting in a ventilation perfusion mismatch. A breakdown of alveolar walls decreases the surface area available for gas exchange, which may result in a decreased oxygen saturation (Ennis 2013). The breakdown of alveolar walls results in hyper-resonance (lower and louder sounds) on auscultation of the lungs. Hence, the impact of age-related changes can affect ventilatory capacity of older people and result in lower ventilatory capacity than younger adults.

Immunological changes include an increase in inflammatory infiltrates (white blood cells, such as neutrophils, eosinophils and lymphocytes) in the blood vessels of the lung, which may be related to life-long exposure to pollutants or age-related changes to inherent immunity (Craft et al 2017). A decrease in the number of cilia reduces the ability of the older person to clear mucus from the lungs, increasing the chance of infection (Craft et al 2017). Ineffective cough and swallowing disorders in older people can allow a build-up of secretions that obstruct airflow and provide an environment in which pathogens can flourish (Cilloniz et al 2016). Moreover, age-related immunological changes decrease the body's ability to defend against infections. These include a diminished antibody response, reduced ability of white blood cells to fight infection, increased cytokine levels and an increased inflammatory response (Cilloniz et al 2016). Together, physiological changes in the respiratory system and a corresponding decrease in the immune efficiency put the older person at increased risk of respiratory infections such as pneumonia and influenza (Ennis 2013).

COMMON CONDITIONS OF THE RESPIRATORY SYSTEM

Chronic Obstructive Pulmonary Disease

Chronic obstructive pulmonary disease (COPD) is a group of irreversible chronic conditions, such as bronchitis and emphysema, which have a progressive decline and result in obstruction to the airways (Charbek et al 2018). It is the fourth leading cause of death and

third leading cause of disability in Australia and New Zealand (Best Practice Journal NZ 2015; Craft et al 2017). As COPD is both preventable and treatable, it is an important public health issue (Global Initiative For Chronic Obstructive Lung Disease [GOLD] 2019). The incidence of COPD increases with age and is expected to rise with the increasing longevity of the population (Craft et al 2017; GOLD 2019). COPD is usually caused by exposure to a significant amount of noxious gases or particles, with the most common irritant being cigarette smoke.

COPD is characterised by chronic airflow limitation and respiratory symptoms caused by a combination of parenchymal destruction and small airways disease. The cause of the airflow limitation varies between people and usually co-exists with other disease. Airflow is limited due to the damage to small airways caused by destruction of the alveoli, decreased elastic recoil or from airway inflammation that produces mucus and remodelling. The changes to the airways results in increased use of the chest respiratory muscles and people with long-term COPD often have a rounding of the chest wall, commonly called barrel chest.

COPD is associated with a range of immunological processes in response to the inflammation and lung damage. The inflammatory process can have systemic consequences and is associated with other co-morbidities (Craft et al 2017). COPD often co-exists with:

- cardiovascular disease
- osteoporosis
- gastro-oesophageal disease
- anxiety and depression
- lung cancer
- infections.

COPD is diagnosed based on lung function tests and history of exposure to noxious inhalants, such as cigarette smoking. Treatment is typically symptom-based and often includes inhaled, long-acting bronchodilator medications and steroids (GOLD 2019). Use of inhalant therapy can be difficult for older people who have decreased dexterity for administering the medication. Inhaler techniques need to be assessed regularly in older people.

Pneumonia

Pneumonia is an infection of the lower respiratory tract, which is associated with increased mortality and morbidity in older people (Cilloniz et al 2016). It is usually caused by a bacterium or virus. Advancing age is a risk factor for pneumonia, with mortality rates in older people reported at up to 25% (Cilloniz et al 2016) due to age-related physiological changes and co-morbid chronic

Research Highlight

A study conducted in the USA focused on hospitalised patients with COPD and investigated the effect of mobility activities on their functional status at discharge. A sample of 111 patients (mean age 67.1 years, 62% female) was included. On admission, half of the patients (55%) could walk without assistance and 31% walked with assistance (cane or walking frame), while the remaining 14% were confined to a wheelchair, bed or chair. Data were extracted from the patients' nursing notes and included the number of times they: ambulated out of their hospital room; got up to go to the bathroom; and sat in a chair or commode by the bed. Researchers also counted the number of days from admission to first time out of bed. Data analysis controlled for age and severity of illness.

Results showed that hospitalised patients with COPD who ambulated outside the hospital room and up to the bathroom more frequently were more likely to be discharged home versus being transferred to residential aged care. For every additional day that a patient remained in bed after admission, he or she was significantly less likely to be discharged home. The authors concluded that early mobilisation was associated with better functional related outcomes in hospitalised patients with COPD.

Shay et al (2020).

diseases. Pneumonia is most commonly caused by the aspiration of oropharyngeal secretions or from inhalation of microorganisms (Craft et al 2017). Often an upper respiratory tract infection precedes the development of pneumonia. Influenza is the most common viral cause of pneumonia in older people and is usually acquired in the community. Viral pneumonia can be severe, but is usually self-limiting.

The main damage from viral pneumonia is to the cilia that function to protect the lower airways from pathogens, which then enables a secondary bacterial infection to develop. The infection causes a build-up of exudate in the alveoli, which decreases the ability of the lungs to exchange gases. This may be seen clinically as either tachypnoea or dyspnoea with associated hypoxaemia and increased exertion with breathing.

Symptoms of pneumonia experienced in older people may be different from that of the general adult population. An older person with pneumonia may present with falls, altered mental status, fatigue, lethargy, delirium, anorexia, tachypnoea and tachycardia, rather than the usual signs of cough and fever (Cilloniz et al 2016). Pneumonia may present as an exacerbation or decompensation of the many co-morbidities, such as heart failure, in older people. Moreover, older people have an increased risk of pneumonia developing into sepsis due to decreasing function of the immune system.

Diagnosis is made based upon:

- physical examination
- white blood cell count
- blood and sputum cultures
- chest X-ray (Craft et al 2017).

Sputum cultures or blood cultures are used to identify the infective organism.

Treatment of pneumonia depends upon the responsible organism. Antibiotics are used to treat bacterial pneumonia. Viral pneumonia is generally only treated with symptom management consisting of:

- adequate hydration
- deep breathing and coughing exercises
- chest physiotherapy.

Antiviral medication is available for treatment of severe cases. As aspiration pneumonia is frequently experienced by older people, assessment of swallowing and oral intake should be standard care. Keeping fit and healthy, along with vaccinations for both influenza and pneumococcal disease, are ways to minimise the risk of developing pneumonia in the older population, although the response to vaccinations may be limited due to the decreased immune response in this cohort (Cilloniz et al 2016).

Influenza

Influenza, usually denoted by its subtypes, is a short-lived virus that infects the respiratory system. It is commonly known as 'the flu' and has a 72-hour incubation period (Craft et al 2017). Seasonal variations affect millions of people worldwide each year. Older people are at a higher risk of developing complications following an influenza episode, such as pneumonia, stroke and myocardial infarction, due to decreased immune responses and existence of co-morbidities (Lapi et al 2019).

The influenza virus is transmitted via airborne secretions that enter the upper airways. The virus is usually immobilised by the body's immune system, but if this does not occur it may infiltrate the respiratory tract lining and multiply. The onset of the condition is usually abrupt and lasts for around 5–10 days. The immune response causes inflammatory mediators to be released resulting in oedema and redness of the mucosal lining and increased mucus secretion. Classic symptoms of influenza include:

- fever
- cough
- muscle pain
- headache
- sore throat.

In susceptible populations, such as older people, influenza may move to the lower respiratory tract and cause pneumonia (Craft et al 2017). Diagnosis is usually based on the symptoms due to the short duration of the condition. Treatment focuses on symptom management, with antiviral therapies available for people at high risk of developing complications. Influenza vaccination is encouraged for those at higher risk, such as healthcare workers and older people, although it is not as effective in older people due to changes to their immune system. The influenza vaccine has an efficacy of between 70% and 90% in adults and children but drops to 30–50% for people over the age of 65 (Ciabattini et al 2018).

Obstructive Sleep Apnoea

Obstructive sleep apnoea (OSA) is the term used for an obstruction of the upper airway, which occurs during sleep. It is usually associated with excessive snoring and multiple apnoeic episodes where the person's breathing stops for between 10 and 60 seconds or more causing a decrease in oxygen saturation (Craft et al 2017). OSA is becoming increasingly common, with up to 25% of middle-aged and older Australians having the condition, and up to 4% of men in New Zealand (Craft et al 2017). Obesity is the leading cause of OSA (Manuel & Hardinge 2016), although other risk factors include male gender, increased age, smoking and alcohol consumption.

OSA is caused by enlargement of the tonsils, adenoids, tongue and soft tissue around the pharynx, often caused by obesity, which reduce the size of the airway. During OSA, pharyngeal tissue completely obstructs the airway preventing the movement of air. Airway obstruction leads to hypoxaemia and causes the person to waken with the increased effort of breathing, interrupting the sleep cycle. People with OSA cycle through obstruction and awakening during the night, resulting in sleep deprivation. Over time, repeated hypoxic episodes eventually lead to polycythaemia (increased number of red blood cells), whereby the body compensates for lower airway

efficiency by increasing the oxygen-carrying capacity in the blood (Manuel & Hardinge 2016).

Symptoms of OSA include snoring and feeling tired and sleepy during the daytime. Chronic tiredness may cause individuals to suffer from neurocognitive impairment (Craft et al 2017). People with OSA are also at a higher risk of death from cardiovascular disease and have an increased mortality from all causes (Manuel & Hardinge 2016; Riaz et al 2019). Diagnosis is often made using sleep studies, which document periods of apnoea by monitoring the older person during sleep for:

- brain, eye and muscle activity
- heart rate
- airflow
- oxygen saturations.

Treatment of OSA focuses on:

- management of obesity
- use of CPAP
- dental devices
- in some cases, surgery on the upper airway to aid in opening the airway.

Practice Points

- Standard dose influenza vaccines, which have been developed for all ages including children, do not have the same efficacy in older people, although new vaccines are being developed that target the older population.
- The presence of co-morbidities increases an older person's susceptibility to respiratory diseases.
- Respiratory disease may present as other co-morbidities in older people.

Australian Government Department of Health (2020).

ASSESSMENT

Assessment of the respiratory system is important for older people, who are at greater risk of developing pulmonary disease. The main objective of undertaking a respiratory assessment is to determine if there are any problems with gas exchange in the lungs related to physiological changes. As the respiratory system is closely connected to the cardiovascular system, changes in one system will have an impact on the other, hence a thorough assessment will cover elements of each system. A detailed history from the older person is needed, which includes:

- current respiratory issues
- medications

- environmental issues
- frequency of respiratory infections
- physical activity
- alterations in activities of daily living (ADLs) due to respiratory limitations.

The physical examination should include an assessment of posture, curvature of the spine and shape of the chest, as they may indicate ageing or disease-related changes that may affect ventilation. Be aware that chest expansion is often decreased in older adults due to general muscle weakness, sedentary lifestyle, general physical disability or calcification of rib articulations. Older people may have difficulty taking deep breaths and holding the breath.

Assessment of respiratory rate and depth, oxygen saturation, blood pressure, pulse and skin colour are needed to provide a determination of the work of breathing. Presence of a cough, whether productive or not, should be noted, including the length of time the cough has been present and the season of the year in which the cough occurs, as this may help determine the cause.

Auscultation of the chest may reveal decreased air entry into the bases of the lungs as part of the normal ageing process, due to the decreased vital capacity and changes to the alveoli. Percussion of the older person's chest may indicate hyperresonance (louder and lower sounds), which is heard when breakdown of the alveoli results in too much air in the lungs. A change in an older person's mental status may indicate oxygen deficiency.

Tips for Best Practice

- Respiratory disease may present as exacerbation of other chronic diseases in older people, so should be considered with any presentation.
- Falls and confusion may be the first signs of respiratory illness in older people.
- Normal changes to lung sounds and air entry may mask the presence of disease, making it harder to pick up changes related to disease processes.

COMMON INTERVENTIONS
Continuous Positive Airway Pressure Therapy

Continuous positive airway pressure/power therapy (CPAP) is a form of external ventilation, in which mild positive air pressure is applied to the respiratory system on a continuous basis to keep the alveoli open in people who are able to breathe spontaneously. A mask is placed over the nose or mouth, or both, and connected to a machine which delivers the CPAP (Manuel & Hardinge 2016). The aim is to prevent collapse of the airway. CPAP has been shown to increase survival and decrease hospitalisations for people experiencing OSA (GOLD 2019). However, CPAP can be difficult for older people to cope with (Riaz et al 2019). For CPAP to work, there needs to be enough pressure to hold the airway open via a well-fitting mask that prevents air leaks. Some people are unable to tolerate the discomfort associated with the high pressures required and noise from the CPAP machine, and find it difficult to fit the mask properly, which results in excessive air leaks.

Inhalation Therapy

Inhalation therapy is used for many respiratory conditions as it enables medication to be delivered directly to the lung tissue. This can be delivered either by metred dose inhalers or through nebulisation with or without oxygen. Due to the decrease in dexterity, vital capacity and muscle strength associated with ageing, some older people find using inhalation devices difficult. The main problems encountered with administration of inhaled medications usually concern inspiratory flow, inhalation duration, coordination, dose preparation, exhalation prior to inhalation and breath-holding during inhalation (GOLD 2019). Therefore, inhalation devices used need to be specifically chosen for each individual to suit their particular needs.

MAXIMISING RESPIRATORY HEALTH

Respiratory health can be maintained and improved through lifestyle modification. Important factors include regular exercise, healthy eating, maintaining influenza vaccinations and a healthy environment. Engaging with multidisciplinary team members to cover all aspects of an older person's health can assist them to be in the best position to maximise their respiratory health.

- **Exercise** – Exercise is one of the most important activities that can maintain and improve respiratory health (Charbek et al 2018). Regular cardiovascular exercise is important in maintaining respiratory muscle strength and mass. Exercise which requires use of the chest wall muscles can increase muscle mass and improve the function of the respiratory system (Casey 2017). Exercises found to be of benefit in improving respiratory health include endurance training, interval training, resistance/strength training, walking, flexibility exercises and inspiratory muscle training (GOLD 2019). Working with physiotherapists and exercise physiologists can assist older people to determine the best exercise routine for their situation.

- **Healthy diet** – Adequate nutrition is required to maintain muscle mass. A diet high in protein, fruits and vegetables is recommended for assisting muscle development and maintaining health. Having a dietitian as part of the healthcare team can ensure the best recommendations are provided regarding healthy food choices.
- **Vaccination** – Yearly influenza and regular pneumococcal vaccination are recommended for older people. Research has been shown this will not only decrease the number of lower respiratory tract infections experienced by older people, but also decrease cardiovascular complications in people with multiple co-morbidities (GOLD 2019).
- **Environment** – Many respiratory diseases are caused due to inhalation of noxious gases, including cigarette smoke and cooking fumes, or exposure to other environmental toxins such as asbestos. Limiting exposure is essential for maintaining healthy lungs. Ensuring well-ventilated rooms and working in a healthy environment will assist in limiting exposure to pollutants.

Promoting Wellness
Maintaining Respiratory Health

- Exercise regularly
- Eat healthy, nutritious food
- Maintain yearly influenza vaccinations
- Maintain a healthy environment

SUMMARY

There are many changes that occur in the respiratory system as people age due to alterations in pulmonary and musculoskeletal tissue and immunological function. As a result, older people are at more risk of respiratory diseases such as pneumonia, chronic obstructive pulmonary disease and obstructive sleep apnoea. Assessment of the respiratory system needs to take into account the common changes in the ageing respiratory system, and the impact of reduced respiratory capacity on other co-morbid conditions. Respiratory care for older people includes encouraging exercise, healthy diet, regular vaccination and ensuring an environment free from toxic causes.

Practice Scenario

Sara Brown is a 72-year-old woman who has presented to the medical clinic for a routine health assessment. She complains of having had a cough for the previous 4 weeks. During the assessment it is noted that she has hyperresonance in her lungs and a pronounced dorsal curvature of her spine. Her respiratory rate is 20 bpm (breaths per minute) and when she is asked to take deep breaths, she appears to use accessory muscles.

MULTIPLE CHOICE QUESTIONS

1. Normal age-related changes to the respiratory system include all of the following, except:
   a. Bilateral hyperresonance of the lungs
   b. Curvature of the spine
   c. Increased use of accessory muscles
   d. Barrel chest
2. Older people often experience a cough due to:
   a. A decrease in the ability of cilia to clear mucus
   b. Chronic infection
   c. Decreased ability to breathe deeply into the lungs
   d. Poor swallowing ability

3. Curvature of the spine in older adults is indicative of:
   a. Development of chronic obstructive airways disease
   b. Normal musculoskeletal changes during ageing
   c. Postural changes that can be improved with exercise
   d. Shortening of the spinal cord
4. Use of accessory muscles for breathing is more common in older people due to:
   a. A decrease in muscle mass in the chest wall causing tiring easily
   b. Increased work of breathing due to chronic disease
   c. Chronic pulmonary disease, which is usually present in older adults
   d. Curvature of the spine, which requires the use of the respiratory muscles
5. Hyperresonance of the lungs is due to:
   a. A decrease in the alveoli due to ageing
   b. Build-up of mucus in the alveoli
   c. Obstruction of the airway due to pulmonary disease
   d. Change in the sound of the airway from increased blood flow

REFERENCES

Australian Government Department of Health (2020) Australian immunisation handbook. Commonwealth of Australia, Canberra. Online. Available: https://immunisationhandbook .health.gov.au/vaccine-preventable-diseases/influenza -flu#vaccine-information

Best Practice Journal NZ (2015) The optimal management of patients with COPD – Part 1: The diagnosis. Issue 66. Online. Available: https://bpac.org.nz/BPJ/2015/February/docs/BPJ66-copd-part1.pdf

Casey G (2017) The biology of ageing. Kia Tiaki Nursing New Zealand 23(10):20–24.

Charbek E, Espiritu JR, Nayak R et al (2018) Frailty, comordidity and COPD. Journal of Nutritional Health and Aging 22: 876–879.

Ciabattini A, Nardini C, Santoro G et al (2018) Vaccination in the elderly: the challenge of immune changes with ageing, Seminars in Immunology 40:83–94.

Cilloniz C, Ceccato A, San Jose A et al (2016) Clinical management of community acquired pneumonia in the elderly patient. Expert Review of Respiratory Medicine 10(11): 1211–1220.

Craft JA, Gordon CJ, Huether SE et al (2017) Understanding pathophysiology, Australia and New Zealand edition, 3rd edn. Elsevier, Chatswood.

Ennis J (2013) The physiology of ageing. Practice Nurse 43(3): 38–42.

Global Initiative For Chronic Obstructive Lung Disease (GOLD) (2019) Global strategy for the diagnosis, management, and prevention of chronic obstructive pulmonary disease. Online. Available: https://goldcopd.org/wp-content/uploads/2018/11/GOLD-2019-v1.7-FINAL-14Nov2018-WMS.pdf

Lapi F, Marconi E, Simonetti M et al (2019) Adjuvanted versus nonadjuvanted influenza vaccines and risk of hospitalizations for pneumonia and cerebro/cardiovascular events in the elderly. Expert Review of Vaccines 18(6):663–670.

Manuel A, Hardinge M (2016) Obstructive sleep apnoea. Medicine 44(6):336–341.

Riaz M, Ravula S, Obesso PD et al (2019) The effect of torso elevation on minimum effective continuous positive airway pressure for treatment of obstructive sleep apnea. Sleep and Breathing 24(2):499–504.

Sanches VS, Santos FM, Fernandes JM et al (2014) Neurodegenerative disorders increase decline in respiratory muscle strength in older adults. Respiratory Care 59(12):1838–1845.

Shay A, Fulton JS, O'Malley P (2020) Mobility and functional status among hospitalized COPD patients. Clinical Nursing Research 29(1):13–20.

CHAPTER 25

Mental Health in Older Age

KAREN HESLOP

LEARNING OBJECTIVES

After reading this chapter, you will be able to:

- identify factors that contribute to good mental health and poor mental health in older people
- describe the prevalence and clinical features of depression, anxiety, psychosis and suicide in older people
- discuss alcohol and other substance use disorders in older people
- outline the care and treatment of older people with mental health problems and mental disorders
- identify cultural factors that contribute to mental disorders in older people.

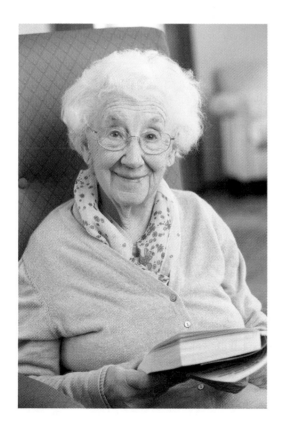

INTRODUCTION

Although most older people (aged 65 years and older) enjoy good mental health and live active and fulfilling lives, some (approximately 10%) suffer high or very high levels of psychological distress or have a diagnosed mental disorder that impacts significantly on their wellbeing and quality of life (Australian Bureau of Statistics [ABS] 2018). Older people may experience mental health problems, such as anxiety, depression, self-harm and alcohol or substance use in response to isolation, loneliness or distress, related to events common in later life, including retirement, bereavement, chronic disease or disability (World Health Organisation [WHO] 2017). If left untreated, these problems can become more problematic and develop into mental disorders, such as major depression, anxiety disorders, bipolar disorder or schizophrenia. An estimated 10–15% of older adults living in the community in Australia experience anxiety or depression (Australian Institute of Health and Welfare [AIHW] 2015). Mental disorders in older people commonly occur alongside other physical conditions or may be a continuation of a mental disorder diagnosed earlier in adulthood. Many older people with mental disorders and/or alcohol and substance use disorders do not get the care they need, as they are reluctant to seek help due to stigma. Then when they

TABLE 25.1 Glossary	
Akathisia	movement disorder characterised by a feeling of inner restlessness and an inability to stay still.
Dysthymia	chronic form of depression that is less acute than a major depressive disorder, but has persistent symptoms that last for at least 2 years.
Mental health	the way a person thinks (cognition), feels (mood and emotions), behaves and relates to others (relationships). www.health.gov.au/health-topics/mental-health
Mental disorder	a clinically recognisable set of symptoms or behaviours that include abnormal thoughts, perceptions, emotions, behaviour and relationships with others that cause distress and interfere with a person's functioning.
Mental disorder classification	mental disorders are classified according to the International Classification of Diseases and Related Health Problems (ICD) and *Diagnostic and Statistical Manual of Mental Disorders* (DSM). There is no way of diagnosing mental disorders using laboratory or medical-imaging diagnostic techniques.
Mental health problem	a temporary state of mental ill health that occurs as a reaction to the stresses of life. Mental health problems are common and interfere with how a person thinks, feels and behaves. A mental health problem may develop into a mental disorder if not effectively managed. www.health.gov.au/mentalhealth
Psychomotor agitation	spectrum of disorders where the person exhibits restlessness and purposeless movements (e.g picking at skin or pacing around the room), which may be accompanied by emotional distress.
Psychomotor retardation	slowing down of thought and physical movements. Can cause a visible slowing of physical and emotional reactions, speech and affect (mood).
Psychosis	severe mental disorder where thoughts and emotions are so impaired that a person loses contact with reality.

do, their symptoms are overlooked or misdiagnosed by health professionals. Regular assessment of mental health status, mental health treatment and management are important aspects of care for the older person. The glossary in Table 25.1 explains the terms referred to throughout the chapter.

MENTAL HEALTH IN OLDER AGE

Good mental health has been described by the WHO (2017) as '… a state of well-being in which the individual realizes his or her own abilities, can cope with the normal stresses of life, can work productively and fruitfully, and is able to make a contribution to his or her community'. For older people, good mental health can also encompass feelings of optimism, satisfaction, self-esteem, a sense of purpose, being in control of their lives and a sense of belonging and support (Wells et al 2014).

Good mental health in older people is characterised by:

- being connected to family and friends, co-workers, community, culture and environment

- having purposeful activity, family or community roles or responsibilities, hobbies, learning and education, volunteering and work
- engaging in new experiences and being involved with the community
- feeling safe, stable and secure financially at home and in the neighbourhood
- having good physical health, being active, eating well and sleeping well.

Good mental health is determined by an older person's resilience and coping skills, their capacity to be productive or to contribute, their social connectedness and provision of basic needs and comfort (Wells et al 2014). There is also a strong link between a person's physical health and their mental health. For example, older people with physical health conditions such as heart disease have higher rates of depression than those who are healthy, and if left untreated, depression in an older person with heart disease can negatively affect the outcome. Thus, encouraging good physical health improves mental health and vice versa. The *Promoting wellness* box provides strategies to promote mental health in older people.

Promoting Wellness
Strategies to Promote Good Mental Health in Older People

- Eat a healthy diet of nutritious food, keep hydrated and maintain a healthy weight to ensure good cognitive functioning and memory and improve wellbeing.
- Be active and keep mobile. Walk and exercise within the older person's ability to increase activity levels, enable social interaction, reduce anxiety and improve mood.
- Get enough sleep and rest to improve mental alertness, concentration and memory formation and to reduce stress and fatigue.
- Have a heathy lifestyle – reduce/stop smoking, alcohol and substance use (including overuse of prescribed medications) to improve cognition, physical health, as well as financial and social situation (reduces stress and social/family disharmony).
- Treat chronic conditions such as diabetes, arthritis and hypertension to reduce pain and discomfort and improve overall health, mood, cognition and sense of wellbeing.
- Maintain good eyesight and hearing – use glasses or hearing aids if necessary to assist communication and confidence in social settings, reduce the risk of falls or injury and maintain hobbies and interests.

Tips for Best Practice
Useful Resources Relating to Mental Health and Wellbeing for Older People

- Wells et al (2014) What works to promote emotional wellbeing in older people: a guide for aged care staff working in community or residential care settings. Beyond Blue Australia
  http://resources.beyondblue.org.au/prism/file?token=BL/1263A
- Head to health – Supporting aged and elderly (Australia)
  https://headtohealth.gov.au/supporting-someone-else/supporting/aged-and-elderly
- Health navigator – New Zealand
  www.healthnavigator.org.nz/healthy-living/s/senior-health/

The *Tips for best practice* box provides useful resources relating to mental health and wellbeing for older people.

MENTAL DISORDERS IN OLD AGE

Although the prevalence of mental health problems generally decreases with age, many older people suffer severe mental disorders that affect quality of life and wellbeing. The most common mental disorders in older age are:

- anxiety
- depression
- alcohol and substance abuse.

Approximately one-quarter of deaths from self-harm are among people aged 60 years and older (WHO 2017). Mental disorders in older age are a risk factor for dementia (Skoog 2011).

Early detection and treatment of mental disorders in older people is important to reduce the impact on the older person, their family and the community. Good quality mental healthcare is needed to reduce the duration and severity of symptoms, prevent recurrence decrease suffering and improve quality of life.

Pathophysiology

Age-related changes to the central nervous system increase the risk of older people developing a mental disorder in later life. Cerebral neurodegeneration (neural death) and cerebrovascular diseases more common in older age, such as stroke, can lead to increased depression, anxiety and psychosis in older people. Post-mortem studies indicate that shrinking of the frontal lobe and hippocampus (areas of the brain related to higher cognitive functioning and memory formation), cerebral ventricular enlargement and changes to the caudate nuclei and putamen are features of anxiety and depression in older people. Subtle changes to the brain from degenerative or vascular changes increase an older person's susceptibility to psychosis (Peters 2006).

As people age, brain volume decreases at a rate of 5% per decade from age 40, with shrinking of grey matter (comprising brain cells – neurons) and white matter (comprising myelinated nerve fibres) increasing after the age of 70 (Peters 2006). Fewer neural connections and signals between brain cells result in slower cognitive processing and cognitive functioning, which are features of most mental disorders. In addition, the ageing brain generates fewer chemical messengers (neurotransmitters). Alterations in neurotransmitter pathways, such as dopamine, acetylcholine, serotonin and noradrenaline, are features of mental disorders, including anxiety, depression, bipolar disorder, psychoses and schizophrenia (Peters 2006).

These age-related changes in the brain occur alongside psychosocial issues and interact to impact on the older person's mental health. Factors that impact on the severity and duration of mental disorders in older people include:

- stressful life events
- physical illness
- disability
- changes in accommodation
- decreased social network and support
- personal or family history of a mental disorder
- low education
- personality factors
- smoking
- alcohol consumption (Skoog 2011).

CULTURE AND OLDER PERSONS' MENTAL HEALTH

Many older people from Indigenous backgrounds (Australian Aboriginal and Torres Strait Islander people and New Zealand Māori), culturally and linguistically diverse (CALD) backgrounds or those born overseas experience poor mental health. Most (88%) Indigenous Australians over the age of 55 years have chronic health conditions, such as diabetes, cardiovascular and respiratory disease. They require more assistance with basic activities of daily living (ADLs), self-care and communication, which impacts on their mental health and wellbeing. Approximately one-quarter of older Indigenous Australians have a mental disorder and at least one co-occurring long-term health condition (McKay et al 2015). Indigenous Australians have a higher mortality rate, with only 5% of the Indigenous population being aged 65 and over.

While mental health professionals conceptualise mental health as a state of wellness, Indigenous Australians see it more holistically as a state of social and emotional wellbeing, encompassing the health of the whole community, cultural identity, a sense of kinship, spirituality and connection to Country.

In this context, the mental health of Indigenous Australians is influenced by a multitude of factors, including:

- the impact of history and politics
- significant experiences of loss and grief
- current physical and functional limitations or impairments
- access to appropriate health care
- stereotyping
- racial discrimination by society and service providers (Beyond Blue 2020b).

Historical social and political issues associated with colonisation and legacies of the Stolen Generation (the forced removal of children from families) continue to have an impact on older Indigenous Australians. Many are living with unresolved trauma and grieve the loss of their culture, land, connections and identity, while also experiencing ongoing social and economic disadvantage and discrimination (Beyond Blue 2020b). Similarly, in New Zealand, lingering effects of colonisation and resultant discrimination impact on the mental health-related quality of life of older New Zealand Māori aged 80 years and over (McKay et al 2015). In both countries, older Indigenous people experience social disparities that negatively affect mental health, related to:

- unresolved trauma from domestic and other violence
- incarceration or imprisonment
- substance abuse
- economic and social disadvantage
- discrimination and racism (Beyond Blue 2020b).

Despite these issues, many protective cultural factors allow older people from Indigenous backgrounds to deal with mental health problems. These include:
- being socially connected
- a sense of belonging, spirituality and ancestry
- being connected to or living on or near traditional land
- having a strong sense of community and self-determination
- holding a respected role within their culture and a responsibility to pass on cultural practices (Beyond Blue 2020b).

Many older Indigenous people have had negative experiences when accessing mental health services, including poor communication, culturally inappropriate care or processes of care, discrimination and stereotyping or lack of confidentiality and privacy. These negative experiences reduce the likelihood of older people accessing the mental health services in the future (Beyond Blue 2020b). It is important that nurses recognise and respect the roles of older Indigenous people and work in partnership to provide culturally appropriate care, incorporating broader concepts of wellbeing in culturally sensitive environments (McKay et al 2015).

Older People From CALD Backgrounds

One in three Australians were born overseas. Almost 20% of people aged over 50 years were born in a non-English speaking country or come from a CALD background. These older people are at higher risk of mental health issues due to trauma experienced prior to migration, a loss of identity or disconnection from their culture and lower socioeconomic status.

Nevertheless, older people from CALD backgrounds tend to underuse mental health services and can delay seeking help for mental health issues due to different understanding or lack of knowledge about mental health, language or communication issues, cultural stigma associated with mental health issues and delayed or incorrect diagnosis.

Other factors influencing the mental health of older people from CALD backgrounds include:

- cultural norms of their country of origin
- extent of acculturation in Australia
- presence of children or other family in adopted country (Australia or New Zealand)
- children or family remaining in the country of origin
- current or previous refugee status
- level of English proficiency
- living in residential aged care.

When caring for older people with mental disorders, nurses must be understanding of and sensitive to the older person's specific cultural needs. Many mental health assessment scales are culturally specific and affected by language and ethnicity. Additionally, a culturally sensitive approach to treatment requires consideration of the older person's beliefs about medications and medical proce-dures, and potential preference for traditional therapies and medicines (Federation of Ethnic Communities' Councils of Australia [FECCA] 2015). The *Tips for best practice* box provides useful mental health resources for older adults from Indigenous and CALD backgrounds.

Tips for Best Practice
Useful Mental Health Resources for Older People From Indigenous and CALD Backgrounds

Beyond Blue – Depression: who does it affect? Aboriginal and Torres Strait Islander people available: www.beyondblue.org.au/who-does-it-affect/aboriginal-and-torres-strait-islander-people

Māori depression and anxiety – https://depression.org.nz/get-better/your-identity/maori/

MENTAL HEALTH ASSESSMENT

Assessment of an older person's mental health involves a mental state examination (MSE). Table 25.2 details the domains assessed in an MSE and questions which identify the type, duration and severity of symptoms. Additional information about the older person's social and physi-cal functioning from friends, family and other health professionals complete the mental health assessment.

The MSE provides information to enable diagnosis of a mental disorder through classification of symptom type, severity and duration against an agreed diagnostic classification system. In Australia and New Zealand, the most commonly used classification systems are The International Classification of Diseases and Related Health Problems (ICD) and the Diagnostic and Statistical Manual of Mental Disorders (DSM). Before confirming the diagnosis of a mental disorder, the doctor may conduct some physical assessments of the brain (e.g. electroencephalogram [EEG]), magnetic resonance imaging [MRI] or blood tests) to exclude other causes for observed changes in the older person's cognition, mood and behaviour.

An important part of a mental state assessment is to determine whether a person is at risk of harm to themselves, to other people or to the community. Older people may pose a non-suicidal risk to themselves through: self-neglect; not eating or drinking; not engaging in treatment for chronic medical conditions (e.g. diabetes; hypertension); or misusing alcohol and other substances.

Older people may also pose a risk of suicide due to social isolation and loneliness, chronic disease or increased depression, anxiety or psychosis.

These issues should be explored during the MSE so that appropriate care and support can be initiated in either the community or the inpatient hospital setting (McKay et al 2015).

Mental Health Care

Much of the mental healthcare provided to older people is by primary care services in the community, such as General Practitioners (GPs) and community support agencies. Care for an older person with a mental disorder depends on the type and severity of symptoms and the older person's social situation. The *Tips for best practice* box provides aspects of general non-specialist mental health care.

For older people with more severe or problematic mental disorders, specialist mental healthcare, treatment and counselling services are available in both hospital and community settings, delivered by a range of mental health workers, including mental health nurses, allied health professionals, care workers, psychiatrists and psychologists (Muir-Cochrane et al 2014). Specialist mental health services include:

- supportive counselling to help the older person address practical problems and conflicts, and to understand the reasons for their illness
- psychological interventions to help the person under-stand their thoughts, behaviour and relationships with other people (e.g. cognitive behavioural therapy)
- medication to address symptoms, restore normal sleep patterns, improve appetite and reduce anxiety.

TABLE 25.2
Components of a Mental State Examination (MSE)

Appearance	• How does the person look? Consider the older person's level of hygiene and grooming, how they are dressed (is their clothing unusual or inappropriate to the climatic conditions?) and apparent level of health.
Behaviour	• How does the person behave? Consider general behaviour, facial expression, eye contact, body movements and gestures. • How is the person reacting? Are they cooperative, withdrawn, hostile, inappropriate, afraid, suspicious, evasive?
Speech and language	• How is the person talking? Consider the rate of speech (rapid, pressured, slow, retarded), the volume (loud, whispering, quiet), tone (monotone, with intonation) quantity of information (little/poverty or pressure of speech, mute/silent) and quality of information (stuttering, slurring). • How does the person express himself or herself? Is the conversation coherent and logical or do the thoughts appear unrelated, loosely connected or tangential? Is speech coherent? Are replies unrelated to the topic or incomplete? Does the speech flow or is it hesitant, interrupted, absent or slow?
Mood and affect (feelings)	• How does the older person describe their emotional state? Do they report feeling happy, sad, depressed, anxious or nervous? • What do you observe? Does the person appear to be low in mood (flat, restricted, tearful, deflated, blunted facial expression), anxious (agitated, fiddly), distressed, fearful, irritable, distracted, angry (hostile, defensive, easily provoked) or excessively happy or over animated? Is their mood constant or labile (rapidly changing), or congruent (consistent with what they are saying, what is observed and the situation)?
Thought content (thinking)	• What is the person thinking about? Consider the amount of thought and rate of production (do their thoughts flow easily, stay on track?). Is there any limitation to their thinking? Do their thoughts have a logical flow or is there repetition of words or gaps? Are there any disturbances in language (is it coherent, organised, are they using correct words)? • Does the person express paranoid, grandiose, bizarre delusional thoughts/false beliefs? Does the person have preoccupations, prominent thoughts (not quite delusional) or overvalued ideas? Are they expressing thoughts of harm to self or others (suicidal or non-suicidal e.g. cutting, hitting, burning)?
Perception	• How does the older person perceive their environment? Does the person have any perceptual disturbance? Does the person report auditory, visual, olfactory, tactile, gustatory hallucinations (perceptions in the absence of stimulus)? Do they have dissociative symptoms such as derealisation (external world seems unreal) or depersonalisation (detached from own thoughts and feelings) or do they have illusions/misinterpret sensory stimuli (e.g. hearing rain on roof as voices)?
Cognition	• What are the older person's thought processes? Assess their level of consciousness (are they alert, sleepy, sedated?), their attention (are they on-task, able to attend to what is being said?), their memory (ability to recall events), orientation (to time, place and person), concentration (ability to focus on a task, follow instructions) and their abstract thinking (ability to identify similarities, plan tasks etc).
Insight and judgement	• What is the person's insight and judgement like? Do they have capacity to recognise their own problems and symptoms and the ability to make sound, reasoned and responsible decisions?

Perth Co-occurring Disorders Capacity Building (2011).

Tips for Best Practice
General Non-Specialist Healthcare

Elements of general non-specialist healthcare include:

- helping the older person to make healthy lifestyle changes, including good nutrition, plenty of exercise and enough rest
- encouraging the older person to make and keep social connections with family, friends and local community groups to reduce social isolation; encouraging the use of telephone or internet communication if the person is immobile or geographically isolated
- treating or managing underlying medical conditions to reduce pain, improve mood and mobility and reduce the older person's perception of ill health
- supporting the older person to access online tools and courses that promote coping skills for mental health problems or functional difficulties.

Tips for Best Practice
Recovery-Focused Care

Principles of recovery-focused care are to:

- recognise the uniqueness of the older person, placing the individual at the centre of their care and accepting that recovery outcomes are personal and unique
- provide the older person with real choices about how to live by building on their strengths, encouraging the taking of responsibility and making the most of new opportunities when possible
- demonstrate recovery-focused attitudes that protect the older person's legal, citizenship and human rights by
  - instilling hope and optimism, and
  - supporting the older person to develop and maintain social, recreational, occupational and vocational activities that are meaningful to them
- promote dignity and respect for older people by being respectful and sensitive to their values, beliefs and culture, and by challenging discrimination and stigma when it exists
- develop partnerships and good communication with older people and their carers in a way that makes sense to them, by sharing important information and working with them in ways that allow them to realise their hope, goals and aspirations
- evaluate recovery and assist older people to track their own progress.

Australian Government Department of Health (2010).

Medications often take time to have a positive effect, but generally people begin to feel better within 3–6 weeks

- support groups run by people with mental health conditions who have developed successful support networks
- tertiary-level inpatient or outpatient treatment for older people with severe mental disorders.

Contemporary mental healthcare for older people is recovery-focused. The focus is recognising that while a cure for the disorder (being free of symptoms) is not always possible, a person can minimise the impact of symptoms, make choices and work towards the goal of a productive and meaningful life. The Australian National Standards for Mental Health Services suggests: 'Recovery means gaining and retaining hope, understanding of one's abilities and disabilities, engagement in an active life, personal autonomy, social identity, meaning and purpose in life, and a positive sense of self'(Australian Government Department of Health 2010). *Tips for best practice: Recovery-focused care* details the principles of recovery-focused mental health care for older people.

Nursing the Older Person With a Mental Disorder

Contemporary mental healthcare is multidisciplinary, ethical, evidence-based, recovery focused and provided in partnership with older people and their families and carers. Nurses are integral to the multidisciplinary care team and provide:

- ongoing assessment and documentation of mental state and risk (potential for self-harm/suicide)
- management planning in partnership with the older person
- treatment (pharmacological and non-pharmacological), ensuring:
  - safe administration of medications
  - assessing adherence
  - monitoring effects of psychotropic medications (medications that act on the central nervous system)
- support to complete ADLs
- guidance to promote structure, routine, social relationships and community engagement
- education relating to mental disorders, including:
  - identification of symptoms and early warning signs
  - medications and treatment

- impact of physical health and social wellbeing on mental state
- support accessing mental health services and treatment.

Legislative Provisions for Involuntary Treatment

Australia and New Zealand have legislative provisions to allow for the involuntary treatment of a person suffering from an acute mental disorder. These provisions ensure access to appropriate mental health care for the person, and protect the person and others from serious harm.

In Australia, this power is vested in each of the states and territories. Box 25.1 provides detail of applicable Acts in Australia and New Zealand. Legislation incorporates the United Nations Principles for the treatment of persons with mental illness and the improvement of mental health care (Office of the United Nations High Commissioner for Human Rights 1991). These principles provide for the basic human right to access to mental health care, in the least restrictive environment, that is appropriate to health needs, with respect for dignity and cultural safety.

Where possible, mental health care should be provided in the community, and consent for treatment must be sought and provided where the person has the capacity to do so. Involuntary admission can only be authorised to treat a person's mental disorder if there is likelihood of serious deterioration in the person's health or risk of imminent self-harm or harm to another person. People treated under the Mental Health Act must be informed of their rights (Royal Australian and New Zealand College of Psychiatrists 2017).

Legislative provisions outline the rights and responsibilities of people receiving treatment under the applicable Act, and responsibilities of nurses and other mental health professionals administering the Act. They also make provisions for the safe transport of people to an authorised mental health facility for treatment, involuntary treatment including electroconvulsive therapy (see below) and the emergency use of seclusion and restraint.

BOX 25.1
New Zealand and Australian State and Territory Mental Health Legislation

NEW ZEALAND

Mental Health (Compulsory Assessment and Treatment) Act 1992
www.legislation.govt.nz/act/public/1992/0046/latest/
DLM262176.html

Mental Health (Compulsory Assessment and Treatment) Amendment Act 1998
www.legislation.govt.nz/act/public/1999/0140/latest/
DLM48972.html?search=ts_act_mental+health
++act+1999_noresel&p=1&sr=1

AUSTRALIA
Australian Capital Territory
Mental Health Act 2015
www.legislation.act.gov.au/a/2015-38

NSW
Mental Health Act 2007
www.legislation.nsw.gov.au/#/view/act/2007/8/full

Northern Territory
Mental Health and Related Services Act 1998
https://legislation.nt.gov.au/en/Legislation/MENTAL
-HEALTH-AND-RELATED-SERVICES-ACT-1998

Queensland
Mental Health Act 2000
www.legislation.qld.gov.au/view/pdf/inforce/2010-07-01/
act-2000-016

South Australia
Mental Health Act 2009
www.legislation.sa.gov.au/LZ/C/A/MENTAL%20
HEALTH%20ACT%202009.aspx

Tasmania
Mental Health Act 2013
www.dhhs.tas.gov.au/mentalhealth/mental_health_act

Victoria
Mental Health Act 2014
www5.austlii.edu.au/au/legis/vic/consol_act/
mha2014128/index.html

Western Australia
Mental Health Act 2014
www.legislation.wa.gov.au/legislation/statutes.nsf/
main_mrtitle_13534_homepage.html

Nurses working in the mental health field must have a good understanding of the applicable Act in their jurisdiction and their role and legal obligations within it.

DEPRESSION IN THE OLDER PERSON

Depression occurs in 7% of the older population worldwide (WHO 2017). Australian figures suggest the rate of depression in older people is 10–15%, increasing to 35% in older people living in residential aged care (Beyond Blue 2020a). In New Zealand, an estimated 2% of older men and 5% of older women live with depression.

Depression in the older person may result in functional decline. Potential consequences include:
- increased care needs
- placement into residential aged care
- increased family stress
- increased likelihood of physical illnesses
- reduced recovery from illness (e.g. stroke)
- premature death due to suicide.

Older people who suffer depressive symptoms have poorer social and physical functioning compared to those with chronic conditions, such as hypertension, diabetes or lung disease. They also suffer higher levels of distress and suffering impacting on quality of life and the use of healthcare services (WHO 2017).

Factors increasing an older person's risk of depression include:
- a previous episode of depression
- family history of depression or suicide attempts
- misuse of alcohol or other substances
- childhood trauma
- social isolation
- responsibilities for caring for others
- chronic or severe physical illness
- experiences of grief or loss (New Zealand Health Navigator 2020).

Common Features of Depression

- Feelings: sadness, hopelessness or emptiness, feeling overwhelmed, worthless or guilty, moodiness or irritability, which may present as anger or aggression.
- Behaviours: general slowing down or restlessness, neglect of responsibilities and self-care, withdrawing from family and friends, decline in day-to-day ability to function, being confused, worried and agitated, inability to find pleasure in any activity, difficulty getting motivated in the morning, behaving out of character, denial of depressive feelings as a defence mechanism.

- Thoughts: indecisiveness, loss of self-esteem, excessive concerns about financial situation, perceived change of status within the family, negative comments like 'I'm a failure', 'it's my fault' or 'life is not worth living', persistent suicidal thoughts.
- Physical symptoms: Sleeping more or less than usual, feeling tired all the time, slowed movement, memory problems, chronic unexplained pain such as headaches or backache, digestive upsets, nausea, changes in bowel habits, agitation, hand wringing, pacing, loss or change of appetite, significant weight loss (or gain) (Beyond Blue 2020a).

Depression is generally underdiagnosed and undertreated in older people, who can be reluctant to seek help due to stigma or encounters with health professionals who overlook or misdiagnose depressive symptoms. Rather than describing sadness or low mood, older people with depression tend to present with physical symptoms, such as poor appetite, difficulty sleeping, headaches, lethargy or increased pain. Older people may also use vague language, for example, complaining of 'bad nerves' rather than describing sadness (Beyond Blue 2020a). Additionally, symptoms of depression often coincide with problems common in later life, such as bereavement, loneliness, financial uncertainty or reduced functioning due to chronic disease or frailty.

Classification of Depression

Depression is classified according to the following:
- *Type of depression* – whether a major depressive disorder that meets the diagnostic classification of the DSM or ICD requiring medical treatment or a dysthymia or low mood that can be managed with modification to lifestyle, financial and social factors.
- *Course of the depression* – whether the depression is a single episode, recurring or cyclical, chronic (long-term with a poor treatment response), unipolar or bipolar. In unipolar depression, the older person experiences only low mood. In bipolar depression, the depressive symptoms are a feature of a bipolar disorder with the older person experiencing periods of low mood and periods of mania (high mood and activity or agitation, racing thoughts, little need for sleep and rapid speech) (Blackdog Institute 2020).
- *Onset of the depression* – whether it is reactive (due to a specific stressor, such as bereavement, or an environmental factor, such as poverty, neglect or abuse) or endogenous (genetic or biological susceptibility to depression and exacerbated by stress).

- *Severity of the depression* – whether the symptoms of depression are mild, moderate or severe (causing marked distress or functional, social or occupational impairment).
- *Features of depression* – or the additional symptoms of the depression:
  - Psychotic depression (where the person experiences all the features of depression and psychotic symptoms, such as hallucinations and delusions).
  - Depressive disorder due to another medical condition (where there is evidence from the history, physical examination or laboratory findings that the depression is a direct pathophysiological consequence of another medical condition).
  - Substance/medication-induced depressive disorder (where the symptoms of depression developed during or soon after intoxication or withdrawal of a substance or medication that is capable of producing the symptoms of depression).

Major Depression

Many older people experience a more severe form of depression and are diagnosed with major depressive disorder. A major depressive disorder according to the DSM-5 (American Psychiatric Association 2013) is when a person presents with at least five of the symptoms listed below (with one being either depressed mood or markedly diminished interest or pleasure) for a two-week period that represents a change from previous level of functioning and causes significant distress or impairment.

- Depressed mood most of the day, nearly every day (e.g. feels sad, empty, hopeless) or observed by others (e.g. appears tearful).
- Markedly diminished interest or pleasure in all, or almost all, activities most of the day, nearly every day.
- Significant weight loss when not dieting or weight gain (e.g. a change of more than 5% of body weight in a month) or decrease or increase in appetite nearly every day.
- Insomnia or hypersomnia nearly every day.
- Psychomotor agitation or retardation nearly every day that is observable by others.
- Fatigue or loss of energy nearly every day.
- Feelings of worthlessness or excessive or inappropriate guilt (which may be delusional) nearly every day.
- Reported or observed diminished ability to think or concentrate, or indecisiveness, nearly every day.
- Recurrent thoughts of death, recurrent suicidal ideation without a specific plan, or a suicide attempt or a specific plan for committing suicide.

These symptoms are not attributable to the physiological effects of substances or another medical condition.

Late-Life Depression

Some older people experience their first episode of depression after the age of 60. Termed 'late-life depression', this disorder is more chronic and has a poorer prognosis with a higher mortality rate than depression experienced in earlier stages of life. It is characterised by recurring bouts of depression with associated cognitive impairment, psychotic symptoms or co-occurring medical or physical health conditions. Factors associated with higher risk of late-life depression are:

- older females (≥ 80 years)
- single (widowed) marital status
- poor physical health or frailty
- cognitive impairment
- neurodegenerative or vascular disease
- nutritional deficits
- multiple medications
- lifestyle factors such as smoking, alcohol use (Van Damme et al 2018).

Mental health assessment must include the older person's medical history and current medications because some medical conditions common in older people can mimic symptoms of depression. These include:

- thyroid disorders
- cerebrovascular disease
- Parkinson's disease
- myocardial infarction
- malnutrition and vitamin B deficiencies.

Side effects of medications such as benzodiazepines, beta-blockers, steroids and anti-parkinsonian drugs can also cause symptoms of depression in older people.

Treatment for Depression

Treatment for depression may include a combination of counselling or other psychological therapy, lifestyle changes and pharmacological approaches, including antidepressants or over-the-counter (OTC) products (e.g. St John's Wort). Useful strategies for some older people include reducing loneliness and isolation, mindfulness, meditation and online tools and courses.

Treatment can also be from traditional or cultural healers, for example, New Zealand tohunga or healers that provide rongoā Māori (Māori healing services) (New Zealand Health Navigator 2020).

Pharmacological approaches

Antidepressant medications are the treatment of choice for depression and are effective in approximately 70% of older people who experience an episode of depression

(Declercq et al 2018). It is common for older people to experience episodic depression and require ongoing or prophylactic antidepressant medications to reduce the frequency and severity of episodes.

Classes of medications used to treat depression are:

- *Selective serotonin reuptake inhibitors* (SSRIs), first-line treatment for depression in older people. Common side effects associated with SSRIs include:
  - nausea
  - dry mouth
  - insomnia
  - somnolence
  - agitation
  - diarrhoea
  - excessive sweating.

  SSRIs have fewer anticholinergic effects, so are useful for older people with cardiovascular disease.
- *Tricyclic antidepressants* (nortriptyline, desipramine) are second-line treatment, due to the number of problematic side effects. Side effects include:
  - postural hypotension, increasing the risk of falls and fractures (see Chapter 16)
  - cardiac conduction abnormalities
  - anticholinergic effects.
- *Atypical antipsychotics* (risperidone and olanzapine) are effective for treatment of severe or refractory depression or for older people who fail to respond fully to antidepressant medications. Low dose atypical antipsychotics are also useful to treat psychotic symptoms associated with depression. Common side effects include:
  - sedation
  - anticholinergic effects
  - extrapyramidal symptoms increasing the risk of falls and injury
  - metabolic effects contributing to weight gain, dyslipidaemia, diabetes and cardiovascular disease (Wiese 2011).

Non-pharmacological approaches

Non-pharmacological approaches can be used alone or in conjunction with pharmacological treatments. Useful strategies for the treatment of mild to moderate depression include:

- supportive counselling (to identify stressors and strategies to reduce depression)
- improving lifestyle factors (improving diet, exercise and reducing substance use)
- improving social situation (addressing issues with housing finance and relationships)
- reducing isolation (encouraging engagement in family and community activities).

Electroconvulsive therapy. For older people with severe depression (or suicidality), electroconvulsive therapy (ECT) is an effective and safe treatment. ECT is particularly useful for treating major depressive disorder and late-life depression when the older person has a medical condition that inhibits the use of antidepressant medications, and when the older person cannot tolerate side effects of antidepressant medication (Dong et al 2018). However, there are many myths and much community stigma surrounding ECT that make older people reluctant to accept this treatment for their depression.

ECT is a medical procedure that induces a modified generalised seizure in an anaesthetised person by passing an electrical stimulus through two electrodes placed on the scalp to the brain (Kavanagh & McLoughlin 2009). ECT is administered as a course of nine to twelve treatments, three times a week. Clinical improvement in depressive symptoms is observable after nine treatments, with optimal treatment effect after 12 weeks. Although the physiological mechanism of ECT is not well understood, the treatment has a demonstrable effect in reducing depressive symptoms in 80–95% of people who receive it, compared to 65–75% of people on antidepressant medication (Dong et al 2018). See *Tips for best practice* box for resources and further reading relating to depressive disorders.

Tips for Best Practice
Useful Resources Relating to Depressive Disorders

Bipolar disorder: www.blackdoginstitute.org.au/
    clinical-resources/bipolar-disorder/
    what-is-bipolar-disorder
Depression – Who does it affect? (Older people):
    www.beyondblue.org.au/who-does-it-affect/
    older-people
Depression in older people (Fact sheet from Black Dog
    Institute): www.blackdoginstitute.org.au/docs/
    default-source/factsheets/depressioninolderpeople.
    pdf?sfvrsn=8

ANXIETY IN OLDER PEOPLE

Anxiety disorders affect approximately 3.8% of the older population (WHO 2017). Between 15% and 50% of community-dwelling older people experience significant anxiety and 12–15% have a formal diagnosis of an anxiety disorder (Koychev & Ebmeier 2016). It is common for older people to experience symptoms of anxiety associated with living alone; changes in social or living situations; financial uncertainty; relationship issues; traumatic events; and changes in physical health, such as increasing frailty and diagnosis of life-threating conditions (e.g. heart attack, stroke, cancer).

The most common anxiety disorders experiences by older people are generalised anxiety disorder (GAD), specific phobias (such as a fear of falling, see Chapter 16), obsessive-compulsive disorder (OCD), panic disorder and post-traumatic stress disorder (PTSD) (Koychev & Ebmeier 2016).

Anxiety is more common in older people than dementia and depression, but more difficult to identify, as the symptoms are similar to symptoms seen in physical disorders (shortness of breath, abdominal and chest pain) or depression (sleep disturbance, restlessness, poor attention, memory and concentration) (Koychev & Ebmeier 2016). Additionally, symptoms of anxiety often develop gradually in older people and alongside other illnesses; therefore, they may be less obvious and are often misdiagnosed and undertreated.

Common features of anxiety in older people include:

- Feelings: feeling overwhelmed, fearful (particularly when facing certain objects, situations or events), worried about physical symptoms (such as fearing the presence of an undiagnosed medical problem), a sense of dread (fearing that something bad is going to happen), constantly tense or nervous and uncontrollable or overwhelming panic.
- Behaviours: not being assertive (i.e. avoiding eye contact), difficulty making decisions, being startled easily, avoiding anxiety-producing objects or situations, urges to perform certain rituals in a bid to relieve anxiety.
- Thoughts: self-talk statements, such as 'I'm going crazy', 'I can't control myself', 'I'm about to die', 'People are judging me'; having upsetting dreams or flashbacks to a traumatic event, finding it hard to stop worrying, thinking unwanted or intrusive thoughts.
- Physical symptoms: increased heart rate/racing heart, vomiting, nausea or abdominal pain, muscle tension and pain. Feeling detached from own physical self or surroundings, having trouble sleeping, sweating, shaking, dizziness, feeling lightheaded or faint, numbness or tingling, hot or cold flushes (Beyond Blue 2020a).

Anxiety Disorders Common in Older People

- *Generalised anxiety disorder (GAD)* is the most common disorder in older people. It is characterised by:
  - excessive worry about common life stressors (e.g. health, relationships, finances)
  - more than 6 months' duration

- accompanying physical symptoms (e.g. fatigue, sleep disturbance, restlessness, agitation, muscle tension).

It is more common for older people to present to a health professional with physical features of anxiety (Koychev & Ebmeier 2016).

- *Fear of falling* (see Chapter 16) is an age-specific anxiety that occurs in approximately 30–77% of older people who have experienced a fall. This anxiety limits the older person's social and physical activity beyond the effect of the fall, reducing overall functioning and quality of life and increasing the risk of further falls (Koychev & Ebmeier 2016).
- *Obsessive-compulsive disorder (OCD)* is common in older people. Older people with OCD experience persistent and distressing thoughts (obsessions) and use rituals or repetitive behaviours (compulsions) to control the consequent anxiety. The rituals or behaviours associated with OCD may interfere with the older person's day-to-day activities and relationships. For example, an obsession with germs may result in the compulsion whereby the older person repeatedly washes their hands until they bleed. Similarly, an obsession with personal security or intruders has the older person undertaking a ritual requiring them to lock and re-lock doors many times before going to bed. Such repetitive behaviours provide temporary relief from the anxiety created by obsessive thoughts, but are generally not pleasurable for the older person and can cause significant long-term functional and social impairment. OCD usually develops in an earlier life stage and is considered a lifelong anxiety disorder. When OCD first occurs in older age, it may signal the onset of Alzheimer's disease or another type of dementia (see Chapter 26).
- *Post-traumatic stress disorder (PTSD)* refers to a set of reactions that develop following a traumatic event that has threatened the person's life or safety, or that of others around them. Common features of PTSD are:
  - feelings of extreme fear or panic
  - physiological responses (sweating, heart palpitations) similar to those experienced at the time of the trauma
  - re-living the traumatic event (flashbacks of distressing images, nightmares of the event)
  - being over-alert or wound up (poor concentration, sleeping difficulties, easily startled, irritated)
  - avoiding reminders of the traumatic event (people, places, events)
  - feeling emotionally numb (emotionally distant from family and friends, losing interest in day-to-day activities)

- feelings of guilt, shame, or self-blame related to the event or having PTSD.

It is estimated that approximately 70% of older people have been exposed to at least one traumatic event during their lifetime. Older men report higher lifetime exposure to trauma (due to more frequent experiences of combat) than older women. PTSD associated with trauma experienced in early life can be severe and lifelong; however, symptom severity generally decreases with age. Additionally, PTSD symptoms related to recent trauma are less severe in older people compared to younger people (Böttche et al 2012).

- *Phobias* are common in older people. A phobia is an extreme or irrational fear of an object or situation that generates an excessive and persistent feeling of fear and anxiety and/or anxiety-related physical symptoms (e.g. tremors, palpitations, sweating, shortness of breath dizziness, nausea). Specific phobias common in older people include:
  - heights
  - enclosed or small spaces
  - animals
  - air travel
  - driving
  - medical procedures (blood, injections, blood tests)
  - illness (Wuthrich et al 2015).

With specific phobias, the emotional response is either irrational or out of proportion to the actual threat. A person with a phobia either tries to avoid the object or situation that triggers the fear or endures it with increasing fear or distress.

Assessment of Anxiety in Older People

Anxiety often occurs alongside other mental health problems or disorders. It is important to conduct an MSE, described earlier in the chapter, to ensure a thorough assessment of the older person's mental state. Anxiety is closely associated with depression and severe anxiety can present as delusion-like experiences (in the absence of dementia) in some older people (Badcock et al 2017), or can be a symptom of an underlying psychosis.

Treatment for Anxiety
Non-pharmacological approaches

Treatment for mild anxiety disorders includes lifestyle changes and supportive counselling. Moderate and severe anxiety require psychological or pharmacological treatment or a combination of both. Lifestyle changes to decrease anxiety symptoms and improve wellbeing in older people include:

- regular physical activity or exercise
- reducing stress

- keeping active
- spending time with family and friends
- participating in enjoyable activities.

Effective strategies or techniques that older people can employ to self-manage anxiety are:

- relaxation
- slow breathing
- progressive muscle relaxation
- challenging self-talk
- meditation
- mindfulness.

These strategies are easily taught to the older person or a carer, inexpensive, and easily accessed online or from health services. These are particularly useful for older people with mild anxiety symptoms.

- *Cognitive Behavioural Therapy (CBT)* is a formal psychological treatment that can help someone recognise the way their thinking (cognition) and actions (behaviour) affect how anxious they feel. CBT teaches the older person to:
  - recognise differences between productive and unproductive worries
  - how to let go of worries
  - use problem-solving approaches
  - use relaxation and breathing techniques (e.g. muscle relaxation) to control or reduce symptoms
  - improve coping skills.

CBT for anxiety generally involves gradually exposing the older person to the stress-producing object or situation so that he or she learns to cope with feeling anxious. CBT encourages older people to engage in pleasant, satisfying and rewarding activities, which tend to reverse patterns of avoidance and worry that increase anxiety (Beyond Blue 2020a).

- *Mindfulness* (see also Chapter 19) is a therapeutic intervention that encourages a person with anxiety to focus on the 'here and now', to be aware of what they see, smell and taste, and how that makes them feel (how are they reacting, responding, how they feel). Mindfulness aims to harmonise the mind and body, particularly through the periods of change or stressful life events common in later life (Subramanyam et al 2018).

Pharmacological Approaches

Pharmacological treatment for anxiety includes antidepressants and benzodiazepines.

- *Antidepressants* – Low-dose antidepressants have proven effective in the treatment and management of anxiety in older people. First-line treatments are the SSRI class (e.g. escitalopram, sertraline) or SNRI class (venlafaxine and desvanlafaxine) and duloxetine.

- *Benzodiazepines* (also called minor tranquillisers, sedative, hypnotic or anxiolytics) – such as diazepam, lorazepam or clonazepam are considered third-line drugs for the short-term (2–3 weeks) treatment of anxiety disorders in older people. Benzodiazepines promote relaxation and reduce tension and agitation. As well as short-term treatment of GAD, benzodiazepines can be used intermittently for acute anxiety. Benzodiazepines are not recommended for long-term use as they can reduce alertness, affect coordination and can be addictive (Subramanyam et al 2018).

PSYCHOSIS IN OLDER PEOPLE

Psychosis is defined by SANE Australia (2020) as a mental disorder where a person loses the capacity to tell what is real from what is not. A person experiencing psychosis may believe or sense things that are not real, and become confused or slow in their thinking (SANE Australia 2020). Symptoms of psychosis include:

- hallucinations
- delusions
- disorganised thinking (illogical or disordered speech)
- behavioural disturbances, such as excitement and overactivity, psychomotor retardation or catatonia (American Psychiatric Association 2013).

As many as 27% of older people living in the community, and between 10% and 62% of residents in residential aged care, develop psychosis in later life. Primary psychosis is related to a mental disorder such as schizophrenia, depression or mania (Karim & Burns 2003). Secondary psychosis occurs as a feature of a neurological a disorder such as dementia; a response to a medical condition (infection, diseases, endocrine or metabolic disturbances, tumours, delirium); a result of intoxication; or a reaction to withdrawal from substances, alcohol or toxins (Reinhardt & Cohen 2015).

Risk factors that make older people more prone to psychosis include:

- sensory deficits
- social isolation
- cognitive decline
- medical co-morbidities
- alcohol and substance intoxication and withdrawal
- comorbid cognitive impairment (e.g. dementia, delirium)
- age-related changes in cerebral structures, such as frontotemporal cortices
- neurochemical changes associated with ageing
- age-related changes in pharmacokinetics and pharmacodynamics (see Chapter 11) (Reinhardt & Cohen 2015).

Symptoms of Psychosis

- Thoughts: in older people, commonly paranoid, grandiose or religious delusional beliefs. They may believe people are following them, talking about them, trying to harm them, or that they have magical powers, or are a God or superior being. They may display problems with poor memory, concentration or attention. Their speech may be illogical or disorganised and the rate of speech disordered due to an increased or decreased number of thoughts. Thought content may be preoccupied with particular concerns or subjects and they may express thoughts of harm to self or others (suicidal or non-suicidal, e.g. cutting, hitting, burning).
- Behaviours: relate to perceptual disturbances (auditory, visual, tactile, olfactory, gustatory hallucinations), such as attending to unseen stimuli, muttering, talking to themselves, preoccupation, inattention and poor eye contact. Other symptoms include poor self-care and grooming; social withdrawal; hostility; inappropriate bizarre or idiosyncratic behaviours; suspicious; evasive or fearful behaviours; and agitation and restlessness.
- Feelings: of derealisation (that one's surroundings are not real), having depressed or low mood (blunted facial expression), feeling anxious (agitated, fiddly), or distressed, fearful, irritable, distracted or angry (hostile, defensive, easily provoked). Mood may be labile (rapidly changing), or congruent (consistent with what they are saying) or excessively happy or overanimated.
- Physical symptoms: neglect of personal self-care resulting in poor nutrition, dehydration, poor hygiene and grooming. Poor adherence to treatment for medical conditions such as diabetes and hypertension.

Types of Psychosis Experienced by Older People

- *Schizophrenia* is a lifelong debilitating psychotic disorder that usually manifests in early adulthood and affects about 1% of the adult population. Late-life onset of schizophrenia (first episode occurs > 65 years) affects approximately 0.1%–0.5% of older people. The most common presentations in older people are delusions and hallucinations that are persecutory in nature. Low-dose antipsychotic medication is useful in treating the psychosis associated with schizophrenia in older people (Reinhardt & Cohen 2015).
- *Medication/substance-induced psychosis* only occurs in the presence of a medication or substance and abates as the medication or substance leaves the body. Any

medication or substance that crosses the blood–brain barrier can cause psychosis. Classes of medications known to have possible psychotic side effects include:

- antiparkinsonian drugs
- anticholinergics
- cimetidine
- digoxin
- antiarrhythmics
- corticosteroids
- interferon.

A psychosis may also occur during intoxication of substances, such as:

- alcohol
- cannabis
- phencyclidine and other hallucinogens
- inhalants
- sedatives
- hypnotics
- anxiolytics.

Psychosis can also occur during withdrawal from alcohol, sedatives, hypnotics or anxiolytics.

- *Bipolar disorder* generally manifests in middle and late adulthood, with approximately 44% of sufferers developing the disorder in later life. Psychosis associated with bipolar disorder may occur in either the depressed or the manic phase. Psychosis during mania is treated with atypical antipsychotic medication (e.g. olanzapine or quetiapine). A combination of antidepressant and antipsychotic medication is most effective in treating psychotic depression.
- *Delusional disorders* are relatively rare in older people (0.03%). A delusional disorder is diagnosed by the presence of one or more delusions occurring for more than a one-month period. Delusions in older people may be erotic, grandiose, persecutory, jealous, somatic or mixed. Delusions may occur in the presence of visual or auditory hallucinations and have been associated with sensory impairment (Reinhardt & Cohen 2015).

Treatment for Psychosis
Pharmacological approaches
Antipsychotic medication (e.g. risperidone, olanzapine) is considered first-line treatment for psychosis in the older person. These medications have demonstrated efficacy and are reasonably safe in older populations.

Common side effects are:

- sedation
- anticholinergic effects (e.g. orthostatic postural hypotension)
- extrapyramidal effects (e.g. tremors, akathisia, which can increase the risk of falls – see Chapter 16).

Many have cardiovascular effects that may increase the risks in people with underlying cardiovascular conditions.

Non-pharmacological approaches
CBT (see above), supportive counselling and psychosocial support are all useful non-pharmacological treatments for psychosis in older people.

These treatments aim to:

- increase physical, emotional and social functioning
- increase independence
- improve quality of life and wellbeing.

Non-pharmacological strategies usually augment pharmacological treatment, but can be useful on their own for older people who have underlying medical conditions or cannot tolerate antipsychotic medications.

SUBSTANCE USE IN OLDER PEOPLE
Substance use problems affect almost 1% of older people worldwide (WHO 2017). Problems that can develop with the use of alcohol and other substances encompass:

- misuse
- dependence
- tolerance
- withdrawal
- overdose
- intoxication.

The most common substances used by older people in Australia are alcohol, cannabis, nicotine and the non-medical use of prescription drugs, particularly benzodiazepines and opioids (AIHW 2020; Searby et al 2016).

Older people who use alcohol and substances tend to have poorer physical and psychological health and quality of life compared with younger people. Older people have a reduced capacity to metabolise, distribute and eliminate chemical agents (see Chapter 11) and are therefore more vulnerable to harms associated with alcohol and substance use. Poor health outcomes include:

- dysfunction in cardiovascular, hepatic, respiratory, endocrine and immune systems
- mental disorder
- cognitive impairment.

Additionally, alcohol and substances may interact with prescribed medications to increase or decrease their effect, cause side effects or injuries from falls that may require medical treatment, or complicate management and treatment of co-occurring medical conditions (Lintzeris et al 2016).

Historically, problematic alcohol or substance use in older people was thought to be less frequent than in younger people. This perception was based on observations that fewer older people accessed substance abuse treatment programs (Kuerbis et al 2014). However, the last decade has seen increases in the reported prevalence of alcohol and substance use disorders and drug-induced deaths among older people (AIHW 2020; Vafeas et al 2018). One reason may be that substance misuse in older people was under-identified in the past. Additionally, the 'baby boomer generation' (born between 1944 and 1964), who consumed alcohol and substances at higher rates during the social upheaval of the 1960s and 1970s, are now entering older age (currently aged between 56 and 76 years). Baby boomers throughout the world remain the largest group of alcohol and substance users (Kuerbis et al 2014; Loscalzo et al 2017), a trend that is expected to continue.

Alcohol

In 2017–18, 19.5% of males and 8.7% of females aged over 70 drank alcohol daily in Australia (AIHW 2020). Age-related changes that tend to exacerbate the effects of alcohol include lower body mass and total body water, decreasing the liver's capacity to process alcohol, and a more permeable blood–brain barrier and increased neuronal receptor sensitivity, resulting in higher blood alcohol concentration and increased impairment.

Older people who drink alcohol at risky levels are therefore vulnerable to the ill effects and likely to experience consequent problems that interfere with everyday function, such as shopping, cooking, self-care and medication management. These older people are also at increased risk of poor health outcomes, such as haemorrhagic stroke and cognitive impairment and adverse effects from interaction between medications and alcohol, even in moderate amounts (Kuerbis et al 2014).

Illicit Drug Use

Illicit drug use among older people in Australia has doubled over the past decade (22% of older people in 2016 compared to 11% in 2001) (AIHW 2020). Drugs most commonly used illicitly by older people are:
- cannabis
- cocaine
- inhalants
- hallucinogens
- methamphetamine
- heroin.

These substances can cause alterations in mental state and cognitive functioning that interfere with social relationships and physical functioning. Additionally, other harms may be encountered when illicit substances interact with prescribed medicines, particularly opioids and sedative hypnotics, increasing the risk of falls (see

Chapter 16) and other injuries in older people (Kuerbis et al 2014).

Cannabis is one of the most commonly misused drugs by older people (Kostadinov & Roche 2017). While cannabis use may be considered less problematic than other drugs, and even beneficial in coping with illness-related side effects (Kuerbis et al 2014), age-related changes may place older cannabis users at considerable risk of harm. Older people who use cannabis regularly tend to experience increased psychosis; cognitive deficits; poorer mental health; poorer social functioning (Kostadinov & Roche 2017); and greater risk of respiratory and cardiovascular diseases.

Prescription Drugs

Older people tend to take more prescribed and OTC medications than younger people, increasing the risk of misuse, abuse and harmful drug interactions. The most commonly misused prescription medications are opioids and benzodiazepines, which are commonly prescribed for pain (see Chapter 19) and emotional disorders. Problems in older people tend to concern dependence related to over-prescription, misdiagnosis or polypharmacy rather than intentional misuse or abuse (Kuerbis et al 2014).

Assessment for Alcohol and Substance Misuse

Screening procedures for older people who use alcohol and other drugs are limited, resulting in low rates of detection of problematic alcohol and drug use (Searby et al 2016). Despite the variety of screening tools available (e.g. the WHO Alcohol, Smoking, Substance Involvement Screening Test [ASSIST, see Fig. 25.1]), these are seldom utilised in routine health assessments of older people. In turn, alcohol and substance use rates in older people tend to be underestimated and there is a scarcity of age-specific treatment options to address the complex physical, mental, cognitive and social problems that result.

Treatment Options

Treatment options currently available for alcohol and substance use disorders (for all age groups) include:
- supportive counselling for those wishing to change substance-taking or -seeking behaviour
- brief interventions that use motivational strategies to reduce use, misuse and dependency
- pharmacotherapy treatment and withdrawal management
- support groups, such as Alcoholics Anonymous
- residential programs for long-term rehabilitation and cessation.

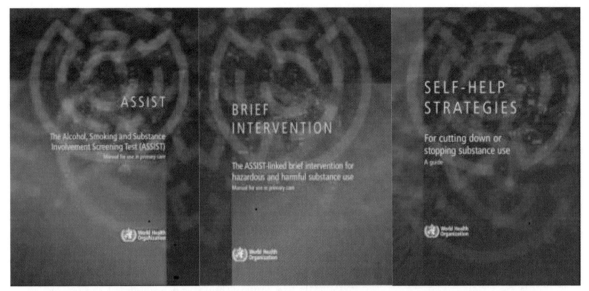

FIG. 25.1 **The WHO ASSIST package comprises three manuals:** (1) The Alcohol, Smoking and Substance involvement Screening Test (ASSIST) (2) The ASSIST-linked brief intervention for hazardous and harmful substance use (3) Self-help strategies for cutting down or stopping substance use: a guide. The WHO ASSIST project facilitates the prevention, early recognition and management of substance use in primary and general medical care settings by promoting screening and brief intervention for alcohol and other substances (e.g. cannabis, amphetamines, cocaine and opiate) use/misuse. (WHO 2010.)

However, older people require a wider range of substance use programs and alternative treatment options. For example, older people who misuse prescription medications have different behaviours and clinical manifestations to those who misuse illicit substances, and people with later-onset misuse tend to have fewer or different dependence characteristics. As the rate of alcohol and substance use among older people is expected to grow substantially in the next few decades, so too is the need for age-specific treatment options (Kuerbis et al 2014).

SUICIDE IN OLDER PEOPLE

Around one-quarter of deaths from self-harm or suicide worldwide are among people aged 60 or older (WHO 2017). In Australia, older males are more likely to die by suicide than older females, and the rates of suicide increase with age, with the highest incidence of suicide in older adults aged 85 years and over (32.8 deaths per 100,000 persons) (ABS 2018) (see Fig. 25.2). Similarly, New Zealand research indicates that older people who died by suicide tended to be male, widowed, living alone or in residential aged care and no longer working

(Cheung et al 2018). Depression and physical illness can both be factors in suicide for older adults.

An older person's vulnerability to suicidal behaviour is due to individual, relationship and community societal factors. Often these factors are cumulative, making suicide in older people hard to predict. International research highlights that society's attitudes towards older people (particularly negative perceptions or effects of ageism) impacts on suicide mortality (AIHW 2015).

Assessment of Suicide Risk

It is important for health professionals to assess the risk of suicide and self-harm in older people. While suicide may be difficult to predict, there are some general warning signs. These include:

- social withdrawal, being isolated or alone
- low mood (dramatic changes in mood)
- feeling trapped
- feeling alone or that they don't belong
- feeling like a burden to other people
- expressing feelings of worthlessness, hopelessness
- expressing no hope for the future
- misuse of alcohol and other drugs (including prescribed medications)

Research Highlight
Alcohol Consumption Patterns of Older People

A study of community dwelling older people in the southwest region of Western Australia was conducted between 2011 and 2014. This study aimed to demonstrate that opportunistic health screening at health promotion events can provide an overall impression of alcohol consumption patterns. A repeated cross-sectional survey design, completed over a four-year period, was used to assess the risk of harmful alcohol consumption. An alcohol screening survey (AUDIT) was used to collect data on alcohol consumption patterns of those aged 65 years and over. A total of 411 surveys were completed. Results found a statistically significant difference in mean risk scores across the four years ($p < 0.001$). Between 6.3% and 22.2% of survey completers presented as 'risky', and a further 3.8% to 12.3% were 'high risk' in terms of alcohol consumption. These findings confirmed that health promotion events designed for the general public present a useful avenue to screen older people's alcohol consumption to aid the identification of at-risk individuals who may require further education or treatment.

REFERENCE
Vafeas C, Graham R, DeJong G et al (2018). Alcohol consumption patterns of older adults: A study in a regional town in Western Australia. Contemporary Nurse 5(6):1–11.

- dramatic changes in behaviour or risky behaviours
- frequently talking about death
- thoughts of suicide
- giving belongings away
- acquiring lethal means (hoarding medications, poisons, guns) (Beyond Blue 2020a).

Preventing suicide in older people involves an ongoing assessment of mental state and risk, and the development of strategies to reduce the risk of self-harm or suicidal behaviour. Developing a safety plan is an evidence-based strategy to reduce the risk of self-harm for people of all ages, including older people. *Tips for best practice* lists strategies to promote the safety of an older person at risk of suicide.

Treatment
Pharmacological
- Antidepressants if low or depressed mood or anxiety
- Short-term sedation for sleep disturbance, if required
- Antipsychotics can be useful if the person is very distressed or has psychotic symptoms.

Non-pharmacological
- Reducing social isolation
- Distraction and activity
- Supportive counselling.

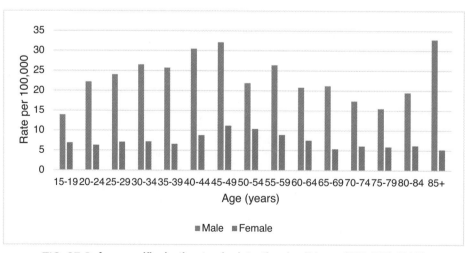

FIG. 25.2 **Age-specific death rates for intentional self-harm 2017** (ABS 2018.)

Tips for Best Practice
Developing a Safety Plan for an Older Person at Risk of Suicide

- Identify the older person's individual warning signs, e.g. feeling low in mood, poor sleep, negative thinking.
- List things important in the older person's life (protective factors) – family, hobbies, roles.
- Ensure a safe environment – remove any means of committing suicide (e.g. medications, poisons, weapons, reduce isolation), keep other people around to observe for risky behaviour.
- Identify ways for the older person to distract themselves from suicidal thoughts – being with friends and relatives, participating in community activities, playing music, watching TV.
- List people who the older person trusts and can talk to when feeling suicidal – friends, family, health professional, GP – and make sure they are able to contact them (provide telephone numbers, online FaceTime accounts).
- Provide emergency contacts – Lifeline, Beyond Blue (Beyond Blue 2020a).

Safety Alert

It is important for health professionals to identify and provide care for an older person who has witnessed or been affected by another person's suicide or suicide attempt.

People who know someone who died by suicide in the past year are:

- 10 times more likely to experience suicidal ideation
- 2.9 times likely to have a plan for suicide
- 3.7 times more likely to attempt suicide within one year
- more likely to develop depression and PTSD after 6 months
- more likely to experience complicated grief (Tal Young et al 2012).

Many people grieving the loss of someone to suicide also experience the effects of trauma that may be immediate, or last for days, weeks, months or even years.

Practice Scenario

Marta is a 72-year-old woman who migrated from Croatia in 1999. Marta's husband died three years ago and she lives alone. Marta is generally in good physical health, but has arthritis, which limits her physical activity, and mild hypertension, which is well controlled with medication. Marta normally enjoys an active social life, is a member of the local Croatian Club and looks forward to attending fortnightly dances with her friends. Over the past 2 months Marta's daughter has noticed that Marta does not seem her usual self. She seems to have withdrawn from her family and friends and no longer attends Croatian Club activities. She is reluctant to venture outside her house and has become very worried about her health. Marta reports that she is not eating or sleeping well and that she has not felt like herself since she had a fall while hanging out her washing approximately 6 weeks ago. At the time, she sustained only minor abrasions that have healed well.

MULTIPLE CHOICE QUESTIONS

1. Which of the following issues put Marta at risk of developing a mental disorder? (tick all that apply)
   a. Fragility
   b. Arthritis
   c. Hypertension
   d. Poor sleep
   e. Living alone
   f. Social withdrawal
   g. Health worries
   h. Minor abrasions
   i. Poor appetite
   j. Being Croatian

2. Which mental disorder is Marta most at risk of developing?
   a. Bipolar disorder
   b. Dementia
   c. Late-life depression
   d. Post-traumatic Stress Disorder
   e. Substance misuse disorder

3. Marta is reluctant to mobilise. This may be due to a 'fear of falling', which is common in older people who have sustained a fall. What type of mental disorder is a 'fear of falling'?
   a. Depressive disorder
   b. Psychotic disorder
   c. Anxiety disorder
   d. Personality disorder

Continued

Practice Scenario—cont'd

4. Which of the following non-pharmacological treatments may be helpful for Marta? (tick all that apply)
   a. Electroconvulsive therapy
   b. Supportive counselling
   c. Lifestyle changes
   d. Hospitalisation to a mental health unit
   e. Treating or managing underlying medical conditions
   f. Support groups
   g. Cognitive behavioural therapy

5. What pharmacological treatment may be helpful for Marta?
   a. Benzodiazepines
   b. Antidepressants
   c. Anxiolytics
   d. Antipsychotics
   e. Analgesics

REFERENCES

American Psychiatric Association (2013) Diagnostic and statistical manual of mental disorders: DSM-5. American Psychiatric Association, Arlington, VA.

Australian Bureau of Statistics (ABS) (2018) National health survey: first results, 2017–18. Cat. 4364.0.55.001. Online. Available: www.abs.gov.au/ausstats/abs@.nsf/Lookup/by%20Subject/4364.0.55.001~2017-18~Main%20Features~Key%20Findings~1

Australian Bureau of Statistics (ABS) (2018) Causes of death, Australia, 2017. Cat. 3303.0. Online. Available: www.abs.gov.au/ausstats/abs@.nsf/Lookup/by%20Subject/3303.0~2017~Main%20Features~Intentional%20self-harm,%20key%20characteristics~3

Australian Government Department of Health (2010) Principles of recovery oriented mental health practice. National standards for mental health services 2010. Online. Available: www1.health.gov.au/internet/main/publishing.nsf/Content/CFA833CB8C1AA178CA257BF0001E7520/$File/servpri.pdf

Australian Institute of Health and Welfare (AIHW) (2015) Australia's welfare 2015. Australia's welfare series no. 12. Cat. AUS 189. AIHW, Canberra.

Australian Institute of Health and Welfare (AIHW) (2020) Alcohol, tobacco and other drugs in Australia. Australian Government. Online. Available: www.aihw.gov.au/reports/alcohol/alcohol-tobacco-other-drugs-australia/contents/priority-populations/older-people.

Badcock JC, Dehon H, Laroi F (2017) Hallucinations in healthy older adults: an overview of the literature and perspectives for future research. Frontiers in Psychology 8:1134.

Beyond Blue (2020a) Signs and symptoms of anxiety and depression in older people. Beyond Blue Ltd. Online. Available: www.beyondblue.org.au/who-does-it-affect/older-people/signs-and-symptoms-of-depression-in-older-people.

Beyond Blue (2020b) Who does it affect? Aboriginal and Torres Strait Islander people. Online. Available: www.beyondblue.org.au/who-does-it-affect/aboriginal-and-torres-strait-islander-people

Blackdog Institute (2020) Depression in older people. Blackdog Institute. Online. Available: www.blackdoginstitute.org.au/clinical-resources/depression/what-is-depression.

Böttche M, Kuwert P, Knaevelsrud C (2012) Posttraumatic stress disorder in older adults: an overview of characteristics and treatment approaches. Int J Geriatr Psychiatry 27:230–239.

Cheung G, Merry S, Sundram F (2018) Do suicide characteristics differ by age in older people? International Psychogeriatrics 30:323–330.

Declercq T, Lemey L, Tandt H et al (2018) Late-life depression: issues for the general practitioner. International Journal of General Medicine 11:113–120.

Dong, M, Zhu X-M, Zheng W et al (2018) Electroconvulsive therapy for older adult patients with major depressive disorder: a systematic review of randomized controlled trials. Psychogeriatrics 18(6):468–475.

Federation of Ethnic Communities' Councils of Australia (FECCA) (2015) Ageing and mental health issues for older people from CALD backgrounds. In: Review of Australian research on older people from culturally and linguistically diverse backgrounds. Deakin, ACT.

Karim S, Burns A (2003) The biology of psychosis in older people. J Geriatr Psychiatry Neurol 16:207–212.

Kavanagh A, McLoughlin DM (2009) Electroconvulsive therapy and nursing care. British Journal of Nursing 18:1370.

Kostadinov V, Roche A (2017) Bongs and baby boomers: Trends in cannabis use among older Australians. Australasian Journal of Ageing 36:56–59.

Koychev I, Ebmeier KP (2016) Anxiety in older adults often goes undiagnosed. Practitioner 260:17–20, 2–3.

Kuerbis A, Sacco P, Blazer DG (2014) Substance abuse among older adults. Clinics in Geriatric Medicine 30:629–654.

Lintzeris N, Rivas C, Monds LA et al (2016) Substance use, health status and service utilisation of older clients attending specialist drug and alcohol services. Drug & Alcohol Review 35:223–231.

Loscalzo E, Sterling RC, Weinstein SP (2017) Alcohol and other drug use in older adults: results from a community needs assessment. Aging Clinical and Experimental Research 29:1149–1155.

McKay R, Casey J, Stevenson J et al (2015) Psychiatry services for older people: A report on current issues and evidence to inform the development of services and the revision of RANZCP Position Statement 22. In: Psychiatry services for older people: a report on current issues and evidence, Royal Australian and New Zealand College of Psychiatrists (eds). Melbourne, Victoria.

Muir-Cochrane E, Barkway P, Nizette E (eds) (2014) Mosby's pocketbook of mental health. 2nd edn. Elsevier Australia, Mosby, NSW.

New Zealand Health Navigator (2020) Depression in later life, New Zealand Government. Online. Available: www .healthnavigator.org.nz/health-a-z/d/depression-later-life/.

Office of the United Nations High Commissioner for Human Rights (1991) Principles for the treatment of persons with mental illness and the improvement of mental health care https:// www.who.int/mental_health/policy/en/UN_Resolution _on_protection_of_persons_with_mental_illness.pdf

Perth Co-occurring Disorders Capacity Building Project (2011) Understanding the mental state examination (MSE): a basic training guide. PCDCBP, Subiaco, WA.

Peters R (2006) Ageing and the brain. Postgraduate Medical Journal 82:84–88.

Reinhardt MM, Cohen CI (2015) Late-life psychosis: diagnosis and treatment. Current Psychiatry Rep 17:1.

Royal Australian and New Zealand College of Psychiatrists (RANZCP) (2017) Mental health legislation – Australia and New Zealand, RANZCP. Online. Available: www.ranzcp.org/ practice-education/guidelines-and-resources-for-practice/ mental-health-legislation-australia-and-new-zealand.

SANE Australia (2020) Psychosis, SANE Australia. Online. Available: www.sane.org/information-stories/facts-and-guides/ psychosis.

Searby A, Maude P, McGrath I (2016) Prevalence of co-occurring alcohol and other drug use in an Australian older adult mental health service. International Journal of Mental Health Nursing 25:151–158.

Skoog I (2011) Psychiatric disorders in the elderly. The Canadian Journal of Psychiatry 56:387–397.

Subramanyam AA, Kedare J, Singh OP et al (2018) Clinical practice guidelines for geriatric anxiety disorders. Indian Journal of Psychiatry 60:S371–S382.

Tal Young I, Iglewicz A, Glorioso D et al (2012) Suicide bereavement and complicated grief. Dialogues in Clinical Neuroscience 14:177–186.

Vafeas C, Graham R, DeJong G et al (2018). Alcohol consumption patterns of older adults: A study in a regional town in Western Australia. Contemporary Nurse 5(6):1–11.

Van Damme A, Declercq T, Lemey L et al (2018) Late-life depression: issues for the general practitioner. International Journal of General Medicine 11:113–120.

Wells Y, Bhar S, Kinsella G et al (2014) What works to promote emotional wellbeing in older people: A guide for aged care staff working in community or residential care settings. Beyond Blue, Melbourne.

Wiese B (2011) Geriatric depression: The use of antidepressants in the elderly. British Columbia Medical Journal 53:341–347.

World Health Organization (WHO) (2017) Mental health of older adults. Online. Available: www.who.int/news-room/ fact-sheets/detail/mental-health-of-older-adults.

World Health Organization (WHO) 2010 The ASSIST project – Alcohol, Smoking and Substance Involvement Screening Test. Online. Available: www.who.int/management -of-substance-use/assist

Wuthrich VM, Johnco CJ, Wetherell JL (2015) Differences in anxiety and depression symptoms: comparison between older and younger clinical samples. International Psychogeriatrics 27:1523–1532.

CHAPTER 26

Neurocognitive Disorders

SHERIDAN READ • SUSAN SLATYER

LEARNING OBJECTIVES

After reading this chapter, you will be able to:

- describe and differentiate delirium and major and minor neurocognitive disorders
- identify tools used to detect dementia and delirium
- discuss the importance of use of language within the context of caring for people living with dementia
- define responsive behaviours and discuss in the context of behaviours and psychological symptoms of dementia
- describe a dementia-friendly environment and identify strategies for a person with dementia to live well.

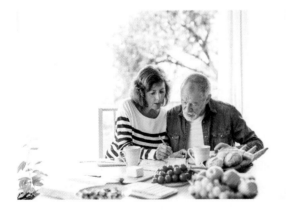

INTRODUCTION

The term neurocognitive disorders (NCDs) describes a group of acquired conditions that result in cognitive impairment. These conditions include delirium and a range of syndromes that are classified as either major or mild in nature. Delirium is an acute change in cognitive function that is usually reversible and occurs in response to one or more contributing factors, such as infection, pain, surgery or metabolic imbalance (Australian Government Department of Health and Ageing 2011; Inouye et al 2014). Conditions classified as major NCDs are compatible with dementia, indicating a significant decline in cognitive function. Mild NCDs have similar symptoms to major NCDs, but the cognitive decline is less severe, meaning that the older person is likely to retain sustained capacity for independence. Some older people with Parkinson's disease develop a mild or major NCD as the disease progresses. While Parkinson's disease primarily causes physical symptoms, older age and increased time since diagnosis are associated with development of cognitive problems termed Parkinson's disease dementia (Jellinger & Korczyn 2018).

Older people diagnosed with a NCD show declining cognitive function in any of the following domains:

- complex attention, including sustained or divided attention
- executive functioning including planning and decision making
- learning and memory
- receptive and expressive language skills

- perceptual motor skills
- social cognition (American Psychiatric Association 2013).

This chapter will focus on the care of older people with delirium and mild and major neurocognitive disorders (including dementia and Parkinson's disease) with a focus on nursing interventions. Within the *Diagnostic and Statistical Manual of Mental Disorders 5th edition* (DSM-5) the term 'dementia' has been replaced with 'major and mild neurocognitive disorders' in an effort to reduce dementia-related stigma, to recognise the continuum of cognitive decline and to facilitate early diagnosis. While recognising this important change, the terms *dementia* and *cognitive impairment* will be used in this chapter.

DELIRIUM

Delirium is a potentially reversible clinical condition that results in acute decline in cognitive function. Delirium is a serious disorder, which, while usually short term, can be fatal for some older people. It is thought to result from the interplay between biological factors that disrupt neuronal networks (Inouye et al 2014). There is not usually a single cause but rather an interaction of predisposing factors that make an older person more vulnerable (e.g. existing cognitive impairment, depression, sensory impairment) and precipitating factors (e.g. infection, surgery, medication, a fall) leading to the development of delirium which represents brain failure. The causes of delirium are potentially reversible, therefore accurate assessment and early identification and intervention are crucial.

Delirium most commonly occurs in older people aged 65 years or over (Australian Commission on Safety and Quality in Health Care [ACSQHC] 2016; Clinical Epidemiology and Health Services Evaluation Unit 2006). Estimates suggest that 10–18% of Australians in this older cohort have delirium on admission to hospital, with another 2–8% developing delirium while an inpatient (ACSQHC 2016). In New Zealand, a study of patients aged 70 years or older admitted to general medical wards reported the prevalence of delirium at 23% and incidence during the hospital stay of 5.7% (Holden et al 2008). While there is little recent evidence from New Zealand, a robust systematic review and meta-analysis of 33 international studies conducted from 1982 to 2018 found that published rates of delirium remained stable at one in four older medical in-patients (Gibb et al 2020). Delirium is also the most common postoperative complication in older people who undergo surgery, with an incidence of 50% after high-risk procedures, such as

hip fracture repair and cardiac surgery (Marcantonio 2017).

An episode of delirium is frequently characterised by the rapid onset of confusion and inattention, which can fluctuate over days or even hours. Symptoms include:
- confusion
- agitation
- restlessness
- anxiety
- hallucinations.

Four sub-types of delirium, differentiated by the level of psychomotor activity, have been identified: hypoactive, hyperactive, mixed and normal psychomotor activity (Albrecht et al 2015). These sub-types can fluctuate from assessment to assessment. An older person presenting with a hypoactive delirium is often passive, inactive, lethargic, drowsy, withdrawn and lacking facial expression (Albrecht et al 2015). In contrast, older people who present with hyperactive delirium have fast or loud speech, aggressive behaviours and perceptual disorders such as hallucinations or delusions.

An older person with the mixed sub-type will present with elements of both hypoactive and hyperactive features, often fluctuating between the two. Older people who have the normal psychomotor sub-type can present with altered cognition (e.g. memory deficit, disorientation, language disturbance) while exhibiting normal levels of activity (Albrecht et al 2015).

The *hypoactive* sub-type of delirium is more common, but often goes undiagnosed and, therefore, undermanaged (Albrecht et al 2015). Indeed, delirium in general is often under-recognised and under-documented in routine clinical care (Rieck et al 2020). This is despite well-established evidence that delirium is strongly associated with poor short-term and long-term health outcomes. Potential consequences of an episode of delirium are serious and include:
- higher risk of mortality (Hapca et al 2018)
- long term cognitive impairment
- longer hospital stay
- admission to residential aged care.

Factors that put an older person at higher risk of developing delirium include:
- increasing age
- a previous history of delirium
- pre-existing cognitive impairment, particularly dementia and depression
- an underlying medical condition
- infection
- sensory impairments, including reduced vision or hearing
- polypharmacy (see Chapter 11)

- certain medications (narcotic pain medication, benzodiazepines, NSAIDs and anticholinergic medications) (Rosen et al 2015)
- the presence of an indwelling urinary catheter
- the use of physical restraint
- health problems related to alcohol consumption.

Assessment

The nurse has an integral role in identifying and addressing the presence of a delirium and ascertaining when an older person may be at high risk of developing delirium. Timely identification of delirium can facilitate early implementation of non-pharmacological strategies for prevention and management, which may improve outcomes for the older person. Nurses can contribute to the early detection of delirium by understanding the risk factors and remaining vigilant for changes in the older person's clinical presentation (Rieck et al 2020). Assessment involves a baseline cognitive screen and the use of a validated delirium screening tool. Furthermore, routine reassessment throughout the delirium episode is required to detect changes in the older person's condition, which may fluctuate rapidly. Validated assessment tools improve the recognition of delirium. The most commonly used tools are:

- The **Confusion Assessment Method (CAM)** (Inouye et al 1990) is the most widely used validated tool to detect delirium. The tool is designed to capture four defining features, including: (1) acute onset and fluctuating course of symptoms, (2) inattention, (3) disorganised thinking, and (4) altered level of consciousness (Wei et al 2008). A positive diagnosis of delirium requires that the older person has both features (1) and (2), with either (3) or (4) present (Inouye et al 1990).
- The **4AT** (Bellelli et al 2014) is a screening instrument designed for rapid initial assessment of delirium and cognitive impairment through assessment of four domains:
  1. level of alertness (score 0–4)
  2. orientation (score 0–2)
  3. inattention (score 0–2)
  4. acute changes or fluctuations in alertness, cognition or other mental functions (score 0–4).

  A score of 4 or more *suggests* delirium (with or without cognitive impairment), while a score of 1–3 *suggests* cognitive impairment. A score of 0 does not exclude delirium or cognitive impairment, as more detailed testing may be required depending on the clinical context.
- **Delirium Rating Scale (DRS)** (Trzepacz et al 2001) is a widely used instrument which reliably measures

delirium symptoms in people with or without dementia. The tool integrates information gathered by the clinician from the older person (interview and mental status examination), medical history, nursing observations and family reports. The revised Delirium Rating Scale (DRS-R-98) has 16 items with a maximum total score of 46 points (Trzepacz et al 2001).

> **Tips for Best Practice**
> *Recommended Resources – Delirium*
>
> Dementia Support Australia, Delirium Screen, available at: https://dementia.com.au/downloads/dementia/Resources-Library/Care-Support-Guides/J0001025RB-Delirium-ScreenFlyer.pdf
>
> Australian Commission on Safety and Quality in Health Care (ACSQHC) (2018) Hospital Acquired Complication 11 – Delirium, available at: www.safetyandquality.gov.au/sites/default/files/migrated/Delirium-detailed-fact-sheet.pdf

Delirium is considered a medical emergency. Treatment aims to correct factors contributing to the onset of the delirium, if known. A thorough assessment comprising a medical history and physical examination is required to identify the underlying cause/s. Table 26.1 details components of the medical history and physical examination. The goal of treatment is to alleviate symptoms and reduce risk of complications. Delirium usually lasts for only a few days but may continue for weeks or months.

Preventing and Treating Symptoms of Delirium

The nurse has a role in implementing environmental and clinical strategies which not only help prevent the onset of delirium, but also alleviate symptoms once a diagnosis has been made.

Environmental strategies

- Reduce noise and promote a quiet, calming environment by avoiding intercom communication systems, ringing telephones and loud voices.
- Accommodate the older person in a single room to reduce risk of disturbance and promote rest and sleep.
- Provide visual prompts and displays to orientate the older person to the surroundings, and reduce confusion with signs, clocks, calendars and appropriate lighting.

TABLE 26.1
Components of Assessment to Identify the Underlying Cause/s of Delirium

Obtain history	Medications – prescribed, over-the-counter, past and present
	Dehydration
	Falls (see Chapter 16)
	Infection
	Bladder and bowel function
	History of diet and fluid intake (include alcohol consumption)
	Past medical and social history
	Sensory impairments
Examination	Vital signs include oxygen saturation
	Mental state examination (see Chapter 25) – decreased arousal/attention – disorientation
	Neurological examination
	Chest auscultation
	Abdomen/bowel/bladder
	Skin – lesions, signs of dehydration

Note: Investigations are dependent upon clinical features and expert consultant advice
Adapted from Australian Government Department of Health (2011).

- Promote a familiar, homelike environment with personal photos and objects.
- Encourage family to visit and assist with care and support as appropriate.

Clinical strategies
- Arrange a medication review.
- Ensure adequate sleep.
- Ensure sufficient food and fluid intake.
- Ensure use of sensory aids (glasses and hearing aids).
- Avoid the use of indwelling urinary catheters where possible.
- Encourage mobility and independence with activities of daily living (ADLs).
- Monitor bowel function.
- Treat pain.

All nurses, healthcare team members and other visitors should introduce themselves (stating their name and role) each time they interact with the older person to help them stay orientated. Additionally, the nurse has a role to access interpreters and other communication aids as required (Clinical Epidemiology and Health Service Evaluation Unit 2006; National Institute for Health and Clinical Excellence 2010).

MILD COGNITIVE IMPAIRMENT (MILD NCD)
Mild cognitive impairment describes a level of cognitive decline that is beyond what might be considered normal ageing, but not so severe that the older person requires assistance with daily living or meets the diagnostic criteria for dementia. Signs of mild cognitive impairment may include:
- forgetting to go to events or appointments
- losing things often
- having more trouble finding words than other people the same age.

Importantly, not all people who receive a diagnosis of mild cognitive impairment go on to develop dementia.

A diagnosis of mild cognitive impairment first requires a medical and social history to be taken to identify the onset of symptoms. This history is taken from the older person and, if required, from a family member. A complete neurological and psychiatric examination is required to identify any causal factors, including, but not limited to:
- vision or hearing impairment
- behavioural or personality changes which may indicate depression (see Chapter 25)
- thyroid disease (Langa & Levine 2014).

A medication review will identify whether the older person has been taking any medications or a combination of medications known to cause cognitive impairment.

While no pharmacological treatment has proven beneficial in reducing mild cognitive impairment, the nurse can encourage older people to maintain good health and implement strategies to improve or maintain cognitive functioning.

Promoting Wellness
Strategies to Promote and Maintain Cognitive Function

- Manage vascular risk factors such as blood pressure, cholesterol and blood glucose levels
- Limit alcohol consumption
- Engage in social interactions (see Chapters 25 and 29)
- Undertake mentally stimulating activity
- Maintain physical exercise (Barnes 2010; Cheng et al 2014; Nagamatsu et al 2013)
- Eat a diet rich in fruits, vegetables and omega-3-rich oils (Barberger-Gateau et al 2007)

DEMENTIA (MAJOR NCD)

Dementia is a collection of symptoms caused by a range of conditions that impact on brain function. A person diagnosed with dementia may experience memory impairment and a limited ability to reason and perform everyday activities (Banerjee et al 2007; World Health Organisation [WHO] 2017). In Australia in 2015, an estimated 316,000 people were living with the condition. By the year 2050, depending upon whether a cure is found, that number is expected to rise to over 942,000 (WHO 2017). In 2016, over 62,000 New Zealanders were living with dementia, representing an increase of 29% over the previous five years (Alzheimer's New Zealand 2017). More than 170,000 people in New Zealand are forecast to have dementia by 2050 (Alzheimer's New Zealand 2017).

Dementia changes the way a person perceives and experiences the world around them. While changes in the brain result in functional decline, older people with dementia are able to experience wellbeing and may retain complex abilities long after first receiving a diagnosis (Power 2017). However, many people living with dementia experience stigma due to others' misunderstanding and misconceptions (Edvardsson et al 2008). The belief that dementia is a disease of the brain and that people with dementia are of little value may cause family and friends to distance themselves from the person and speak over rather than directly to them in conversation.

These attitudes stem from the predominance of the biomedical model that conceptualises dementia as a disease and calls for active, primarily pharmacological, treatment (Vernooij-Dassen et al 2020). While this understanding has driven scientific research progress, it focuses on pathology and deficits rather than capabilities, and overlooks concepts of brain resilience and social health. Social health refers to the person being able to fulfil obligations, manage life with some independence and continue social activities (Vernooij-Dassen et al 2020). Currently, there is no cure on the horizon for dementia. However, there are emerging indications that lifestyle factors contribute to prevention (Salinas & Schwamm 2017), and that higher levels of social participation can reduce progression of cognitive impairment (Vernooij-Dassen et al 2020).

An alternative to the biomedical model is the experiential model (Power 2017). In this model, the experience of the person with dementia is central and helps to determine the person's needs. While the biomedical model conceptualises dementia as a progressive, irreversible disease process, the experiential model defines dementia as a shift in the way a person perceives the world and recognises that neuroplasiticity can enable learning to occur. It assumes the person's potential for growth, autonomy and satisfaction, which shape the goals and focus of care.

PARKINSON'S DISEASE (MILD OR MAJOR NCD)

Parkinson's disease (PD) is defined as 'a progressive multi-system neurodegenerative disease affecting people mainly in later years of life' (Sveinbjornsdottir 2016: 318). Globally, it is the second most common neuro-degenerative disease after Alzheimer's disease. In Australia, approximately 1 in every 308 people is living with a diagnosis of PD, with these people five times more likely to live in residential aged care facilities than people without PD (Parkinson's Australia 2020). In New Zealand, the number of people with PD has increased from approximately 7000 in 2006 to nearly 11,000 in 2017, with that number expected to double over the next 25 years as more people move into the higher risk age group (above 60 years) (Myall et al 2017). While the cause is unknown, several genetic risk factors have been identified, which may be influenced by environmental factors, including smoking, exposure to pesticides and consumption of caffeine (Kouli et al 2018). The strongest risk factor for development of PD is age, with the median age of onset being 60 years, and incidence rising to 93.1 people per 100,000 between 70 and 79 years (Kouli et al 2018).

Typically, PD progresses slowly as cells in the brain are destroyed by toxic clumps of alpha-synuclein, a protein normally found in the brain that malfunctions. Large accumulations of alpha-synuclein are known as Lewy bodies. Lesions initially occur in the medulla oblongata in the brainstem and progress to the midbrain, in particular the substantia nigra, which produces the neurotransmitter dopamine, and then to the higher order neocortex (Braak et al 2003).

Dopamine has a number of important roles in the body, including control of movement, moderating the release of various hormones, influencing kidney and gastrointestinal function and playing a central role in motivation and reward behaviours (Sveinbjornsdottir 2016). While most of the symptoms seen in PD relate to impaired motor function, there are also a number of common non-motor symptoms, which include:

- orthostatic hypertension (fall in blood pressure upon standing)
- constipation
- urinary frequency, urgency and incontinence

- nocturia (waking at night to urinate)
- erectile dysfunction in males
- excessive sweating
- sleep disturbances (frequent waking at night, daytime sleepiness)
- rapid eye movement (REM) sleep behaviour disorder (acting out dreams, thrashing and kicking during sleep)
- visual hallucinations and illusions
- cognitive deterioration (mild cognitive impairment progressing to dementia)
- depression and anxiety
- loss of sense of smell
- pain (Sveinbjornsdottir 2016).

Motor Symptoms of PD

Evidence suggests that up to 80% of dopamine-producing cells are lost before the typical motor symptoms of PD appear (Sveinbjornsdottir 2016). The four major signs are:

- bradykinesia (slow to start voluntary movements)
- resting tremor ('pill rolling' tremor where thumb and finger contact make circular motions; arm, leg and head less affected; may worsen with anxiety)
- muscular rigidity
- postural instability.

A prerequisite for a diagnosis of PD is bradykinesia and at least one of the other three signs. Symptoms usually start on one side of the body with the other side becoming involved several years later. Before making the diagnosis, other potential causes must be excluded. Then the diagnosis is confirmed with a 'challenge', which involves giving the older person a dose of the medication 'levodopa', a precursor to dopamine which crosses the blood–brain barrier and is converted to dopamine. If the symptoms rapidly improve, PD is thought to be confirmed.

The rate at which PD progresses and the intensity of symptoms varies greatly between individuals. Early in the disease course, the older person may experience only mild symptoms occurring on one side of body and have a good response to treatment. However, as the disease progresses, the symptoms spread to both sides of the body and treatment becomes less effective (Sveinbjornsdottir 2016). Muscle movements in the trunk, extremities and face may be affected, leading to lack of facial expression and difficulties chewing, swallowing and speaking. As the bradykinesia and muscle rigidity worsen, the older person may remain still for long periods, increasing the risk of pressure injury. The older person will develop the characteristic gait seen in PD, which includes:

- shuffling steps that become progressively smaller
- no arm movement
- hesitancy starting to walk
- a forward lean
- difficulty turning around, which may require many small steps
- poor balance, and difficulty correcting if the person loses balance.

There is no cure for PD, and pharmacological treatment aims to rebalance dopamine levels. Treatment options include:

- dopamine replacement therapy: levodopa (as above) addresses muscle rigidity and bradykinesia and is considered gold standard to treat PD; it may be combined with carbidopa to promote transmission across the blood–brain barrier
- dopamine agonists: medications that mimic dopamine; may be used alone or together with levodopa (Rodriques 2017).

Medications are usually given on a set schedule to prevent fluctuations in symptoms. The nurse has a role to closely monitor the older person for side effects of medications and/or the PD itself, which include:

- hypotension
- dyskinesia (involuntary movements)
- dystonia (lack of control of movements)
- hallucinations
- sleep disorders
- depression (Jett 2018).

The symptoms of PD will always increase over time. As they increase, the older person will require more assistance with ADLs and positioning. Nursing interventions are directed to promoting the older person's safety as he or she becomes increasingly at risk of:

- falls from disturbances in gait and balance (see Chapter 16)
- pressure injury from lack of movement (see Chapter 15)
- poor dietary intake from difficulty chewing and swallowing (see Chapter 12).

PD is commonly thought of as a movement disorder; however, as shown here, its effects on the person and impacts on quality of life are far more wide-ranging (Sveinbjornsdottir 2016), including the development of Parkinson's Disease Dementia which is so common in the later stages.

Types of Dementia

Commonly occurring types of dementia include Alzheimer's disease, vascular dementia, dementia with Lewy bodies and several diseases that encompass frontotemporal dementia. Table 26.3 summarises the four main types

TABLE 26.2
Types of Dementia and Defining Characteristics

Type of Dementia	Detail
Alzheimer's disease	Most common type of dementia Accounts for up to 80% of all dementia diagnoses Pathological changes within the brain include accumulation of amyloid plaques and neurofibrillary tangles (Weller & Budson 2018) Short-term memory loss is usually the first indication (Bondi et al 2017)
Vascular dementia	Cognitive impairment results from cerebrovascular disease or reduced blood-flow to the brain Symptoms are progressive, and depend upon the affected region of the brain May have stroke-related/stroke-like deficits Affects cognitive abilities, especially executive functioning (Venkat et al 2015)
Lewy body disease Similar features to Parkinson's disease (see below)	Occurs most commonly in people aged between 60 and 90 years Caused by an accumulation of alpha-synuclein protein within neurons within the brain Core symptoms include fluctuations in cognition, recurrent visual hallucinations and sleep behaviour disorder Extrapyramidal motor features are common, but not essential for the clinical diagnosis (Grand et al 2011; Outeiro et al 2019)
Frontotemporal dementia	A group of neurodegenerative diseases which is divided into behavioural and language sub-types Occurs most commonly in people aged between 45 and 65 years Most commonly reported symptoms include executive functioning behavioural disinhibition and language impairment (Bang et al 2015; Young et al 2018)

of dementia and their defining characteristics. People can be diagnosed with dementia at any age, although it is more common in those aged 65 years or older. People who develop dementia before the age of 65 years are said to have 'younger onset dementia' (Dementia Australia 2020).

While there is currently no cure for dementia, several other treatable conditions have very similar symptoms, including, but not limited to:

- depression
- delirium
- sleep apnoea
- thyroid conditions
- medication side effects
- vitamin B deficiency (Tripathi & Vibha 2009).

Before confirming a diagnosis of dementia, it is important to rule out underlying conditions that may present with dementia-like symptoms. Box 26.1 summarises the cognitive function tests used by medical physicians to differentiate between dementia and other potentially correctable conditions (Tripathi & Vibha 2009). In summary, a diagnosis of dementia should only be made following a comprehensive assessment by a medical practitioner, including:

- history from the person
- history from someone who knows the person well (if possible)
- cognitive assessment (see Box 26.1) and mental state examination (see Chapter 25)
- physical examination
- review of medications (including over the counter products) to identify and minimise medications that might affect cognitive functioning
- consideration of other causes, e.g. depression, delirium (NHMRC Guideline Adaptation Committee 2016).

Only a medical practitioner should communicate a diagnosis of dementia to the person with dementia. The nurse has a role to provide the person who has dementia and their family with written and verbal information in an accessible format about:

- signs and symptoms of dementia
- the course of the condition and how it may progress
- treatments
- where to obtain financial and legal advice and advocacy
- medico-legal issues, such as about driving
- sources of community support (NHMRC Guideline Adaptation Committee 2016).

BOX 26.1
Cognitive Function Assessment Instruments

- Montreal Cognitive Assessment (MoCA)

  A tool developed to screen people who present with mild cognitive impairment (Nasreddine et al 2005)

  www.mocatest.org/pdf_files/test/MoCA-Test-English_7_1.pdf

- Mini-Cog Test

  A brief three-minute, easy-to-use assessment tool designed to detect cognitive impairment (Borson et al 2003)

  https://mini-cog.com/

- Mini-Mental State Examination

  A commonly used screening test for cognitive impairment in older people (Folstein et al 1975; Molloy & Standish 1997)

  www.onlinejacc.org/content/accj/69/12/1609/DC1/embed/media-1.pdf?download=true

- Dementia Severity Rating Scale (DSRS)

  An informant-based, multiple-choice questionnaire designed to assess dementia severity in the functional and cognitive domains affected in Alzheimer disease (Clark & Ewbank 1996)

  www.alz.org/media/documents/dementia-severity-rating-scale.pdf

- Clock drawing test

  Used for screening for cognitive impairment and dementia and as a measure of spatial dysfunction (Rouleau et al 1992)

  www.sralab.org/sites/default/files/2017-07/Clock%20Drawing%20Test%20Instructions.pdf

---

SYMPTOMS OF DEMENTIA

Dementia is a syndrome that commonly presents with symptoms that are classified as either cognitive symptoms or neuropsychiatric symptoms.

Cognitive Symptoms
Memory impairment

Memory impairment is a common symptom of dementia and often the primary presenting symptom of Alzheimer's disease. People experiencing memory impairment are unable to store new information, orientate to time and place or recall recent events (Sandilyan & Dening 2015). People with dementia may confabulate (fill in a memory gap by inventing something they believe to be true) or unintentionally respond to a question or tell a story inaccurately because they cannot remember the details

of an event (Dalla Barba & La Corte 2015; Grand et al 2011). Over time, as the condition progresses, a person diagnosed with dementia will have difficulty recalling both long- and short-term memories.

Apraxia

Apraxia is the inability to carry out learned patterns of behaviour and occurs when:
- the brain is unable to coordinate required actions to complete the task (e.g. walking)
- the person cannot remember the correct sequence of events (e.g. socks go on before shoes)
- the person forgets the purpose of required objects (e.g. a comb is used to groom the hair).

In some cases, the older person with dementia may know what they have to do to complete a task but are unable to execute the action (Chandra et al 2015; Chen & Bailey 2016; Sandilyan & Dening 2015).

Aphasia

Aphasia, defined as the impaired ability to produce or understand speech, is a common symptom of dementia. When a person has expressive aphasia, he or she has difficulty finding the correct word and difficulty speaking clearly enough to be understood. A person with dementia who has receptive aphasia displays an impaired ability to comprehend information (Grand et al 2011; Sandilyan & Dening 2015).

Agnosia

Agnosia is the inability to recognise familiar stimuli and occurs because the brain is unable to correctly interpret information from within the environment. Visual agnosia is the most common form, although the disorder can occur in any sensory modality. People with agnosia may not be able to recognise familiar household objects or familiar faces (Sandilyan & Dening 2015; Tranel & Damasio 2001).

Executive dysfunction

Executive dysfunction is the disruption of higher-order thinking and processes, such as the ability to plan, problem solve, perform sequential actions and respond appropriately when interacting with others. Executive dysfunction occurs due to damage in the frontal lobes of the brain, which impairs the older person's ability to function effectively on a day-to-day basis.

Attention, concentration, thinking, judgement and mental capacity

People with dementia are often easily distracted, unable to concentrate and become easily confused when completing familiar tasks. An inability to concentrate is a common early presenting symptom of dementia and often means that a person has difficulty completing work roles effectively. Autonomous decision-making may be affected in various ways by dementia, given that decision-making requires a person to understand and retain information, process verbal information and communicate a response.

Neuropsychiatric Symptoms

Neuropsychiatric symptoms are non-cognitive disturbances, also known as behavioural and psychological symptoms of dementia (BPSD) (Mushtaq et al 2016), a term introduced by the International Psychogeriatric Association (IPA) (2012). Such behavioural symptoms may include:

- agitation
- aberrant motor behaviour, such as pacing, wandering, fidgeting
- elation
- irritability
- aggression
- abnormal vocalisations (Cerejeira et al 2012).

Some specialists working in the field have come to understand that a person with dementia may express an unmet need through behaviours in response to something within their environment. Use of the term 'responsive behaviours' is preferred by people living with dementia and is suggested as an alternative to the term BPSD. This is explored later in this chapter (see section on nursing assessment below).

Along with behavioural symptoms, people with dementia can also experience the following psychological symptoms:

- Delusions and hallucinations
  Delusions and hallucinations are common symptoms of dementia. A delusion is a firm, fixed, false belief that presents after the onset of dementia and cannot be explained by medication side effects. A common delusion experienced by people with dementia is the idea of persecution, embodied in a sense that someone will harm them or steal their belongings. Hallucinations are altered sensory perceptions. People living with dementia may often report both visual and auditory hallucinations. Mood disturbances, such as anxiety and depression, are also common in people diagnosed with dementia (Cerejeira et al 2012).
- Apathy
  Apathy, an early indicator of Alzheimer's disease, is characterised by a loss of motivation, reduced goal-directed behaviour, low social engagement and poor insight (Cerejeira et al 2012; Mortby et al 2012). While

an apathetic person may lack motivation to complete a task, this does not mean they lack the capacity to accomplish it.

- Disruption to circadian rhythms or sleep wake cycles
  Sleep disturbance is common in dementia and most commonly manifested as disruption to circadian rhythms or sleep wake cycles. The cause of sleep disturbance in dementia is multifaceted. Possible causes include:
  - neurological changes in the brain
  - breakdown in the neural pathways that initiate and maintain sleep
  - reduced daytime activity (Rose & Lorenz 2010; Sandilyan & Dening 2015).
- Changes to appetite and eating behaviour
  People with dementia often experience reduced appetite, problems with eating and weight loss. Several factors underpin these nutritional changes, including:
  - swallowing difficulties, known as dysphagia, caused by the neurological disease processes
  - diminished oral motor function which reduces chewing ability
  - changed sensory awareness that affects the experience of eating
  - problems in the teeth and gums that cause oral discomfort (Kai et al 2015).

People with dementia can also lose weight due to physiological changes, including hypermetabolism (increased metabolic activity), inflammatory processes and hormonal disturbances (Cerejeira et al 2012). The nurse can promote the maintenance of a healthy weight by ensuring the person with dementia has access to healthy and appetising foods and good oral health that makes eating enjoyable. See *Promoting wellness: Maintaining nutrition and oral health*.

Promoting Wellness
Maintaining Nutrition and Oral Health

- Provide a healthy and balanced diet to ensure adequate nutrition.
- Assess appetite
- Monitor weight
- Consult dietitian or speech therapist if undernutrition identified
- Arrange dental appointment for dental assessment and development of long-term oral healthcare plan.

NHMRC (2016).

Nursing Assessment

Assessment of the person with dementia focuses on understanding behavioural expressions of distress that communicate unmet needs. These may include pain, hunger, lack of privacy, need to use the toilet, lack of meaningful activities and inability to communicate (NHMRC 2016).

Identifying the individual's needs and how to sustain their wellbeing is complex. To determine what the person with dementia is trying to communicate through behaviours requires that the nurse has a relationship with the person, an understanding of who they are, knowledge of their life history and familiarity with how the person relates to their environment.

Nursing assessment focuses on the nurse's ability to gain an understanding of the person, including skilled observation to identify physical, psychosocial and environmental factors that may be causing the person distress. There are several nursing models of care and frameworks that can be used to help the nurse recognise and respond to unmet needs.

Need-driven dementia-compromised behaviour model

The need-driven dementia-compromised behaviour model is a framework for understanding that the way a person behaves has meaning and is a form of communication (Algase et al 1996). Behaviours may result from interaction between pathological changes in the brain and the person's cultural background, level of education, personality factors and response to stress. Stressors can include:

- physiological factors such as hunger or pain
- alterations in mood
- disturbances in the physical environment (e.g. lighting or temperature)
- the social environment, including the nature of interactions with others.

The nurse observes what the person with dementia is doing and interprets the observed behaviour using knowledge of the person to identify, and then address, the source of the person's stress (Algase et al 1996).

Progressively lowered stress threshold model

The progressively lowered stress threshold model (Hall & Buckwalter 1987; Smith et al 2006) evaluates how much support a person with dementia requires as the ability to withstand stress decreases with the progression of the dementia. The model categorises presenting symptoms of dementia into four groups encompassing:

- cognitive impairment

- personality changes
- decreased ability to communicate and plan, which leads to functional decline
- lower stress threshold.

The model suggests that symptoms of dementia result from the person's inability to cope with stress. To counter this experience, the focus is on using the person's remaining skills and structuring care to avoid unnecessary triggers and provide a safe, predictable environment (Smith et al 2006).

Newcastle model

The Newcastle model is a framework based on the premises that:

- knowing the person with dementia helps determine what their beliefs about a particular situation might be
- behaviours are an attempt to communicate an unmet need in that situation (Jackman & Beatty 2015).

For example, a person with dementia may feel threatened when a nurse tries to assist them to shower and dress, particularly if the person had previously experienced sexual abuse. In this situation, the person with dementia may perceive the nurse's actions as invasive, rather than helpful, provoking anxiety and defensive behaviours. Using the Newcastle model, the nurse collects a range of information about the person with dementia and their background, hobbies, health status, prescribed medications and significant relationships. Understanding the context helps the nurse consider how the person with dementia may be feeling and why, and how to identify and address the person's unmet need (Jackman & Beatty 2015).

Nursing Interventions

Nurses provide care for people with dementia across the care continuum, in the community, in hospitals and in residential aged care settings. They work with families and healthcare staff to provide evidence-based approaches to care, while providing education and support. The goals of nursing care for a person with dementia are to maintain function, prevent excess disability and structure the physical and social environment to nurture the personhood of the individual and promote wellbeing. The foundational principle of care for people with dementia and their families is person-centred care. Nursing interventions aim to promote functional and social independence through daily activities that engage the person with dementia and focus on their abilities (NHMRC 2016). Strategies to enhance communication, maintain wellbeing and create enabling environments are detailed below. Support for caregivers of people with

Tips for Best Practice
Use of Mnemonics to Assess Need

A mnemonic (pattern of letters that helps you remember information) is useful to structure an assessment of what a person with dementia may need and potential factors contributing to the person's responsive behaviours. The PIECES acronym is one such tool. Each letter prompts assessment questions in a different domain of experience for the person living with dementia:

P: physical cause – basic physical needs, medications or medical conditions

I: intellectual capacity – memory loss and loss of ability to communicate

E: emotional health – mental health, general mood, recent experience of loss

C: capability

E: environment

S: social self.

The nurse or support person can use the PIECES tool to identify strategies that target the triggers for, and consequences of, the person's responsive behaviour. For further detailed information, refer to *Tips for Best Practice: Resources to support person-centred care.*

dementia is an essential nursing role and is discussed in Chapter 28. Other care concerns, such as continence (Chapter 13), falls (Chapter 16) and nutrition (Chapter 12), are addressed in earlier chapters.

Person-Centred Care

Person-centred care is a philosophy underpinning support provided to people with dementia that challenges the traditional disease-focused medical model while emphasising the uniqueness of the individual (Fazio et al 2018). Person-centred care has an understanding of the person with dementia at its core. Kitwood (1997) postulated that a number of elements influence how the person with dementia experiences the world and his or her wellbeing. These factors are the person's:

- biography (the person's personal history)
- personality
- physical health
- neurological impairment
- social psychology, including the person's interactions with people providing care as part of the wider social environment (Jackman & Beatty 2015).

Person-centred care conceptualises a person's experience of dementia as not only determined by the degree of neurological impairment but by a combination of these factors. Nurses can positively affect the wellbeing of a person with dementia by ensuring that the person is physically well, by understanding his or her personal history and by ensuring a positive social environment.

Person-centred care takes a communication- and relationship-focused approach to care. Nurses provide person-centred care by identifying and responding to the individual needs and preferences of the person with dementia. Allowing people diagnosed with dementia to be as self-directed as possible, and to initiate social contact, help others and show affection can promote wellbeing. Person-centred care highlights the need to provide people with dementia with opportunities for meaningful engagement and a sense of purpose (Kitwood & Bredin 1992).

Tips for Best Practice
Resources to Support Person-Centred Care

CHOPS SUNFLOWER TOOL
The Sunflower tool summarises and displays information about a person's life and preferences in an engaging visual way. Designed for use in acute care, the Sunflower tool helps staff get to know the hospitalised older persons with cognitive impairment or dementia.

www.aci.health.nsw.gov.au/__data/assets/pdf_file/
0017/401930/CHOPS-sunflower.pdf

FOCUS ON THE PERSON FORM
The Focus on the Person form is an evidence-based tool that has been designed to assist families and health professionals to be allies in providing person-centred care. The form is designed to be completed by family members in the community ready to give to staff should the person with dementia become unwell and require hospital care. It contains comprehensive information about the person's routines, needs, preferences, pain and previous experiences of hospitalisation.

www.alzheimerswa.org.au/wp-content/uploads/2019/
02/Focus-on-the-Person-Form.pdf

PIECES-ABC TOOL
Frameworks to systematically assess factors causing the person with dementia to experience stress and exhibit responsive behaviours as an expression of unmet needs, and to establish the timeline of behavioural events

www.interiorhealth.ca/sites/Partners/SeniorsCare/
DementiaPathway/MiddleDementiaPhase/
Documents/PIECES-ABCtool.pdf

Communication

Older people living with dementia may have retained the capacity to provide answers to questions about what they feel they need and what constitutes a good quality of life for them. Each person's perceived needs are unique and likely to change throughout his or her life. For people living with dementia, the ability to communicate needs may be dependent upon the type of dementia they have been diagnosed with. In the early stages of dementia, a person may have trouble finding words and keeping track of conversations. As the person's cognitive function declines, the nurse must consider how to support his or her ability to communicate their needs into the future. The nurse should consider:

- referral to a speech therapist to advise on suitable person-centred communication strategies (see *Tips for best practice: Strategies for communicating* with a person with dementia)
- implementation of an advance care plan (see Chapter 17) stating the person's wishes, which serves to preserve their decision-making autonomy even when their capacity to communicate has diminished.

Older people living with dementia depend on supportive relationships with skilled and caring nurses. Communication becomes problematic when the person with dementia finds it difficult to select the correct word to convey a meaning and remember what has been said or fails to detect nuances and abstract ideas in the conversation. The inability to communicate their needs can be frightening for older people who live with dementia, as well as anxiety-producing for their caregivers, resulting in frustration for both parties.

Nurses can employ a range of verbal and non-verbal strategies to determine what the person with dementia is trying to communicate and respond accordingly. Furthermore, the nurse has a role to educate others (family, health professionals and support workers) in these strategies, so that people with dementia remain included in conversations and decision-making about matters that affect their lives for as long as possible. The *Tips for best practice: Strategies for communicating with a person with dementia* box provides strategies for communicating with people living with dementia.

Use of Language and Stigma

Nurses need to consider the importance of language when talking to an older person with dementia and when providing information to families, carers and other health professionals. The choice of words can impact on how other people perceive and respond to a person with dementia.

> **Tips for Best Practice**
> *Strategies for Communicating With a Person With Dementia*
>
> - Talk directly to the person with dementia, not their family member, care partner or friend
> - Smile and use positive body language
> - Make eye contact and speak clearly
> - Position yourself at the person's eye level
> - Call the person by their name to engage their attention
> - Use short, simple questions and sentences. Use sensitivity and repeat if necessary.
> - Provide information in smaller chunks
> - Talk about one topic at a time
> - Allow time for the person to answer a question
> - Eliminate background noise and other distractions
> - Use verbal and or visual prompts to help the person remember a time, place or person (e.g. 'I really enjoyed our picnic at the park yesterday. Here are the photos I took')
> - Use clear simple signage
> - Provide people with dementia from culturally and linguistically diverse backgrounds, and their family, with information in their preferred language and use professional interpreters if required.

Dementia Australia (2018).

> **Tip for Best Practice**
>
> For more comprehensive information regarding communication, use of language and considering dementia-related stigma, access Alzheimer's WA resource, Communication and Engagement. Available at: www.alzheimerswa.org.au/wp-content/uploads/2019/04/Alzheimers-WA-Communicating-and-Engaging.pdf

---

Language with negative connotations is often stigmatising, causing a person with dementia to lose self-esteem and potentially withdraw from interactions with others. Instead, it is important to use language to empower and enable. An example is to support and encourage the older person's independence by talking about what a person with dementia can do, rather than the capacity they have lost.

EVIDENCE-BASED COMMUNICATION THERAPIES

Reminiscence Therapy

As people with dementia experience increasing short-term memory impairment, they tend to speak more frequently of past events, particularly as the ability to interpret their surroundings diminishes. Reminiscence therapy involves the discussion of previous experiences using memory aids such as photographs, cards, music or other recordings (Woods et al 2018). The person with dementia benefits through the experience of engaging with another person and the emotions that are raised. It is not important that the person with dementia remembers accurate detail. Additionally, the aim is to create positive engagement and wellbeing for the person with dementia, so memories of negative experiences should be avoided. Reminiscence therapy can be helpful when the person with dementia is experiencing anxiety or agitation or has a diagnosis of depression (Woods et al 2018).

Validation Therapy

Validation is a form of communication therapy that affirms the reality of the person with dementia and in doing so strengthens relationships with the person, builds trust and ameliorates any distress he or she may experience (Feil 1993). For example, validation therapy may be useful when an older person with dementia has the altered perception that he or she is a young parent, expressing concern for their children and is extremely anxious. It is important to respond by acknowledging how the person feels and then explore their fond memories of their children while providing reassurance that their children are safe. Validation therapy is about responding to the emotions expressed by the person with dementia rather than trying to correct the facts. It provides an opportunity to shift negative emotions that a person with dementia may be experiencing to a more positive outlook and enhance quality time together (Feil 1993).

MAINTAINING WELLBEING

Domains of Wellbeing

A model of seven domains of wellbeing, termed the 'Eden Alternative Domains', provides a proactive, strengths-based approach to the care of people with dementia (Power 2014). Based on the experiential model of dementia, the domains of wellbeing encompass seven factors that are essential to maintaining the identity of the person with dementia and his or her relationships with others. With these in place, the

person is more likely to sustain a sense of wellbeing. Nursing care is informed by an understanding of the person's unique individuality, attitudes and values, and the living environment is structured to support the person's wellbeing. Understanding a person's unique individuality, attitudes and values means the person's identity and their relationship with other people are maintained.

The seven domains of wellbeing are:

1. Security – the person has freedom from fear, anxiety and doubt, they feel safe, and have privacy, dignity and respect.
2. Growth – an environment that nurtures a sense of something to do that enables personal development and enrichment.
3. Autonomy – an environment that provides the person with choice so they are in control and can have the freedom to take risks.
4. Connectedness – an environment that offers a sense of belonging, engagement, involvement and meaning-ful relationships.
5. Identity – being well-known, promoting individuality gives a connection to life stories and what matters to the person.
6. Meaning – identifies a person's values and self-esteem, supports purpose, validating what a person can still do for themselves.
7. Joy – happiness, enjoyment, pleasure and content-ment, grows from the other six elements of wellbeing (Power 2014).

Tips for Best Practice
Utilising a Person's Life Story

Reminiscing with a person living with dementia about his or her life story can be a very effective way to connect with the person and help to calm any distress or low mood they may be experiencing. Strategies to enhance reminiscence include:

- producing a life story album or book that collects and records the person's past experiences
- where possible, involving the person with dementia in the creation of their life story book by sharing their knowledge, significant events and achievements
- producing the life story in other formats, such as auditory albums, DVDs and digital devices (e.g. iPad).

Promoting Wellness

An online interactive resource is available to inform healthcare staff about implementing a wellness approach to care for people living with dementia. This 'talking book' titled *Prescription for Life!* applies the seven Eden Alternative Domains to the care of people with younger onset dementia (diagnosed prior to the age of 65 years), but is relevant to the care of people living with dementia of any age. The resource is available at: https://content. ecu.edu.au/yod/mobile/index.html

Vafeas et al (2016, rev. 2020).

Promoting Independence

Research suggests that people who are diagnosed with dementia often express a desire to stay connected to their pre-diagnosis lifestyle (Read et al 2016). This encompasses a desire for sustained independence and the ability to carry out day-to-day activities without dependency on others. When engaging with people with dementia, it is important to focus on the person's remaining functional capacity rather than their functional decline. See *Tips for best practice: Promoting functional independence* in people with dementia.

Tips for Best Practice
Promoting Functional Independence in People With Dementia

- Ensure flexibility in daily activities to accommodate fluctuating abilities
- Provide support to participate in meaningful and enjoyable activities tailored to the person's ability and preferences
- Promote stability in the living environment
- Ensure consistency in care staff (whether community-based or in residential aged care)
- Promote independence in self-care skills and minimise disability, with particular attention to retaining continence (see Chapter 13)

NHMRC 2016.

Exercise and Psychosocial Activities

Person-centred psychosocial therapies are designed to promote wellbeing and self-esteem for people with dementia while reducing the incidence of responsive behaviours. Individualised activities can include light housework tasks, such as dusting or folding laundry or helping to prepare a meal, gardening or other recreational activities.

Research has indicated that physical activity may enhance cognition (Barber et al 2012) and can improve physical function in people diagnosed with dementia (Potter et al 2010).

Multisensory therapies are also reportedly beneficial for people with dementia, particularly those who present with apathy (Verkaik et al 2005). Creative therapies, as well as being enjoyable, are also helpful for people with dementia. Music therapy can reduce anxiety (Sung et al 2010), and art therapy provides an opportunity for the older person to focus on a pleasant activity, while promoting self-expression and a sense of control (Manthorpe et al 2008). Animal-assisted therapies involve introducing a visiting pet (most commonly a dog), resident pet, toy animal or robotic pet to the person with dementia. Studies have demonstrated reductions in behavioural disturbances and greater social interactions in people with dementia when the therapeutic animal is present (Filan & Llewellyn-Jones 2006). Implementation of intergenerational programs for people with dementia have proved effective in improving mood and quality of life (Gerritzen et al 2019).

Addressing Pain

The experience of pain will limit the extent to which a person with dementia can move and mobilise, and commonly underlies responsive behaviours. The nurse, therefore, has an essential role to address pain to maximise the person's ability to function and consequent independence.

Many people with dementia who have mild to moderate cognitive impairment are still able to report experiences of pain (see Chapter 19). Self-report is the most reliable indicator of the presence and severity of pain. If the older person can talk about their pain, it is important to ask simple and direct questions, listen to the answers and document the conversation. If the person with dementia cannot describe their pain, the nurse can use an observational pain assessment tool, such as the Abbey Pain Scale (see Chapter 19). Non-pharmacological approaches, such as massage, positioning, distraction and music, may be helpful. Do not use heat or cold therapies for people who cannot feel high or low temperatures or report how they are feeling (see Chapter 19, Safety alert). Pain medication can be trialled using a stepped approach with small incremental doses and regular reassessment, for a defined period of time.

Creating Enabling Environments

The physical and social environments in which a person lives are key to their safety and quality of life. There are strategies that can be implemented to help promote the independence and wellbeing of a person with dementia for as long as possible. These include:

* adapting the environment

  A well-designed environment for a person with dementia can help to sustain their abilities and enhance meaningful engagement through use of prompts to aid accessibility and reduce risks. In contrast, a poorly designed environment can lead to confusion, disorientation and further dependency on others. For this reason, a set of ten evidence-based 'dementia enabling environment principles' has been developed (Fleming & Bowles 1987; Fleming et al 2003). These principles can be used to inform the environmental designs in home, residential aged care and hospital settings (Alzheimer's WA 2020). Examples of environmental strategies that enable people with dementia and promote wellbeing include:

  * use of simple visual signage to help the person locate facilities such as the toilet
  * painting door frames or handrails in contrasting colours assist wayfinding
  * personalising spaces with the person's familiar objects
  * reducing clutter so the person can move around easily, safely and securely.

  For further information, see *Promoting wellness: Resources for environmental strategies to aid people with dementia*.

* implementing the use of assistive technology

  Use of assistive technology can support the independence and wellbeing of people living with dementia and reduce risk. There are a range of technologies available to people with dementia from sensor lights to satellite positioning systems to reduce the risk of someone becoming lost while walking. See *Promoting wellness: Resources for environmental strategies to aid people with dementia* for a guide to websites providing further information and resources.

* promoting dementia-friendly communities

  Encourage communities to foster a culture that enables the lives of people living with dementia by ensuring that outdoor and built environments are safe, and that organisations are inclusive of people with dementia. Strategies to achieve these aims include:

  * educating people within the community about what it means to live with dementia
  * encouraging business owners to ensure services are accessible to people with dementia.

* encouraging a citizenship and human rights focused approach in the support of people living with dementia

Encourage people with dementia to remain active decision-makers for as long as possible and to give back to the community in which they live, if possible. In this approach, support for people with dementia is underpinned by values of respect, dignity, autonomy, inclusion and freedom from discrimination.

* considering cognitive rehabilitation

  Cognitive rehabilitation is an individual goal-oriented program where people with dementia (and their support people if required) work with health professionals to identify personal goals and aim to achieve these with the implementation of strategies. Goals may include remembering recent events or re-establishing how to use the cooktop (Clare et al 2011).

Promoting Wellness
Resources for Environmental Strategies to Aid People With Dementia

DEMENTIA ENABLING ENVIRONMENTS
www.enablingenvironments.com.au/

This interactive website is very useful for people with dementia, care partners and staff to seek out ways in which the environment can be adapted to accommodate the needs and promote the independence of people living with dementia.

ASSISTIVE TECHNOLOGY
Information about assistive technology is available from Alzheimer's WA and Dementia Australia at the following websites:

Alzheimer's WA Assistive Technology Help Sheets
www.alzheimerswa.org.au/about-dementia/living-well-
   dementia/assistive-technology-help-sheets/

Dementia Australia – Assistive Technology
www.dementia.org.au/resources/assistive-technology

Consider sustaining the independence of a person with dementia by accessing suitable assistive technology. In Australia, approach Alzheimer's WA or Dementia Australia for advice and suggestions. In New Zealand, approach Dementia New Zealand at: https://dementia.nz/get-information/

PHARMACOLOGICAL MANAGEMENT

There are some medications available that alleviate symptoms of Alzheimer's disease and delay the progression of the condition. The medication class cholinesterase inhibitors may help people with mild to moderate Alzheimer's disease. The most commonly prescribed cholinesterase inhibitors are donepezil, rivastigmine and

Promoting Wellness
Case Snapshot – Living Well With Dementia

Vince was diagnosed with Alzheimer's disease at the age of 62. When giving Vince this diagnosis, the general practitioner told him very little other than to go home and get his affairs in order. Vince recalled memories of his aunt living with dementia many years before and her experience of residential aged care and consequently reported feeling extremely depressed. Vince's wife was becoming extremely concerned about his wellbeing and, on a friend's suggestion, phoned the local dementia support organisation. The organisation responded quickly and provided Vince and his wife with counselling, education sessions and access to support groups. Vince appreciated hearing of the experiences of other people who also had a diagnosis of dementia, who were living meaningful and connected lives. The dementia support organisation organised for Vince to take on some voluntary work at the local community garden centre. Vince was more optimistic about his future and much happier. With this support, he came to accept his diagnosis of dementia and was able to speak of it to others. Staff at the dementia support organisation invited Vince to speak about his experiences to student doctors and nurses at a Dementia Awareness forum. Vince willingly accepted this invitation and was pleased that he could give back to the community despite living with dementia.

galantamine. The mechanism of action is to inhibit the enzymes responsible for breaking down the neurotransmitter acetylcholine, thereby safeguarding availability to assist with memory and cognitive functions (Massoud & Gauthier 2010). Not all people with dementia benefit from cholinesterase inhibitors and the effect may only be temporary. Side effects of cholinesterase inhibitors include:

- loss of appetite
- nausea and vomiting
- diarrhoea
- falls
- muscle cramps
- headache
- dizziness
- fatigue
- bradycardia (Ali et al 2015; Alzheimer's Society 2018).

The common gastrointestinal side effects may mean the drug is not well tolerated. An alternative option is memantine, an NMDA receptor antagonist which protects the brain's nerve cells and works by targeting the neurotransmitter, glutamate (Molinuevo et al 2005; Salomone et al 2012). Memantine may improve memory, awareness and functional ability in people with moderate to severe symptoms of dementia. Common side effects include:

- dizziness
- headache
- fatigue
- constipation
- hypertension (Alzheimer's Society 2018).

Practice Scenario

You are the registered nurse at an aged care facility and have recently become quite concerned about the wellbeing of one of the residents.

Mr Smith is 75 years of age and was born in Perth, WA. Mr Smith had six brothers and three sisters. He reports having had a good relationship with his mother but not his father. He recalls that when he was in his early 20s, he had many disputes with his father, centred around when he was able to socialise and drive his car. Throughout his school years, Mr Smith played the trumpet and was a keen sportsman. He recalls being particularly good at Australian Rules football. He married and had five children of his own. He reports having had a good relationship with his wife until he developed dementia about five years ago. Six months ago, he moved into a residential aged care facility and has found this transition difficult.

Mr Smith sees himself as a person who likes to keep busy through gardening and socialising with others. However, he has not been able to get to know many other residents despite having lived in the facility for six months. Also, he feels that the staff don't know him as not many have asked about his life, his interests or what is important to him. He feels he lacks privacy as he is required to share his room with another person, and often feels annoyed at mealtimes. This is because the evening meal is served at 5 pm, while Mr Smith has always eaten dinner at 7 pm. Overall, he reports feeling very lonely. He wishes that he had the freedom to go shopping and buy gifts for his grandchildren with his own money, but this doesn't seem to be allowed.

Using a person-centred care approach and domains of wellbeing, what strategies can the nurse put in place to improve and sustain Mr Smith's wellbeing?

CONSIDERING THE DOMAINS OF WELLBEING

Identity

Mr Smith has expressed a lot of personal information about himself, including his relationship with his father, which helps to define his uniqueness as a person. Additionally, he wants to socialise with others. He feels that not many residents or staff are aware of his story. Creating a book telling Mr Smith's life story is one way that his identity can be shared with others.

Connectedness

Mr Smith reports having had a good relationship with his wife until he developed dementia and entered residential aged care. He states that he does not know many people in the nursing home, despite having lived there for six months. His reported loneliness indicates his lack of connectedness to other people in his new home. Strategies are required to connect him to his environment, both the physical (the building) and social (relationships with people) environment. He may feel more connected to his room if he is able to personalise the space with his familiar objects and will become more connected to other people within the facility if he is encouraged to attend groups with the other residents. He may also appreciate the opportunity to participate in intergenerational activities (such as with children from a playgroup if they were to visit the facility) if this could be organised by the facility.

Autonomy

Mealtimes are one time where Mr Smith feels he lacks autonomy as he cannot choose what food he eats or when he can eat it. He also feels a lack of privacy in that he shares a room with another person. If possible, consider a single room for Mr Smith if one is available, and involve him in personalising it with photos and other personal items.

Simple signage and use of colour to help Mr Smith locate his room and other areas will assist him to more independently navigate the facility. Consider opportunities for Mr Smith to assist with meal planning, and the potential for staggered mealtimes to increase resident choice.

Meaning

The despondence in Mr Smith's voice may indicate how much he is missing elements of life prior to entering the residential aged care facility, which were important to him. Find quiet moments to sit with Mr Smith, giving him opportunity to talk about these. Depending on Mr Smith's preferences, consider opportunities for him to engage in these again. These may include opportunities for him to take shopping trips to buy gifts for his grandchildren, either with staff support or with arranged family support. Acknowledging Mr Smith's love of music, strategies may include displaying photos of him with his trumpet or other visual mementos to communicate this interest to other staff and residents. Family could bring Mr Smith a CD player and CDs so he can play these in his room. Encourage staff to reminisce with Mr Smith about what it meant to be a trumpet player when he was younger, what and when he played and for whom.

Joy

Take time to sit with Mr Smith and ask him about his life and significant life events. Note events that he is particularly proud of and likes to discuss. Find ways to enable Mr Smith to share these events with the people he mixes with on a day-to-day basis. For example, display photos of Mr Smith holding a football trophy or receiving an award for trumpet playing. Encourage family to bring his grandchildren to visit, and provide a comfortable private meeting space, suitable for children, where the family can relax together.

SUMMARY

Neurocognitive disorders are acquired conditions that result in cognitive impairment. They include delirium and a range of syndromes classified as major or mild in nature. Delirium is a serious yet potentially reversible condition that presents with acute cognitive decline and fluctuating symptoms, and has poor health outcomes. Nurses are well placed to identify delirium and implement early treatment to alleviate symptoms and reduce complications. Mild cognitive impairment is a level of cognitive decline beyond what is considered normal ageing but not meeting diagnostic criteria for dementia. Parkinson's disease is a neurodegenerative disease, in which cells in the brain that produce the neurotransmitter

dopamine are progressively destroyed. Dementia is a collection of symptoms caused by pathology in the brain, including Alzheimer's disease, Lewy-body dementia, vascular dementia and frontotemporal dementia. Nursing assessment of a person with dementia focuses on understanding behavioural expressions of distress communicating unmet needs, which are known as 'responsive behaviours'. The philosophy of person-centred care informs contemporary care for people with dementia and emphasises the uniqueness of the individual. When caring for a person living with dementia, choice of language is important to avoid the stigma that can cause that person to lose self-esteem and withdraw from interactions with others. It is better to talk about what the person with dementia can do, rather than the capacity they have lost. Enabling environments help people with dementia feel safe and included through adaption of the environment, assistive technologies, dementia-friendly communities, a citizenship and human rights approach and cognitive rehabilitation.

REFERENCES

Albrecht JS, Marcantonio ER, Roffey D et al (2015) Stability of postoperative delirium psychomotor subtypes in individuals with hip fracture. Journal of the American Geriatrics Society 63(5):970–976.

Algase DL, Beck C, Kolanowski A et al (1996) Need-driven dementia-compromised behaviour: an alternative view of disruptive behaviour. American Journal of Alzheimers Disease and other Dementias 11:10–19.

Ali TB, Schleret TR, Reilly BM et al (2015) Adverse effects of cholinesterase inhibitors in dementia. PloS one 10(12). Online. Available: https://doi.org/10.1371/journal.pone.0144337

Alzheimer's New Zealand (2017) Dementia economic impact report 2016. Online. Available: www.alzheimers.org.nz/news/dementia-economic-impact-report-2016

Alzheimer's Society (2018) Effects of Alzheimer's disease drugs. Online. Available: www.alzheimers.org.uk/about-dementia/treatments/drugs/effects-of-alzheimers-drugs#content-start

Alzheimer's WA (2020) Dementia Enabling Environments Principles. Online. Available: www.enablingenvironments.com.au/dementia-enabling-environment-principles.html

American Psychiatric Association (2013) Diagnostic and statistical manual of mental disorders: DSM-5 (5th edn). American Psychiatric Association Publishing, Arlington, VA.

Australian Commission on Safety and Quality in Health Care (ACSQHC) (2016) Delirium clinical care standard. ACSQHC, Sydney.

Australian Government Department of Health and Ageing (2011) Delirium Care Pathways. Online. Available: www1.health.gov.au/internet/main/publishing.nsf/Content/FA0452A24AED6A91CA257BF0001C976C/$File/D0537(1009)%20Delirium_combined%20SCREEN.pdf

Banerjee S, Willis R, Matthews D et al (2007) Improving the quality of care for mild to moderate dementia: An evaluation of the Croydon Memory Service Model. International Journal of Geriatric Psychiatry 22:782–788.

Bang J, Spina S, Miller BL (2015) Frontotemporal dementia. The Lancet 386(10004):1672–1682.

Barber SE, Clegg AP, Young JB (2012) Is there a role for physical activity in preventing cognitive decline in people with mild cognitive impairment? Age and Ageing 41:5–8.

Barberger-Gateau P, Raffaitin C, Letenneur L et al (2007) Dietary patterns and risk of dementia: the three-city cohort study. Neurology 69(20):1921–1930.

Barnes DE (2010) The mental activity and exercise (MAX) trial: A randomized, controlled trial to enhance cognitive function in older adults with cognitive complaints. Alzheimer's & Dementia: The Journal of the Alzheimer's Association: Supplement 6(4):S145–S146.

Bellelli G, Morandi A, Davis DH et al (2014) Validation of the 4AT, a new instrument for rapid delirium screening: a study in 234 hospitalised older people. Age and ageing 43(4):496–502.

Bondi MW, Edmonds EC, Salmon DP (2017) Alzheimer's disease: past, present and future. Journal of the International Neuropsychological Society 23(9–10):818–831.

Borson S, Scanlan JM, Chen P et al (2003) The Mini-Cog as a screen for dementia: validation in a population-based sample. Journal of the American Geriatrics Society 51(10):1451–1454.

Braak H, Del Tredici K, Rüb U et al (2003) Staging of brain pathology related to sporadic Parkinson's disease. Neurobiology of Aging 24(2):197–211.

Cerejeira J, Lagarto L, Mukaetova-Ladinska EB (2012) Behavioral and psychological symptoms of dementia. Frontiers in Neurology 3:73.

Chandra SR, Issac TG, Abbas MM (2015) Apraxias in neurodegenerative dementias. Indian Journal of Psychological Medicine 37(1):42–47.

Chen CK, Bailey RW (2016) Episodic memories of relationship quality, procedural knowledge of attachment scripts, and the experience of daughters caring for a parent with dementia. Dementia 17(1):61–77.

Cheng S-T, Chow PK, Song Y-Q et al (2014) Mental and physical activities delay cognitive decline in older persons with dementia. The American Journal of Geriatric Psychiatry 22(1):63–74.

Clare L, Evans S, Parkinson C et al (2011) Goal-setting in cognitive rehabilitation for people with early stage Alzheimer's disease. Clinical Gerontologist 34(3):220–236.

Clark C, Ewbank D (1996) Performance of the Dementia Severity Rating Scale: A caregiver questionnaire for rating severity in Alzheimer disease. Alzheimer Disease and Associated Disorders 10:31–39.

Clinical Epidemiology and Health Service Evaluation Unit (2006) Clinical practice guidelines for the management of delirium in older people. Victorian Government Department of Health and Human Services, Melbourne.

Dalla Barba G, La Corte V (2015) A neurophenomenological model for the role of the hippocampus in temporal consciousness. Evidence from confabulation. Frontiers in Behavioral Neuroscience 9:218.

Dementia Australia (2020) Types of dementia. Online. Available: www.dementia.org.au/information/about-dementia/types-of-dementia

Dementia Australia (2018) Let's Talk: Good communication tips for talking with people with dementia. Online. Available: www.dementia.org.au/sites/default/files/resources/2019-Lets-Talk-Booklet.pdf

Edvardsson D, Winblad B, Sandman PO (2008) Person-centred care of people with severe Alzheimer's disease: current status and ways forward. Lancet Neurology 7:362–367.

Fazio S, Pace D, Flinner J et al (2018) The fundamentals of person-centered care for individuals with dementia. The Gerontologist 58:S10.

Feil N (1993) The validation breakthrough: Simple techniques for communicating with people who have Alzheimers and other dementias. Health Professions Press, Baltimore.

Filan SL, Llewellyn-Jones RH (2006) Animal-assisted therapy for dementia: a review of the literature. International Psychogeriatrics 18(4):597–611.

Fleming R, Bowles J (1987) Units for the confused and disturbed elderly: Development, Design, Programming and Evaluation. Australian Journal on Ageing 6(4):25–28.

Fleming R, Forbes I, Bennett K (2003) Adapting the ward for people with dementia. NSW Department of Health, Sydney.

Folstein MF, Folstein SE, McHugh PR (1975) 'Mini-mental state': A practical method for grading the cognitive state of patients for the clinician. Journal of Psychiatric Research 12(3):189–198.

Gerritzen EV, Hull MJ, Verbeek H et al (2019) Successful elements of intergenerational dementia programs: a scoping review. Journal of Intergenerational Relationships 18(3):1–32.

Gibb K, Seeley A, Quinn T, Najma S, Shenkin S, Rockwood K, Davis D. (2020) The consistent burden in published estimates of delirium occurrence in medical inpatients over four decades: a systematic review and meta-analysis study, Age and Ageing, 49(3):352–360.

Grand JHG, Casper S, MacDonald SWS (2011) Clinical features and multidisciplinary approaches to dementia care. Journal of Multidisciplinary Healthcare 4:125–147.

Holden J, Jayathissa S, Young G (2008) Delirium among elderly general medical patients in a New Zealand hospital. Internal Medicine Journal 38(8):629–634.

Hall GR, Buckwalter KC (1987) Progressively lowered stress threshold: A conceptual model for the care of adults with Alzheimer's disease. Archives of Psychiatric Nursing 1:399–406.

Hapca S, Guthrie B, Cvoro V et al (2018) Mortality in people with dementia, delirium, and unspecified cognitive impairment in the general hospital: prospective cohort study of 6,724 patients with 2 years follow-up. Clinical Epidemiology 10:1743–1753.

Inouye SK, van Dyck CH, Alessi CA et al (1990) Clarifying confusion: the confusion assessment method. A new method for detection of delirium. Annals of Internal Medicine 113(12):941–948.

Inouye SK, Westendorp RG, Saczynski JS (2014) Delirium in elderly people. Lancet (London, England) 383(9920):911–922.

International Psychogeriatric Association (2012) The IPA Complete Guides to Behavioral and Psychological Symptoms of Dementia: Specialists Guide. Online. Available: www.ipaonline.org/publications/guides-to-bpsd

Jackman L, Beatty A (2015) Using the Newcastle Model to understand people whose behaviour challenges in dementia care. Nursing Older People 27(2):32–39.

Jellinger KA, Korczyn AD (2018) Are dementia with Lewy bodies and Parkinson's disease dementia the same disease?. BMC Med 16(34).

Jett K (2018) Neurological disorders. In Touhy TA, Jett K (eds) Ebersole and Hess' Gerontological Nursing and Healthy Aging, 5th edn. Elsevier, St Louis.

Kai K, Hashimoto, M, Amano K et al (2015) Relationship between eating disturbance and dementia severity in patients with Alzheimer's disease. PloS one 10(8):e0133666.

Kitwood T (1997) Dementia reconsidered: The person comes first. Open University Press, Buckingham.

Kitwood T, Bredin K (1992) Towards a theory of dementia care: personhood and well-being. Ageing and Society 12(3):269–287.

Kouli A, Torsney KM, Kuan WL (2018) Parkinson's disease: etiology, neuropathology, and pathogenesis. In: Stoker TB, Greenland JC (eds). Parkinson's disease: pathogenesis and clinical aspects. Codon Publications, Brisbane.

Langa KM, Levine DA (2014) The diagnosis and management of mild cognitive impairment: a clinical review. JAMA 312(23):2551–2561.

Manthorpe J, Moniz-Cook E, Droes R et al (2008) Early psychosocial interventions in dementia: Evidence-based practice. Jessica Kingsley Publishers, London.

Marcantonio E (2017) Delirium in hospitalized older adults. New England Journal of Medicine 377:1456–1466.

Massoud F, Gauthier S (2010) Update on the pharmacological treatment of Alzheimer's disease. Current Neuropharmacology 8:69–80.

Molinuevo JL, Lladó A, Rami L (2005) Memantine: Targeting glutamate excitotoxicity in Alzheimer's disease and other dementias. American Journal of Alzheimer's Disease and other Dementias 20:77–85.

Molloy DW, Standish TI (1997) A guide to the Standardized Mini-Mental State Examination. International Psychogeriatrics 9(S1):87–94.

Mortby ME, Maercker A, Forstmeier S (2012) Apathy: a separate syndrome from depression in dementia? A critical review. Aging Clinical and Experimental Research 24(4):305–316.

Mushtaq R, Pinto C, Tarfarosh SF et al (2016) A comparison of the Behavioral and Psychological Symptoms of Dementia (BPSD) in early-onset and late-onset Alzheimer's Disease – A study from South East Asia (Kashmir, India). Cureus 8(5):e625.

Myall DJ, Pitcher TL, Pearson JF et al (2017) Parkinson's in the oldest old: impact on estimates of future disease burden. Parkinsonism and Related Disorders 42:78–84.

Nagamatsu LS, Chan A, Davis JC et al (2013) Physical activity improves verbal and spatial memory in older adults with probable mild cognitive impairment: a 6-month randomized controlled trial. Journal of Aging Research 2013(12):861893.

Nasreddine ZS, Phillips NA, Bédirian V et al (2005) The Montreal Cognitive Assessment, MoCA: A brief screening tool for mild cognitive impairment. Journal of the American Geriatrics Society 53(4):695–699.

National Health and Medical Research Council (NHMRC) Guideline Adaptation Committee (2016) Clinical practice guidelines and principles of care for people with dementia. NHMRC Partnership Centre for Dealing with Cognitive and Related Functional Decline in Older People, Canberra.

National Institute for Health and Clinical Excellence (NICE) (2010) Delirium: diagnosis, prevention and management. NICE, London.

Outeiro TF, Koss DJ, Erskine D et al (2019) Dementia with Lewy bodies: an update and outlook. Molecular Neurodegeneration 14(1):5–5.

Parkinson's Australia (2020) Statistics on Parkinson's. Online. Available: www.parkinsons.org.au/statistics

Potter R, Ellard D, Rees K et al (2010) A systematic review of the effects of physical activity on physical functioning, quality of life and depression in older people with dementia. International Journal of Geriatric Psychiatry 26:1000–1011.

Power GA (2017) Dementia beyond drugs: Changing the culture of care (2nd edn). Health Professions Press, Baltimore.

Power GA (2014) Dementia beyond disease: Enhancing wellbeing. Health Professions Press, Baltimore.

Read ST, Toye C, Wynaden D (2016) Experiences and expectations of living with dementia: A qualitative study. Collegian 24(5):427–432.

Rieck KM, Pagali S, Miller DM (2020) Delirium in hospitalized older adults. Hospital Practice 48(sup1):3–16.

Rodriques J (2017) Parkinson's disease: A general practice approach (3rd edn). Parkinson's Western Australia. Online. Available at www.drjulianrodrigues.com.au/wp-content/uploads/2017/03/Parkinsons-disease-GP-Manual-20171.pdf

Rose KM, Lorenz R (2010) Sleep disturbances in dementia. Journal of Gerontological Nursing 36(5):9–14.

Rosen T, Connors S, Clark S et al (2015) Assessment and management of delirium in older adults in the emergency department: literature review to inform development of a novel clinical protocol. Advanced Emergency Nursing Journal 37(3):183–196.

Rouleau I, Salmon DP, Butters N et al (1992). Quantitative and qualitative analyses of clock drawings in Alzheimer's and Huntington's disease. Brain and Cognition 18(1):70–87.

Salinas J, Beiser A, Himali JJ et al (2017) Associations between social relationship measures, serum brain-derived neurotrophic factor, and risk of stroke and dementia. Alzheimer's & Dementia: Translational Research & Clinical Interventions 3:229–237.

Salomone S, Caraci F, Leggio GM et al (2012) New pharmacological strategies for treatment of Alzheimer's disease: focus on disease modifying drugs. British Journal of Clinical Pharmacology 73(4):504–517.

Sandilyan MB, Dening T (2015) Signs and symptoms of dementia. Nursing Standard (Royal College of Nursing (Great Britain) 29(41):42–51.

Smith M, Hall GR, Gerdner L et al (2006) Application of the Progressively Lowered Stress Threshold Model across the continuum of care. Nursing Clinics of North America 41(1):57–81.

Sung H, Chang AM, Lee W (2010) A preferred music listening intervention to reduce anxiety in older adults with dementia in nursing homes. Journal of Clinical Nursing 19:1056–1064.

Sveinbjornsdottir S (2016) The clinical symptoms of Parkinson's disease. Journal of Neurochemistry 139:318–324.

Tranel D, Damasio AR (2001) Agnosia. In: NJ Smelser, PB Baltes (eds) International Encyclopedia of the Social & Behavioral Sciences. Pergamon, Oxford.

Tripathi M, Vibha D (2009) Reversible dementias. Indian Journal of Psychiatry 51 Suppl 1(Suppl1):S52–S55.

Trzepacz PT, Mittal D, Torres R et al (2001) Validation of the Delirium Rating Scale-Revised-98. The Journal of Neuropsychiatry and Clinical Neurosciences 13(2):229–242.

Trzepacz P, Meagher D, Franco J (2016) Comparison of diagnostic classification systems for delirium with new research criteria that incorporate the three core domains. Journal of Psychosomatic Research 84:60–68.

Vafeas C, Jacob E, White S (2016, rev. 2020) Prescription for Life! Edith Cowan University and Lovell Foundation. Online. Available: https://content.ecu.edu.au/yod/mobile/index.html

Venkat P, Chopp M, Chen J (2015) Models and mechanisms of vascular dementia. Experimental Neurology 272:97–108.

Verkaik R, van Weert JCM, Francke AL (2005) The effects of psychosocial methods on depressed, aggressive and apathetic behaviors of people with dementia: a systematic review. International Journal of Geriatric Psychiatry 20(4):301–314.

Vernooij-Dassen M, Moniz-Cook E, Verhey F et al (2019). Bridging the divide between biomedical and psychosocial approaches in dementia research: The 2019 INTERDEM Manifesto. Aging & Mental Health 1–7.

Wei LA, Fearing MA, Sternberg EJ et al (2008) The Confusion Assessment Method: A systematic review of current usage. J Am Geriatr Soc 56(5):823–830.

Weller J, Budson A (2018) Current understanding of Alzheimer's disease diagnosis and treatment. F1000Res 2018; 7: F1000 Faculty Rev-1161.

Woods B, O'Philbin L, Farrell EM et al (2018) Reminiscence therapy for dementia. The Cochrane Database of Systematic Reviews (3):CD001120.

World Health Organisation (WHO) (2017) Global action plan on the public health response to dementia 2017–2025. Geneva, Switzerland, Online. Available: https://apps.who.int/iris/bitstream/handle/10665/259615/9789241513487-eng.pdf?sequence=1

Young JJ, Lavakumar M, Tampi D et al (2018) Frontotemporal dementia: latest evidence and clinical implications. Therapeutic Advances in Psychopharmacology 8(1):33–48.

Relationships in Later Life

DAVID BETTS

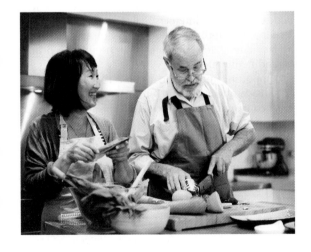

INTRODUCTION

This chapter explores the importance of relationships in later life. From exploring the nature of intimacy, sexuality and sexual diversity, to examining how relationships change and develop through life transitions, this chapter

will cover why it is important for nurses and healthcare professionals to be aware of the value of relationships for older people. The first part of this chapter explores the nature of intimacy and sexuality by challenging the idea that older people are non-sexual, non-physical and cease to be interested in romantic relationships. Next, the chapter addresses some of the challenges and obstacles that may emerge in relationships in later life, such as loneliness, divorce and elder abuse, before briefly covering some common life transitions in later life, including moves to retirement and aged care.

RELATIONSHIPS

Relationships are important for the wellbeing of all individuals, but especially so for older people as they age and engage with healthcare and nursing services. It is important for nurses and healthcare professionals to recognise the role that relationships have in supporting the wellbeing of older people generally, but also for promoting positive and healthy ageing.

Relationships can operate as a strong source of personal, social and economic support for all individuals, and this is equally so for older people (Oxoby 2009; Touhy 2016b). These relationships can take many forms, with common examples being in the form of friendships, families, children and between neighbours. Depending on an individual's circumstance, these relationships can also encompass healthcare professionals and, potentially, other residents of aged care facilities and services (Jang et al 2014; Touhy 2016c). Positive relationships can provide a range of resources, from psychological support, emotional and personal connections, to practical and financial resources. As a result, these relationships help support a wide range of factors associated with positive wellbeing (Blieszner 2014). Positive relationships also provide access to stimulation, socialisation opportunities and have been demonstrated to have a direct impact on the self-rated emotional, psychological and physical wellbeing of older people (Blieszner 2014; Touhy 2016c).

Maintaining positive relationships has a direct impact on the independence of older people, the ability to age in place and the likelihood of recovery after illness or injury (Arnold 2020). The notion of ageing in place, which emphasises that healthcare services and professionals aim to support older people to live independently in their own homes for as long as possible, is an important part of healthy and sustainable ageing (Meehan 2018). Recognising and supporting the relationships older people have in later life is one strategy nurses can use to assist older people to maintain their independence for longer, and to support ageing in place policies and procedures.

While the term relationship covers a broad scope of interpersonal connections and interactions, there is one concept that is closely tied to the notion of positive and beneficial relationships. That is the idea of intimacy, which continues to be important for relationships in later life.

Practice Points

- Relationships with others are a source of personal, social and economic support for older people.
- Relationships with others are vital for maintaining physical and psychological wellbeing.
- Relationships with others have a direct relationship on the independence of older people and an ability to age healthily.

INTIMACY

Intimate personal relationships are almost universally recognised as important to the wellbeing of individuals, including older people (Hughes & Heycox 2010). Intimacy is a broad term and can encompass a wide range of definitions, behaviours and attitudes. Commonly, intimacy is understood as a sense of closeness, companionship, support, safety, sexual and romantic satisfaction, as well as personal validation within relationships (Bratt et al 2017; Hughes & Heycox 2010; Wilson 2006).

It is important to note that despite many common cultural depictions, intimacy is not inherently tied to sexual relationships or sexual desire. Rather, these represent just one aspect of a broader range of feelings, social connections and personal links (Touhy 2016b). Intimacy can be understood as a sense of closeness and comfort that a person feels from their connections with others, regardless of the form of that connection (Syme 2014; Touhy 2016c; Youngkin 2004).

For older people, intimacy is an important component of late life satisfaction (Hughes & Heycox 2010; Youngkin 2004); therefore, it is imperative that nurses can articulate the importance of intimacy and support it in practice. Nurturing intimacy for older people may be difficult to achieve in certain healthcare settings due to restrictions and limitations on visitors, the ability of healthcare providers to spend adequate time with clients and the nature of clinical settings (Di Napoli et al 2013; Syme 2014). However, there are a few ways in which intimacy can be supported through best practice principles.

Intimacy for older people, that is a sense of closeness and comfort from interpersonal relationships, can best be supported through:

- facilitating close personal contact with loved ones and family members
- supporting interpersonal contact with individuals outside of clinical care settings
- encouraging the participation of friends, family members and close personal connections in healthcare plans and delivery (Touhy 2016b).

However, it is important to note that intimacy should always be measured from the older person's perspective – including both where intimacy comes from and whether intimacy is needed. Assumptions about the nature of intimacy, or the perceived need for intimacy in healthcare settings, can lead practitioners to pressure clients into unwanted contact, or inadvertently undervalue their connections with others (Di Napoli et al 2013; Touhy 2016b). Therefore, discussions around the nature of intimacy and relationships in later life in general require an open and constant dialogue with older people, as both patients and healthcare users.

A similar topic that requires the same level of open and honest dialogue with older adults is the area of sexuality.

Tips for Best Practice

- Intimacy is not about sexuality or sexual desire; intimacy is about closeness, comfort and connection.
- Intimacy can be nurtured by allowing older people to have close contact with loved ones and supporting interpersonal contact and interactions.
- The need for intimacy is subjective and determined by an individual's personal needs and desires.

Promoting Wellness
Suggestions for Encouraging Open Dialogue About Intimacy With Older Persons

- Use open and non-assuming questions about romantic relationships, partners and connections with others.
- Frame conversations around the needs of the older person, such as 'Who is important to you?' or 'Is there anyone you would like us to contact and support on your behalf?'
- Negative reactions to an older person's comments and responses about intimacy can inhibit an open and supportive dialogue. It is important to create spaces where older persons can discuss their needs regarding intimacy without these reactions.

SEXUALITY

A topic related to the nature of intimacy is sexuality. Sexuality and sexual desire are not often associated with older people, primarily due to a belief that older people are not sexually active or interested in sex, or that sexuality is no longer important for their wellbeing (Chandler et al 2004; Hughes & Heycox 2010). However, sexuality is important for the wellbeing of older people for a variety of reasons. It is essential that nurses recognise and support the role sexuality has in the lives of older people.

Sexuality and sexual relationships can be important for people as they age. As with any age group, not all older people will express a sexual desire, but for those who do, sexual relationships are a way of maintaining personal relationships, expressing intimacy and desire and maintaining a holistic form of wellbeing (Hughes & Heycox 2010; Syme 2014; World Health Organisation [WHO] 2014). For many older people, sexual identity is important as part of their sense of self; one that is often

denied, reduced or ignored by others as they age (Bach et al 2013). Recognising the importance of sexual identity can help support older people to express themselves, to fulfil their desires and to support their wellbeing as they age (Touhy 2016b, 2016c). This may be challenging in certain healthcare settings, which historically have not readily recognised sexual desire or sexual identity in older people (Touhy 2016b). It is therefore important for nurses to challenge systems, services and procedures that do not support the inclusion of sexuality.

Promoting Wellness

- Sexuality and sexual relationships are important for older people as they age.
- Sexual identity does not diminish with age.
- Recognising sexuality as an important subject for older people and their identities is necessary in promoting their wellbeing and recognising individuality.

The importance of recognising sexual identity is particularly salient for individuals with diverse sexual desires and experiences. Older people are not often regarded as sexual beings. When they are, however, they are often assumed to be heterosexual, with assumptions made about partners, sexual practice, family systems and children (Jablonski et al 2013; Syme 2014). Sexual identity is important for older people to maintain a positive sense of self and to express their identity. Sexually diverse older people face extra challenges in having their identities recognised and supported in many institutional settings and services.

SEXUAL AND GENDER DIVERSITY

A cohort of older adults that are frequently underacknowledged when it comes to considering relationships in later life are members of the lesbian, gay, bisexual, transgender, queer and intersex (LGBTQI+) community.

LGBTQI+, or sexual and gender diversity, can refer to a broad range of sexual and gender identities that are often grouped together due to their non-heterosexual and non-cisgender characteristics (Cronin & King 2010) (see Table 27.1). Both demographics contain a diverse and varied set of experiences, identities and potential needs as they age (Cronin & King 2010).

Broadly, however, there are some similar potential considerations that nursing professionals need to be

TABLE 27.1
Glossary of terms

Word	Meaning
LGBTQI+ community	people who identify as lesbian, gay, bisexual, transgender, queer or intersex.
Non-heterosexual	individuals who do not have sole sexual interest in individuals of the opposite sex.
Non-cisgender	individuals who do not identify as the gender they were assigned at birth

Tips for Best Practice

Older members of the LGBTQI+ community may be less open or willing to divulge their identity to nursing and healthcare professionals due to previous negative experiences from professional services.

- Terminology such as 'close friends', 'special friend' or 'housemate' may be used to avoid disclosure.
- Nurses can use open and gender-neutral language to inquire about relationships.
- The use of the term partner, avoidance of gender-based language and visual signs that LGBTQI+ identities are accepted in care settings can signal to older LGBTQI+ persons that they are welcome in clinical and healthcare practices.

aware of when supporting older LGBTQI+ individuals. When compared to older heterosexual and older cis-gender adults, members of the LGBTQI+ community are more likely to have experienced stigma and discrimination throughout their lives, have a higher rate of mental health concerns and are less likely to be able to rely on their biological family as they age (Fredriksen-Goldsen et al 2014; Hash & Rogers 2013; Mink et al 2014). While there is significant diversity in the experiences of older LGBTQI+ people, the increased likelihood of these factors mean that all healthcare professionals need to be mindful that older LGBTQI+ individuals may require additional support and assistance to navigate healthcare systems in older age.

Practice Points

- Sexual and gender diversity refers to a broad range of sexual and gender identities.
- LGBTQI+ individuals are more likely to have experienced discrimination and stigma throughout their lives.
- LGBTQI+ individuals are more likely to express fear of future discrimination and stigma from aged care professionals and aged care services.

Older LGBTQI+ individuals may be less willing to engage with healthcare services, and specifically aged care services, due to concerns about discrimination and stigma (Gratwick et al 2014). Many older LGBTQI+ people have expressed fears about experiencing discrimination from healthcare professionals as they age, and linked this concern to stigmatising experiences throughout their lifetime (Fronek 2012; Hughes 2009). A commonly expressed concern by older LGBTQI+ people is the perceived need to hide their sexual and gender identity

if they have to enter aged care services or facilities due to the potential stigma from either professionals or other residents (Hughes et al 2011; Johnson et al 2005). This hesitancy can place older LGBTQI+ people at risk if they abstain from seeking support or regular check-ups. It is therefore important that nurses are mindful of this potential concern and take all efforts to create and display an open and supportive environment that is inclusive of diverse sexual and gender identities.

Open Environments

Nurses can create and support inclusive environments by:
- using gender-neutral language on clinical forms and instruments.
- displaying visual images and examples of relationships that are non-heterosexual; for example, displaying the rainbow flag and having same-sex couples on visual information provided to patients.
- challenging colleagues' heteronormative and cisnormative behaviours.

While acknowledging that diversity of relationships in later life is important, it is equally valuable to consider what happens when older people do not have access to these close forms of personal connection, and the impact this can have on their wellbeing.

LONELINESS

One area of potential concern for older people that nursing professionals need to consider is the impact of loneliness. Loneliness and social isolation have been reported as being among the biggest concerns impacting older people (Pettigrew et al 2014; Touhy 2016c). This has ramifications for their wellbeing as they age and engage with healthcare services.

Loneliness is closely linked to a variety of physical and psychological conditions, including depression, dependence and a heightened risk of accidents (Jang et al 2014; Machielse 2015; Nyqvist et al 2013). It is one of the more common causes for distress in older people and can be exacerbated or influenced by a variety of factors. Loneliness has been found to be highly influenced by health status, with more physically independent and healthy older people reporting higher rates of satisfactory social connections and reduced feelings of loneliness (Nyqvist et al 2013). In contrast, loneliness has been found to be more common for older people who live in residential aged care facilities, compared to those living in their own homes or community settings (Nyqvist et al 2013). This means that nurses are more likely to engage with older people who are more vulnerable to feelings of loneliness and have reduced social connections.

Promoting Wellness

- Loneliness has a direct impact on physical and psychological wellbeing.
- Loneliness is one of the most common causes of distress for older people.
- Loneliness can be a result of a lack of interpersonal and community connections. Supporting and promoting connections with others within healthcare settings is vital in combating loneliness and supporting older people.

Nurses might recognise loneliness in older persons by picking up on the following indicators:

- Expression of a lack of social contact or diminishing social contact over time.
- Increased forms of psychological distress, such as depression or anxiety.
- Apathy towards previously enjoyed daily tasks or activities.

Most suggested strategies for supporting older people with loneliness focus on increasing the size and scope of their social networks. When achievable, this is a valuable objective, however, it is not necessarily a realistic goal for all socially isolated older people, especially when their feelings of loneliness and isolation relate to other social and physical problems (Machielse 2015). Nevertheless, there are supportive strategies reported to be successful, which could be utilised by nursing professionals. These include:

- making small and incremental advances in social connections tailored specifically to the individual

- offering or supporting others to provide personal assistance, so the older person can be more embedded in social networks
- focusing on and emphasising the importance of building empathetic connections with existing social and personal connections (Pettigrew et al 2014).

These strategies will not necessarily be practical in all contexts, but can provide basic guidance on how to offer support, suggestions and advice for older people who are feeling lonely.

DIVORCE, SEPARATION AND RELATIONSHIP LOSS

Related to the concept of loneliness, and highlighting the importance of relationships in later life, are the impact of divorce, separation and relationship loss on older people. Those who have a relationship breakdown in later life typically report higher rates of physical, psychological and economic distress (Bennett & Soulsby 2012; Touhy 2016c). These discrepancies mean that older people who encounter relationship losses are more likely to present to healthcare and social services and are more likely to require support with recovery and maintaining their social, physical and psychological wellbeing (Blieszner 2014).

Relationship losses can impact older people in diverse and varied ways. The effects of divorce, separation and relationship losses tend to differ based on gender. In general, older men report more psychological and financial distress following a relationship loss, while older women tend to report lower levels of social and personal distress (Touhy 2016a). Additionally, older people are less likely to have personal or social supports in their own home or community after a relationship breakdown and, therefore, more likely to rely on aged care and residential services (Hughes 2010; Hughes & Kentlyn 2011). This means that nurses need to be mindful of how older people respond to the loss of a relationship, the impact these losses can have on their physical, social and psychological wellbeing (see Chapter 29), and the role these relationships used to play in forming and maintaining broader social connections.

ELDER ABUSE

An area that nurses need to be trained to recognise when working with and supporting older people is the possibility of elder abuse.

Elder abuse is defined as either deliberate action, or a lack of action, which can cause harm and hurt to an older person (Arendts & Rawson 2019). This form of abuse is often unrecognised by those around an older person, and in some cases will not be acknowledged or identified by older people themselves (Arendts & Rawson 2019; Arnold 2020). Elder abuse can present in many forms, including financial, physical, psychological and sexual abuse, and can occur within many different relationships, including between children and parents, within wider families, between friends, neighbours and partners and from professional carers (Arendts & Rawson 2019).

The impacts of elder abuse are broad, and can include serious consequences for older adults, their wellbeing and their quality of life. Common impacts of long-term and unaddressed elder abuse can include a decline in functional abilities, severe impact on mental health and wellbeing, social withdrawal and isolation, as well as premature death (Arnold 2020).

It is important that nurses are aware of, and can recognise, indications that an older person is being abused. Warning signs of potential elder abuse include:
- visible signs on the body, in the case of physical abuse
- changes in behaviour and personality, in the case of emotional abuse
- malnutrition, dehydration and poor hygiene, in the case of neglect (Robinson et al 2019).

Financial abuse is a common but more subtle form of elder abuse. Potential indicators include:
- an increase in withdrawals from bank accounts
- missing items or objects
- unpaid service expenses (Robinson et al 2019).

Older people most at risk of abuse include those who:
- live alone
- are reliant on others for care
- live with a carer
- are living with dementia
- have a mental illness
- have a functional impairment.

Nurses play an important role in recognising and supporting individuals who may be victims of elder abuse. Older people make frequent visits to medical professionals and services, and therefore nurses are often an intermediary between older people and their engagement with social and healthcare services (Arendts & Rawson 2019).

Nurses and other professionals in this context have a responsibility to be aware of the warning signs and potential impacts of elder abuse, to support older adults to have a voice in their own decision-making and advocate for their needs over the needs of others, and, if appropriate, to report concerns to suitable authorities (Arendts & Rawson 2019). New Zealand has no legislation dictating the mandatory reporting of elder abuse; however, there are specific organisational guidelines and frameworks that support nurses in cases of elder abuse (New Zealand Nurses Organisation 2013). The Ministry of Health NZ has issued family violence intervention guidelines on the topic of elder abuse and specifies that nurses should always report cases of elder abuse – either to their official workplace reporting body, or to the local District Health Board, or to the Health and Disability Commissioner (Ministry of Health NZ 2007). Australia similarly has no mandatory reporting laws regarding elder abuse; however, compulsory reporting requirements within the *Aged Care Amendment (Security and Protection) Act 2007* stipulate that employers, staff and residents of aged care services should report such claims to the Office of Aged Care Quality and Compliance (Raghunathan 2017). Mandatory reporting to protect vulnerable individuals or individuals at risk of harm is also a requirement of the Australian Health Practitioner Regulation Agency (Raghunathan 2017). In Australia there are state-specific specialised units dedicated to investigating claims of elder abuse, while hospital-based social workers also take referrals of suspected elder abuse (Arendts & Rawson 2019). It is important that nurses are aware of their responsibilities under these institutions and can recognise and react accordingly to cases of elder abuse with older people in their care.

Mandatory Reporting (see Box 27.1)

Mandatory reporting is the professional and legal obligation to report misconduct and harmful activity. In Australia, registered health practitioners, including registered nurses, are legally and professionally obligated to make a mandatory report if a health practitioner has breached their code of conduct and practice as per the requirements of their profession (Australian Health Practitioner Registration Agency [AHPRA] 2020a, 2020b).

In Australia, mandatory notifications were legislated in 2010. Notifiable conduct includes: engaging in practice while intoxicated, sexual misconduct and placing the public at risk either due to the practitioner's own health difficulties or because of practice that is unacceptable to the profession.

The *Aged Care Act 1997* contains provisions for compulsory reporting to police and the Aged Care Quality and Safety Commission (the Commission) of any allegations that a resident of an approved aged care provider has been subject to a reportable assault (Australian Government Aged Care Quality and Safety Commission 2020). A reportable assault is defined as either unreasonable use of force, being deliberate and violent physical force including kicking, hitting and pinching, or unlawful sexual assault. The report must be made within 24 hours of the allegation being made. Responsibility for investigating the alleged assault will fall to the police, while the Commission will record the report, which may be used as part of its regulatory functions (Australian Government Aged Care Quality and Safety Commission 2020).

New Zealand does not have any legal requirements for mandatory notifications for registered nurses (Nursing Council of New Zealand 2020a). However, quality safe patient care is a professional standard and expectation (Nursing Council of New Zealand 2020b). The Nursing Council of New Zealand has a mandate to keep the public safe and expects registered nurses to practise accordingly and be fit to practise.

BOX 27.1
Elder Abuse Support Services

AUSTRALIA – NATIONAL

1800 ELDERHelp
Telephone: 1800 353 374 (national free call phone number that automatically redirects callers seeking information and advice on elder abuse to existing phone line service in their jurisdiction).

NEW ZEALAND – NATIONAL

Age Concern New Zealand National Office
Telephone: 04 801 9338
Email: national.office@ageconcern.org.nz

AUSTRALIAN STATES AND TERRITORIES
Australian Capital Territory

Older Persons Abuse Prevention Referral and Information Line (APRIL)
Telephone: 02 6205 3535
Email: oma@act.gov.au

New South Wales

NSW Ageing and Disability Abuse Helpline
Telephone: 1800 628 221
Email: nswadc@adc.nsw.gov.au

Northern Territory

Elder Abuse Information Line
Telephone: 1800 812 953
Email: info@dcls.org.au

Queensland

Elder Abuse Prevention Unit
Telephone: 1300 651 192
Email: eapu@uccommunity.org.au

Rural and Remote Peer Support Network
Email: eapu.psn@uccommunity.org.au

South Australia

Elder Abuse Prevention Phone Line
Telephone: 1800 372 310
Email: stopelderabuse@sa.gov.au

Tasmania

Tasmanian Elder Abuse Helpline
Telephone: 1800 441 169
Email: eahelpline@advocacytasmania.org.au

Victoria

Senior Rights Victoria
Telephone: 1300 368 821
Email: info@seniorsrights.org.au

Western Australia

WA Elder Abuse Helpline
Telephone: 1300 724 679
Freecall: 1800 655 566 (country callers)
Email: rights@advocare.org.au

Australian Institute of Family Studies (2020).

LATER LIFE TRANSITIONS

Older people go through a variety of later life transitions, which may impact on their wellbeing and relationships with others. Nurses are in a prime position to support older people during these transitions, and to recognise the value of relationships during this time.

One common transition for older people is the move to retirement. Many older people work less as they age, with a significant number choosing to forgo formal paid employment altogether (Touhy 2016b). A transition into retirement may be predictable and planned, or it can occur due to unforeseen circumstances. Events such as illness, loss of employment, permanent disability or a change in family circumstances may necessitate a change in retirement plans (Touhy 2016b). Research has shown that retirees who have ceased work due to ill-health, loss of employment or adverse family circumstances reported higher levels of psychological distress than those who prepared for this transition (Vo et al 2015).

The notion of successful retirement is based on the needs of the older individual, and can include their socialisation needs and connections, physical health and independence, financial security, social support and ability to adapt to their new circumstances (Touhy 2016b). Nurses may have the opportunity to work alongside older people who are transitioning into retirement and can help the transition by recognising and supporting the role and value of various interpersonal relationships during this life stage (Touhy 2016b).

Promoting Wellness

- Unexpected or unplanned transitions in later life can negatively impact on the wellbeing of older people.
- Successful transitions in later life are based on the needs of the individual, and relationships with others can help support these needs as older people enter later life.
- Nurses often support older people throughout their life transitions and can provide support by recognising and supporting the inclusion of relationships with others during this time.

Practice Scenario

Rowan is an 85-year-old transgender woman who recently decided to pursue gender reassignment surgery. Rowan has a wife, Judy, and they have been married for 33 years. After Rowan reaffirmed their gender identity as a transgender woman, Judy and Rowan mutually decided to separate. After this separation Rowan has been experiencing incidents of depression, increased anxiety and social isolation. Rowan has become distant from close friends and connections and has been displaying signs of malnutrition. Rowan's children have suggested that home-based support might be appropriate, or even residential care if Rowan continues to de-condition. Rowan has expressed concerns about both options.

MULTIPLE CHOICE QUESTIONS

1. Why might Rowan be displaying signs of depression, anxiety and social isolation?
   a. Rowan was already depressed, anxious and isolated, and these are unrelated to any recent life changes and should not be acknowledged when supporting Rowan.
   b. Rowan has recently gone through a relationship loss, and despite it being an amicable separation has lost a close form of personal support.
   c. Rowan is expressing typical signs of ageing.
   d. Rowan does not want gender reassignment surgery.

2. How might people supporting Rowan attempt to encourage social contact and connection?
   a. Rowan should be strongly encouraged to attend new events and activities, even if they are psychologically and physically unable to participate.
   b. Rowan should be slowly supported to reconnect with pre-existing social relationships, with a focus on building empathetic connections.
   c. Rowan should be encouraged to incrementally increase social contact that is both physically and socially appropriate to Rowan's current needs and desires.
   d. A combination of B and C.

3. Why might Rowan be expressing concerns for formal support either at home or within residential care services?
   a. Rowan does not want strangers entering the home.
   b. Rowan believes that such services are a waste of time and money.
   c. Rowan has concerns that carers and professional services might not acknowledge or support their gender identity.
   d. Both A and B.

Another later life transition that older people may experience is the move into aged care services and facilities. Many older people can remain in either their own or shared home as they get older, with only a relatively small percentage of the aged population requiring support from an aged care facility or service (Meehan 2018). Reasons for entering residential aged care vary, and can include reduced physical independence, illness and chronic conditions and the need for ongoing rehabilitative or restorative support (Meehan 2018). For older people, the transition into aged care can impact on their wellbeing, and may be associated with feelings of isolation, loss and frustration (see Chapter 29). A common concern is the impact of this move on relationships with others in the community. Nurses and other healthcare professionals can help to support an older person during this transition by recognising the importance of relationships in later life, and by facilitating the involvement of these relationships in the planning, delivery and evaluation of these transitions.

SUMMARY

Relationships in later life are important for the wellbeing of older people. These relationships can be diverse and varied, involving connections with friends, family and members of the community. Types of relationships in later life can vary greatly, and can include various forms of intimacy, sexual desire, connection and identity. However, relationships in later life are not static, with many older people encountering obstacles, challenges and transitions in their relationships with others. Nurses have an important role in supporting older people through periods of illness, recovery and rehabilitation. To do this successfully it is vital that nurses articulate the diverse and varied relationships older people can have as they age, and the role of these relationships in supporting wellbeing during the challenges and transitions encountered in later life.

REFERENCES

Arendts G, Rawson H (2019) The older person. In: K Curtis, C Ramsden, RZ Shaban et al (eds) Emergency and trauma care for nurses (3rd edn). Elsevier, Sydney.

Arnold EC (2020) Communicating with older adults. In: EC Arnold & KU Boggs (eds) Interpersonal relationships, 8th edn. Elsevier, St Louis, Missouri.

Australian Government Aged Care Quality and Safety Commission (2020) Compulsory reporting for approved providers of residential aged care services. Online. Available: www.agedcarequality.gov.au/providers/compulsory-reporting-approved-providers-residential-aged-care-services

Australian Government Australian Institute of Family Studies (2020) Elder abuse support services. Online. Available: aifs.gov.au/elder-abuse-support-services

Australian Health Practitioner Registration Agency (AHPRA) (2020a) Guidelines for mandatory notifications. Online. Available: www.aphra.gov.au/Notifications/mandatorynotifications/Revised-guidelines.aspx

Australian Health Practitioner Registration Agency (AHPRA) (2020b) Revised Guidelines for mandatory notifications. Online. Available: www.ahpra.gov.au/Notifications/mandatorynotifications/Revised-guidelines.aspx

Bach LE, Mortimer JA, VandeWeerd C et al (2013) The association of physical and mental health with sexual activity in older adults in a retirement community. The Journal of Sexual Medicine 10(11):2671–2678.

Bennett KM, Soulsby LK (2012) Wellbeing in bereavement and widowhood. Illness, Crisis & Loss 20(4):321–337.

Blieszner R (2014) The worth of friendship: can friends keep us happy and healthy? Generations 38(1):24–30.

Bratt AS, Stenstrom U, Rennemark M (2017) Effects on life satisfaction of older adults after child and spouse bereavement. Aging & Mental Health 21(6):602–608.

Chandler M, Margery M, Maynard N et al (2004) Sexuality, older people and residential aged care. Geriaction 22(4):5–11.

Cronin A, King A (2010) Power, inequality and identification: Exploring diversity and intersectionality amongst older LGB adults. Sociology 44(5):876–892.

Di Napoli EA, Breland GL, Allen RS (2013) Staff knowledge and perceptions of sexuality and dementia of older adults in nursing homes. Journal of Aging & Health 25(7):1087–1105.

Fredriksen-Goldsen KI, Cook-Daniels L, Kim H-J et al (2014) Physical and mental health of transgender older adults: An at-risk and underserved population. The Gerontologist 54(3):488–500.

Fronek P (2012) Issues in ageing for lesbian, gay, bisexual, transgender and intersex (LGBTI) people.Online. Available: www.podsocs.com/podcast/issues-in-ageing-for-lesbian-gay-bisexual-transgender-and-intersex-people/

Government of Western Australia, Department of Communities, Adocare, Blundell B (2017) Elder abuse protocol: Guidelines for action. A 5-step approach to responding to Elder Abuse. Government of Western Australia, Dept of Communities.

Gratwick S, Jihanian LJ, Holloway IW et al (2014) Social work practice with LGBT seniors. Journal of Gerontological Social Work 57(8):889–907.

Hash KM, Rogers A (2013) Clinical practice with older LGBT clients: Overcoming lifelong stigma through strength and resilience. Clinical Social Work Journal 41(3):249–257.

Hughes AK, Harold RD, Boyer JM (2011) Awareness of LGBT aging issues among aging services network providers. Journal of Gerontological Social Work 54(7):659–677.

Hughes M (2009) Lesbian and gay people's concerns about ageing and accessing services. Australian Social Work 62(2):186–201.

Hughes M (2010) Expectations of later life support among lesbian and gay Queenslanders. Australian Journal on Ageing 29(4):161–166.

Hughes M, Heycox K (2010) Older people, ageing and social work: knowledge for practice. Allen & Unwin, Melbourne.

Hughes M, Kentlyn S (2011) Older LGBT people's care networks and communities of practice: A brief note. International Social Work 54(3):436–444.

Jablonski RA, Vance DE, Beattie E (2013) The invisible elderly: lesbian, gay, bisexual, and transgender older adults. Journal of Gerontological Nursing 39(11):46–52.

Jang Y, Park NS, Dominguez DD et al (2014) Social engagement in older residents of assisted living facilities. Aging & Mental Health 18(5):642–647.

Johnson MJ, Jackson NC, Arnete JK et al (2005) Gay and lesbian perceptions of discrimination in retirement care facilities. Journal of Homosexuality 49(2):83–102.

Machielse A (2015) The heterogeneity of socially isolated older adults: a social isolation typology. Journal of Gerontological Social Work 58(4):338–356.

Meehan S (2018) Health and aged care services in Australia and New Zealand. In: K. Scott, M Webb, C Kostelnick (eds) Long-term caring: residential, home and community aged care, 4th edn. Elsevier: Sydney.

Ministry of Health NZ (2007) Family violence intervention guidelines: Elder abuse and neglect. MOH, Wellington.

Mink MD, Lindley LL, Weinstein AA (2014) Stress, stigma and sexual minority status: The intersectional ecology model of LGBTQ health. Journal of Gay & Lesbian Social Services 26(4):502–521.

New Zealand Nurses Organisation (2013) Reporting abuse – actual or suspected: Frequently asked questions. New Zealand Nurses Organisation, Wellington.

Nursing Council of New Zealand (2020a) Keeping the public safe. Online. Available: www.nursingcouncil.org.nz/Public/concerns/Keeping_the_public_safe/NCNZ/concerns-section/Keeping_the_public_safe.aspx?hkey=89fd89dd-681a-4d3a-a0b6-91efe858c809

Nursing Council of New Zealand (2020b) Standards and guidelines for nurses. Online. Available: www.nursingcouncil.org.nz/Public/Nursing/Standards_and_guidelines/NCNZ/nursing-section/Standards_and_guidelines_for_nurses.aspx?hkey=9fc06ae7-a853-4d10-b5fe-992cd44ba3de

Nyqvist F, Cattan M, Andersson L et al (2013) Social capital and loneliness among the very old living at home and in institutional settings: A comparative study. Journal of Aging and Health 25(6):1013–1035.

Oxoby R (2009) Understanding social inclusion, social cohesion, and social capital. International Journal of Social Economics 36(12):1133–1152.

Pettigrew S, Donovan R, Boldy D et al (2014) Older people's perceived causes of and strategies for dealing with social isolation. Aging and Mental Health 18(7):914–920.

Raghunathan K (2017) Professional nursing practice: Legal and ethical frameworks. In: G Koutoukidis et al (eds) Tabbner's nursing care: theory and practice, 7th edn. Elsevier, Sydney.

Robinson L, de Benedictis T, Segal J (2019) Elder abuse and neglect: warning signs, risk factors, prevention, and help. Online. Available: www.helpguide.org/articles/abuse/elder-abuse-and-neglect.htm

Syme ML (2014) The evolving concept of older adult sexual behavior and its benefits. Generations 38(1):35–41.

Touhy TA (2016a) Mental health. In: TA Touhy, K Jett (eds) Ebersole & Hess' toward healthy aging: human needs and nursing response, 9th edn. Elsevier, St. Louis, Missouri.

Touhy TA (2016b) Long-term care. In: TA Touhy, K Jett (eds) Ebersole & Hess' toward healthy aging: human needs and nursing response, 9th edn. Elsevier, St. Louis, Missouri.

Touhy TA (2016c) Relationships, roles and transitions. In: TA Touhy, K Jett (eds) Ebersole & Hess' toward healthy aging: human needs and nursing response, 9th edn. Elsevier, St. Louis, Missouri.

Vo K, Forder PM, Tavener M et al (2015) Retirement, age, gender and mental health: findings from the 45 and Up Study. Aging and Mental Health 19(7):647–657.

Wilson L (2006) Developing a model for the measurement of social inclusion and social capital in regional Australia. Social Indicators Research 75(3):335–360.

World Health Organisation (WHO) (2014) Sexual and reproductive health: defining sexual health. Online. Available: www.who.int/reproductivehealth/topics/sexual_health/sh_definitions/en

Youngkin EQ (2004) The myths and truths of mature intimacy: mature guidance for nurse practitioners. Advance for Nurse Practitioners 12(8):45–48.

CHAPTER 28

The Caregiver

DAVINA POROCK

LEARNING OBJECTIVES

After reading this chapter, you will be able to:

- describe the changing role and recognition of family caregivers within the context of Australian and New Zealand health systems and policy
- analyse family caregiving from multiple perspectives in order to identify positive and negative impacts and develop strategies to improve outcomes and manage barriers
- develop knowledge and skills in assessing family caregiving and provide training and education to support the caregivers, ensuring good outcomes for the older person requiring care and the family caregiver.

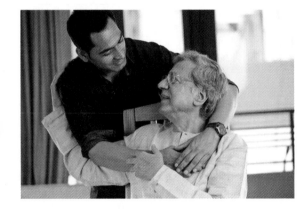

INTRODUCTION

Families have always been the first-line caregivers for older people as a natural part of social organisation. The changing picture of chronic illness and longevity means that family members are now providing care for more complex conditions, for longer periods of time, often requiring mastery of tasks that were previously the province of registered health professionals. This shift has occurred within the context of a much-changed society where both men and women are in the paid workforce, the family size is smaller and there may be greater geographic distance between family members, thereby reducing the number of available family caregivers. These circumstances create a new paradigm for how we understand, assess and support family members as vital members of the healthcare team. This chapter provides a guide to understanding family members as caregivers from the perspective of the older person requiring care, the family members, health professionals and policymakers.

In this chapter, the term family caregiver is used to refer to unpaid care and support provided to older family members and friends who have a physical disability, mental illness, chronic condition or terminal illness. They may provide assistance with activities of daily living (ADLs) and/or nursing and medical tasks (Carers Australia 2019; Carers New Zealand n.d.). The terms family caregiver, carer, caregiver are used interchangeably.

So who are family caregivers, what do they do, how much time is spent providing care and where does it

TABLE 28.1
Statistics Describing Australian and New Zealand Family Caregivers

Descriptor	Australian Caregivers	New Zealand Caregivers
Number of caregivers in country	2.65 million caregivers (ABS 2018) 861,000 (32.5%) are primary carers – those who provide the most informal assistance to another individual (ABS 2018) 1:11 Australians are family caregivers	431,649 caregivers (Infometrics 2014) 12.8% or 1:8 New Zealanders are family caregivers (Infometrics 2014)
Hours of caregiving	1.9 billion hours of unpaid care (Deloitte Access Economics 2015) 1:2 caregivers provide 20+ hours of care each week (ABS 2018) 1:3 provide 40+ hours of care each week (ABS 2018)	672 million hours of unpaid care Average of 30 hours per week (Infometrics 2014)
Estimated replacement value of caregiving if provided by paid workers	AU$60.3 billion (Deloitte Access Economics 2015)	NZ$10.8 billion (5% of GDP in 2013) (Infometrics 2014)
Profile of caregivers	7:10 caregivers are women Average age of primary caregiver is 54.3 years 1:11 caregivers are under 25 years old (over 235,000) Median income of working age primary carers is 42% lower than non-carers (ABS 2018)	2:3 caregivers are women Median age of caregivers is 49 years. NZ caregivers are increasingly older than the typical New Zealander (Infometrics 2014) In 2013, households of unpaid caregivers earn 10% less income than households without caregiving responsibilities (Infometrics 2014)

Australian Bureau of Statistics (2018); Deloitte Access Economics (2015); Infometrics (2014).

happen? Table 28.1 provides summary descriptive statistics profiling caregivers in Australia and New Zealand using available sources of data. The message from the summary is that family caregivers provide significant amounts of unpaid care that contributes economically and socially to Australian and New Zealand societies and healthcare systems. In fact, without family caregivers our healthcare systems would be hard pressed to cope with the volume of work to be done.

Family caregivers provide the lion's share of care for older people in our society. With the unprecedented epidemiological shifts in the age of the population and with most growth happening in the over 85 years age group (the oldest old), there is a greater need for family caregiving than ever before. However, the pool of family caregivers is shrinking due to family sizes being smaller, an increase in the number of single people, long distances between older people and their children

or younger relatives, along with both men and women being in the paid workforce (Carers Australia 2019). Despite the immense sociocultural changes of the 20th century, the typical caregiver is still female, but is now more likely to be employed and to need employment income than in previous times (Carers New Zealand n.d.). With this fact comes the likelihood of limited schedule flexibility to juggle caring, work and other responsibilities.

The data certainly paint a clear picture of the role of family caregivers in our society. The use of data in this way over the past few years has been very effective in persuading politicians and policymakers to see the major contribution that family caregivers make to the healthcare system. In recent times, significant changes have been made by governments to recognise and support the work that family caregivers make to the healthcare system and to society in general.

THE CHANGING ROLE AND RECOGNITION OF FAMILY CAREGIVERS

As noted, families have been and always will be the mainstay for support and care of older people in our society. For much of the time, the type and amount of support is quite sustainable within the usual give and take of family life. When the older person has more complex or multiple chronic conditions, is becoming frail, has dementia or serious life limiting conditions such as cancer or a progressive neurodegenerative disease, then occasional support and assistance becomes more intense, long-lasting and the family may well be heavily relied upon to gain technical skills as the health systems come under increasing pressure (Mair & May 2014; May et al 2014). Furthermore, the role of family caregiving was transformed when de-institutionalisation of people with mental health problems, young people with disability and ageing in place were encouraged and promoted (Jorgenson et al 2010). As a result, family caregiving has become more likely to result in significant physical, mental and emotional stress for the family caregiver, particularly when care is required over a number of years.

The demands of long-term caregiving began to receive greater attention in the nursing literature from the early 1980s with an article published in *The Canadian Nurse Journal* by Mary Vachon (1980). Before this, research on family caregiving was pretty much confined to child-rearing and mother–infant bonding. It is interesting to note that as the 'boomer' generation were hitting their 40s during the 1980s, and parents were beginning to require more assistance, the rise of interest in family caregiving took off, demonstrating the close connection between changes in society and nursing's response to societal need.

Research in nursing, psychology and the social sciences gradually began to reveal the full impact of long-term, skilled family caregiving. Caregiver burden, strain or stress became an issue of great concern, with descriptions of burnout and fatigue building a large evidence base. The impact on family caregivers' mental and physical health was the next focus in the literature and most recently the economic discrimination, when caregivers need to reduce hours of paid employment or stop working altogether in order to meet the demands of caregiving. This places family caregivers at greater risk of economic and social hardship for their own futures as they have less income and face the prospect of reduced independence in retirement.

In parallel to the increasing evidence base growing from academic researchers, caregivers themselves were becoming organised, forming peak bodies and actively lobbying politicians for change in recognition. Carers New Zealand was established in the early 1990s by and for family caregivers, and now acts as the national peak body providing information, advice, learning and support for caregivers in New Zealand (Carers New Zealand n.d.). Australia can trace the beginnings of political development for caregivers to the early 1970s when a grant was awarded to explore the care given by family and friends of frail-aged and disabled Australians. The Carers Association of Australia was formed in 1993 and ultimately became Carers Australia. It is through the persistent and persuasive work of these voluntary organisations, using research evidence and telling personal caregiving stories, that significant changes to policy in both Australia and New Zealand have recently occurred. There is, of course, a long history of policy implications for family caregivers, but for this chapter we will focus on the recent, most relevant policy.

Australia

In October 2019, following an extensive two-year consultation process with caregivers, caregiver and disability organisations and professionals, and utilising research evidence, the Australian Government launched the Integrated Carers Support Service (ICSS) Model, which is accessed via the Carer Gateway. Box 28.1 summarises the services available. In this model, Regional Delivery Partners (RDPs) deliver front-line support and information services to carers. The development of the new ICSS signifies a shift away from crisis emergency response (e.g. emergency respite), which is costly and reactive, to early intervention and support for carers. As health professionals, it is important to know how to access these services to support and guide older people and families.

New Zealand

New Zealand has an inclusive definition of family, recognising the cultural differences of the First Nations peoples, in particular Māori and Samoans. Whānau is the Māori language word for extended family, and Aiga is the Samoan language word. Aiga refers not just to the immediate family or members of the direct generations, but also to the wider group who are connected by blood or marriage. Aiga will include people 'adopted' into the group; all of whom acknowledge the Matai (head of family) as the leader/chief. These important terms are used in all New Zealand policy related to family caregivers and represent a significant recognition of diversity in the definition of family.

BOX 28.1
Australian Integrated Carer Support
Services Model

ONLINE SERVICES

- Peer support to assist connection with and learn from other carers. The community forum helps carers share their stories, knowledge and experience with others.
- Self-guided coaching to support and teach skills useful to the caring situation. Coaching modules cover a range of topics and can be completed online at the carer's own pace.
- A phone-based counselling service to provide short-term emotional and psychological support for carers.
- Practical skills courses to improve general skills and knowledge.

TAILORED SUPPORT

- Carer support planning – to help identify what areas of support will best help in the caring role and to develop a simple plan for ongoing support and service.
- Tailored financial packages – to give carers practical assistance. Packages are arranged by service providers and can be one-off practical support in the form of equipment or an item to assist in the caring role; or ongoing practical supports, such as respite or transport, provided over a 12-month period.
- In-person counselling – for one-on-one support with a professional counsellor if the carer is feeling stressed or overwhelmed.
- In-person peer support – where carers can meet with people in similar caring situations and share stories, knowledge and experience.
- In-person coaching – where carers can work one-on-one with a qualified coach to gain skills and resilience.
- Emergency respite care – to make sure the person being cared for will be looked after if an urgent or unplanned event stops the carer from being there.

Adapted from Australian Government Department of Social Services (2020).

In December 2019, the New Zealand Government launched its third Carers Strategy Action Plan for Family Carers, Whānau and Aiga 2019–2023 (Ministry of Social Development [MSD] 2019). The renewal of the strategic plan, which has been in place since 2008, once again followed extensive consultation with carer groups in New Zealand. One significant difference between Australian and New Zealand policy is the greater initiative to support carers financially in response to the evidence that women, Māori and Pacific Islanders are more likely to be caregivers and therefore less likely to be able to participate in education or employment. This stance arose following a claim in 2010, called the Atkinson Case, which was taken by a group of families against the New Zealand Government, citing discrimination for not paying family members for undertaking care (NZ Human Rights n.d.). Since this class action, New Zealand policy has taken a lead in acknowledging the negative impacts of caregiving on family carers and recognising the important contributions they make. The plan includes particular attention to the ongoing issues of the need for respite, support when things are not going well, assistance with the increasing financial pressures of caring and a desire for greater carer choice and flexibility (New Zealand MSD 2019).

The four main areas of focus in this latest iteration of the strategy are:

- recognising – ensuring that carers are recognised, valued and acknowledged for the important work they do
- navigating – ensuring carers receive support and services by helping to navigate systems and services
- supporting – ensuring carers are cared for including financial support and carer wellbeing
- balancing – ensuring carers are supported to balance caring with paid work, study and other responsibilities.

Each of these four areas has action plans with leadership expected from carer organisations as well as the government. This approach recognises the knowledge and skill of voluntary and not-for-profit organisations.

As with all initiatives and developments, as indicated in these latest Australian and New Zealand policies, the proof will be in how the services and supports actually provide what is needed for family caregivers. Do the early intervention supports and training reduce the strain on caregivers and support resilience over the long term? Nursing, health and carer organisations will be monitoring the situation, and evaluation has been outlined by both the Australian and the New Zealand governments. Globally, the need to monitor and measure progress has been noted, in particular by the International Alliance of Carer Organisations (IACO).

Globally

The IACO released a report on government support of carers from nine countries in 2018. The *Global State of Care* report reinforces the growing carer movement and recognises advancements around the world (IACO

2018). Despite the enormous impact of family caregivers' work, few countries have policies and systems in place to reduce the economic and social discrimination that many family caregivers encounter. To support the growing movement of caregiver recognition, the IACO has endorsed the development of measures to assess the quality of caregiver support and to make it possible to compare across countries; Australia and New Zealand are two of the 17 IACO member countries. There are six assessment areas:

- Legislation – to ensure rights of caregivers
- Financial support – while caregiving
- Working arrangements – to support flexibility and fair work practices
- Pension credits – to prevent discrimination due to restricted employment
- Respite care – planned and emergency respite
- Information and training – to improve care standards and upskill the family caregivers for care as well as personal health and resilience.

VIEWS OF CAREGIVING

Despite the recent changes in policy and support at government level, daily provision of care for older people remains challenging and sometimes just plain hard, monotonous work. The increasing prevalence of dementia in older Australians and New Zealanders (see also Chapter 26) is a case in point of the demands on family caregivers. This section of the chapter will focus on the research literature that explores family caregiving from multiple perspectives, from family caregiver experience to interventions tested by nurses and other health professionals. The literature will focus wherever possible on Australian and New Zealand studies for context, although all developed countries are experiencing similar issues.

The Family Caregiver Experience

Research uncovering the experiences of family caregivers from their own perspective helps nurses and other health professionals strategise on how best to provide help and support at an individual and family level. Although there is evidence to support the positive elements of family caregiving, such as reciprocation for prior caregiving or keeping one's marriage vows (Morris et al 2015), it can still be hard physical, mental and emotional work.

A landmark study conducted in 1999 demonstrated that primary caregivers were at greater risk for mortality than their non-caregiving counterparts (Schultz & Beach 1999). The research in carer burden, strain and stress

that has burgeoned in the 20 years since this study has continued to confirm that carer strain is significant and has negative impacts on both the caregiver and the care-receiver (Family Caregiver Alliance 2006a). Although subsequent research and meta-analysis disputes the claim that long-term caregiving increases the risk of premature death (Roth et al 2015), there is still considerable evidence that caregiving is challenging, affecting physical, mental, emotional, financial and social outcomes in the caregiver. This phenomenon is most often found in caregivers who do not have sufficient support from other family members, health professionals or the healthcare system. Older carers are particularly vulnerable to social isolation as they look after a partner or spouse. The demands on older carers reduces their ability to take part in social activities, which can result in a lack of social connectedness and loneliness. They are also more likely to be managing their own health conditions and require support themselves, alongside dealing with the demands of being a carer (New Zealand MSD 2019).

A well-conducted meta-analysis on caregiver interventions by Adelman and colleagues (2014) summarised which people are at greatest risk for caregiver strain:

- women
- low educational attainment
- living with the care recipient
- higher number of hours spent caregiving
- depression
- socially isolated
- financial stress
- lack of choice in being a caregiver.

Given the importance and essential contribution of family caregiving to healthcare, it is imperative that nurses and other health professionals partner with family caregivers to ensure they have the knowledge and skills to provide care to their older relative. Supporting and coaching others, rather than being direct caregivers, is something of a shift away from the way nurses are currently educated. Nurses' knowledge and skills need to be adapted to educate, train, support and coach carers to provide direct care. Results of the Adelman and colleagues (2014) meta-analysis demonstrated that most improvements in caregiver strain (such as mood, coping, self-efficacy) were achieved with multi-component interventions focused on support and psycho-educational strategies. This kind of evidence has been applied in the Australian and New Zealand implementation policies for carers.

There are risk factors that increase the potential for caregiver strain, but there are also crisis points that make caregiving more complicated and emotionally stressful. Two examples of this are hospitalisation and being a family caregiver to an older relative in a residential aged care facility.

Acute Care Setting

Much interaction with health professionals of all kinds occurs when the older person is admitted to hospital for acute medical or surgical care, where health professionals are least likely to specialise in gerontology or the intricacies of family caregiving. This is further complicated when the older person has dementia and/or is experiencing delirium. Findings from a grounded theory study in an acute hospital in the UK found that all those involved – the person with dementia, family caregivers, co-patients (those sharing the ward but without dementia) and staff – found the presence of a person with dementia to be disruptive to their usual practice and routine (Clissett et al 2013a; Porock et al 2015). This often resulted in a poor experience for family carers, who had difficulties in communicating and interacting with staff, trying to help where co-patients were affected, and trying to help with direct caregiving (Clissett et al 2013b). Staff often found family carers demanding. Family carers felt excluded and their knowledge of the older person overlooked, making discharge planning difficult (Clissett et al 2013a).

Fetherstonhaugh and McAuliffe's (2019) qualitative study of surrogate decision-makers eloquently describes the frustrations and anxieties around making decisions for the older person with dementia. This was particularly evident in the hospital setting where they described family caregivers as needing to challenge healthcare professionals. They called for professionals to be empathic guides on the caregiving journey.

Moyle and colleagues (2016) found that family carers wanted to be involved with direct care when a family member with dementia was admitted to hospital. However, as the article title succinctly reports, staff 'rush you and push you ... and you can't really get a good response off them'. Staff did not consider the ways in which care was routinely provided at home, but expected the family caregiver to provide care how, when and where it was done in the hospital. This study recommended that family carers in the acute setting need:

- a central source of information
- educated staff
- guidelines on the rules and processes in the hospital

- positive communication
- respect from staff for the carer's knowledge
- to be included in medical discussions about treatment and care.

It does not seem much to ask, and it looks logical, but unfortunately the hospital machine of protocols, timings and expectations of behaviour are very rigid. Nurses are as much a part of the problem here, but they are potentially a large part of the solution.

Residential Aged Care Setting

Another stressor for family caregivers is the decision to change caregiving arrangements, particularly where placement of the older person into residential aged care is required. Decision-making on behalf of another is difficult in itself (Fetherstonhaugh & McAuliffe 2019) and known to be frightening and frustrating. The decision to place someone in long-term care is even more complex and difficult. Couture and colleagues' (2020) comprehensive systematic review found that the process is fraught with anxiety and guilt and extremely value-laden, where the family caregiver has to first evaluate the current living arrangements and come to terms with their own inability to care for the older person at home. The process of finding an acceptable placement in residential aged care then becomes possible, but again appraisal and evaluation is arduous and interpreted through a highly value-laden lens, including what others might think.

Even when relocation to aged care has occurred, family carers report varying degrees of feeling included in care and decision-making. Family inclusion is presented in the marketing for aged care as something that is natural and occurs easily (Verleye et al 2011). The nursing literature reports that increased family inclusion leads to more family satisfaction with care provided to residents and an enriched sense of wellbeing for themselves (Cohen et al 2014; Nguyen et al 2017). Furthermore, there are advantages for staff members from family members providing help (Roberts 2020). Despite these glowing benefits, studies testing family inclusion interventions portray a different situation. Puurveen and colleagues (2018) found that family members were marginalised in case conferences and where 'expert one-way communication' from staff to family was documented. A study by Maas and colleagues (2004) found that staff felt judged and monitored by families, constantly under scrutiny and that it was difficult for them to feel relaxed with the residents.

These are very difficult circumstances, particularly given that aged care facilities see their residents as being at home – yet both family caregivers and staff caregivers can feel quite uncomfortable. This is certainly an area for further research and staff development.

CARING FOR FAMILY CAREGIVERS

As nurses and health professionals, we need to carefully assess our attitudes to family caregivers and where they fit in the multidisciplinary healthcare team. Two quotes from a keynote speech given by a family caregiver illustrate the things that healthcare workers forget about family caregivers and reinforce what is needed. The first quote comes from a caregiver whose friend had suffered a brain aneurysm and spent the last 20 years of their life in a residential aged care facility:

> Will you remember what I said about my dear friend in his nursing home and think only of a 50-year-old who will spend each and every remaining day of his life dependent on others for all of his basic daily needs? Or will you please remember his elderly mother too? Will you think of her needs and how she is his lifeline to his sanity and to his emotional wellbeing and who without fanfare has spent the last 20 years of her life re-parenting a man she already raised? (Family Caregiver Alliance 2006b:10).

In the second quote, the family caregiver challenges audience members to reconsider their attitude to family caregivers and asks health professionals to commit themselves to genuine partnering:

> Will you leave this conference and view caregivers as being extraordinary people who happened to be dealt a tough hand? You see, that's not what caregivers want from you. What caregivers want and need is the formal recognition that is the commitment of your intelligence, your resources, and your acknowledgment that without family caregivers, we have missed the real truth to this whole caregiving agenda (Family Caregiver Alliance 2006b:10).

Nurses can commit their collective intelligence and resources, and acknowledge the necessity of partnership with family caregivers, to:

- ensure a thorough and comprehensive assessment of needs
- provide training and encouragement in skills and resilience
- offer tangible support so the carer can be successful in the role.

Florence Nightingale once claimed that 'there is no such thing as amateur nursing' (Monteiro 1985). If that is the case, then by extending the nursing ranks to the family caregiver, the profession has a duty to recognise the family caregiver and to guide and coach them with nursing knowledge and skills. See *Promoting wellness: Caring for the caregiver* for strategies to support caregivers.

Promoting Wellness
Caring for the Caregiver

Caring for an older person can be an immensely satisfying and meaningful experience. However, caregivers can experience stress and fatigue, which can lead to poor health outcomes. The Australian Government Carer Gateway website emphasises the need for caregivers to care for their own mental and physical health. Not only is this important for caregivers' wellbeing, it also recognises that mentally and physically healthy caregivers can provide better care to the older person and potentially care for longer. Here are some suggested strategies.

SUPPORTING CAREGIVER MENTAL HEALTH

1. If the caregiver is very stressed or requires urgent help: In Australia, contact Lifeline on 131144 or lifeline.org.au; or BeyondBlue on 1300 224 636 or www.beyondblue.org.au/get-support/get-immediate-support. In New Zealand, contact Lifeline New Zealand on 0800 543 354 or www.lifeline.org.nz/

2. Caregivers may find that talking with someone can help to relieve worry and stress:
   - Professional counselling can help the caregiver talk through worries. See counselling resources for details of how to obtain phone- and web-based support.
   - Caregivers can also find local services for counselling at home or in a private clinic. The option to obtain a mental health care plan that will fund up to 20 appointments with mental health services is available through Medicare (in Australia).
   - Some caregivers may like to join a carer support group, either in the community or online. Groups are usually free and meet at a public place, such as a community hall or hospital.

Continued

Promoting Wellness
Caring for the Caregiver—cont'd

3. Using relaxation and mindfulness have been shown to help with preventing and managing stress:
   - Practise meditation and breathing techniques to promote relaxation.
   - Mindfulness is about focusing on the present rather than thinking about the past or worrying about the future. It can help the caregiver to enjoy day-to-day pleasures. Mindfulness can be learnt from instructors. Also organisations such as the Black Dog Institute (www.blackdoginstitute.org.au/resources-support/wellbeing/) have tips on mindfulness.

4. Encourage the caregiver to think of their own needs. This might include:
   - taking a break from caring to keep up their own social activities and interact with other people
   - staying physically healthy (see Supporting caregiver physical health, opposite)
   - asking for help when needed (see point 1 above).

5. Getting help with stress
   - Self-guided coaching can help the caregiver to learn to deal with stress. Organisations such as This Way Up (https://thiswayup.org.au/) and Mindspot Clinic (https://mindspot.org.au/) run online courses on many topics including stress, anxiety and depression (see also Chapter 25).
   - Caregivers can talk to their General Practitioner about ways to manage stress.
   - Other organisations providing help to deal with stress include:
     - Healthdirect (www.healthdirect.gov.au/stress)
     - Beyond Blue (www.beyondblue.org.au/get-support/get-immediate-support)
     - Black Dog Institute (www.blackdoginstitute.org.au/resources-support/depression/)
     - Head to Health (https://headtohealth.gov.au/).
   - Utilise respite care: respite care is when someone else takes care of the older person so that the caregiver can have time to themselves to rest and recharge, take care of daily activities and deal with stress. To organise emergency respite care, call Carer Gateway on 1800 422 737. Otherwise, My Aged Care may be able to organise community or residential respite care. This requires that both the older person and the caregiver are assessed to determine which services are most suitable. Contact My Aged Care on 1800 200 422 or www.myagedcare.gov.au/short-term-care/respite-care

SUPPORTING CAREGIVER PHYSICAL HEALTH

1. Maintain an adequate nutritious diet. A guide to choosing healthy foods is available at The Australian Guide to Healthy Eating (www.eatforhealth.gov.au/guidelines/australian-guide-healthy-eating) (see also Chapter 12).

2. Sleep well. Most adults need 7–9 hours of sleep per night, but caregivers can find this difficult. Tips for a better night's sleep are available at Healthdirect (www.healthdirect.gov.au/healthy-sleep-habits) (see also Chapter 14).

3. Exercise: Caregivers should aim to have some exercise every day. This can range from a regular walk to going to the gym. Tips for how to get active are available at Healthdirect (www.healthdirect.gov.au/tips-for-getting-active).

4. Don't smoke. One of the best things a caregiver, and indeed all people, can do for their health is not to smoke. Tips and tools to help with quitting smoking are available at Quit Now (www.health.gov.au/health-topics/smoking-and-tobacco/how-to-quit-smoking).

5. Maintain a moderate alcohol intake. Healthy adults should drink no more than two standard drinks of alcohol per day. The Australian Government Department of Health website provides information on how to reduce or quit drinking alcohol (www.health.gov.au/health-topics/alcohol/about-alcohol/how-much-alcohol-is-safe-to-drink?).

Adapted from Australian Government Carer Gateway (2020).

> **Tips for Best Practice**
> *Support for Carers Experiencing Stress*
>
> **AUSTRALIA**
>
> Carer Gateway Counselling Service: Phone 1800 422 737. Or request a callback by visiting www.carergateway.org.au/s/
>
> Lifeline (Australia): Call on 131144 or lifeline.org.au
>
> BeyondBlue: Call on 1300 224 636 or www.beyondblue.org.au/get-support/get-immediate-support
>
> Black Dog Institute: www.blackdoginstitute.org.au/resources-support/depression/
>
> **NEW ZEALAND**
>
> Carers NZ Helpline: Call on 0800 777 797 or http://carers.net.nz/services/
>
> Lifeline New Zealand: Call on 0800 543 354 or www.lifeline.org.nz/

> **Tips for Best Practice**
> *Principles of Caregiver Assessment*
>
> 1. Because family caregivers are a core part of healthcare and long-term care, it is important to recognise, respect, assess and address their needs.
> 2. Caregiver assessment should embrace a family-centred perspective, inclusive of the needs and preferences of both the older person and the family caregiver.
> 3. Caregiver assessment should result in a plan of care (developed collaboratively with the caregiver) that indicates the provision of services and intended measurable outcomes.
> 4. Caregiver assessment should be multidimensional in approach and periodically updated.
> 5. Caregiver assessment should reflect culturally competent practice.
> 6. Effective caregiver assessment requires assessors to have specialised knowledge and skills. Practitioners' and service providers' education and training should equip them with an understanding of the caregiving process and its impacts, as well as the benefits and elements of an effective caregiver assessment.
> 7. Government and other third-party payers should recognise and pay for caregiver assessment as a part of care for older people and adults with disabilities.

Family Caregiver Alliance (2006a:12).

ASSESSMENT

Adelman and colleagues' (2014) meta-analysis concluded that one of the most important interventions for caregiver burden was assessment of caregiver needs and addressing those individually. Significantly, both the Australian and the New Zealand caregiver strategies place assessment of need at the centre of plans. Caregiver assessment refers to a systematic process of gathering information that describes a caregiving situation and identifies the particular problems, needs, resources and strengths of the family caregiver. It approaches issues from the caregiver's perspective and culture, focuses on what assistance the caregiver may need and the outcomes the family member wants for support and seeks to maintain the caregiver's own health and wellbeing (Family Caregiver Alliance 2006a). The *Tips for best practice: Principles of caregiver assessment* summarises the principles of the caregiver assessment that should apply across healthcare service settings. It should be noted that periodic reassessment is also necessary, partly as an evaluation of previous assessments and to ensure adaptation to changing care requirements of the care receiver.

Table 28.2 lists all the domains for assessment, some of which are clearly needed at the initial assessment and others that are suitable for reassessment. It is important to note that these assessment content areas need to be developed in collaboration with others in the healthcare team. A decision needs to be made in the team about who conducts all or parts of the assessment (e.g. nurse, social worker), what triggers assessment and reassessment and how frequently reassessment takes

place. A system also needs to be put in place about where and how the assessment is documented and communicated with the healthcare team, caregiver and the older person receiving the care.

For much of the time during interactions, health professionals simply need to check in with family caregivers and provide an opportunity for expression of concerns, changes and small victories. Quickly assessing how the family is doing, including the family caregiver and older person, could be achieved by asking: 'Are you satisfied with the way you and your family share time together?' (Takenaka & Ban 2016). Alternatively, the reliable and valid three-item dementia caregiver burden screening tool (Liew & Yap 2018) directs the nurse to ask:

- 'Are you afraid what the future holds for your relative?'
- 'Do you feel your health has suffered because of your involvement with your relative?'
- 'Do you feel you have lost control of your life since your relative's illness?'

TABLE 28.2
Domains of Caregiver Assessment

Domain	Assessment Content
Context	• Caregiver relationship to care recipient • Physical environment (home, facility) • Household status (number in home etc.) • Financial status • Quality of family relationships • Duration of caregiving • Employment status (work/home/volunteer)
Caregiver's perception of health and functional status of care recipient	• ADLs and need for supervision • Instrumental ADLs (managing finances, using the phone) • Psychosocial needs • Cognitive impairment • Behavioural problems • Medical tests and procedures
Caregiver values and preferences	• Caregiver/care recipient willingness to assume/accept care • Perceived filial obligation to provide care • Culturally based norms • Preferences for scheduling and delivery of care and services
Well-being of the caregiver	• Self-rated health • Health conditions and symptoms • Depression and other emotional distress • Life satisfaction/quality of life
Consequences of caregiving	Perceived challenges • Social isolation • Work strain • Emotional and physical health strain • Financial strain • Family relationship strain Perceived benefits • Satisfaction of helping family member • Developing new skills and competencies • Improved family relationships
Skills/abilities/knowledge to provide needed care	• Caregiving confidence and competencies • Appropriate knowledge of medical care tasks (e.g. wound care)
Potential resources that caregiver could choose to use	• Formal and informal helping network and perceived quality of social support • Existing or potential strengths (e.g. what is going well now) • Coping strategies • Financial resources (e.g. benefits) • Community resources and services (e.g. caregiver support programs, volunteer agencies, religious organisations)

ADLs: activities of daily living
Family Caregiver Alliance (2006a:16).

However assessment is done, the key to successful support of the family caregiver is good communication, along with multi-component training and support interventions.

Several recent studies and meta-analyses have been conducted, demonstrating, in various settings:

• the importance of communication (e.g. Aoun et al 2018; Nguyen et al 2019),
• preparedness for caregiving (Mason et al 2019) and training (Aksoydan et al 2019),
• multi-component interventions (Adelman et al 2014; Abrahams et al 2018).

These and other similar studies have provided the evidence for the policy changes in Australia and New Zealand that set global standards in caring for family caregivers. More research is needed to further develop the evidence base for family caregiving as an expanding area of nursing practice. For those particularly interested in this area refer to the International Family Nursing Association.

Research Highlight

The Further Enabling Care at Home (FECH) program was developed and trialled with family carers of older people after discharge from an Australian hospital. The FECH program is a phone-based nursing intervention, in which a registered nurse, who is experienced in older person's healthcare, guides carers to identify and address their own needs for support during a series of phone contacts in the weeks following the older person's hospital discharge. The FECH nurse then supports the carer to access information and resources to sustain home-based caregiving. The FECH program was evaluated in a randomised controlled trial with carers of older patients discharged from the Medical Assessment Unit at a Western Australian Hospital. Results showed that carers who received the FECH program in addition to usual post-discharge care (intervention, $n = 62$) were more prepared to care compared to carers who received only usual care (controls, $n = 79$), both soon after receiving the FECH program (effect size = 0.52; $p = 0.006$), and at follow-up (effect size = 0.43; $p = 0.019$). Small but significant positive impacts were observed in other outcomes, including caregiver strain.

Toye et al (2016).

SUMMARY

In this chapter, the most recent policy and implementation strategies to recognise and support the essential work of family caregivers in Australia and New Zealand have been introduced and discussed. An overview of the issues facing family caregivers, with a particular focus on assessing caregiver needs in order to individualise training and support, has been presented. It is most important even when providing direct nursing care to an older person, that the nurse considers the family caregiver, recognises them for the knowledge and expertise they have in caring for the older person, and ensuring that communication is clear and positive. After all, successful care in the community relies almost entirely on the family caregiver.

Practice Scenario

Jane is the 55-year-old daughter of Vera, aged 78 years who has been living with Jane's family since she was widowed 2 years ago. Jane is married to Allen and they have two children living at home – Amy aged 26, a newly graduated lawyer working in a large city law practice, and Jeremy aged 23, studying at university. Jane enjoys having her mother with her and provides daily support, as well as running her own interior design business. Vera has mild cognitive impairment (see Chapter 26), a heart condition, and osteoarthritis in her left hip and knee. However, she is usually mobile with a walking frame, able to manage her showering and toileting, and enjoys some gentle gardening. Three weeks ago, Vera scraped her right ankle in the garden and developed a venous ulcer, which became infected and is being treated by her GP. Jane brings Vera to you as the practice nurse for weekly wound dressings.

At their second visit, Jane tells you that Vera seems to have a lot of pain from the leg ulcer. Vera is not sleeping and is very restless at night and, while she takes her antibiotics, has little appetite. Jane thinks Vera looks exhausted and is finding that she can't do much for herself now. Jane has noticed that Vera has more trouble finding words and often forgets to use her walking frame. She wonders whether Vera has more pain from the arthritis in her hip and knee because she quite quickly becomes restless when sitting in her chair, calling out and trying to get up.

REVIEW QUESTIONS

1. What might be the impacts on Jane of the changes in Vera's condition?
2. Using a family-centred and multidimensional approach, how could you assess Jane's current caregiving needs?
3. What might a plan of care, developed collaboratively with Jane, include?
4. Where could you guide Jane to find more information and supportive resources?

ADDITIONAL RESOURCES

Carers Australia: www.carersaustralia.com.au/
Carer Gateway: www.carergateway.gov.au/
Carers NZ: carers.net.nz/
International Carers: https://internationalcarers.org/
International Family Nursing Association: https://internationalfamilynursing.org/
New Zealand Carers Strategy and Action Plan: https://msd.govt.nz/about-msd-and-our-work/work-programmes/policy-development/carers-strategy/

REFERENCES

Abrahams R, Liu K, Bissett M et al (2018) Effectiveness of interventions for co-residing family caregivers of people with dementia: Systematic review and meta-analysis. Australian Occupational Therapy Journal 65(3):208–224.

Adelman RD, Tmanova LL, Delgado D et al (2014) Caregiver burden: a clinical review. JAMA 311(10):1052–1060.

Aksoydan E, Aytar A, Blazeviciene A et al (2019) Is training for informal caregivers and their older persons helpful? A systematic review. Archives of Gerontology and Geriatrics 83(201907):66–74.

Aoun SM, Stegmann R, Slatyer S et al (2019) Hospital post-discharge intervention trialled with family caregivers of older people in Western Australia: Potential translation into practice. Health and Social Care in the Community 27(4):926–935.

Associated Press-NORC Center for Public Affairs Research (2018). Long-term caregiving: the true costs of caring for aging adults. AP-NORC, University of Chicago.

Australian Bureau of Statistics (2018) Disability, ageing and carers, Australia: Summary of Findings, 2018. Online. Available: www.abs.gov.au/ausstats/abs@.nsf/mf/4430.0

Australian Government Carer Gateway (2020), Looking after yourself. Online Available: www.carergateway.gov.au/help-advice/looking-after-yourself

Australian Government Department of Social Services (2020) New services for carers. Online. Available: www.dss.gov.au/sites/default/files/documents/02_2020/dac_new-services-carers_20200220.pdf

Carers Australia (2019) Annual report 2018–2019. Care Australia, Melbourne.

Carers New Zealand (n.d.) Carers New Zealand. Online. Available: http://carers.net.nz/

Clissett P, Porock D, Harwood RH et al (2013a) Experiences of family carers of older people with mental health problems in the acute general hospital: a qualitative study. Journal of Advanced Nursing 69(12):2707–2716.

Clissett P, Porock D, Harwood RH et al (2013b) The responses of healthcare professionals to the admission of people with cognitive impairment to acute hospital settings: an observational and interview study. Journal of Clinical Nursing 23:1820–1829.

Cohen LW, Zimmerman S, Reed D et al (2014) Dementia in relation to family caregiver involvement and burden in long-term care. Journal of Applied Gerontology 33(5):522–540.

Couture M, Ducharme F, Sasseville M et al (2019) A qualitative systematic review of factors affecting caregivers' decision making for care setting placements for individuals with dementia. Geriatric Nursing 41(2):172–180.

Deloitte Access Economics (2015) The economic value of informal care in Australia. Online. Available: www2.deloitte.com/au/en/pages/economics/articles/economic-value-informal-care-Australia-2015.html

Donelan K, Hill CA, Hoffman C et al (2002) Challenged to care: Informal caregivers in a changing health system. Health Affairs 21:222–231.

Family Caregiver Alliance (2006) Caregiver assessment: principles, guidelines and strategies for change. Report from a National Consensus Development Conference (Vol. I). San Francisco: Author.

Family Caregiver Alliance (2006) Caregiver assessment: principles, guidelines and strategies for change. Report from a National Consensus Development Conference (Vol. II). San Francisco: Author.

Fetherstonhaugh D, McAuliffe L (2019) Did I make the right decision?: The difficult and unpredictable journey of being a surrogate decision maker for a person living with dementia. Dementia 18(5):1601–1614.

Infometrics (2014). The economic value and impacts of informal caregivers in New Zealand. Online. Available: https://cdn.auckland.ac.nz/assets/auckland/about-us/equity-at-the-university/equity-information-staff/information-for-carers/The%20economic%20value%20of%20informal%20care%20in%20New%20Zealand%20Final%20copy.pdf

International Alliance of Carer Organisations [IACO] (2018) Global state of care. Online Available: https://internationalcarers.org/publications/

Jorgensen D, Parsons M, Jacobs S et al (2010) The New Zealand informal caregivers and their unmet needs. The New Zealand Medical Journal 123(1317):9.

Liew TM, Yap P (2019) A 3-item screening scale for caregiver burden in dementia caregiving: Scale development and score mapping to the 22-item Zarit burden interview. Journal of the American Medical Directors Association 20:629–633.

Maas ML, Reed D, Park M et al (2004) Outcomes of family involvement in care intervention for caregivers of individuals with dementia. Nursing Research 53(2):76–86.

Mason N, Hodgken S (2018) Preparedness for caregiving: A phenomenological study of the experiences of rural Australian family palliative carers. British Medical Journal Open Access 8(11):e022747.

Mair FS, May CR (2014) Thinking about the burden of treatment. British Medical Journal 349:g6680

May CR, Eton DT, Boehmer K et al (2014) Rethinking the patient: using Burden of Treatment Theory to understand the changing dynamics of illness. BMC Health Services Research 14:281.

Ministry of Social Development [MSD] (2019) Carers Strategy Action Plan for Family Carers, Whānau and Aiga 2019-2023. Online. Available: https://msd.govt.nz/about-msd-and-our-work/work-programmes/policy-development/carers-strategy/

Monteiro L (1985) Florence Nightingale on public health nursing. American Journal of Public Health 75(2):181–218.

Morris SM, King C, Turner M et al (2015) Family carers providing support to a person dying in the home setting: A narrative literature review. Palliative Medicine 29(6):487–495.

Moyle W, Bramble M, Bauer M et al (2016) 'They rush you and push you too much … and you can't really get any good response off them': A qualitative examination of family involvement in care of people with dementia in acute care. Australasian Journal on Ageing 35(2):E30–E34.

NZ Human Rights (n.d.) Caring for disabled adult family members. Online. Available: www.hrc.co.nz/enquiries-and-complaints/faqs/caring-disabled-adult-family-members/

New Zealand Ministry of Social Development (2019) Mahi Aroha. Carers Strategy and Action Plan 2019–2023. Online. Available: https://msd.govt.nz/about-msd-and-our-work/work-programmes/policy-development/carers-strategy/

Nguyen M, Beattie E, Fielding E et al (2017) Experiences of family–staff relationships in the care of people with dementia in residential aged care: a qualitative systematic review protocol. JBI database of systematic reviews and implementation reports 15(3):586–593.

Nguyen H, Terry D, Phan H et al (2019) Communication training and its effects on carer and care-receiver outcomes in dementia settings: A systematic review. Journal of Clinical Nursing 28(7–8):1050–1069.

Porock D, Clissett P, Harwood RH et al (2015) Disruption, control and coping: responses of and to the person with dementia in hospital. Ageing & Society 35:37–63.

Puurveen G, Cooke H, Gill R et al (2018) A seat at the table: The positioning of families during care conferences in nursing homes. The Gerontologist 59(5):835–844.

Roberts AR, Ishler KJ, Adams KB (2020) The predictors of and motivations for increased family involvement in nursing homes. The Gerontologist 60(3):535–547.

Roth DL, Fredman L, Haley WE (2015) Informal caregiving and its impact on health: a reappraisal from population-based studies. The Gerontologist 55(2):309–319.

Schulz R, Beach SR (1999) Caregiving as a risk factor for mortality: the caregiver health effects study. Journal of the American Medical Association 282(23):2215–2219.

Takenaka H, Ban N (2016) The most important question in family approach: the potential of the resolve item of the family APGAR in family medicine. Asia Pacific Family Medicine 15(3) online DOI: 10.1186/s12930-016-0028-9

Toye C, Parsons R, Slatyer S et al (2016) Outcomes for family carers of a nurse-delivered hospital discharge intervention for older people (the Further Enabling Care at Home Program): Single blind randomised controlled trial. International Journal of Nursing Studies 64:32–41.

Vachon ML (1980) Care for the caregiver. The Canadian Nurse Journal 76(10):23–33.

Verleye K, Gemmel P, Rangarajan D (2011) Why indirect customers deserve managers' attention: a quantitative and qualitative study on indirect customer engagement behaviour. In 12th Annual International Research Symposium on Service Excellence in Mangement (QUIS12-2011).

CHAPTER 29

Loss, Grief and Bereavement in Later Life

MARGARET SEALEY

LEARNING OBJECTIVES

After reading this chapter you will be able to:

- differentiate between loss, grief, mourning and bereavement
- explain the cultural influences on loss and grief
- describe the main factors that influence an older person's risk of developing complicated, prolonged or persistent grief
- describe nursing responses to assist older people experiencing ambiguous loss
- describe communication strategies to support a bereaved older person.

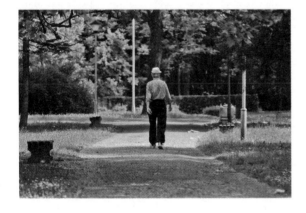

INTRODUCTION

Dominating the landscape of later life includes change, loss and grief. As Humphrey and Zimpfer (1996) state, events involving change are losses that may provoke grief and often require '… that some part of the individual be left behind and grieved before the process of transition and rebuilding can occur' (p. 1). However, while change necessitating transition is a given in later life, rebuilding may not be as easy as it was in younger adulthood. Generally, ongoing losses encountered in transitional periods are overlooked, with loss and grief usually only associated with death and dying. However, all losses have the potential to shatter what one understands as a just world, but grief provides the means to mend that shattered world (Winokuer & Harris 2016). We should also be mindful that the encounter of loss is very much an individual experience, whereby two people may interpret the same event differently – one negatively, one positively (Murray 2016).

Grief

Grief is defined as a reaction to loss; often it is painful and creates suffering. There is no prescribed or 'correct' way to grieve, rather grief responses are unique to the individual. Grief affects one's physical, cognitive, psychological, social and spiritual domains, which all influence behaviour. All domains may be involved, others may be affected in part, or not be affected at all (DeSpelder & Strickland 2015). Examples of responses across the psychosocial spiritual domains can include (but are not limited to):

- heart palpitations, headaches, fatigue, irritability, anxiety, sadness, crying
- difficulty concentrating
- forgetfulness
- disorientation
- withdrawal
- altered sleeping patterns
- difficulty accommodating the changes (Murray 2016).

In the event of a death, those who are newly bereaved typically report a sense of disbelief or numbness, yet experience intense emotional pain; a yearning for the deceased accompanied by searching for their loved one, knowing that he or she is no longer present; sadness and an inability to engage in enjoyable activities or interests; and/or a sense of meaninglessness or purpose in life without the deceased. Despite the intense suffering following a loss, most bereaved people have internal resources and support to eventually adjust to life without their deceased loved one (Lundorff et al 2017).

The experiences of loss and grief are universal; that is, they affect everyone at some point in time. People generally interpret the idea of loss and grief as painful events and transition periods in life that can be commonly understood by all; however, loss and grief are very much individually experienced and, as such, there is no 'one-size-fits-all' or right way to react to loss and grief (Murray 2016).

Mourning

The idea that grief responses follow certain patterns and are expressed in obvious ways may stem from confusion with the concept of mourning. Mourning refers to the socially sanctioned expression of grief, which includes customs that are common to a culture (Stroebe, Hanseson et al 2010). Examples include periods of time where the bereaved person is expected to show signs of grief (such as not attending to work); to wear particular clothing; and participate in rituals such as a funeral or body disposal. Mourning can also be thought of as the internal process of adjusting to the loss, a necessary process if the individual is to integrate the loss into his or her life (Murray 2016).

Mourning and grief are therefore easily confused. It is often impossible to say whether someone who is crying is responding to an emotional grief reaction or responding to a societal requirement to express grief (Stroebe, Hanseson et al 2010). What is observed may not have any bearing on the individual's internal experience, emphasising the need to try to understand the nature of the loss and change, as well as the impact of such events on each individual.

Bereavement

Bereavement is the tangible condition of having lost someone significant. It encompasses the pain and suffering of grief, which enables one to integrate the loss and heal (Stroebe, Hanseson et al 2010). Parkes and Prigerson (2010) suggest that in bereavement what is lost is not obvious; for example, the loss of a husband may mean the loss of a sexual partner, confidant or handyman, or any number of things. With any loss there are usually secondary losses which add to distress, such as loss of income or loss of home.

CHANGE AND LOSS IN OLDER AGE

While change across the entire life span brings about inevitable challenges, transitions and losses, in the later stage of life the very process of ageing and accompanying disability in many cases add to the individual's sense of loss. Some examples of ageing are changes in appearance, e.g. wrinkled skin, greying hair, physical changes, such as impaired eyesight and hearing; and cognitive changes, i.e. decline in explicit memory and information processing speed (Santrock 2014).

Chronic Disease

Today, with an increased average life expectancy, many older people now live with chronic illness. It is expected that approximately 60% of Australians aged 65 years and older are living with at least two of eight chronic health conditions: arthritis, back pain (Chapter 22), asthma and other pulmonary disease (Chapter 24), cardiovascular disease (Chapter 23), cancer, diabetes (Chapter 9), mental health conditions (Chapter 25), and dementia (Chapter 26). Similarly, in New Zealand people are living longer but are also living with the same co-morbid chronic health conditions that affect Australians. For New Zealanders, neuropsychiatric disorders are the leading cause of health issues, while musculoskeletal disorders and cardiovascular disease continue to cause disability (Ministry of Health NZ 2016). Health system approaches to care focus on 'recovery' within a person-centred framework (see Chapter 26); however, in an ageing population, mental health disorders such as depression and anxiety co-exist with organ dysfunction such as dementia and cancer, presenting challenges for health professionals (McKenna et al 2014). Additionally, care of chronic disease is increasingly managed in outpatient settings requiring family carers to undertake complex tasks for which they have little or no training

(May et al 2014). When also considering the carer's emotional ties to the older person, carers are vulnerable to distress, which generally has a negative impact on the carer's emotional and physical health, particularly with advancing age (Slatyer et al 2019).

Retirement

Adjusting from an active work life to retirement is also characteristic of this stage of life and can be a source of stress and loss as people transition socially and financially to a changing lifestyle (see Chapter 27). In Australia and New Zealand, typical patterns of work and retirement have changed with the baby boomer generation now reaching retirement age. While there is no official retirement age in New Zealand (New Zealand Government 2018), people are currently eligible for the age pension at 66 years in Australia (Australian Government Department of Human Services 2019). The Australian 2016–17 Multipurpose Household Survey (MPHS) indicated that 64% of those aged between 65 and 69 years of age were retired, while 82% of those aged over 70 were retired. Following retirement in both countries, individuals report their main sources of income as stemming from the government pension/allowance and superannuation (Australian Bureau of Statistics [ABS] 2017). This means that for many people finances may be of concern.

Global financial problems have prevented many older people from retiring, with research showing that despite being loyal employees and productive workers, ageism and stereotyping negatively affect employability (Radford et al 2018). For those approaching retirement who have identified strongly with their work, and for those who experience health issues, financial problems and/or stresses, such as the death of a spouse, adjustment to retirement can be very difficult and creates a sense of loss and grief that is difficult to reconcile (Santrock 2014).

COPING AND ADJUSTING TO CHANGE AND LOSS

Such losses are cumulative and come from a multitude of different sources, which may or may not be within the individual's control (Boerner & Jopp 2007). As postulated by Erikson (1963), when confronted by change or loss, some individuals respond with remarkable resilience, while others develop ongoing problems. A number of theories help explain why this might be so. Central to such theories is the idea that development is an ongoing process of adapting to physical and psychosocial changes; however, the theories vary on the underlying mechanisms of coping with change (Boerner & Jopp 2007).

Dual-Process Model of Assimilative and Accommodative Coping

This model proposes two mechanisms people use to cope with change. The *assimilative mode* requires an active effort to adapt to the given circumstances in order to achieve one's goals. This may involve knowledge or skill acquisition, the use of aids or a change in lifestyle to help compensate the loss. In the *accommodative mode*, the individual readjusts by reviewing and renegotiating goals considering current limitations. When change and loss occur, the individual is likely to employ assimilative strategies to close the gap; however, with irretractable loss or change, accommodative strategies tend to be more effective (Brandtstädter & Renner 1990). Recent research on this model confirms the usefulness of this theory, but shows that it can take several months before older people adapt to their age-related losses (Loidl & Leipold 2019).

Model of Selection, Optimisation and Compensation (SOC)

Based on the premise that resources are limited across the life span, people will adapt to their circumstances by minimising losses and maximising gains, particularly as they age. *Selection* refers to the setting of goals, which may be intentional or subconscious. This may be an elective decision based on choice, or a loss-centred decision to compensate for a loss in resources. *Optimisation* refers to the ability one has to acquire and maintain resources needed for a desired outcome. *Compensation* refers to acquiring or activating resources as substitutes to compensate for the loss or change (Baltes et al 2014).

Life-Span Theory of Control

Behaviour aimed at gaining control in the face of loss or change may be either primary or secondary. Primary control is aimed towards controlling the external environment, while secondary control is focused on how one might adapt one's self to accommodate the changes (Heckhausen & Schulz 1995).

CULTURAL INFLUENCES ON LOSS AND GRIEF

From cradle to grave, life is a continuous series of changes, often stimulating a loss response in the individual. Erikson (1963) believed that the individual's readiness to interact with a broadening social radius was the condition necessary to successfully negotiate each life stage. Regardless of how healthy an individual is, or how well she or he adapts, loss features prominently in older age, yet it is often only acknowledged when it occurs with death. To understand why this is, we need to be aware of the role culture plays in one's response to death, loss and grief, and how it is shaped by whether the society in question is death-denying, death-accepting or death-defying (Murray 2016).

According to Klass and Chow (2011), culture can be defined as how a group of people interpret and make sense of their world. Culture regulates grief with rules about how grief should be expressed, and how bonds with the deceased should be handled. Multicultural societies, such as Australia and New Zealand, will therefore have a vast range of rules and rituals relating to dying, death and bereavement. Many cultures place great importance on continuing bonds with the deceased, while some societies believe that breaking bonds is necessary. Many Australian Aboriginal cultures participate in 'sorry business' in bereavement and the name of the deceased person is not spoken again as a sign of respect. In New Zealand, Māori people come together as family units to support each other and observe practices across the period from death into bereavement (Santrock 2014). Other cultures observe ancestor rituals that define the identity and values of the family (Klass & Chow 2011). While a culture may have imperatives about death, dying and grief, it is worth remembering that individuals will also be influenced by family rules and may not adhere to the cultural group's norms.

Like many Western societies, Australia and New Zealand also have a curious and perhaps ambiguous relationship with death. Mostly, death is quarantined so as not to contaminate life. Euphemisms such as 'kicked the bucket' or 'passing on' are often used rather than 'dying'. Death avoidance is particularly common in healthcare, where some studies show that ill patients overestimate life expectancy while others have unrealistic expectations about their treatment and survival, indicating that people are poorly prepared for death (Broom 2014). Despite this sanitisation of death narratives, many people buy life insurance, presumably on the understanding that one day they will die. Television and radio advertise life insurance, funeral insurance and services; the media regularly deliver the bad news on loss of life due to natural disasters, road trauma, drug abuse and homicide (Corr 2015).

Death System

Every society has cultural rules and mores surrounding death, loss and grief, in what Robert Kastenbaum (1973) referred to as a *death system*. A death system is made up of numerous interrelated components such as: places to do with death and dying (hospitals, funeral homes); contexts (memorialisation and remembrance); occasions (anniversaries, ANZAC day); objects (coffins, arm bands, flowers); symbols (skull and crossbones); and rituals (last rites) applied to the people who are dying (or have died) and those affected by their loss. Given that dying is individually unique and affects numerous people close to the dying person, as well as the community in which people live and work, death is an important aspect of any community or society. A death system therefore provides a society with warning systems about threat to life, preventative measures against death, care for the dying and disposal of the dead, making sense of death and strengthening social connection in the face of the inevitability of death (Corr 2015).

GRIEF AND BEREAVEMENT

Given the cultural influence on death, loss and grief, it remains that responses to loss are as individual as the people who grieve; that is, there is no 'correct' way to grieve. Apart from the losses to aspects of self, identity and declining health, older people increasingly contend with the deaths of others in their cohort while drawing closer to their own deaths (Corr 2015; DeSpelder & Strickland 2015).

Terror management theory suggests that awareness that one's own death is nearing creates existential fear (Greenberg et al 1986); yet studies show that death anxiety decreases with age (De Raedt et al 2013). Yalom (2008) states that an awareness that death is on the horizon can be an awakening, stimulating a desire for intimacy and connection.

Whether death of spouse/partner, friends and relatives of their own cohort, bereavement itself is an additional source of stress for this age group, often precipitating other losses (Parkes & Prigerson 2010). Older people not only encounter more bereavements than individuals in other phases of the life span, but they also experience the greatest variety of bereavements in respect of types of relationships lost (Shah & Meeks 2012).

Spousal Loss

While death of a spouse is common in the older population, it remains one of the most stressful events, with the potential to negatively affect the survivor's quality of life and wellbeing (Lundorff et al 2019). At this stage in life, the relationship has probably been an intimate partnership that has endured over many decades requiring major adjustment to the survivor's social identity and financial situation, as well as requiring other physical and practical readjustments. Additionally, research shows that bereaved people generally experience high rates of depression, loneliness, morbidity and mortality (Spahni et al 2015; Stroebe & Schut 2010a).

The loss of a life partner may coincide with the older person's own health issues, cognitive impairment or weakened physical status, chronic or acute illness or disability, and/or the necessity to relocate from the shared home, thus separating them from familiar sources of support. These changes may be in addition to previous losses, such as employment, or a long period of caregiving that has affected their own health. Despite these considerations, studies show that individuals respond in a wide variety of ways, from experiencing short-lived minor symptoms to debilitating, long-lasting symptoms (Carr & Jeffreys 2011).

As Carr and Jeffreys (2011) suggest, a combination of numerous factors unique to each individual influence how a person adjusts to the death of their partner. However, research has shown that there are four main influences on adjustment:

1. **The nature of the lost relationship** – relationships founded on affection, dependence and low conflict bring about increased grief symptoms in the first 6 months, but such relationship traits are protective in the longer term. This is possibly due to the ease in which the bereaved partner can continue bonds with the deceased.

2. **The nature of the death and conditions surrounding the death** – expected deaths can allow husband and wife to prepare for the death by dealing with financial and legal matters and addressing any emotional issues. In the lead-up to an expected death, there may have been a long, difficult period of care where the carer's health had suffered, or the carer now struggles with images of their loved one's ongoing suffering. At times, the end of the suffering (death) may provide relief to the surviving spouse and a sense of satisfaction for a caring job well done.

3. **Social support and the person's ability to access it** – women are more likely than men to have developed more varied and close relationships socially across their lifetime. Women tend to derive support from friendships, whereas men tend to look for support in re-partnering. Social isolation is a major factor in poor adjustment to loss. For older people, it can be brought about by systems problems, such as re-location to a new home, lack of transport or poor mobility. It is also worth keeping in mind that as their cohort of friends and siblings are dying, older people are at risk of becoming isolated from people who share their own age-related cultural values.

4. **Losses and stressors** – the loss of a life partner in older age is frequently associated with other stressors. These include (but are not limited to):
   - financial pressures
   - changing roles and identity within the community
   - possible relocation
   - deteriorating health and vitality
   - declining vision and hearing
   - change in daily routine which may have given life meaning.

Additionally, the loss of a partner is likely to also be the loss of a best friend, confidante and helpmate. The higher mortality and morbidity rates associated with bereavement probably stem from the fact that partners provide meals, remind the individual to take their medication and prompt them to visit the doctor when unwell.

Women are more likely than men to suffer financially following the death of their spouse and this can lead to poverty, triggering a great deal of stress and anxiety. At this point in time, older women have had fewer years in paid employment, have generally not received equal pay to men and, as a result, have not built up superannuation to fund living in widowhood (United Nations 2017). If seeking to re-enter the workforce, they are likely to face discrimination. The costs of funeral and legal expenses on the estate and health-related costs also compound the economic worries for many widows.

Life expectancy is higher for women than men, in both Australia and New Zealand. On average, women live about four years longer than men (Ministry of Health NZ 2016). As a result, more women than men are widowed and the likelihood of re-partnering and forming new and lasting friendships is also less likely for women (Carr & Jeffreys 2011). In spite of what may seem negative repercussions to spousal loss in later life, research shows that there are three broad patterns relating to bereavement outcome:
- time-limited disruption to function comprising increased sadness and depression, cognitive disruption and health issues which may last between several months up to two years
- chronic long-term disruption to function lasting several or more years
- absence of depression or disruption to function (Bonanno et al 2004).

It seems that for most adults, positive emotions can be experienced, thus ameliorating the stress of bereavement. The factors leading to better adjustment relate to personality factors, such as resilience, and the capacity of the individual to engage in active coping strategies. As suggested earlier, adjustment is also linked to the nature of the relationship (Ong et al 2010), with the greatest challenges stemming from the emotional and practical interdependency inherent in long-term intimate relationships (Kosminsky & Jordan 2016).

Attachment theory

Individual differences in the ways in which people respond and adjust to loss partly depend on one's attachment to the deceased person (LeRoy et al 2020). Following World War II, John Bowlby studied the effects of early parental separation on child development and later found similar responses in grieving adults. Bowlby believed that infants are driven to attach to significant caregiver figures to ensure survival. This need for attachment endures throughout life as adults continue to be influenced by pre-verbal experiences stored in the memory, which can have a negative impact on emotional regulation. Separation distress at the time of a partner's death includes yearning and searching for the deceased, anxiety about how they will cope without their loved one and a general sense of disorientation (Kosminsky & Jordan 2016).

Assisting older people whose spouse has died

Health professionals wishing to assist individuals bereaved by the loss of their partner should first assess if intervention is warranted, or what type of support may be needed. While findings show that the majority of older people have minimal disruption from bereavement, a minority, particularly those who have cared for a loved one in the lead-up to death, suffer consequences that impair their emotional, physical and social function (Shah & Meeks 2012). For many, loneliness, chronic grief and, for some, pre-existing depression or anxiety (see Chapter 25) may be exacerbated by bereavement. Bereaved older males are at the greatest risk of attempted and completed suicide (Parkes & Prigerson 2010) (see Chapter 25). Bereavement in late adulthood therefore should be taken seriously by health professionals with the aim of providing the most appropriate type of support an older person might need. Before moving on to assessment and support, the different ways grief may be experienced or labelled need to be considered.

Anticipatory Grief

There is a widely held assumption that grieving begins from the moment one knows a loved one is going to die, implying that grief after the death will be easier to deal with (Murray 2016). This may stem from earlier theories suggesting that grief was a process of stages to be worked through. First proposed by Lindemann in 1944, research on anticipatory grief over the years

has been beset by methodological issues, particularly how anticipatory grief is operationalised and researched. Understanding anticipatory grief has therefore been elusive. More recently terms such as pre-death or pre-loss grief are more likely to be used to describe the ongoing living losses experienced in the lead-up to death (Nielsen et al 2016).

Forewarning that death is likely to ensue following illness does give people an opportunity to prepare for the death by addressing emotional issues and getting one's affairs in order (Parkes & Prigerson 2010). Indeed, research shows that lack of preparedness for the death is associated with difficult bereavement outcomes. By the same token, research consistently shows that caregiving is stressful for carers, both psychologically and physically, and is associated with depression, anxiety and complicated grief reactions in bereavement (Nielsen et al 2016). A recent Singaporean study found there is a distinction between prolonged or complicated grief responses and caregiver burden responses in carers of people with dementia, which supports the idea that grief associated with ongoing living losses should be addressed (Liew et al 2018). Across the period of caregiving, which can be lengthy for chronic disease in the older population, non-death losses are a constant. Just some of the losses faced at this time include:

- deterioration in the older person's condition
- loss of support networks and friendships
- loss of function
- loss of role (or loss of self).

These are living losses or non-finite losses that keep occurring and have no endpoint (Murray 2016).

Non-Finite and Living Losses

Bruce and Schultz (2001) state that the main features of non-finite losses are those losses which develop, are ongoing and are out of step with hopes and expectations of those affected. Triggered by a negative life event – for example, a cardiovascular accident (or stroke) with ensuing paralysis or weakness, dysphagia, dysphasia and/or vision impairment – such living or non-finite losses are ongoing as a part of everyday life. Accompanied by uncertainty about the future progression of the disease, this constant daily reminder of loss can lead those affected to a sense of being overwhelmed and disempowered by their circumstances and because loss is a constant, the sadness is often set aside. Life can settle into a seemingly 'normal' pattern, but the sadness is continually present, building and intensifying over time. Unrecognised by others, support systems are often inadequate or missing, resulting in individuals feeling disconnected and isolated (Murray 2016; Winokuer & Harris 2016).

Chronic Sorrow

The grief response to these ongoing living, non-finite losses is referred to as chronic sorrow. 'Chronic sorrow' was first proposed by Olshanski in 1962, who studied the unique and ongoing form of grief experienced by parents of children with disabilities. Research has been conducted since in relation to chronic conditions such as neurodegenerative disease, dementia and mental illness. The grief intensifies over time as, in the case of many older people, the ongoing loss of chronic disease takes hold, changing one's functional ability and health, relationship with self, and with others. The main features of chronic sorrow are that it is:

- ongoing
- recurring with no predictable end
- may be elicited externally or internally
- escalates in intensity over time.

Feelings associated with chronic sorrow may fluctuate between overwhelming sadness and crippling numbness accompanied by an underlying anxiety and trauma. Progressive in nature, chronic sorrow is disenfranchised or unrecognised by others (Winokuer & Harris 2016).

Disenfranchised Grief

Doka (1999) defines disenfranchised grief as a loss '… that is not, or cannot be, openly acknowledged, publicly mourned or socially supported' (p. 37). Typical cases of disenfranchised grief relate to stigmatised situations, such as death by suicide or homicide, certain diseases such as HIV/AIDS and disability. These situations relate to the grieving 'rules' put in place by a society's death system. Therefore, relationships such as extra-marital affairs, cohabiting adults, homosexual partnerships or divorced couples, for example, are less likely to be recognised and provided with support. In other situations, the loss itself may be deemed unimportant, such as, for example, the loss of a pet. With technological medical advancements, people are now living longer; the ongoing loss associated with chronic disease, the nature of relationships and the lack of psychosocial, physical or financial support mean that these disenfranchised scenarios are increasingly common in the world of the older adult (Boss et al 2011). The enigma is that disenfranchised grief itself exacerbates the experience of grief (Doka 1999).

Ambiguous Loss

Disenfranchised grief also results from situations where a person is physically alive but regarded as dead; for example, institutionalised persons, or those with mental health conditions such as addiction or dementia (Doka 1999). Boss (1999) refers to this form of disenfranchised grief as ambiguous loss. There are two forms of ambiguous loss:

- the person may be *physically absent*, but very much to the forefront of one's mind psychologically, as in the case of missing persons, or
- the person is physically present, but *psychologically absent*, as in the case of dementia or severe mental illness.

Ambiguous loss is particularly stressful. Apart from the pain of the ongoing living losses mentioned earlier, there is no likelihood of closure and there is a lack of clarity about whether the person is dead or alive, present or absent (Boss et al 2011). Furthermore, family members experience ambiguity in feelings: possibly angry about the demands of caring, sad about the losses (Boss 1999). Boss and colleagues (2011) suggest that individuals in this situation experience role confusion due to the constant uncertainty with no end in sight.

Ambiguous loss becomes problematic when decisions are often put off, leading to immobilisation and further crises. Grief and support needs are unacknowledged and family boundaries blur; people are ignored, celebrations or rituals are no longer held. Ambivalence, depression, hopelessness and helplessness are quick to set in and often lead to feelings of guilt, anxiety and being overwhelmed. Both chronic sorrow and ambiguous loss are similar to complicated grief (CG) or prolonged grief disorder (PGD), with symptoms of anxiety and depression accompanied by somatic symptoms and relationship problems (Boss et al 2011).

Given the increasing prevalence of dementia in the elderly population and the challenges this will inevitably bring to the health system (Australian Institute for Health and Welfare [AIHW] 2018), health professionals will need to address these stressful forms of grief that occur for older people and their carers. It is essential that healthcare professionals understand these phenomena to ultimately help clients. See *Tips for best practice* in providing support for an older person experiencing ambiguous loss.

DISTURBED GRIEF
Complicated Grief, Prolonged Grief Disorder, Persistent Complex Bereavement Disorder

Past models of bereavement suggesting that grief occurs in stages, following a set process from bereavement to recovery, are unhelpful. Research over the past two to three decades has shown that the majority of people adapt to their loss over time. Acute grief is a normal response to loss, which brings symptoms of tearfulness,

Tips for Best Practice
Responding to Ambiguous Loss and Chronic Sorrow

The overall goal is to strengthen the older person's resilience. As the loss is relational, the response should also be relational. Following are important considerations and examples of things the nurse might say to gently guide the older person:

- Validating the individual nature of experiences and naming grief as the culprit that results from ambiguous loss. This is reaffirming and can bring about some relief. The person can now see the problem does not reside within him or herself.

  Example:

  'You have been carrying a heavy load caring for your husband as he has become more unwell. I can see that you have coped with many changes that may feel like losses of important parts of your life at times; connections with friends, time to yourself, a good night's sleep, financial security. It is not unusual to grieve for these things and for the life you used to have.'

- Finding meaning in the situation and beginning to accept the ambiguity of opposing circumstances allows people to reconnect with others and engage with life once more.

  Example:

  'You have told me that your husband has been becoming frailer and more forgetful over the past three years. What do you think is ahead for you both? Considering how much care he needs now, how do you see yourself managing if he needs more help in the future?'

- Tempering mastery by becoming realistic about what gains can be made in the face of the situation.

  Example:

  'Now that your husband has moved into a residential facility, are there other ways that you can care for him, for example, by helping him with his meals?'

- Reconstructing one's personal identity as being more than the ambiguous loss has reduced it to; for example, being more than a carer.

  Example:

  'You have been married for over 50 years. Can you tell me about the many different things you have done together over the years?'

- Normalising ambivalence and tolerance for opposing feelings such as anger and sadness.

  Examples:

  'I understand that it must have been very difficult for you caring for your husband when you have no nursing experience and have had to learn so many new skills. While caring for someone you love can be satisfying, it can also be difficult. I expect you felt frustrated and even angry at times.'

  'As your husband has become more and more unwell, you must have experienced lots of change that has felt like losses over the years. Do you think that has contributed to how you have been feeling?'

- Revising attachment by connecting with the loved one's present capabilities, while letting go of what is no longer possible.

  Example:

  'When you visit your husband in the care facility, you might like to reminisce with him about the joy you shared when you were courting and going out to dance. Perhaps you could take some photo albums and music from those days to enjoy together?'

- Reconstructing one's personal identity as being more than the ambiguous loss has reduced it to; for example, being more than a carer.

  Example:

  'Your life has been so full. Can you tell me about your role in the family business, and how you managed that while bringing up three children?'

- Reconnection with hope occurs when attachment is revised, and people begin to feel less isolated.

  Example:

  'You mentioned that you lived in the country for many years of your marriage. That must have been a busy time. What was the community like where you lived, and what did you enjoy most?'

- Connect with resources and available support in the community. Assist clients to learn self-care strategies and take responsibility for their health.

  Examples:

  'You may find it helpful to connect with a carer support group where others are dealing with similar situations to yours. Would you like me to give you the details of several carer groups that might be suitable?'

  'You may be eligible for some assistance in your own home. Would you like me to help you organise an assessment for a care package?'

Boss et al (2011).

sadness and insomnia. However, a minority of people struggle to integrate the loss into life. For this significant minority, initial acute symptoms persist over many months and/or years, adversely affecting the grieving person's health, quality of life and relationships (Boelen & Smid 2017). The typical acute symptoms of grief continue to be painful, intense and unremitting as time goes by, experienced as:

- intense yearning for the deceased
- emotional numbness
- a sense of confusion
- disorientation
- lack of meaning (Aoun et al 2015).

These individuals are at heightened risk of morbidity and mortality. However, as grief is a painful but normal life event, demarcating when grief is disrupted to the point of needing intervention is difficult and controversial (Boelen & Smid 2017).

The *Diagnostic and Statistical Manual of Mental Disorders 5th edition* (DSM-5) and *International Classification of Diseases 11th Revision* (ICD-11) provide clinicians with definitions and guidance to identify grief that does not follow a 'normal' trajectory. The DSM-5, published in 2013, describes criteria for persistent complex bereavement disorder (PCBD) diagnosable 12 months after bereavement. The ICD-11, published in 2018, describes criteria for prolonged grief disorder (PGD) diagnosable 6 months following a significant loss. Boelen and Smid (2017) suggest that these terms may be used interchangeably, given that research has demonstrated the two conditions are very similar. The focus in diagnosis is on the pervasiveness of the distress and disability that fails to ameliorate with time.

Risk Factors for Complicated, Persistent or Prolonged Grief

Complicated and prolonged grief reactions are complex and multifactorial. Burke and Neimeyer (2013) state that identifying individuals with prospective risk factors is critical to support these people; however, the complexity and wide variety of factors contributing to problematic grief make this difficult. A full discussion of risk factors is outside the scope of this chapter; however, the most common risk factors may be grouped into the following broader themes:

- *Relationship:* As mentioned earlier, the relationship to the deceased plays a major role in adjusting to bereavement. The loss of a close, long-term relationship, common among older people, can be difficult to come to terms with. People with insecure attachment, particularly those who experienced adversity during childhood, have an elevated risk of complicated

bereavement (LeRoy et al 2020). Higher dependency on the deceased, whether practical or emotional, is also a risk factor. Moreover, a history of other losses can complicate grief and, as discussed earlier, multiple losses are common in older adulthood (Tofthagen et al 2017).

- *Interpersonal:* Most studies show that having social support protects against complicated grief (Burke & Neimeyer 2013).
- *Disposition, resilience and coping:* Optimistic individuals seem to take a more flexible approach to difficulties, solve problems actively and seek assistance and social support. The death of a significant other can challenge one's self-narrative and assumptive worldview linking past, present and future. Those who lack adaptive coping skills often struggle with the meaning of the loss (Neimeyer 2014).
- *Cognition:* Repetitive continuous thinking about negative feelings (depressive rumination) is linked to depression following a loss and is a predictor of complicated grief. Rumination about injustice and relationships associated with the loss are linked to complicated grief. Such unhelpful cognition blocks healthy adaptation to the loss and may influence the bereaved individual's behaviour, such as avoiding places associated with the deceased, which has a further impact on integrating the loss (Eisma et al 2014).
- *Co-morbid or previous mental health conditions:* Caregiving throughout a loved one's illness increases the risk for complex grief responses, given the high emotional toll and fatigue associated with caring. An Australian study by Thomas and colleagues (2014) found that 44% of family caregivers in palliative care had higher levels of anxiety and depression, with 15% meeting criteria for pre-loss grief.
- *Environment and conditions relating to death:* Dissatisfaction with care provided to the dying older person or circumstances related to the death also negatively influence bereavement outcomes, along with concurrent stressful life events and perceived lack of support. As stated earlier, for many in this age group, financial matters can be a secondary stressor that outstrip the older person's coping resources (Thomas et al 2014).

Prevalence of Complicated, Persistent or Prolonged Grief

An Australian population-based cross-sectional survey by Aoun and colleagues (2015) found that approximately 7% of bereaved people may be in this high-risk category of people with disturbed, complicated or persistent grief. The presence of prolonged grief was measured by use

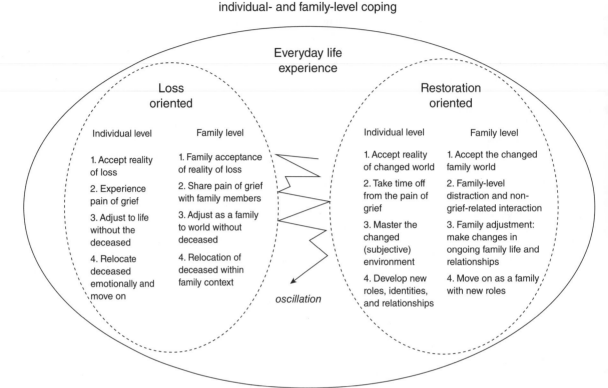

FIG. 29.1 **Dual Process Model of Coping with Bereavement – Revised (2015).** (Stroebe & Schut 2015. Copyright 2015 by SAGE Publishing. Reprinted with permission.)

of the PG-13 instrument, which evaluates social and functional impairment, as well as symptoms present at least 6 months after bereavement. A further 35.2% were found to be in a sub-threshold group of moderate risk. These individuals did not require psychological intervention, but a support group or peer-led assistance would be helpful to prevent them from moving into a complicated grief response in time (Aoun et al 2015).

For this minority of bereaved people, nurses have a role in identifying those at risk and providing a culturally appropriate response. However, understanding the processes that people undergo when coping with bereavement is necessary in order to be helpful.

COPING WITH BEREAVEMENT

Stroebe and Schut (1999) propose a model to account for the coping processes that occur following a significant loss (see Fig. 29.1). The Dual Process Model of Coping with Bereavement (DPM) consists of two co-occurring processes: loss orientation (LO) and restoration orientation (RO); each is used to address different types of

bereavement stressors. Drawing on Cognitive Stress Theory (Lazarus & Folkman 1984) and the Stress Response Syndrome (Horowitz 1986), bereavement integrates avoidance and confrontation on a number of different circumstances relating to the loss; for example, events leading to the death; the death itself; thoughts about the deceased; changes brought about by the death.

Grief is at the centre of loss orientation and focuses on the relationship with the deceased, including rumination about life before the death and the events leading up to and surrounding the death. Symptoms include (but are not limited to) searching, yearning and pining for the deceased, tears and sorrow. The emotional responses can be mixed, from having pleasurable memories to utmost despair. Adapting to the loss is at the centre of restoration orientation. While the loss orientation is most commonly experienced around the time of the death, the griever must also focus on other secondary activities needing attention. Adjustment to the loss is pressing, whereby the bereaved person may need to fill the gap usually attended to by the deceased, such as deal with finances, return to work, provide care for others and develop a new identity as a widow/widower. The DPM holds that the bereaved person must oscillate between these two foci – loss and restoration. Both are stressful, but dealing with one gives temporary respite from the other. In time, the dynamic changes as the bereaved person accommodates the loss and adjusts to a changed life (Stroebe & Schut 1999).

Since its introduction in 1999, the DPM has been widely researched; for example, studies have looked at the role of attachment patterns in complicated grief; gender differences in coping with bereavement in terms of health outcomes; cultural differences in coping with bereavement; bereavement responses in older people; and efficacy of interventions for complicated grief (Stroebe & Schut 2010b).

RESPONDING TO COMPLEX BEREAVEMENT OUTCOMES

By using the DPM, health professionals can gain an understanding of how various risk factors and predictors of complex grief are dealt with in relation to available resources. Some bereaved individuals become stuck in their loss, others focus on restoration and become stuck there. For others, the difficulty may lie in the oscillation process, where switching between loss and restoration does not run smoothly; for example, when one continues to have intrusive thoughts or goes to great lengths to avoid reminders of the deceased. The use of the DPM can facilitate a plan for problem-solving or emotional-focused approaches to support those bereaved at elevated risk of complicated or prolonged grief.

As mentioned earlier, the challenge is if, when and how to intervene with older people who are at risk of poor bereavement outcomes (Boelen & Smid 2017). Given the many individual, cultural and situational variables that contribute to complex grief responses, assessment and management can also pose problems, particularly for older people with complex health and social circumstances. Often clinicians must make their own judgements about an individual's stress and impairment (Burke & Neimeyer 2013).

Assessment

As Boelen and Smid (2017) identify, assessment should be focused on the degree of distress and disability. Over the past 50 years, numerous bereavement risk assessment measures have been used; however, it should be kept in mind that the majority of people integrate their loss and adjust to life without their loved one over time (Sealey et al 2015). A functional assessment of ability, coping, distress and support may be more practical than using a measure.

Intervention

For those individuals in the high-risk category for complicated grief, referral to a general practitioner (GP) or mental health professional for a thorough assessment is key. These include older people:

- with co-morbid mental or physical health problems
- with social or financial difficulties
- with lack of support networks
- who have experienced multiple losses.

For the remainder, supporting identified needs on an individualised basis is more helpful.

Social Connection and Positive Ageing

Research shows that being socially engaged in later life supports positive outcomes. Importantly, social engagement is also a protective factor against cognitive decline (see Chapter 26). Older people, particularly those in the oldest old group (above 80 years), tend to have reduced levels of social activity due to:

- deteriorating health and mobility
- reduced social networks because of the deaths of family and friends
- low socioeconomic circumstances – they may live in disadvantaged neighbourhoods that may not provide a sense of safety or support.

Furthermore, these older people are more likely to need to make a transition from living independently at home to a residential aged care facility, a potentially stressful transition. Given the economic challenges of the ageing population, programs to reduce social isolation in older people are essential to promote positive ageing. Research shows that programs based on a theoretical approach that include education and are targeted towards specific groups, such as widowed people or carers, are the most effective (Windsor et al 2016).

Advance Care Planning

A lack of preparedness for the death, and trauma from lengthy bouts of caring for family loved ones, has negative impacts on bereavement outcomes, so health professionals should promote preparation for end of life by encouraging advance care planning to ensure an individual's wishes regarding healthcare can be made (see also Chapter 17). Such plans can be formalised through an advance care directive, which is a legal document in both Australia and New Zealand. Requirements and documentation differ from state to state or territory in Australia. More information can be sought from Advance Care Planning Australia and the Health Quality and Safety Commission New Zealand. Advance care planning not only gives people peace of mind, but it gives back some sense of control at a stage in life when people do

Promoting Wellness
Communication Strategies to Support a Bereaved Older Person

- Acknowledge the situation.

  This could be as simple as saying 'I am sorry that your wife died'. Using the word 'died' shows the person that you can talk openly about how he or she really feels.

- Let the bereaved older person talk about how their loved one died.

  An older person who is grieving may need to tell the story over and over again, which helps them to process and accept the death. With each retelling, the pain lessens. Try to be patient and listen compassionately.

- Ask the bereaved person how he or she feels.

  Do not assume that you know how the older person is feeling as the emotions of grief can change rapidly. Grief is an intensely personal experience. Focus on listening, and how *they're* feeling.

- Accept the bereaved person's feelings.

  Let the grieving person know that it's okay for them to cry in front of you or to express their anger. Allow the bereaved person to feel free to show their feelings without fear of judgement or argument.

- Be genuine in your communication.

  Just listen to the bereaved person. You can simply admit: 'I'm not sure what to say, but I want you to know I care.' Don't try to minimise the loss or give unsolicited advice.

- Be willing to sit in silence.

  Comfort can come from you simply being in their company. Try to make eye contact, and if appropriate, touch the bereaved person's hand.

- Understand that everyone responds differently.

  Some people may not be tearful or want to talk; others may be resentful, while others cope best by directing their attention elsewhere.

WHAT NOT TO SAY TO A BEREAVED OLDER PERSON

If you are finding it difficult to know what to say, then just being with the older person is comforting. It is better to sit in comfortable silence and be genuine in your communication (as above), than to make simplistic statements such as:

- 'It's part of God's plan.'

  This may make the older person angry. He or she may answer: 'What plan? Nobody told me there was a plan'.

- 'Look at what you have to be thankful for.'

  While the bereaved person may know they have positives in their life, these are not important to them at this moment.

- 'He's in a better place now.'

  The bereaved person may not believe this.

- 'This is behind you now. It's time to get on with your life.'

  The bereaved person may feel that 'getting on with life' means forgetting their deceased loved one.

Adapted from The American Hospice Foundation (2000).

not always feel they have any control due to deteriorating health.

SUMMARY

More than any other phase in the life span, older adulthood features change and loss. Inevitably grief comes along with the many challenges and losses faced; whether it is loss of one's health and vitality, sense of identity and purpose, or the loss of meaningful relationships. These people often experience multiple, ongoing, living losses and due to the range of change and loss across a variety of domains, this group is at higher risk for complicated or prolonged grief. Most people adjust in time, integrating the loss into the fabric of their altered

lives; however, a small number of people struggle to adjust. For these people, their health and quality of life are severely affected, and they are at heightened risk of mortality and morbidity.

Overall, it needs to be understood that people deal with change, loss and grief in individual ways and that their responses to bereavement will be variable. Such grieving practices are culturally entrenched. While some with unremitting or complex grief issues may require mental health care or social work intervention, many may benefit from individualised assistance, once their needs have been identified. The Dual Process Model (Stroebe & Schut 1999) provides a culturally sensitive framework for assessing where people may be stuck in their bereavement. Understanding the individual's sense of loss and the meaning they attribute to the loss is also important if nurses are to assist them appropriately. Support should be put in place in response to the individual's needs.

Health professionals need to be comfortable discussing topics related to ageing, dying, death and bereavement, and should also be up-to-date with professional development in this area. Research has shown that university training on these topics for health professionals is often outdated and that many do not access continuing professional development to remain knowledgeable about current research on loss, grief and bereavement (Breen et al 2013). Additionally, to maximise client care, health professionals working in this area should also keep in mind their own care to avoid vicarious trauma and burnout.

Practice Scenario

Joan (70) has been caring for her husband of 50 years (Ron), who was diagnosed with vascular dementia four years ago. Over the past 6 to 12 months Ron has had a series of small strokes, each one impairing his cognitive abilities and physical function. His deterioration has increased the strain on Joan's own health. She has hypertension, back problems and arthritis requiring a hip replacement. Ron's care needs escalated to the point that the geriatrician suggested he should go into residential care following his last hospitalisation where he also had a fall. Joan is struggling with this decision, believing that Ron is deteriorating because he's not receiving 'proper care' in the facility. While she is exhausted from caring for Ron and understands that she can't continue the carer role, she also feels like a failure as a wife and feels guilty about having to place Ron in a care facility. She finds herself in tears more than usual, fatigued and in constant pain. She is overwhelmed by the decisions she needs to make and is angry about the situation. Her friends and relatives have also found Joan to be 'impossible' and they are beginning to withdraw, leaving Joan feeling even more isolated than previously.

REVIEW QUESTIONS

1. Why might Joan be experiencing symptoms such as frequent crying, fatigue and pain?
2. What features of Joan's situation might suggest that she is experiencing ambiguous loss?
3. How could the nurse gently assist Joan to accept the ambiguity of her feelings and consider what gains she can still make in the face of the situation?
4. What strategies could the nurse suggest to assist Joan to connect with resources and support available in her community?
5. What could the nurse say to Joan to help her reconstruct her own identity as more than the ambiguous loss has reduced it; that is, a carer for Ron?

Research Highlight

A recent Australian study explored the perceptions of older people who were dying about their family members' need for bereavement support. A purposive sample of inpatients being treated at a palliative care unit participated in an individual semi-structured interview. All participants were aware of the life-limiting nature of their illness and provided informed consent for the interview. Nineteen patients were interviewed. Most were female ($n = 11$) and the mean age was 71 years (range 52–88 years). The majority of participants (73%) had a diagnosis of cancer. When asked who they were most concerned about following their death, many participants nominated someone other than their documented next-of-kin, including their adult children (particularly those with a disability), siblings, parents and friends.

The findings generated three themes. Firstly, it was suggested that families that were close and supportive of each other may not always require bereavement follow-up. Some participants who felt they had a cohesive family expressed comfort that their loved ones would be well supported, making it easier to think about the future. Secondly, family members who had extenuating circumstances or 'lived more complex lives' were thought to be more likely to need bereavement support. This was despite family support and systems already in place, particularly if they had experienced other losses. Lastly, this study demonstrated that it is possible to ask older people who are dying to consider who in their support networks may require bereavement support.

Factors that led participants to feel concerned for family members after their death included: lack of family cohesion; a difficult relationship with the dying person; a negative world view; low self-esteem; a previous history of depression; or avoidance of emotional problems. The authors concluded that there is value in supporting nurses to involve older people who know they are dying to, where possible, help identify loved ones who may benefit from bereavement follow-up.

REFERENCE

Phillips JL, Lobb EA, Bellemore F et al (2019) 'Through the eyes of the dying' – Identifying who may benefit from bereavement follow-up: a qualitative study. Collegian 26:615–620.

REFERENCES

Aoun SM, Breen LJ, Howting DA et al (2015) Who needs bereavement support? A population-based survey of bereavement risk and support need. PLoS ONE 10:1–14.

American Hospice Foundation (2000). Available: https://americanhospice.org/working-through-grief/helping-your-bereaved-friend/

Australian Bureau of Statistics (ABS) (2017) Retirement and retirement intentions, Australia. July 2016 to June 2017. Cat no. 6238.0. Online. Available: www.abs.gov.au/ausstats/abs@.nsf/mf/6238.0

Australian Government Department of Human Services (2019) Age pension. Online. Available: www.humanservices.gov.au/individuals/services/centrelink/age-pension/who-can-get-it

Australian Institute of Health and Welfare (AIHW) (2018) Australia's health 2018. Australia's health series no. 16. AUS 221. Canberra: AIHW. Online. Available: www.aihw.gov.au/reports/australias-health/australias-health-2018/

Baltes BB, Wynne K, Sirabian M et al (2014) Future time perspective, regulatory focus, and selection, optimization, and compensation: Testing a longitudinal model. Journal of Organizational Behaviour 35:1120–1133.

Boelen PA, Smid GE (2017) Disturbed grief: Prolonged grief disorder and persistent complex bereavement disorder. BMJ 357:j2016.

Boerner K, Jopp D (2007) Improvement/maintenance and reorientation as central features of coping with major life change and loss: Contributions of three life-span theories. Human Development 50:171–195.

Bonanno GA, Wortman CB, Nesse RM (2004) Prospective patterns of resilience and maladjustment during widowhood. Psychology and Aging 19(2):260–271.

Boss P (1999) Ambiguous loss: Learning to live with unresolved grief. Harvard University Press, Cambridge, MA.

Boss P, Roos S, Harris DL (2011) Grief in the midst of ambiguity and uncertainty: An exploration of ambiguous loss and chronic sorrow. In: RA Neimeyer, DL Harris, HR Winokuer et al (eds) Grief and bereavement in contemporary society: Bridging research and practice. Routledge, New York, NY.

Brandtstädter J, Renner G (1990) Tenacious goal pursuit and flexible goal adjustment: Explication and age-related analysis of assimilative and accommodative strategies of coping. Psychology and Aging 5(1):58–67.

Breen LJ, Fernandez M, O'Connor M et al (2013) The preparation of graduate health professionals for working with bereaved clients: An Australian perspective. Omega: The Journal of Death and Dying 66:313–332.

Broom A (2014) Before you go … are you in denial about death? The Conversation, 27 November 2014. Online. Available: theconversation.com/before-you-go-are-you-in-denial-about-death-34056

Bruce EJ, Schultz CL (2001) Nonfinite loss and grief: A psychoeducational approach. Paul H. Brookes, Baltimore, MD.

Burke LA, Neimeyer RA (2013) Prospective risk factors for complicated grief. In M Stroebe, H Schut, & J van den Bout. Complicated grief: Scientific foundations for health care professionals. Routledge, New York, NY.

Carr D, Jeffreys JS (2011) Spousal bereavement in later life. In: RA Neimeyer, DL Harris, HR Winokuer et al (eds) Grief and bereavement in contemporary society: Bridging research and practice. Routledge, New York, NY.

Corr CA (2015) The death system according to Robert Kastenbaum. Omega 70(1):13–25.

De Raedt R, Koster EHW, Ryckewaert R (2013) Aging and attentional bias for death related and general threat-related information: less avoidance in older as compared with middle-aged adults. The Journals of Gerontology, Series B: Psychological Sciences and Social Sciences 68(1):41–48.

DeSpelder LA, Strickland AL (2015) The last dance: Encountering death and dying (10th ed.) McGraw-Hill Education, New York, NY.

Doka KJ (1999) Disenfranchised grief. Bereavement Care 18(3):37–39.

Eisma M, Schut H, Stroebe M et al (2014) Adaptive and maladaptive rumination after loss: A three-wave longitudinal study. British Journal of Clinical Psychology, 1–18.

Erikson EH (1963) Childhood and society. WW Norton & Company, New York, NY.

Greenberg J, Pyszczynski T, Solomon S (1986) The causes and consequences of a need for self-esteem: A terror management theory. In: RF Baumeister (ed.) Public self and private self. Springer-Verlag, New York, NY.

Heckhausen J & Schulz R (1995) A life-span theory of control. Psychological Review 102(2):284–304.

Horowitz MJ (1986) Stress response syndromes, 2nd edn. Aronson, New York, NY.

Humphrey GM, Zimpfer DG (1996) Counselling for grief and bereavement. Sage, London.

Kastenbaum R (1973) On the future of death: Some images and options. Omega – Journal of Death and Dying 3(4): 307–318.

Klass D, Chow AYM (2011) Culture and ethnicity in experiencing, policing and handling grief. In: RA Neimeyer, DL Harris, HR Winokuer et al (eds) Grief and bereavement in contemporary society: Bridging research and practice. Routledge, New York, NY.

Kosminsky PS, Jordan JR (2016) Attachment informed grief therapy: The clinician's guide to foundations and applications. Routledge, New York, NY.

Lazarus RS, Folkman S (1984) Stress, appraisal, and coping. Springer, New York.

LeRoy AS, Gabert T, Garcini L et al (2020) Attachment orientations and loss adjustment among bereaved spouses. Psychoneuroendocrinology 112:104401.

Liew TM, Tai BC, Yap P et al (2018) Contrasting the risk factors of grief and burden in caregivers of persons with dementia: Multivariate analysis. International Journal of Geriatric Psychiatry 34:258–264.

Loidl B, Leipold B (2019) Facets of accommodative coping in adulthood. Psychology and Aging 34(5):640–654.

Lundorff M, Holmgren H, Zachariae R et al (2017) Prevalence of prolonged grief disorder in adult bereavement: A systematic review and meta-analysis. Journal of Affective Disorder 212:138–149.

Lundorff M, Thomsen DK, Damkier A et al (2019) How do loss- and restoration-oriented coping change across time? A prospective study on adjustment following spousal bereavement. Anxiety, Stress & Coping 32(3):270–285.

May CR, Eton DT, Boehmer K et al (2014) Rethinking the patient: using Burden of Treatment Theory to understand the changing dynamics of illness. BMC Health Services Research 14:281.

McKenna B, Furness T, Dhital D et al (2014) Recovery-oriented care in older-adult acute inpatient mental health settings in Australia: An exploratory study. JAGS 62:1938–1942.

Ministry of Health NZ (2016) Health loss in New Zealand 1990–2013: A report from the New Zealand burden of diseases, injuries and risk factors study. Online. Available: www.health.govt.nz/nz-health-statistics/health-statistics-and-data-sets/new-zealand-burden-diseases-injuries-and-risk-factors-study

Murray J (2016) Understanding loss: A guide for caring for those facing adversity. Routledge, New York, NY.

Neilsen MK, Neergaard MA, Jensen AB et al (2016) Do we need to change our understanding of anticipatory grief in caregivers? A systematic review of caregiver studies during end-of-life caregiving and bereavement. Clinical Psychology Review 44:75–93.

Neimeyer RA (2014) The changing face of grief: Contemporary directions in theory, research, and practice. Progress in Palliative Care 22(3):125–130.

New Zealand Government (2018) Retirement age. Online. Available: www.govt.nz/browse/work/retirement/retirement-age/

Olshanski, S (1962) Chronic sorrow: a response to having a mentally defective child, Social Casework 43(4):190–193.

Ong AD, Fuller-Rowell TE, Bonanno GA (2010) Prospective predictors of positive emotions following spousal loss. Psychology and Aging 25(3):653–660.

Parkes CM, Prigerson HG (2010) Bereavement: Studies of grief in adult life, 4th edn. Routledge, New York, NY.

Radford K, Chapman G, Bainbridge et al (2018) The ageing population in Australia: Implications for the workforce. In: S Werth & C Brownlow (eds) Work and identity: Contemporary perspectives on workplace diversity. Palgrave Macmillan, Basingstoke, UK.

Santrock JW (2014) Life span development Australia/New Zealand. McGraw-Hill Education, North Ryde, NSW.

Sealey M, Breen LJ, O'Connor M et al (2015) A scoping review of bereavement risk assessment measures: Implications for palliative care. Palliative Medicine 29(7):577–589.

Shah SN, Meeks S (2012) Late-life bereavement and complicated grief: A proposed comprehensive framework. Aging & Mental Health 16(1):39–56.

Slatyer S, Aoun SM, Hill KD et al (2019) Caregivers' experiences of a home support program after the hospital discharge of an older family member: A qualitative analysis. BMC Health Services Research 19:220.

Spahni S, Morselli D, Perrig-Chiello P et al (2015) Patterns of psychological adaptation to spousal bereavement in old age. Gerontology 61:456–468.

Stroebe MS, Hansson RO, Stroebe W et al (2010) Introduction: Concepts and issues in contemporary research on bereavement. In MS Stroebe, RO Hanson, W Stroebe et al (eds) Handbook of bereavement research: Consequences, coping, and care. Washington, DC: American Psychological Association.

Stroebe W, Schut H (2010a) Risk factors in bereavement outcome: A methodological and empirical review. In MS Stroebe, RO Hanson, W Stroebe et al (eds) Handbook of bereavement research: Consequences, coping, and care. American Psychological Association, Washington, DC.

Stroebe W, Schut H (2010b) The dual process model of coping with bereavement: A decade on. Omega 61(4):273–289.

Stroebe MS, Schut H (1999) The dual process model of coping with bereavement: Rationale and description. Death Studies 23(3):197–224.

Thomas K, Hudson PL, Trauer T et al (2014) Risk factors for developing prolonged grief during bereavement in family carers of cancer patients in palliative care: A longitudinal study. Journal of Pain and Symptom Management 47(3):531–541.

Tofthagen CS, Kip K, Witt A et al (2017) Complicated grief: Risk factors, interventions, and resources for oncology nurses. Clinical Journal of Oncology Nursing 21(3):331–337.

United Nations (June 2017) Population ageing and sustainable development. Online. Available: www.un.org/en/development/desa/population/publications/pdf/popfacts/PopFacts_2017-1.pdf

Windsor TD, Curtis RG, Luszcz MA (2016) Social engagement in late life. In H Kendig, P McDonald, J Piggott (eds) Population ageing and Australia's future. ANU Press, Acton, ACT.

Winokuer HR, Harris DL (2016) Principles and practice of grief counselling, 2nd edn, Springer, New York, NY.

Yalom ID (2008) Staring at the sun: Overcoming the terror of death. Jossey-Bass, San Francisco, CA.

Practice Scenario Multiple Choice Answers

CHAPTER 3

1 A, B, C, D
2 A, B, C
3 A, B, C, D

CHAPTER 4

1A, 2D, 3A, 4B, 5D

1 Detailed responses
   a. **Pre-contemplation – correct response**. Mable is not yet ready to make a change, due to lack of awareness of the need for and benefits of change
   b. Contemplation – **incorrect response**. Mable is not yet aware of the problem or considering the pros and cons for change; she is in the pre-contemplation stage, lacking awareness of the need for and benefits of change
   c. Preparation – **incorrect response**. Mable is not yet planning for or taking steps towards an actual change, she is in the pre-contemplation stage, lacking awareness of the need for and benefits of change
   d. Action – **incorrect response**. Mable has not yet made the required change, she is in the pre-contemplation stage, lacking awareness of the need for and benefits of change
2 Health literacy strategies to assist the nurse progress Mable from one stage to another:
   a. Assume low health literacy level and provide universal precautions with all written and verbal communication delivered in plain English – **incorrect response**. While this strategy will promote health literacy levels, the most correct response is all of the above
   b. Provide clear, correct and evidenced-based health information – **incorrect response**. While this strategy will promote health literacy levels, the most correct response is all of the above
   c. Encourage Mable to ask questions when in doubt – **incorrect response**. While this strategy will promote health literacy levels, the most correct response is all of the above
   d. **All of the above – Correct response**

3 Stage of readiness for change Mable was in in June:
   a. **Preparation – correct response**. Mable is planning and taking some steps taken towards change
   b. Action – **incorrect response**. Mable has not yet made the required change, she is in the preparation stage, planning and taking some steps towards change
   c. Maintenance – **incorrect response**. Mable has not yet made the required change and converting it into routine habit. She is in the preparation stage, planning and taking some steps towards change
   d. Termination – **incorrect response**. Mable has not yet made the required change, which is now a routine behaviour with no temptation for relapse. She is in the preparation stage, planning and taking some steps towards change
4 Known modifiable risk factors for dementia that Mable also knows about to reduce her risk:
   a. Hypertension; obesity and old age – **incorrect response**. While hypertension and obesity of known modifiable risk factors – old age is a non-modifiable risk factor
   b. **Smoking, alcohol overuse, mental inactivity – correct response**. Smoking, alcohol overuse and mental inactivity are all known modifiable risk factors for dementia.
   c. High blood cholesterol, being female, hypertension – **Incorrect response**. While high blood cholesterol and hypertension are known modifiable risk factors – female sex is a non-modifiable risk factor
   d. Diabetes, carrying mutated BRCA1 gene and obesity – **Incorrect response** – While diabetes and obesity are known modifiable dementia risk factors, a mutated BRCA1 gene is a non-modifiable risk for breast cancer and ovarian cancer in woman.
5 Actions the nurse could take to assist Mable with a relapse in September:
   a. Facilitate self-re-evaluation to identify strengths and weaknesses at the time of relapse – **incorrect response**. While this action will assist with relapse the most correct response is all of the above
   b. Raise health literacy level of falls risk and risk reduction – **incorrect response**. While this action will assist with relapse the most correct response is all of the above

c. Refer to falls prevention program – **incorrect response**. While this action will assist with relapse the most correct response is all of the above

d. **All of the above – correct response**

CHAPTER 5
1D, 2B, 3E

CHAPTER 6
1C, 2B, 3D

CHAPTER 7
1C, 2B, 3B

CHAPTER 9
1B, 2E, 3D

CHAPTER 10
1B, 2D, 3B, 4A, 5D

CHAPTER 11
1A, 2D, 3C, 4B, 5B

CHAPTER 12
1C, 2B, 3D, 4D

CHAPTER 13
1B, 2C, 3A, 4D, 5C

CHAPTER 14
1C, 2C, 3C

CHAPTER 15
1A, 2C, 3A, 4C

CHAPTER 19
1C, 2B, 3C

CHAPTER 21
1 A, C

2 A, D

3 B, C, D

CHAPTER 22
1B, 2C, 3A, 4B, 5A

CHAPTER 23
1D, 2A, 3B, 4A

CHAPTER 24
1D, 2A, 3B, 4A, 5A

CHAPTER 25
1A, B, E, G, I
2C
3C
4B, C, E, F
5C

CHAPTER 26
Suggested answers

Considering the Domains of Wellbeing
Identity

Mr Smith has expressed a lot of personal information about himself, including his relationship with his father, which helps to define his uniqueness as a person. Additionally, Mr Smith wants to socialise with others. He feels that not many residents or staff are aware of his story. Creating a book telling Mr Smith's life story is one way that his identity can be shared with others.

Connectedness

Mr Smith reports having had a good relationship with his wife until he developed dementia and entered residential aged care. Mr Smith states that he does not know many people in the nursing home, despite having lived there for six months. Mr Smith's reported loneliness indicates his lack of connectedness to other people in his new home. Strategies are required to connect Mr Smith to his environment, both the physical (the building) and social (relationships with people) environment. Mr Smith may feel more connected to his room if he is able to personalise the space with his familiar objects and will become more connected to other people within the facility if he is encouraged to attend groups with the other residents. Mr Smith may also appreciate the opportunity to participate in intergenerational activities (such as with children from a playgroup if they were to visit the facility), if this could be organised by the facility.

Autonomy

Mealtimes are one time where Mr Smith feels he lacks autonomy as he cannot choose what food he eats or when he can eat it. Mr Smith also feels a lack of privacy in that he shares a room with another person. If possible, consider a single room for Mr Smith if one is available, and involve him in personalising it with photos and other personal items. Simple signage and use of colour to help Mr Smith locate his room and other areas will assist him to navigate the facility more independently. Consider opportunities for Mr Smith to assist with meal planning, and the potential for staggered mealtimes to increase resident choice.

Meaning

The despondence in Mr Smith's voice may indicate how much he is missing elements of life prior to entering the residential aged care facility, which were important to him. Find quiet moments to sit with Mr Smith, giving him an opportunity to talk about these. Depending on Mr Smith's preferences, consider opportunities for him to engage in these again. These may include opportunities for Mr Smith to take shopping trips to buy gifts for his grandchildren, either with staff support or with arranged family support. Acknowledging Mr Smith's love of music, strategies may include displaying photos of Mr Smith with his trumpet or other visual mementos to communicate this interest to other staff and residents. Family could bring Mr Smith a CD player and CDs so he can play these in his room. Encourage staff to reminisce with Mr Smith about what it meant to be a trumpet player when he was younger, what and when he played and for whom.

Joy

Take time to sit with Mr Smith and ask him about his life and significant life events. Note events that he is particularly proud of and likes to discuss. Find ways to enable Mr Smith to share these events with the people he mixes with on a day-to-day basis. For example, display photos of Mr Smith holding a football trophy or receiving an award for trumpet playing. Encourage family to bring his grandchildren to visit, and provide a comfortable private meeting space, suitable for children, where the family can relax together.

CHAPTER 27

1B, 2D, 3C

Index